MW01200573

FIFTH EDITION

Intrapartum Management Modules

A PERINATAL EDUCATION PROGRAM

FIFTH EDITION

Intrapartum Management Modules

A PERINATAL EDUCATION PROGRAM

EDITORS

BETSY BABB KENNEDY PhD, RN, CNE

Associate Professor, Director of Faculty Development
Vanderbilt University School of Nursing
Nashville, Tennessee

SUZANNE McMURTRY BAIRD DNP, RN

Founder, Clinical Concepts in Obstetrics, Inc.
Brentwood, Tennessee
Adjunct Faculty
Vanderbilt University School of Nursing
Nashville, Tennessee

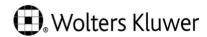

Philadelphia • Baltimore • New York • London
Buenos Aires • Hong Kong • Sydney • Tokyo

Executive Editor: Shannon W. Magee
Product Development Editor: Maria M. McAvey
Production Project Manager: Marian Bellus
Design Coordinator: Joan Wendt
Manufacturing Coordinator: Kathleen Brown
Senior Marketing Manager: Mark Wiragh
Prepress Vendor: Aptara, Inc.

5th edition

Copyright © 2017 Wolters Kluwer

Copyright © 1996 (2e) Lippincott Williams & Wilkins; 2002 (3e) Lippincott Williams & Wilkins; 2008 (4e) Lippincott Williams & Wilkins.

All rights reserved. This book is protected by copyright. No part of this book may be reproduced or transmitted in any form or by any means, including as photocopies or scanned-in or other electronic copies, or utilized by any information storage and retrieval system without written permission from the copyright owner, except for brief quotations embodied in critical articles and reviews. Materials appearing in this book prepared by individuals as part of their official duties as U.S. government employees are not covered by the above-mentioned copyright. To request permission, please contact Wolters Kluwer at Two Commerce Square, 2001 Market Street, Philadelphia, PA 19103, via email at permissions@lww.com, or via our website at lww.com (products and services).

9 8 7 6 5 4 3 2 1

Printed in China

Library of Congress Cataloging-in-Publication Data

Names: Kennedy, Betsy Babb, editor. | Baird, Suzanne McMurty, editor.
Title: Intrapartum management modules : a perinatal education program /
   [edited by] Betsy Babb Kennedy, Suzanne McMurtry Baird.
Description: Fifth edition. | Philadelphia : Wolters Kluwer, [2017] |
   Preceded by Intrapartum management modules : a perinatal education program
   / editors, Betsy B. Kennedy, Donna Jean Ruth, E. Jean Martin. 4th ed.
   2009. | Includes bibliographical references and index.
Identifiers: LCCN 2016002806 | ISBN 9781451194630
Subjects: | MESH: Labor, Obstetric | Delivery, Obstetric–nursing |
   Maternal-Child Nursing–methods | Prenatal Care–methods | Programmed
   Instruction
Classification: LCC RG951 | NLM WY 18.2 | DDC 618.4–dc23
LC record available at http://lccn.loc.gov/2016002806

This work is provided "as is," and the publisher disclaims any and all warranties, express or implied, including any warranties as to accuracy, comprehensiveness, or currency of the content of this work.

This work is no substitute for individual patient assessment based upon healthcare professionals' examination of each patient and consideration of, among other things, age, weight, gender, current or prior medical conditions, medication history, laboratory data, and other factors unique to the patient. The publisher does not provide medical advice or guidance and this work is merely a reference tool. Healthcare professionals, and not the publisher, are solely responsible for the use of this work including all medical judgments and for any resulting diagnosis and treatments.

Given continuous, rapid advances in medical science and health information, independent professional verification of medical diagnoses, indications, appropriate pharmaceutical selections and dosages, and treatment options should be made and healthcare professionals should consult a variety of sources. When prescribing medication, healthcare professionals are advised to consult the product information sheet (the manufacturer's package insert) accompanying each drug to verify, among other things, conditions of use, warnings and side effects, and identify any changes in dosage schedule or contraindications, particularly if the medication to be administered is new, infrequently used, or has a narrow therapeutic range. To the maximum extent permitted under applicable law, no responsibility is assumed by the publisher for any injury and/or damage to persons or property, as a matter of products liability, negligence law, or otherwise, or from any reference to or use by any person of this work.

LWW.com

CCS0416

This text will always be dedicated to

the readers, dedicated professionals

who render care that touches not only

the body, but also the soul. On behalf

of the women, babies, and families

you care for in a sensitive, safe, and

knowledgeable manner,

thank you.

CONTRIBUTORS

Diane J. Angelini, EdD, CNM, NEA-BC, FACNM, FAAN
Clinical Professor
College of Nursing
Medical University of South Carolina
Charleston, South Carolina

Julie M. R. Arafeh, MSN, RN
Senior Simulation Specialist
Center for Advanced Pediatric and Perinatal Education
Stanford University
Palo Alto, California

Susan L. Baudhuin, Esq.
Attorney at Law
Peachtree City, GA

Meghan Bertani-Yang, MA, CCLS, CIMI
Certified Child Life Specialist
Houston, Texas

Sarah Branan, MSN, RN
Senior Instructor in Nursing
University of South Carolina, Upstate
Spartanburg, South Carolina

Michelle R. Collins, PhD, CNM, FACNM
Professor, Director, Nurse-Midwifery Program
Vanderbilt University School of Nursing
Nashville, Tennessee

Jennifer Dalton, MSN, RN
Nursing Supervisor of Maternal Fetal Medicine
  Outpatient Clinics
Texas Children's Hospital
Houston, Texas

Susan Drummond, RN, MSN, C-EFM
Associate in Obstetrics
OB-GYN, Vanderbilt University Medical Center
Nashville, Tennessee

Donna R. Frye, RN, MN
Perinatal Consultant
Nashville, TN

Jennie G. Hensley, EdD, CNM, WHNP, LCCE
Associate Professor of Nursing
Vanderbilt University School of Nursing
Nashville, Tennessee

Sharon L. Holley, DNP, CNM
Associate Professor of Nursing
School of Nursing
Vanderbilt University School of Nursing
Nashville, Tennessee

Elisabeth D. Howard, CNM, PhD, FACNM
Clinical Assistant, Professor
Department of Midwifery
Women and Infants Hospital
Providence, Rhode Island

Valerie Yates Huwe, RNC-OB, MS, CNS
Perinatal Outreach Educator
Benioff Children's Hospital
University of California San Francisco
San Francisco, California

Maribeth Inturrisi, RN, BSN, MSN, CNS, CDE
Perinatal Diabetes Educator
Maternal Fetal Medicine
Sutter Pacific Medical Foundation
San Francisco, California

Frances C. Kelly, PhD(c), MSN, RNC-OB, NEA-BC, CPHQ
Director, Quality and Safety, Pavilion for Women
Texas Children's Hospital
Houston, Texas

Cynthia F. Krening, MS, RNC-OB, C-EFM, CNS
Perinatal Clinical Nurse Specialist
Women's Services, St. Joseph's Hospital
Denver, Colorado

E. Jean Martin, RN, MS, MSN, CNM
Professor Emeritus
College of Nursing, Graduate Nurse-Midwifery
Medical University of South Carolina
Charleston, South Carolina

Lisa A. Miller, CNM, JD
Founder
Perinatal Risk Management & Education Services
Portland, Oregon

Heather M. Robbins, MSN, MBA, RN
Instructor
Vanderbilt University School of Nursing
Nashville, Tennessee

Erin Rodgers, DNP, RN, CPN
Assistant Professor of Nursing
Vanderbilt University School of Nursing
Nashville, Tennessee

Donna J. Ruth, MSN, RN-BC
Director of Educational Services
Association of Women's Health, Obstetric and
    Neonatal Nurses
Washington, DC

Lucinda Steen Stewart, MSN, RN
Assistant Professor of Nursing
Vanderbilt University School of Nursing
Nashville, Tennessee

Dinez Swanson, DNP, RN, FNP
Associate Dean of Faculty Professor
Chamberlain College of Nursing
Houston, Texas

Susan C. Swart, B-Cur (RN, Registered Midwife, Psychiatric
and Community Health Nursing)
House Supervisor
Texas Children's Hospital
Houston, Texas

Patricia M. Witcher, MSN, RNC-OB
Clinical Specialist, Labor and Delivery
Labor and Delivery, Northside Hospital
Atlanta, Georgia

PREVIOUS EDITION CONTRIBUTORS

Angel Carter, MSN, APRN, NNP

Elizabeth Fritz, RN, MSN

Kelly Gee, MSN, RNC, WHNP

Mary Jo Gilmer, PhD, MBA, RN

Marcella T. Hickey, RN, MSN, CNM

Anne Moore, MSN, RNC, FAANP

Mary Copeland Myers, CNM, MSN, CDE

Judith H. Poole, PhD, RNC

Nancy Webster Smith, RN, MSN, CNM

Francilla Thomas, RNC, MSN, EFMC

Penny Spencer Waugh, MSN, RNC

Ann Mogabgab Weathersby, RN, MSN, CNM

Kimberly Yeager, RN, BSN

PREVIOUS EDITION REVIEWERS

Carol Abrahams, RN, MS

Joanne E. Foresman, RNC, MSN

Ann C. Holden, RN, BScN, MSc, PNC

Mary Lou Moore, PhD, RNC, FACCE, FAAN

Virginia Bradford Pearson, RN, MSN

Kathleen Simpson, PhD, RNC, FAAN

PREVIOUS EDITION
REVIEWERS

While the phenomenon of birth has not changed, our knowledge base continues to expand exponentially, and the clinical challenges facing those who provide intrapartum care are increasingly and uniquely complex. Provision of the "best" and individualized care for women and their families during childbearing involves compassion, safety, accuracy, and sensitivity. It is our sincere wish for this text to support those who support others during this critical time.

The fifth edition of Intrapartum Management Modules has undergone significant changes in content, authorship, and editorial leadership. Content revisions reflect the most current evidence and best practices in the care of women and infants. The topics presented should be relevant for anyone in an intrapartum setting: staff nurses, educators, nurse midwives, nurse practitioners, clinical nurse specialists, physician assistants, and health professions students. Content and skill sets are presented along with review questions/answers for validation of comprehension of the material. The modules may be used as an adjunct to unit orientation, and completed within the orientation framework.

Jean Martin was the founding editor of this text 25 years ago, and we owe her an enormous debt of gratitude. She created an enduring voice and established a standard of excellence we strive to uphold. She is forever present in these pages. We gratefully acknowledge all past editors and contributors to the text for their tremendous commitment, passion, and scholarship. We extend deep and sincere thanks to all the new contributing authors for sharing their expertise and time. They are valued friends, colleagues, and experts from around the country. The spectacular image from the last edition that still graces the cover of this edition was created by the talented Lana Feole, who now has her own beautiful baby boy, Des. The team at Lippincott Williams & Wilkins has been tremendous in its guidance, assistance, and patience in the development of this edition. To all those who contributed to this work, a heartfelt "thank you."

Care provided during the intrapartum period has profound and lasting effects upon the woman and her family. You will be remembered for your actions, your interactions, and perhaps preserved in images to be viewed again and again. As Jean acknowledged, "the dynamics of such interactions work both ways . . . the gratitude is ours for being allowed to participate in one of life's most incredible events!" It is indeed a privilege.

Betsy Babb Kennedy, PhD, RN, CNE
Suzanne McMurtry Baird, DNP, RN

CONTENTS

Contents

xvi

Overview of Labor

BETSY BABB KENNEDY, E. JEAN
MARTIN, AND HEATHER M. ROBBINS

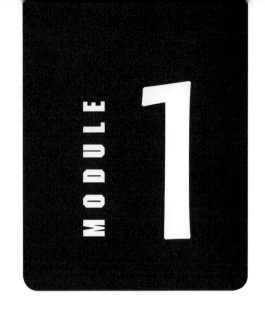

MODULE 1

Key Terms

When you have completed this module, you should be able to recall the meaning of the following terms. You should also be able to use the terms when consulting with other health professionals. The terms are defined in this module or in the glossary at the end of this book.

cervix
contraction
corticotropin-releasing factor (CRF)
cultural competence
cytokines
decidua
endogenous

gap junctions
macrophages
parturition
placenta
progesterone
prostaglandins

Physiology of Labor and Birth

Identifying Features of Labor

• What is labor?

Labor can be defined medically as regular, progressively intense uterine contractions that, over time, produce cervical effacement and dilation, leading to the development of expulsive forces adequate to move the fetus through the birth canal against the resistance of soft tissue, muscle, and the bony structure of the pelvis.

NOTE: *Uterine contractions in the absence of cervical change are not labor.*

A number of integrated and sequential biochemical, physiologic, and pharmacologic pathways are thought to exist; it is through these pathways that the term labor is initiated and maintained. The exact mechanism for the onset and maintenance of labor has not yet been fully revealed. Improved experimental laboratory techniques and increasingly sophisticated research approaches *in humans* are leading to better understanding of the numerous hormonal interactions in human labor and birth; however, these are processes that are not able to be directly investigated.

NOTE: *Ancient civilizations believed that the fetus was delivered head first so that it could kick its legs against the top of the uterus and propel itself through the birth canal!*[1]

There is no doubt that, under hormonal influences, the uterus is maintained in a quiescent state throughout most of pregnancy. Certainly, a dramatic physiologic change is involved in taking a pregnancy from the state of relatively low-level antepartum uterine contractility to the coordinated, intense uterine contractility of labor. However, rather than an active process initiated by uterine stimulants, labor may be promoted as a result of the removal of the inhibitory effects of pregnancy on the myometrium.[1] In addition, there is substantial evidence from the research that indicates the fetus plays an important role in the timing of labor. In fact, there may be a "parturition cascade" that involves the fetus, the mother, and the placenta.[1]

Labor Initiation and Maintenance

- During quiescence, the uterus is maintained by inhibitors such as progesterone, prostacyclin, relaxin, nitric oxide, adrenomedullin, and other substances.
- In the weeks and days before term, all parts of the uterus undergo preparation for labor and delivery (*parturition*).[2]
- Hormonal mediators from the placenta and maternal and fetal endocrine glands are believed to affect the regulation of the uterine musculature (myometrium).
- In pregnancy, the lining of the uterus (the endometrium) is referred to as the *decidua*. Experiencing marked change in thickness and vascularity, the decidua has the capacity to alter hormonal proportions (e.g., estrogen increases over progesterone content) and enzymes and to nourish the embryo. Special decidual cells called macrophages synthesize prostaglandins and another group of compounds called cytokines.[3]
- Direct tissue-to-tissue communication occurs among uterine musculature, the decidua, and fetal membranes.[3]
- The uterine myometrium consists of thick and thin contractile fibers grouped in bundles. Few intracellular contacts between them exist until late in pregnancy. At that time, areas between muscle fiber cells develop pathways for communication (cell to cell). These pathways are called gap junctions. They are clearly present in great numbers as parturition nears. These efficient cell-to-cell gap junctions serve as channels for the transfer of chemical and electrical signals from one muscle fiber cell to another. Simultaneous contractions of a majority of cells are needed to make an effective contraction. This synchronization of the uterine muscle fibers leads to efficient, coordinated *contractions,* which soften, thin, and dilate the cervix.[2]
- A placental hormone called *corticotropin-releasing factor* (*CRF*) is released into maternal circulation early in the second trimester, with concentrations rising significantly as pregnancy advances. CRF production increases the strength of contractions and stimulates production of oxytocin and prostaglandins.[4]

- *Prostaglandins* are chemicals derived from the fetus, amniotic membranes, decidua, and other sources. These prostaglandins, particularly PGF and PGE$_2$, cause smooth muscle contraction and vasoconstriction, soften ("ripen") cervical tissue, and modulate hormonal activity.[3,5]
- *Cytokines* are an important group of compounds. These compounds have numerous functions in labor physiology, which act either synergistically or antagonistically.
- Calcium (the calcium ion) is vital for the contractile process in myometrial cells, which depends on the influx of extracellular free calcium. The calcium ion also plays a critical role in transmitting signals of excitation from the myometrial cell membranes to the contractile complex inside the cell.[2]

NOTE: Agents that block this movement of calcium, called calcium channel blockers (e.g., nifedipine), are in fact used as tocolytic agents for the purpose of suppressing uterine contractility.

- Once the uterus has been prepared, myometrial activity may be initiated by the fetoplacental unit and the mother, through the secretion of hormones and mechanical stretch of the uterus.[1]
- The nonpregnant or very early gravid uterus is not sensitive to oxytocin. However, oxytocin is secreted in pulses of low frequency throughout pregnancy.[2]
- As the uterus gradually approaches term, it is thought that the myometrium becomes increasingly responsive to oxytocic hormones, mainly PGE and PGF. Toward the end of pregnancy, the number of oxytocin receptors increases, peaking in the myometrium and decidua in early labor.
- Secretion of oxytocin seems to be in a pulsatile fashion, even in labor (Figs. 1.1 and 1.2).[2]
- Maternal plasma concentrations of endogenous oxytocin are equivalent to a range of 4 to 6 mU/min during the first stage of labor.[6]

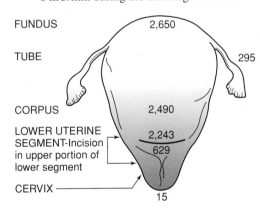

FIGURE 1.1 Distribution of oxytocin receptors in a pregnant human uterus, removed in preterm labor at 34 weeks. Numbers denote oxytocin receptors (OTRs) per unit measurement (fmol/mg DNA). (Reprinted with permission from Fuchs, A. R., & Fuchs, R. [1996]. Physiology and endocrinology of parturition. In Gabbe, S. G., Niebyl, J. R., & Simpson, J. L. [Eds.], *Obstetrics: Normal and problem pregnancies* [3rd ed., p. 123]. New York: Churchill Livingstone.)

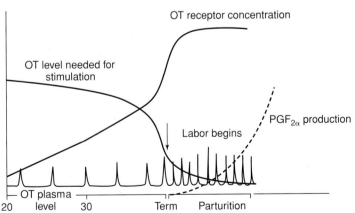

FIGURE 1.2 Diagrammatic representation of the concentration of myometrial oxytocin, the level of oxytocin needed to elicit contractions, and maternal plasma oxytocin levels at the end of gestation and during labor. Oxytocin is secreted in pulses of low frequency. During labor, pulse frequency increases. Fetal secretion of oxytocin can be considerable and may contribute to the oxytocin level reaching the myometrium. PGF production does not increase significantly until labor is in progress and then increases progressively throughout the third stage of labor. OT, oxytocin. (Reprinted with permission from Fuchs, A. R., & Fuchs, R. [1996]. Physiology and endocrinology of parturition. In Gabbe, S. G., Niebyl, J. R., & Simpson, J. L. [Eds.], *Obstetrics: Normal and problem pregnancies* [3rd ed., p. 124]. New York: Churchill Livingstone.)

Identifying Stages and Phases of Labor

• How are the parts of the labor process described?[1-5]

For the sake of description, labor is divided into the following four stages:

Stage I   Stage I begins with the onset of regular uterine contractions and lasts until full dilatation of the cervix is achieved. Dilation is the *gradual opening of the cervical entrance* to the uterus. Stage one may be further divided into two phases:
Early phase—extends from the onset of regular contractions that cause cervical change to the beginning of the active phase, when dilation occurs more rapidly. It usually extends over hours.
Active phase—begins when the laboring woman reaches approximately 6 cm, and ends when the cervix is 10 cm or completely dilated.

Stage II   Stage II begins with full cervical dilation (10 cm) and lasts until the baby is born. During this phase, the presenting part of the fetus descends through the maternal pelvis. Stage II may be accompanied by an increase in bloody show, feelings of pressure in the rectum, nausea and vomiting, and desire to push or bear down.

Stage III   Stage III is that part of the process after the birth of the baby during which the placenta is delivered.

Stage IV   Stage IV is that part of the process after the delivery of the placenta in which the uterus effectively contracts, preventing excessive bleeding. This is a period of adjustment as the mother's body functions begin to stabilize.

NOTE: A thorough description of the stages of labor may be found in Module 5.

Uterine Contractions

• How is the uterus suited to accomplish labor and birth?

The uterus is composed of *three* layers of tissue. These layers are arranged as shown in Figure 1.3.

1. **Perimetrium**—a thick outer membrane covering the uterus.
2. **Myometrium**—the middle layer that contains special muscle cells called myometrial cells.
3. **Endometrium**—the innermost layer containing glands and nutrient tissue.

Figure 1.4 illustrates the changes in the uterus and cervix as normal labor progresses.

Under the influence of myometrial contractions, labor progresses with the uterus becoming separated into *two distinct parts*. The upper portion becomes *thicker* and more powerful because of shortening and thickening of the myometrial fibers. This prepares the uterus to exert the effort necessary to push the baby out at birth. The lower portion of the uterus becomes *thinner, softer,* and *more relaxed* as the myometrial fibers relax and become longer. As a result, the baby can more easily be pushed out at birth.

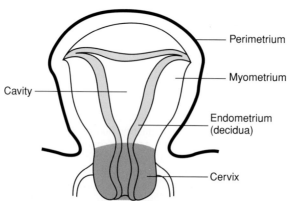

NOTE: The endometrium is altered through hormonal influences during pregnancy to become what is called the decidua, which functions to maintain the pregnancy.

FIGURE 1.3   The three major tissue layers of the uterus.

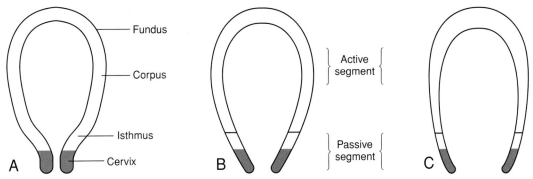

FIGURE 1.4 Changes in the uterus and cervix as normal labor progresses. **A.** Uterus and cervix at term. **B.** Uterus and cervix early in stage I. **C.** Uterus and cervix in stage II.

Downward pressure caused by the contraction of the fundal segment is gradually transmitted to the passive lower segment or cervical portion, causing effacement (thinning of the cervix) and dilatation. The cervix is drawn upward and over the baby, allowing the baby to descend into the passageway. The cervix is made up of an inner part called the internal os and an outer part called the external os. Figure 1.5 demonstrates how the internal and external os change position as effacement occurs.

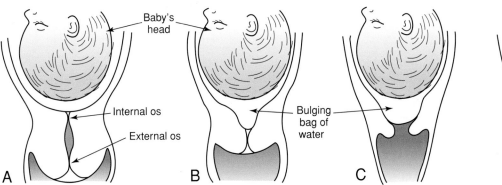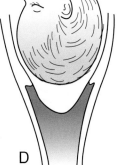

FIGURE 1.5 **A.** Cervix before effacement begins. **B.** Effacement in its early phase. **C.** Effacement with some dilation. **D.** Complete effacement and dilation.

• How are uterine contractions described?

Contractions have a wave-like pattern that can be divided into segments (Fig. 1.6).
- Increment—usually makes up the *longest* part of the contraction.
- Acme—the *shortest,* but most intense, part of the contraction.
- Decrement—a fairly rapid diminishing of the contraction.

Four characteristics of a contraction have been identified:
1. **Frequency**—This is how often the contractions are occurring. Contractions can begin 10 to 15 minutes apart, but get closer together as labor progresses. They can occur as frequently as 2 to 3 minutes apart late in the labor process. It is important to remember that the frequency of contractions does not reflect the intensity.
2. **Regularity**—As labor becomes well established, contractions occur with a rhythmic pattern.

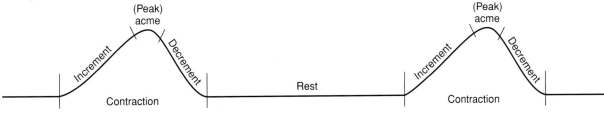

FIGURE 1.6 The segments of a contraction.

3. **Duration**—The length of contractions increases as labor progresses. Contractions in early labor can be as short as 30 seconds and gradually increase to as long as 90 seconds.

4. **Intensity**—This characteristic can be assessed as mild, moderate, or strong. The strength of contractions increases as labor intensifies. Other variables that affect the intensity (strength) of contractions include parity, the condition of the cervix, pain medication, and the use of exogenous oxytocin. To obtain an estimate of the intensity, you can palpate the mother's abdomen with your hand. A true assessment of the contraction's intensity can be obtained only by using an internal uterine monitor, which is described in detail in Module 6.

NOTE: In physiologic labor, the intensity (or amplitude) of the contraction varies from 30 to 55 mm Hg and the frequency is two to five contractions every 10 minutes. During the second stage of labor, peak intensity of contractions may reach 65 mm Hg. In prolonged labor, the intensity of the contractions is less than 25 mm Hg and the frequency is fewer than two contractions every 10 minutes. No labor is occurring if the intensity is less than 15 mm Hg.

The duration and frequency of a contraction can be diagrammed as in Figure 1.7.

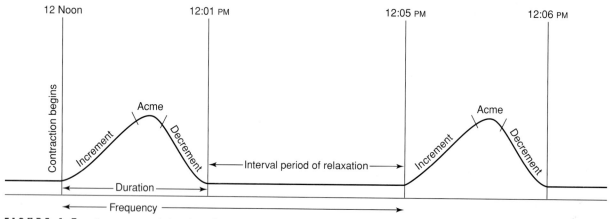

FIGURE 1.7   Frequency and duration of contractions.

Notice that the duration of a contraction is timed from the beginning of the increment to the end of the decrement. The frequency of a contraction is timed from the beginning of one contraction to the beginning of the next.

Although the interval between contractions is referred to as a period of relaxation, in fact, the uterus never entirely relaxes between contractions. It maintains what is called a resting tone, a result of increased tension and thickening of muscle fibers in the upper portion of the uterus. Contractions are assessed in three basic ways:

1. **Subjectively**—This is a description given by the patient. She will respond to questions such as "When did they start?" "How often are they coming?" "How long do they last?" and "Are they getting stronger?"

2. **Palpation**—This is an efficient method of assessment using the palmar surface of the fingertips. Fingertips should be kept moving throughout the contraction to continually palpate the changing uterus through the abdominal wall (Fig. 1.8).

The intensity of the uterine contraction can be described as follows:
- Mild—The uterus can be indented with gentle pressure.
- Moderate—The uterus indents only with firm pressure at the peak of a contraction.
- Strong—The uterus feels firm or hard and cannot be indented at the peak of a contraction.

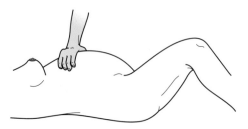

FIGURE 1.8   Palm or surface of the fingers palpates for intensity and duration of a contraction.

NOTE: Your moving fingertips pick up the changes within a contraction as it gains in intensity and then recedes. Do this carefully so that you do not cause discomfort to the laboring woman.

3. **Electronic fetal monitoring**—This type of fetal monitoring can be either external or internal. The external method involves the use of electronic equipment that measures and records the frequency and duration of contractions. The intensity of contractions can be truly measured only with the internal method. True representation of heart rate variability is obtained only with the internal method (fetal spiral electrode).

When assessing contractions, the nurse typically stays at the bedside for 20 to 40 minutes (depending on the general frequency of contractions), with fingertips lightly placed over the fundal portion of the mother's abdomen (Fig. 1.9). This enables an accurate detection of the beginning and end of the contraction. Do not depend solely on signals from the mother such as restlessness or a statement that the contraction is beginning because she is often unaware of the initial changes in the uterine muscle. Fingertips are placed near the top of the uterus because the uterus has pacemakers located there. These pacemakers are a group of highly excitable myometrial cells that are responsible for starting contractions (Fig. 1.10). They are located on either side of the uterus near the oviducts or fallopian tubes: *The contraction begins at the top of the uterus and sweeps down over the main body of the uterus.*

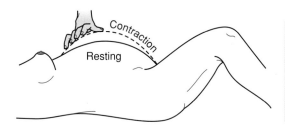

When feeling for the general intensity and duration of a contraction, the best area of the mother's abdomen on which to place your fingertips is near the top of the uterus.

FIGURE 1.9   The palpating fingers are placed near the top of the uterus.

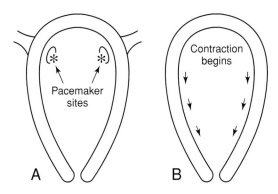

FIGURE 1.10   **A.** Sites where the uterine contraction begins (pacemaker sites). **B.** Contraction pathway.

NOTE: Further description of assessment of labor and uterine contractions may be found in Modules 5 and 7.

Each contraction wave has three components:
1. **Propagation** of the wave starts at the pacemaker site. The wave starts above and moves downward toward the lower part of the uterus.
2. **Duration** of the contraction lessens progressively as the wave moves away from the pacemaker. Throughout any contraction the upper portion of the uterus is in action for a longer period than the lower portion.
3. **Intensity** of the contraction decreases from the top to the bottom of the uterus; that is, the upper segment of the uterus contracts more strongly than the lower.

NOTE: Analysis of wave properties of the uterine contraction indicates that the full impact of the contraction is not felt at the cervix until the last half of the contraction.

A Different View of Labor: Promotion of Physiologic and Family-Centered Birth

"Birth is not only about making babies. Birth is also about making mothers—strong, competent, capable mothers who trust themselves and know their inner strength."[7]

The experience of pregnancy and childbirth, although shared with husbands, partners, or family members is uniquely female. It is life altering, one of nature's most powerful events. The manner in which a woman experiences birth has profound implications, possibly affecting the quality of her immediate infant interaction and subsequent parenting. Research shows that childbirth affects a woman's self-esteem and can also affect her emotional availability to her infant.[8]

The birth setting and its participants powerfully influence the childbirth experience, shaping roles and the amount of control held by the woman herself, those who support her, and her caregivers.[9] Supporting the woman and her family in any birth setting, through any type of birth, and providing sensitive care is the nurse's privilege and honor.

Supporting the Laboring Woman

A partner, family member, friend, doula, nurse midwife, or labor nurse may provide primary labor support. Families are diverse in nature and it is important to remember that the woman is the only one who can determine who is important to her, and who she wants to support her during this experience. Respect the woman's preferences and needs in support of the family. The labor nurse is a powerful and influential presence wherever labor and birth are occurring.[10] Effective nursing labor support involves emotional support, physical comfort, advocacy and includes the following[10]:

- Understanding of the physiologic and anatomic adaptations involved in labor and birth.
- Compassion for the enormous but individualized adaptive responses required on the part of the woman and her family in the birth process.
- Knowledge of the woman's (and her support person's) preparation, understanding, and goals for the birth experience.
- Commitment to provide continuous support for the woman and her family, and to *work at advancing this philosophy of care.*

A detailed discussion of labor support interventions for comfort and pain relief is presented in Module 6.

NOTE: The continuous presence of a support person reduces the likelihood of medication for pain relief, operative vaginal delivery, cesarean delivery, and a 5-minute Apgar score of less than 7.[11]

The Coalition for Improving Maternity Services, Lamaze International, The World Health Organization (WHO), The Association for Women's Health, Obstetric, and Neonatal Nurses (AWHONN), and The Association of Certified Nurse Midwives (ACNM) support evidence-based, healthy birth practices. Philosophical premises for the global effort to promote normal childbirth include the following[12–18]:

- Birth is a normal, healthy, natural process which takes place in a variety of settings, including homes, birth centers, and hospitals.
- Women should be empowered and confident in their ability to give birth and care for their new baby. The encounters and experiences that occur during this time may have profound and long-lasting effects.
- Every woman should have the opportunity to have a positive birth experience in her choice of setting. Her personal preferences, well-being, right to information and autonomy, and privacy should be respected.
- Interventions should not be routinely applied. Any necessary interventions should be based on the most up-to-date, quality evidence.
- Caregivers are responsible for the quality of care provided. Individuals (mothers and their families) are responsible for making informed choices about their health care.

All those who care for laboring or pregnant women should make provision of patient-centered, evidence-based, quality, safe, culturally sensitive care the primary priority.[15]

It is something to be able to paint a particular picture, or to carve a statue, and so to make a few objects beautiful; but it is far more glorious to carve and paint the very atmosphere and medium through which we look, which morally we can do. To affect the quality of the day, that is the highest of the arts.

—Henry David Thoreau, *Walden*

Specific practices that provide support for the laboring woman, her unborn baby, and support person(s) include the following[12–18]:

1. Assist women in the transition from home to the birth setting.
   - Education for the woman and her family prior to admission should emphasize physiologic labor, or labor beginning on its own.
   - Recognize that this is a vulnerable time and the mother may not know the "right" time to arrive at the birth setting, hospital, or birthing center.
   - Welcome the woman into the new environment. A medical facility environment can be unfamiliar and can be overwhelming.
   - Encourage the presence of a trusted support person (as described above) so that the woman feels protected and comforted.
2. *Make the woman and her unborn baby the central focus in the situation* and include her coach through all phases of labor and birth.
   - Introduce yourself and others who might be providing care.
   - Inform the woman and support person of her progress.
   - Include the woman and support person in conversations with others.
   - Offer choices when possible.
   - Actively involve and coach the support person in efforts to help the woman.
   - Think of the unborn baby as a sensing, responsive, and social being as you give care. Use touch, sound, and light as soothing, even therapeutic, elements.
   - Keep the woman and baby together to maximize physiologic benefits for both.
3. Ensure the woman's privacy.
   - Try to provide a private environment.
   - Orient the woman to her surroundings.
   - Keep the woman draped adequately.
   - Request the woman's permission for procedures and examinations and keep the support person updated and involved.
   - Control the environment according to the woman's wishes (e.g., a darkened or bright room, open or closed door, quiet atmosphere).
4. Promote preparedness.
   - Assess the woman's knowledge level and preparedness. Give information about labor and birth that addresses where she is in labor. Use simple, direct terminology appropriate to her level of understanding and ability to take it in at the time. Orient the woman and support person to the expected time frame for labor. Update as necessary.
   - Instruct the woman and support person in relaxation, breathing, and pushing techniques. For women who have attended childbirth education classes, these techniques may need to be reviewed. Give brief, practical instructions to women who have not attended childbirth education.
   - Assist and support the woman for movement in labor, encouraging walking and position changes to facilitate comfort and labor progress.
5. Instill confidence.
   - Praise the efforts of the woman and support person.
   - Speak positively about labor and delivery events. For example, when giving a sedative, tell the woman that the medication will help her to relax.
   - Stay with the woman if she is without a support person. If you must leave her for a brief time, tell her why and when you will return.
   - Provide a call light or buzzer when you are out of the room.
   - Inform the woman and support person in advance of special procedures or examinations.
   - Use vocabulary that is suited to the needs of the woman and support person and ensure that they understand.
   - Encourage a support person or family member to remain with the woman throughout labor and include this person in your explanations and care. Remember, those providing labor support are in need of reassurance, too.
6. Apply culturally aware and sensitive care to each woman and family.

• What is culturally sensitive care?

Diversity is the norm in our society, with 1 in every 10 people in the United States an immigrant.[19] The majority of these immigrants are women and for many of them the first exposure to health care may be maternity care.[19] Cultural groups might also include the homeless, migrants, refugees, or same-sex couples. These women and their families approach childbirth within their cultural context, that is, a set of core values, cultural beliefs, and practices. Language, dietary practices, and childbirth traditions including positioning, support behaviors, and newborn care represent examples of cultural influences that may significantly affect healthcare needs. It is essential for healthcare providers to provide care that is sensitive, responsive, individualized, and congruent.[20] Without cultural knowledge, delivery of appropriate, respectful care is difficult.[21]

Becoming culturally sensitive and/or responsive is generally viewed a process of developing cultural awareness, knowledge, skill, and appreciation.[20] It is the motivation of the care provider that initiates the process. Adapting skills for providing care in a culturally responsive and congruent manner is a progressive and developmental, but conscious, process that should be a focus for the clinically responsive care provider.

Behaviors and attitudes of providers, and institutional policies enable a system, agency, and/or individual to function effectively with culturally diverse patients and communities. Display 1.1 describes traits of the culturally responsive provider.[21]

A cultural assessment should be done to ensure the caregiver has adequate knowledge of beliefs about labor support, drug therapies, and taboos. The use of a tool ensures consistency in that all women are asked the same questions. Questions to consider for a cultural assessment tool[20]:
- Where were you born?
- How long have you lived in the United States?
- Who are your major support people?
- What languages do you speak and read?
- What are your religious practices?
- What are your food preferences?
- What is your economic situation?
- What does childbearing represent to you?
- How do you view childbearing?
- Are there any maternal precautions or restrictions?
- Is birth a private or social experience?
- How would you like to manage labor pain?
- Who will provide labor support?
- Who will care for the baby?
- Do you use contraception?

DISPLAY 1.1 CHARACTERISTICS OF A CULTURALLY RESPONSIVE PROVIDER

Moves from cultural unawareness to an awareness of and sensitivity to own cultural heritage.
Recognizes own values and biases and is aware of how he or she may affect patients from other cultures.
Demonstrates comfort with cultural differences that exist between self and patients.
Knows specifics about the particular cultural group(s) with which he or she works.
Understands the historical events that may have caused harm to particular cultural groups.
Respects and is aware of the unique needs of patients from diverse communities.
Understands the importance of diversity within as well as between cultures.
Endeavors to learn more about cultural communities through patient interactions, participation in cultural diversity workshops and community events, readings on cultural dynamics, and consultations with community experts.
Makes a continuous effort to understand the other's point of view.
Demonstrates flexibility and tolerance of ambiguity; is nonjudgmental.
Maintains a sense of humor and an open mind.
Demonstrates a willingness to relinquish control in clinical encounters; to risk failure; and to look within for the source of frustration, anger, and resistance.
Acknowledges that the process is as important as the product.

Adapted with permission from Rorie, J. L., Paine, L. L., & Barger, M. K. (1996). Cultural competence in primary care services. *Journal of Nurse Midwifery, 41*(2), 99.

It is important to ask these questions in a conversational, nonjudgmental tone. Open-ended questions should be used. If the mother does not speak English, then a medical interpreter should be used if available. The use of a female interpreter is best; remember too that a member of the woman's family, especially another child, should not be used as an interpreter. Address questions to the woman, not the interpreter, in short, but clear sentences.

The care of the laboring woman is addressed further in Module 5.

PRACTICE/REVIEW QUESTIONS

After reviewing this module, answer the following questions.

1. Define *labor* in your own words. Compare your definition with that presented in the text.

   _____

   _____

2. There is probably one predominant factor that results in rhythmic contractions leading to labor initiation and birth.

   a. True

   b. False

3. Current evidence shows that the functions of the uterus during labor are controlled by hormonal mediators from the placenta and the maternal and fetal glands.

   a. True

   b. False

4. Match the actions listed in Column B with the description of probable hormones, chemicals, or functions in labor listed in Column A.

   Column A

   1. _____ Calcium ions

   2. _____ Decidua

   3. _____ Increased number of oxytocin receptor sites in the myometrium

   4. _____ Prostaglandins

   5. _____ Oxytocin

   6. _____ Both maternal and fetal signals

   Column B

   a. Part of the endometrium; in pregnancy plays an important role in increasing estrogen content and synthesizing prostaglandins

   b. Secretion is pulsatile even during labor

   c. Results in increasing uterine sensitivity to oxytocin

   d. Derived from the fetus, decidua, and amniotic membranes

   e. Initiation of labor

   f. Vital for the contractile process in myometrial cells

5. When does Stage I begin and end?

6. Describe each of the two phases of Stage I.

   Early phase:_____

   Active phase:_____

7. When does Stage II begin and end?

8. Describe what occurs in Stage III.

9. Describe what occurs in Stage IV.

10. Briefly describe why it is important to assess what stage of labor a woman is in.

    _____

    _____

11. What are the three layers of tissue that make up the uterus?

    a. _____

    b. _____

    c. _____

12. Which layer of the uterus contains special muscle cells that aid in expulsion of the baby at birth?

    _____

13. What does *effacement* mean when referring to the labor process?

    _____

    _____

14. Describe the changes that take place in the uterus as labor progresses.

    Upper portion: _____

    Lower portion: _____

15. Label the following diagram of the uterus.

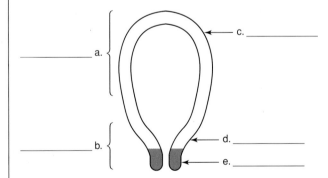

16. Which group of women is likely to experience effacement before labor actually begins?

    _____

17. The longest part of a contraction is the _____ segment.

18. The shortest and the most intense part of a contraction is the _____ segment.

11

19. The contraction diminishes in the _____ segment.

20. List the four characteristics of a contraction.

    a. _____

    b. _____

    c. _____

    d. _____

21. For each of the following statements, identify the characteristics of a contraction that is described.

    a. Contractions last for 15 seconds: _____

    b. An internal electronic monitor is needed to assess this characteristic: _____

    c. Contractions are 6 minutes apart: _____

    d. There is an established, predictable pattern: _____

22. Match the appropriate labor description in Column A with the contraction intensity described in Column B.

    Column A

    1. _____ Normal labor

    2. _____ No labor

    3. _____ Prolonged labor

    Column B

    a. The intensity of the contraction is less than 15 mm Hg.

    b. The intensity of the contraction is less than 25 mm Hg (and the frequency is fewer than two contractions every 10 minutes).

    c. The intensity of contractions varies from 30 to 55 mm Hg (and the frequency is 2 to 5 contractions every 10 minutes).

23. Refer to the following diagram below to answer questions a through d.

    a. What is the duration of the contractions?

    _____

    b. What is the frequency?

    _____

    c. How long can the woman relax?

    _____

    d. At what time will the next contraction begin?

    _____

24. List three ways to assess contractions.

    a. _____

    b. _____

    c. _____

25. What is the most efficient method of assessing contraction intensity?

    _____

26. What part of the hand is used to assess contractions?

    _____

27. Approximately how long would you need to remain at the bedside to assess contractions?

    _____

28. Where should you palpate the mother's abdomen and why?

    _____

29. a. To obtain a true assessment of cervical dilation, when is the best time to perform a vaginal examination?

    _____

    b. Why?

    _____

30. State three evidence-based outcomes when a laboring woman has a continuous supportive person with her.

    a. _____

    b. _____

    c. _____

4:00 AM   4:01 AM   4:03 AM   4:04 AM

31. Which is *not necessarily* effective in providing support for the laboring woman?

    a. Telling her in advance about special procedures, even though the procedure might be uncomfortable for her

    b. Protecting her privacy

    c. Keeping the visit of family members limited

    d. Including her in conversations when speaking with others in the room about her progress

32. In general, effective support during labor depends on which of the following?

    a. The health professional's interest and compassion

    b. The health professional's understanding of the physiologic and anatomic aspects of the birth process

    c. The health professional's appreciation of the psychological aspects of the birth process

    d. Knowledge of the level of preparation and the goals of the couple

    e. All of these

33. One of the first steps in becoming culturally competent is to increase awareness and sensitivity to one's own cultural heritage.

    a. True

    b. False

34. Relinquishing control in clinical situations does not play any role in culturally competent care.

    a. True

    b. False

35. When working with a non–English-speaking client, the nurse should address all questions directly to an interpreter.

    a. True

    b. False

36. The use of a cultural assessment tool increases consistency of care.

    a. True

    b. False

PRACTICE/REVIEW ANSWER KEY

1. *Labor* is a process involving a series of integrated uterine contractions occurring over time, leading to the development of expulsive forces adequate to propel the fetus through the birth canal against the resistance of soft tissue, muscle, and the bony structure of the pelvis.
2. b, False
3. a, True
4. 1. f
   2. a
   3. c
   4. d
   5. b
   6. e
5. Stage I begins with true labor and ends with full dilation of the cervix.
6. The *early phase* begins with regular contractions and *lasts until* rapid cervical *dilation begins.*

   The *active phase* begins with rapid cervical *dilation* and lasts until *full dilation* of the cervix occurs.
7. Stage II begins with full dilation of the cervix and lasts until the baby is born.
8. In Stage III, the placenta is delivered.
9. In Stage IV, the uterus contracts and the mother's body functions begin to stabilize.
10. Assessment of a woman's progress through the stages of labor is helpful in detecting problems.
11. a. Perimetrium
    b. Myometrium
    c. Endometrium
12. Myometrium
13. In labor, *effacement* refers to the thinning of the cervix.
14. The upper portion of uterus becomes thicker because of shortening and thickening of the myometrial fibers.
    The lower portion of uterus becomes thinner, softer, and more relaxed as myometrial fibers become longer.
15. a. Active fundal segment
    b. Passive segment
    c. Fundus
    d. Isthmus
    e. Cervix
16. Mothers experiencing their first labor
17. Increment
18. Acme
19. Decrement
20. a. Frequency
    b. Regularity
    c. Duration
    d. Intensity
21. a. Duration
    b. Intensity
    c. Frequency
    d. Regularity
22. 1. c
    2. a
    3. b
23. a. 1 minute
    b. every 3 minutes
    c. 2 minutes
    d. 4:06 AM
24. a. Subjectively
    b. By palpation
    c. With the use of electronic fetal monitoring
25. Internal electronic monitoring
26. Palmar surface of fingertips
27. At least 30 minutes

28. Fingertips should be placed lightly over the fundal portion of the abdomen, which is near the top of the uterus. This is an appropriate area because this is where contractions begin and end.
29. a. Throughout the entire contraction
    b. Because of the nature of the contraction wave, the full effects of the contraction forces on cervical dilatation will be appreciated only at the peak and toward the end of the contraction.
30. Any three of the following:
    a. Less likelihood of medication need for pain relief
    b. Less likelihood of need for vaginal operative delivery
    c. Less likelihood of need for cesarean delivery
    d. Less likelihood of Apgar score of less than 7 at 5 minutes
31. c, Keeping the visit of family members limited
32. e, All of these
33. a, True
34. b, False
35. b, False
36. a, True

REFERENCES

1. Liao, J. B., Buhimschi, C. S., & Norwitz, E. R. (2005). Normal labor: Mechanism and duration. *Obstetrics and Gynecology Clinics of North America, 32*, 145–164.
2. Kilpatrick, S., & Garrison, E. (2012). Normal labor and delivery. In Gabbe, S. G., Niebyl, R., Galan, H., et al. (Eds.), *Obstetrics: Normal and problem pregnancies* (6th ed.). New York: Churchill Livingstone.
3. Cunningham, F. G., Leveno, K. J., Bloom, S., et al. (Eds.). (2014). *Williams obstetrics* (24th ed.). New York: McGraw-Hill.
4. Lund, K., & McManamam, J. (2008). Normal labor, delivery newborn care, and puerperium. In Gibbs, R., Karlan, B., Haney, A., et al. (Eds.), *Danforth's obstetrics & gynecology* (10th ed., pp. 22–42). Philadelphia, PA: Lippincott Williams & Wilkins.
5. Author. (2013). Guidelines for care of patients requiring induction of labor with oxytocin. In Troiano, N. H. (Ed.), *AWHONN's high-risk and critical care obstetrics* (3rd ed., p. 397). Philadelphia, PA: Lippincott Williams & Wilkins.
6. Simpson, K. R. (2008). *Cervical ripening and induction and augmentation of labor* (Practice Monograph, 3rd ed.). Washington, DC: Association of Women's Health, Obstetric and Neonatal.
7. Rothman, B. K. (1996). Women providers and control. *Journal of Obstetric, Gynecologic, and Neonatal Nursing, 25*(3), 254.
8. Peterson, G. (1996). Childbirth: The ordinary miracle—effects of childbirth on women's self-esteem and family relationships. *Pre- and Perinatal Psychology Journal, 11*(2), 101–109.
9. McKay, S. (1991). Shared power: The essence of humanized childbirth. *Pre- and Perinatal Psychology, 54*(4), 283–296.
10. Barrett, S., & Stark, M. (2010). Factors associated with labor support behaviors of nurses. *The Journal of Perinatal Education, 19*(1), 12–18.
11. Hodnett, E. D., Gates, S., Hofmeyr, G. J., et al. (2007). Continuous support for women during childbirth. *Cochrane Database of Systematic Reviews, 18*(3), CD003766.
12. Lothian, J. (2009). Healthy birth: What every pregnant woman needs to know. *The Journal of Perinatal Education, 18*(3), 48–54.
13. American College of Nurse-Midwives, Midwives Alliance of North America, National Association of Certified Professional Midwives. (2012). Supporting healthy and normal physiologic childbirth: A consensus statement by the American College of Nurse-Midwives, Midwives Alliance of North America, and the National Association of Certified Professional Midwives. *Journal of Midwifery and Women's Health, 57*(5), 529–532.
14. Association of Women's Health, Obstetric and Neonatal Nurses. (2011). *Position statement: Nursing support of laboring women.* Washington, DC: Author.
15. JOGNN. (2011). Quality patient care in labor and delivery: A call to action. *Journal of Obstetric, Gynecologic, & Neonatal Nursing, 41*(1), 151–153.
16. Association of Women's Health, Obstetric and Neonatal Nurses. (2014). *Position statement: Non-medically indicated induction and augmentation of labor.* Washington, DC: Author.
17. Moore, J. E., Low, L. K., Titler, M. G., et al. (2014). Moving toward patient-centered care: Women's decisions, perceptions, and experiences of the induction of labor process. *Birth, 4*, 138–146.
18. Low, L. K., & Moffat, A. (2006). Every labor is unique, but "call when your contractions are 3 minutes apart." *Maternal Child Nursing, 31*(5), 307–312.
19. March of Dimes. (2010). *Cultural competence: An essential journey for perinatal nurses.* White Plains, NY: March of Dimes Birth Defects Foundation Education Services.
20. American College of Obstetricians and Gynecologists Committee on Health Care for Underserved Women. (2011). Cultural sensitivity and awareness in the delivery of health care. Committee Opinion No. 493. *Obstetrics & Gynecology, 117*, 1258–1261.
21. Rorie, J. L., Paine, L. L., & Barger, M. K. (1996). Cultural competence in primary care service. *Journal of Nurse Midwifery, 4*(2), 99.

Maternal and Fetal Response to Labor

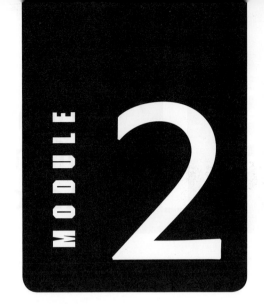

MODULE 2

E. JEAN MARTIN, BETSY BABB KENNEDY,
AND HEATHER M. ROBBINS

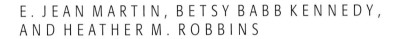

Part 1

Identifying Features of the Pelvis That Make it Adequate for Labor

Part 2

Identifying Relationships Between the Fetus and Pelvis

Part 3

Evaluating for Fetal Malpresentation

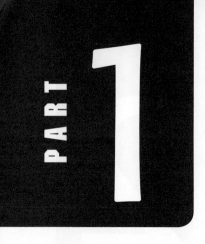

Identifying Features of the Pelvis That Make It Adequate for Labor

Objectives *As you complete Part 1 of this module, you will learn:*

1. Critical factors involved in labor
2. The significance of each type of pelvis to the birth process
3. Features of the pelvis that affect labor
4. Limitations of pelvic evaluation methods

Key Terms *When you have completed Part 1 of this module, you should be able to recall the meaning of the following terms. You should also be able to use the terms when consulting with other health professionals. The terms are defined in this module or in the glossary at the end of this book.*

fetal attitude fetal presentation
fetal lie molding
fetal position pelvic planes

Features of the Pelvis That Make It Adequate for Labor

There are four factors, often referred to as the "four Ps," that affect the progress of labor.

Passage involves
- the size of the pelvis
- the shape of the pelvis
- the ability of the cervix to dilate and the vagina to stretch

Passenger involves
- fetal size, particularly the fetal head
- fetal attitude, which describes the relation of the fetal head, shoulder, and legs to one another
- fetal lie, which refers to the relationship of the long axis ($\updownarrow$) of the fetus to the long axis ($\updownarrow$) of the mother
- fetal presentation, which describes that part of the fetus entering the pelvis first
- fetal position, which refers to the direction toward which the presenting part is pointing—front, side, or back of the maternal pelvis

Powers involve
- the frequency, duration, and intensity of uterine contractions
- abdominal pressures resulting from pushing, which occur in stage II of labor

Psyche involves
- the mother's physical, emotional, and intellectual preparation
- her previous childbirth experiences
- her cultural attitude
- support from significant people in the mother's life

For labor to progress smoothly there must be adaptations of both fetal and maternal factors. Abnormalities of any of these critical factors can mean risk for baby, mother, or both.

16

• **What makes a pelvis adequate for labor?**

The size and the shape of the pelvis make it adequate for labor. The female pelvis is uniquely suited to the demands of childbearing. However, not all women possess the same type of pelvis. The following four classic types of pelves are based on differences in shapes, diameters, and angles (Display 2.1).[1-3] In clinical practice, consistent prediction of a successful vaginal delivery cannot be done based on pelvis shape classification.[4]

DISPLAY 2.1	CLASSIC TYPES OF PELVES

TYPE	**FEATURES**
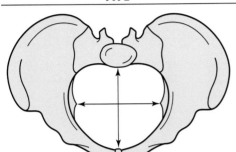 **A.** Gynecoid pelvis	• Typical female pelvis • Adequate for labor and birth • Found in 50% of women
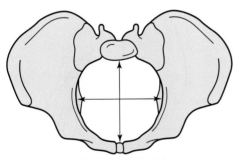 **B.** Android pelvis	• Typical male pelvis • Narrow dimensions • Slow descent of fetal head • Associated with the halting of labor • Forceps delivery often required • Found in 20% of women
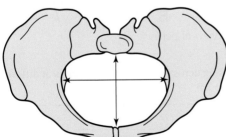 **C.** Anthropoid pelvis	• Apelike pelvis • Adequate for labor and birth • Found in 25% of women
D. Platypelloid pelvis	• Unfavorable for labor • Frequent delay in descent • Found in 5% of women

A woman can have a pelvis that has a combination of characteristics from these classic types. Mixed architectural features are encountered frequently in clinical practice.[5]

In obstetrics, the pelvis is divided into the following parts (Fig. 2.1):
1. *False pelvis*—where there is ample room
2. *True pelvis*—which contains important narrow dimensions through which the fetus must pass

There is a ridge that provides an imaginary dividing line between the two areas. This ridge is the boundary for the inlet to the true pelvis.

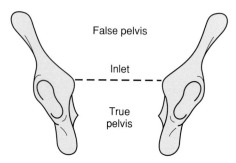

FIGURE 2.1 False pelvis and true pelvis.

NOTE: *The false pelvis has no obstetric significance, whereas the true pelvis has great significance.*

The *true pelvis* can be divided into three key areas (Fig. 2.2):
1. Inlet
2. Pelvic cavity, which extends from the inlet to the outlet
3. Outlet

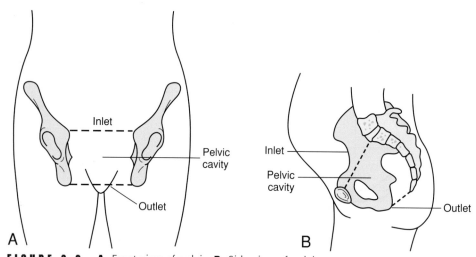

FIGURE 2.2 **A.** Front view of pelvis. **B.** Side view of pelvis.

The *pelvic planes* are imaginary flat surfaces passing across parts of the true pelvis at different levels. Three important planes are shown in Figure 2.3.

• How is the adequacy of the pelvis evaluated?

The relationship of the fetal size to the pelvis must be evaluated. This relationship changes depending on the forces and stages of labor, and positioning of the mother can bring about subtle changes in one or two pelvic dimensions (e.g., the McRoberts maneuver). Dynamic changes

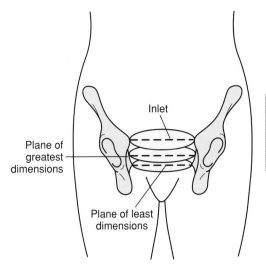

Inlet

Plane of greatest dimensions

Plane of least dimensions

The plane of least dimensions is the narrowest section of the pelvis. Occasionally, labor stops because the fetus cannot descend past this area.

FIGURE 2.3 Pelvic planes.

in the fetal head, thorax, and abdomen occur as the pelvic passageway is negotiated during descent. Efforts to predict cephalopelvic disproportion have included the following[1]:

Clinical pelvimetry	• Estimation of pelvic shapes and dimensions by the examiner • Wide margin of error depending on the examiner's skill
X-ray pelvimetry	• Potential fetal exposure to low-dose radiation • Can provide critical pelvic diameters not otherwise obtainable • Sometimes used in breech presentations • Has been replaced by other pelvic imaging methods
Ultrasonography	• Uses sound waves, not ionizing energy • Not useful for evaluating maternal pelvic measurement • Useful for precisely measuring fetal biparietal diameters and fetal head circumference
Computed tomographic (CT) pelvimetry (CT scanning)	• Has replaced x-ray pelvimetry at many institutions • Accuracy is improved over conventional x-ray pelvimetry • Involves a lower fetal radiation exposure than x-ray • Maternal movement during procedure needs to be minimal to prevent distortion • Expense is comparable to that of conventional x-ray
Magnetic resonance imaging	• Offers accurate pelvic measurements and complete fetal imaging • Has the potential to aid in diagnosing soft tissue dystocia and obstructed labor • Use is limited by expense, length of time needed to obtain the study, and availability of equipment

Imaging studies, although readily defining values for the parameters of the true bony pelvis, have not been shown to consistently predict women at risk for cephalopelvic disproportion.[5] Radiographic studies are generally avoided during pregnancy because of the theoretical risk of radiation exposure to the fetus. Clinical pelvimetry is a skill, yet still may not allow prediction of the course or outcomes of delivery. A trial of labor is commonly used to determine if the woman's pelvis is adequate for delivery of the baby.

Additional considerations include the following:

• Except for some relaxation of the pelvic joints because of hormonal influences, the bones of the pelvis cannot expand.
• The soft tissues of the birth canal (the cervix and pelvic floor musculature) provide resistance during labor. The cervix undergoes biochemical changes that increase its elasticity. The musculature of the pelvic floor facilitates rotation and flexion for the fetal head.
• The relationship of the fetal head size to the pelvis is important.
• The fetal head has the ability to change shape to fit through the pelvis. This ability of the head to change shape is called *molding.*

• Because of the tilt of the pelvis, the fetus descends through this pathway during labor and birth, as shown in Figure 2.4.

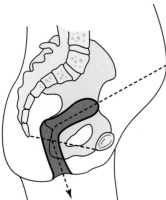

FIGURE 2.4 Pathway of fetal descent.

PRACTICE/REVIEW QUESTIONS

After reviewing Part 1, answer the following questions.

1. List four critical factors involved in the labor process.

   a. _____

   b. _____

   c. _____

   d. _____

2. Match the definition in Column B with the correct term in Column A.

   Column A

   1. _____ Lie

   2. _____ Attitude

   3. _____ Position

   4. _____ Presentation

   Column B

   a. Relationship of the long axis of the fetus to the long axis of the mother
   b. That part of the fetal body that is entering the pelvis
   c. The relationship of fetal parts to one another
   d. The direction toward which the presenting part is pointing with respect to the front, side, or back of the mother's pelvis

3. List the four main types of pelves.

   a. _____

   b. _____

   c. _____

   d. _____

4. The pelvis best suited for labor and birth is the

   _____ pelvis. This type of pelvis is found in

   _____ % of women.

5. The pelvis that has narrow dimensions and is likely to result in labor stopping or a forceps delivery is the

   _____ pelvis. This type of pelvis is found in

   _____ % of women.

6. Match the areas of the pelvis with the correct numbers in the diagram.

   _____ a. Inlet

   _____ b. False pelvis

   _____ c. True pelvis

   _____ d. Outlet

   _____ e. Plane of least dimensions

7. The true pelvis is made up of three key planes called:

   a. _____

   b. _____

   c. _____

8. The planes of the true pelvis are critical because: _____

   _____

9. Name two ways in which the female pelvis is evaluated for adequacy.

   a. _____

   b. _____

10. Explain how it is possible for the fetal head to fit through the rigid, bony pelvis.

   _____

   _____

PRACTICE/REVIEW ANSWER KEY

1. a. Passage
   b. Passenger
   c. Power
   d. Psyche
2. 1. a
   2. c
   3. d
   4. b
3. a. Gynecoid
   b. Android
   c. Platypelloid
   d. Anthropoid
4. Gynecoid; 50
5. Android; 20
6. a. 1
   b. 2
   c. 5
   d. 3
   e. 4
7. a. Least dimensions
   b. Greatest dimensions
   c. Pelvic inlet
8. The fetus must pass through these areas, some of which are narrow.
9. a. X-ray
   b. Pelvic examination
10. The head flexes and the bones of the scalp mold somewhat.

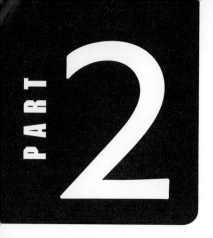

PART 2

Identifying Relationships Between the Fetus and Pelvis

As you complete Part 2 of this module, you will learn:

1. Relationships of the fetal position and presenting part to the outcome of labor
2. Landmarks used to identify the position of the fetus
3. Features of the pelvis that affect labor
4. How to determine and describe fetal lie, presentation, attitude, and position

When you have completed Part 2 of this module, you should be able to recall the meaning of the following terms. You should also be able to use the terms when consulting with other health professionals. The terms are defined in this module or in the glossary at the end of this book.

biparietal diameter	mentum
denominator	occiput
fetal anencephaly	placenta previa
fetal hydrocephaly	prematurity
fontanelle	sinciput
grand multiparity	suture
hydramnios	vertex

Relationships Between the Fetus and Pelvis

- **How does the fetal passenger accommodate to the pelvis during labor?**

The position of the fetus as the mother is ready to go into labor largely determines how smoothly the labor and delivery will progress. The fetal head is the largest part of the baby and is composed of both fixed and flexible parts. Becoming familiar with the parts of the fetal skull is essential because the identification of certain landmarks will assist you when performing vaginal examinations to determine the mother's labor progress. The skull consists of three major divisions (Fig. 2.5):

1. Face
2. Back of the skull
3. Cranium, or top of the skull

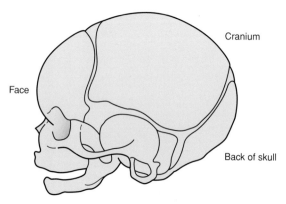

FIGURE 2.5 Major divisions of the fetal skull.

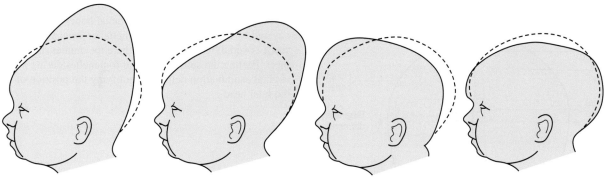

FIGURE 2.6 Molding of the fetal head in different cephalic presentations.

The bones of the face and the back of the skull are fused and fixed, but the cranium consists of several large bones that are not fused together at the time of birth. This permits the shape of the head to change somewhat as the fetus passes through the narrow, rigid pelvis (Fig. 2.6).

The force of uterine contractions on the fetal head can cause overlapping of the cranial bones; this is called *molding* and can be felt during a vaginal examination.

• What other landmarks of the fetal skull are used in describing the fetal head?

There are four landmarks that are important in describing the general areas of the fetal head (Fig. 2.7):
1. *Sinciput*—brow area
2. *Vertex*—area between the anterior and posterior fontanelles
3. *Occiput*—area beneath the posterior fontanelle where the occipital bone is located
4. *Mentum*—fetal chin

NOTE: *These terms are used later in this module to denote which part of the fetal head is leading as the fetus descends.*

If looking down at the fetal cranium, you would see the divisions between the bones of the head, as depicted in Figure 2.8.

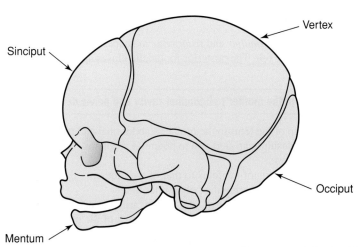

FIGURE 2.7 Bony landmarks used in describing areas of the fetal head.

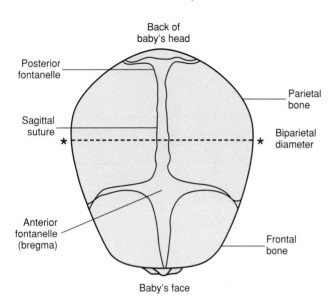

A *suture* is a space between the cranial bones that is covered by a membrane. A *fontanelle,* or *fontanel,* is a space covered by a membrane where the cranial sutures meet. Feeling the suture lines and fontanelles during a vaginal examination helps in identifying the position of the fetal head.

FIGURE 2.8 Suture, fontanelle, and bony landmarks used in describing the position of the fetal head.

There are two important *landmarks* formed by the sutures that are useful in identifying the position of the fetal head in the pelvis.

1. *Anterior fontanelle* (Fig. 2.9)—is *diamond-shaped* and measures 2 × 3 cm. This is sometimes referred to as the *bregma.* When the head is *moderately* flexed or hyperextended, this fontanelle can be palpated. It remains open approximately 18 months after birth to allow for brain growth.

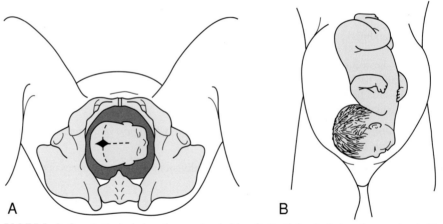

FIGURE 2.9 **A.** Vaginal view (hyperextended head). **B.** Abdominal view (hyperextended head).

2. *Posterior fontanelle* (Fig. 2.10)—is *smaller* and *triangular* in shape. When the head is well flexed, this fontanelle can be felt. The posterior fontanelle closes approximately 12 weeks after birth.

• How is the position of the fetus in the mother's abdominal cavity and pelvis described?

You must understand the relationship of the fetus to the mother's abdominal and pelvic cavities as careful observation of these relationships can alert you to potential problems. To review, four aspects of this relationship are as follows:

1. *Lie*—the relationship of the long axis of the fetus to that of the mother
2. *Presentation*—that part of the fetus entering the pelvic inlet first
3. *Attitude*—the relationship of the fetal parts (e.g., chest, chin, arms) to each other
4. *Position*—the relationship of the presenting part to a specific area of the mother's pelvis

***NOTE:** Station also describes a relationship between the presenting part of the fetus and the maternal pelvis. This is discussed in Part 3.*

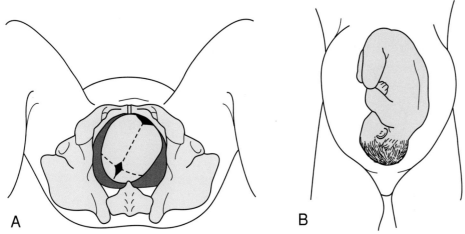

FIGURE 2.10 **A.** Vaginal view (normal flexed head). **B.** Abdominal view (normal flexed head).

Types of Fetal Lie

Figure 2.11 illustrates types of fetal lie. Display 2.2 illustrates longitudinal and transverse lies.

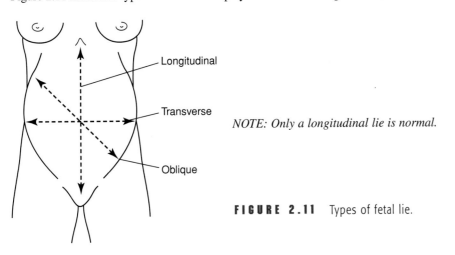

Longitudinal

Transverse

Oblique

NOTE: Only a longitudinal lie is normal.

FIGURE 2.11 Types of fetal lie.

DISPLAY 2.2 ILLUSTRATIONS OF FETAL LIE

A longitudinal lie, occurring in 99.5% of pregnancies, is when the long axis of the fetal body is parallel to the mother's spine.

A longitudinal lie can be either *cephalic* or *breech*.

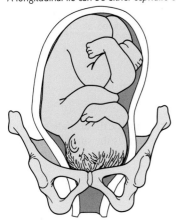

When the head is leading, it is called a *cephalic lie.*

A. Cephalic lie

display text continues on page 26

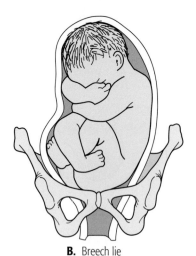

If the buttocks are coming first, it is called a *breech lie.*

B. Breech lie

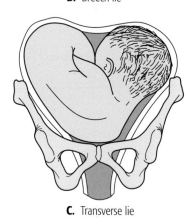

The fetus can assume a *transverse lie,* in which the long axis of the fetus lies directly across the mother's spine. It occurs in approximately 0.3% of pregnancies.

C. Transverse lie

Transverse lie is often associated with the following[6]:
1. *Grand multiparity* (having five or more pregnancies)
2. A small (contracted) pelvis
3. Placenta previa
4. Polyhydramnios
5. Fetal prematurity
6. Uterine anomalies

Most women at 37 weeks' gestation with a transverse lie convert to a longitudinal lie, but the risk of morbidity from cord prolapse and uterine rupture is great. Therefore, **vaginal delivery is not possible with a transverse lie**. External version may be attempted; if it fails, a cesarean delivery is planned.

Types of Fetal Attitude

Attitude refers to the relationship of the fetal parts to each other. Normally, the attitude is one of *flexion* or *extension* in relation to the fetal spine. Adequate flexion creates the smallest cephalic diameter to facilitate delivery (Display 2.3).

DISPLAY 2.3 ILLUSTRATIONS OF FETAL ATTITUDE

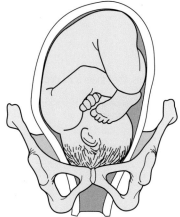

A. Attitude of flexion

Flexion is when the chin is near the chest, the arms and legs are folded in front of the body, and the back is curved.

This position of the fetus presents the smallest possible fetal head measurements in relation to the pelvic passageway and is the only normal attitude.

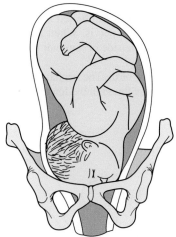

B. Attitude of extension

Extension occurs when the head is bent back and the chest and abdomen are slightly curved.

In the extreme of this position, the fetal face is the leading part as it descends through the pelvis. It is traumatic for the baby, who is often not deliverable vaginally because a larger diameter of the fetal head presents, unlike when the head is well flexed.

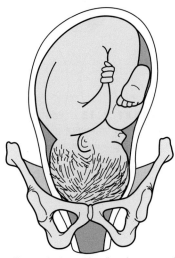

C. Military attitude (neither flexed nor extended)

Military attitude occurs when the fetal position is not one of flexion or extension.

display text continues on page 28

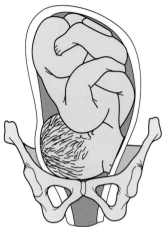

Partial extension occurs when there is moderate extension of the head.

D. Attitude of partial extension.

The *cephalic prominence* describes that part of the fetal head that can be felt by placing both hands on the sides of the uterus and feeling down toward the pelvis. When the head is in normal flexion, the cephalic prominence is felt on the opposite side of the fetal back; in Figure 2.12, it is found in the lower left of the mother's abdomen.

Hyperextension of the head results in the face presenting for birth. The cephalic prominence is felt on the same side as the fetal back; in Figure 2.13, it is found in the lower right of the mother's abdomen.

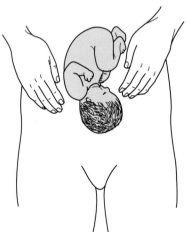

FIGURE 2.12 Position of the cephalic prominence in normal flexion.

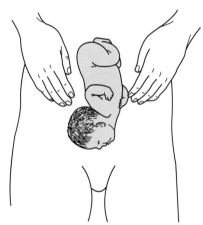

FIGURE 2.13 Position of the cephalic prominence in hyperextension.

The location of the cephalic prominence can aid in diagnosing the attitude of the fetus and any malpositions.

Types of Fetal Presentation

Presentation refers to that part of the fetus entering the pelvic inlet first. The main presentations are as follows (Table 2.1):

- Shoulder
- Breech
- Cephalic

TABLE 2.1	TYPES OF FETAL PRESENTATION	
Shoulder	Either shoulder leads	Fortunately, shoulder presentation rarely occurs.
Breech	Buttocks lead	Breech presentation occurs in 3–4% of pregnancies and is more common in preterm pregnancies.[1]
Cephalic	Head leads	Cephalic presentation occurs in 96–97% of term pregnancies.[1]

***NOTE:** The term "compound presentation" is used when there is more than one fetal part presenting at the pelvic inlet. If the umbilical cord is present at the inlet, it is known as a funic presentation.*

Shoulder Presentation

The shoulder is entering the pelvis first (Fig. 2.14). This presentation occurs infrequently.

Breech Presentation

The buttocks or breech enters the pelvis first (Figs. 2.15 to 2.17). Breech presentation can be complete, frank, or footling. The prevalence of breech presentation depends on gestational age, occurring more frequently in earlier gestations.

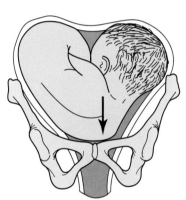

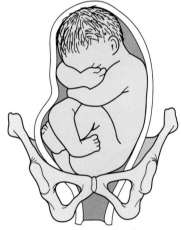

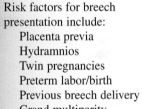

Risk factors for breech presentation include:
   Placenta previa
   Hydramnios
   Twin pregnancies
   Preterm labor/birth
   Previous breech delivery
   Grand multiparity
   Fetal hydrocephaly
   Fetal anencephaly
   Uterine anomalies

FIGURE 2.14 Shoulder presentation.

FIGURE 2.15 Complete breech presentation.

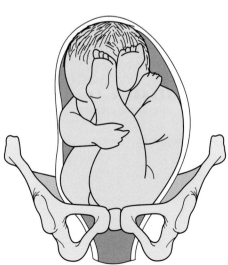

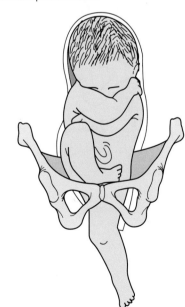

FIGURE 2.16 Frank breech presentation.

FIGURE 2.17 Footling breech presentation.

Cephalic Presentation

Cephalic presentation (96% to 97% of term pregnancies) can occur[1]:

When the head is *well flexed* and the vertex presents first, as in Figure 2.18.
When the head is *poorly flexed* and the brow presents first, as in Figure 2.19.
When the head is *poorly flexed* and the face presents first, as in Figure 2.20.

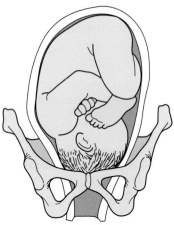

This presentation is optimal for delivery.

FIGURE 2.18 Vertex presents in cephalic presentation.

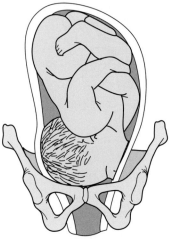

FIGURE 2.19 Brow presents in cephalic presentation.

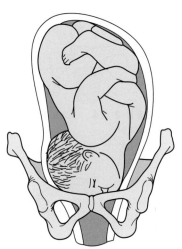

FIGURE 2.20 Face presents in cephalic presentation.

Types of Fetal Position

• How are the fetal positions described?

"Position" refers to the relationship of the presenting part to a specific area on the woman's pelvis. In describing fetal position, certain landmarks on the fetus, called *denominators,* are used.

In *vertex* presentations, the *occiput* is the denominator (Fig. 2.21).

In *face* presentations, the *mentum* (chin) is the denominator (Fig. 2.22).

In *breech* presentations, the *sacrum* is the denominator (Fig. 2.23).

In *shoulder* presentations, the *scapula,* or the *acromial process,* is the denominator (Fig. 2.24).

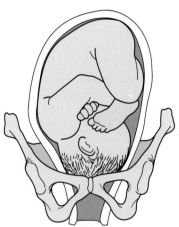

FIGURE 2.21 Vertex presentation with occiput as the denominator.

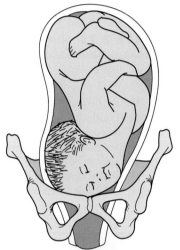

FIGURE 2.22 Face presentation with chin as the denominator.

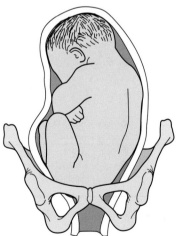

FIGURE 2.23 Breech presentation with sacrum as the denominator.

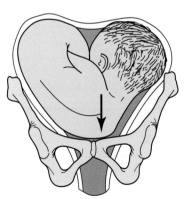

FIGURE 2.24 Shoulder presentation with the scapula (acromial process) as the denominator.

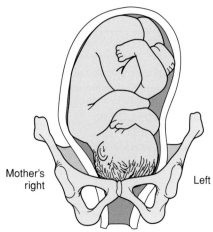

FIGURE 2.25 Occiput leading and pointing to mother's right.

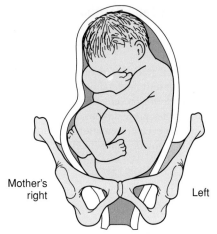

FIGURE 2.26 Sacrum leading and pointing to mother's left.

Having determined which denominator is the leading part of the fetus, its *position* can be described further. Note whether the denominator is pointing to the left (**L**) or right (**R**) side of the mother's pelvis. For example:

The *occiput* of the fetus leads and points to the mother's *right* (Fig. 2.25).

The *sacrum* of the fetus leads and points to the mother's *left* (Fig. 2.26).

Finally, in describing position, note whether the denominator is in the front (anterior), directly to the side (transverse), or in the back (posterior) of the *mother's* pelvis (Display 2.4).

DISPLAY 2.4 EXAMPLES OF DENOMINATOR POSITIONS IN CEPHALIC PRESENTATION

A

Occiput is in the **A**nterior (front) of the pelvis.
R   Right
O   Occiput
A   Anterior

B

Occiput is **T**ransverse (to the side) of the pelvis.
R   Right
O   Occiput
T   Transverse

C

Occiput is in the **P**osterior (back) of the pelvis.
R   Right
O   Occiput
P   Posterior

Display 2.5 shows breech positions.
Display 2.6 shows a face presentation with the *mentum* (chin) leading.

DISPLAY 2.5 EXAMPLES OF DENOMINATOR POSITIONS
IN BREECH PRESENTATION

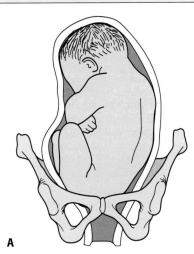 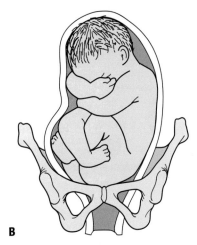

A

Sacrum is in the **A**nterior (front)
of the pelvis.
L Left
S Sacrum
A Anterior

B

Sacrum is in the **P**osterior (back)
of the pelvis.
L Left
S Sacrum
P Posterior

DISPLAY 2.6 EXAMPLE OF DENOMINATOR POSITION IN
CEPHALIC PRESENTATION WITH FACE PRESENTING

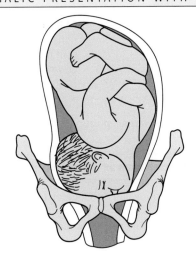

The **M**entum (chin) is in the **L**eft **A**nterior of
the pelvis.
L Left
M Mentum
A Anterior

Vertex Position

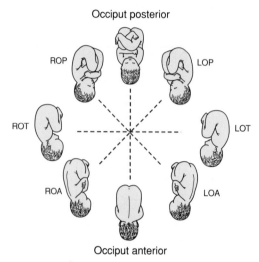

Occiput posterior

ROP   LOP

ROT   LOT

ROA   LOA

Occiput anterior

NOTE: The occiput is the denominator.

FIGURE 2.27 Variety of fetal positions with vertex presentations. (Adapted with permission from Oxorn, H. [1986]. *Oxorn-Foote human labor & birth* [5th ed., p. 59]. New York: Appleton-Century-Crofts.)

Breech Positions

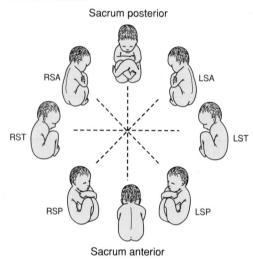

Sacrum posterior

RSA   LSA

RST   LST

RSP   LSP

Sacrum anterior

NOTE: The sacrum is the denominator.

FIGURE 2.28 Variety of fetal positions with breech presentations. (Adapted with permission from Oxorn, H. [1986]. *Oxorn-Foote human labor & birth* [5th ed., p. 59]. New York: Appleton-Century-Crofts.)

Figures 2.27 and 2.28 illustrate how various positions for vertex and breech presentations can be described.

• How can fetal position and presentation be determined?

It is important to determine fetal position and presentation to predict the course of labor. Several methods are available:
- Combined abdominal inspection and palpation (Leopold's maneuvers)
- Vaginal examination
- Ultrasonography
- CT scanning
- X-ray examination

Because x-rays are known to be harmful to the fetus if used frequently or in early pregnancy, they are used rarely, and only when fetal position cannot be determined in any other way.

PRACTICE/REVIEW QUESTIONS

After reviewing Part 2, answer the following questions.

1. Label the following diagrams.

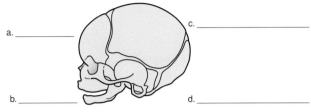

a. _____   c. _____

b. _____   d. _____

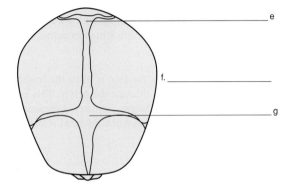

e _____

f. _____

g _____

2. The posterior fontanelle closes approximately _____ months after birth. It is _____ shaped and can be felt when the head is _____ flexed.

3. The anterior fontanelle closes approximately _____ months after birth. It is shaped and can be felt when the head is flexed.

4. The only normal lie is _____.

5. A longitudinal lie can be, when the head leads, or _____, when the buttocks come first.

6. Why is vaginal delivery impossible with a transverse lie?

_____

_____

7. The only normal attitude is one of _____

_____

8. Why is a fetus positioned in extreme extension often not deliverable vaginally?

_____

_____

9. Locating the cephalic prominence is helpful in diagnosing fetal _____ and malpositions.

10. The three primary types of presentations are:

a. _____ (approximately 96%)

b. _____ (3% to 4% of pregnancies)

c. _____ (infrequent)

11. The only normal presentation is _____ , when the _____ presents first.

12. Prematurity, placenta previa, and/or grand multiparity can be associated with a _____ presentation.

13. State the denominator used to describe the fetal position in each of the following presentations.

Fetal Position   Denominator

a. Vertex   _____

b. Face   _____

c. Breech   _____

d. Shoulder   _____

14. Fully describe each of the following according to fetal lie, presentation, and position.

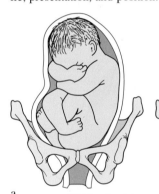 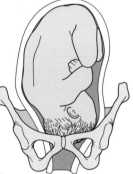

a. _____   b. _____

_____   _____

_____   _____

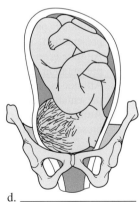

c. _____   d. _____

_____   _____

_____   _____

15. State five ways in which fetal position and presentation can be determined.

    a. _____

    b. _____

    c. _____

    d. _____

    e. _____

16. The term *position* refers to which of the following?

    a. The relationship of the long axis of the fetus to that of the mother

    b. The part of the fetus that first enters the inlet of the pelvis

    c. The degree of descent of the fetus through the maternal pelvis

    d. The relationship of a specific point of the fetus to one of the four quadrants of the mother's pelvis

17. Which statement accurately describes the fetal attitude, lie, presentation, and position in the following illustration?

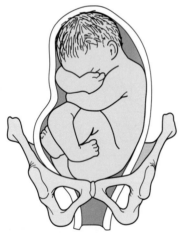

    a. Attitude is one of extension, longitudinal lie, breech presentation, and position is LSP.
    b. Attitude is one of flexion, longitudinal lie, breech presentation, and position is LSA.
    c. Attitude is one of flexion, longitudinal lie, breech presentation, and position is LSP.
    d. Attitude is one of extension, longitudinal lie, cephalic presentation, and position is RSP.

PRACTICE/REVIEW ANSWER KEY

1. a. Sinciput
   b. Mentum
   c. Vertex
   d. Occiput
   e. Posterior fontanelle
   f. Sagittal suture
   g. Anterior fontanelle (bregma)
2. 3; triangular; well
3. 18; diamond; moderately
4. longitudinal
5. cephalic; breech
6. Vaginal delivery is not possible with a transverse lie because the long axis of the fetus lies across the mother's spine.
7. Flexion
8. In extreme extension, the face is often the leading part as the fetus descends through the pelvis. This is traumatic for the baby. A larger diameter is presented to the vaginal passageway than when the head is well flexed.
9. Attitude
10. a. Cephalic
    b. Breech
    c. Shoulder
11. Cephalic; vertex
12. Breech
13. a. Occiput
    b. Mentum
    c. Sacrum
    d. Scapula or acromial process
14. a. Longitudinal (breech) lie
       Breech presentation
       LSP
    b. Longitudinal (cephalic) lie
       Cephalic presentation
       ROA
    c. Longitudinal (cephalic) lie
       Cephalic presentation
       ROP
    d. Longitudinal (cephalic) lie
       Cephalic presentation
       LMT (you may interpret the diagram to be LMA)
15. a. Abdominal inspection and palpation
    b. Vaginal examination
    c. Ultrasonography
    d. CT scanning
    e. X-ray examination
16. d. The relationship of a specific point of the fetus to one of the four quadrants of the mother's pelvis.
17. c. Attitude is one of flexion, longitudinal lie, breech presentation, and position is LSP.

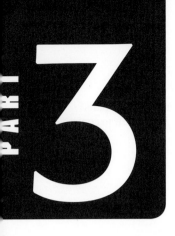

Evaluating for Fetal Malpresentation

Objectives — *As you complete Part 3 of this module, you will learn:*

1. What is meant by fetal malpresentation
2. To identify maternal and fetal conditions that can lead to fetal malpresentation
3. What to do if you suspect a fetal malpresentation

Key Terms — *When you have completed Part 3 of this module, you should be able to recall the meaning of the following terms. You should also be able to use the terms when consulting with other health professionals. The terms are defined in this module or in the glossary at the end of this book.*

anoxia
dystocia
prolapsed cord

Fetal Malpresentation

• What is fetal malpresentation?

Malpresentation means that some other part of the fetus, such as buttocks, shoulder, or face, is presenting at or near the pelvic inlet.

Maternal and Fetal Conditions That Can Lead to Fetal Malpresentation

Maternal factors leading to malpresentation include the following:
- Contracted (small) pelvis (the most commonly occurring factor)
- Lax abdominal muscles so that the uterus and fetus fall forward, preventing good fetal descent
- Uterine tumors (fibroids), which can block the entry to the pelvic passageway
- Uterine malformations, which can prevent efficient labor
- Abnormalities of placental size or location that lead to the fetus assuming a position unfavorable to labor and/or descent

Fetal factors leading to malpresentation include the following:
- Breech presentation or transverse lie
- Abnormal fetal attitude (e.g., hyperextension)
- Multiple pregnancy
- Fetal abnormalities (e.g., hydrocephalus)
- *Polyhydramnios* (excessive amounts of fluid permit greater freedom for fetal movement and, therefore, abnormal positions)

Effects of Malpresentation on Labor
- Weak and irregular contractions that are inefficient
- Prolonged labor
- Slow and incomplete cervical dilatation
- Failure of presenting part to descend
- Increased need for operative delivery
- Increased risk of uterine rupture

Effects of Malpresentation on the Mother

- Maternal exhaustion because of prolonged labor
- Greater chance of lacerations along the birth canal because of wider presenting parts
- Heavier bleeding because of lacerations and/or an exhausted uterus, which fails to contract after delivery
- Increased risk of infection caused by the following:
  - Early rupture of membranes
  - Increased blood loss
  - Tissue damage because of lacerations and bruising
  - Prolonged labor
- Decreased peristalsis of the bowel and bladder

Effects of Malpresentation on the Fetus

- Difficult fit through the pelvis, which leads to edema of the presenting part and excessive molding
- Long labor, which can be hard on the fetus, increasing the possibility of anoxia and intrauterine death
- Increased incidence of forceps and cesarean birth
- More frequently occurring prolapsed cord

• What should you do if you suspect fetal malpresentation?

The nurse is often the first person to recognize a malpresentation such as breech presentation. Fetal malpresentation is detected through careful abdominal palpation and vaginal examination. If you suspect malpresentation during your nursing assessment, take the following steps:

1. Alert the primary care provider immediately.
2. Monitor the baby closely until the primary care provider arrives.
3. Closely assess the mother's status and progress in labor. Do not leave her alone.

For all patients who have a breech presentation or any presentation that does not fit the pelvis well or is not settled well into the pelvis, it is essential to inspect the perineum, listen to fetal heart tones, and conduct a vaginal examination as soon as the membranes rupture.

> When the presenting part fails to fit the pelvic inlet closely, the danger of a prolapsed cord exists.

A vaginal examination should be performed in the following situations:

- There is unexplained fetal distress (this is especially true when the presenting part is high).
- The membranes rupture with a high presenting part.
- The membranes rupture in a woman presenting with a malpresentation.
- The baby is premature.
- There is a twin gestation.

• Why is it necessary to be able to recognize a breech presentation?

A prolapsed cord can occur in a breech presentation because the pelvic cavity is not well filled when the feet or buttocks are coming first. Once the cord is out of the uterus or vagina, the fetal blood and oxygen supply can be blocked because of (a) a drop in temperature, (b) spasm of the blood vessels, or (c) compression between the pelvic brim and the presenting part. When a prolapsed cord occurs, a delay of more than 30 minutes in delivering the baby increases fetal mortality fourfold.[2] (Prolapsed cords are discussed further in Module 16.)

NOTE: *For more information on describing fetal descent during labor, refer to Module 5.*

PRACTICE/REVIEW QUESTIONS

After reviewing Part 3, answer the following questions.

1. Define malpresentation. _____

2. State at least four maternal or fetal factors that can lead to malpresentation. _____

   _____

3. Why is it critical that you be able to recognize a breech

   presentation? _____

   _____

PRACTICE/REVIEW ANSWER KEY

1. *Malpresentation* means that a part other than the vertex, such as buttocks, shoulder, or face, is presenting at or near the pelvic inlet.
2. Maternal factors are a contracted pelvis, lax abdominal muscles, uterine tumors blocking entry to the pelvic passageway, uterine malformations preventing efficient labor, and abnormalities of placental size or locations. Fetal factors are breech or transverse lie, abnormal fetal attitude, multiple pregnancy, fetal abnormalities, and polyhydramnios.
3. A prolapsed cord can occur in a breech presentation. The prolapsed cord can result in blockage of blood supply to the fetus, which could result in fetal death.

REFERENCES

1. Cunningham, F. G., Leveno, K. J., Bloom, S. L., et al. (Eds.). (2014). *Williams obstetrics* (24th ed.). New York: McGraw-Hill.
2. Oxorn, H. (1986). *Oxorn-Foote human labor & birth* (5th ed.). New York: Appleton-Century-Crofts.
3. King, T. L., Brucker, M. C., Kreibs, J. M., et al. (Eds.). (2013). *Varney's midwifery* (5th ed.). Burlington, MA: Jones & Bartlett.
4. Yeomans, E. R. (2006). Clinical pelvimetry. *Clinical Obstetrics and Gynecology, 49*(1), 140–146.
5. Liao, J. B., Buhimschi, C. S., & Norwitz, E. R. (2005). Normal labor: Mechanism and duration. *Obstetrics and Gynecology Clinics of North America, 32*, 145–164.
6. Stitely, M. L., & Gherman, R. B. (2005). Labor with abnormal presentation and position. *Obstetrics and Gynecology Clinics of North America, 32*, 165–179.

Admission Assessment of the Laboring Woman

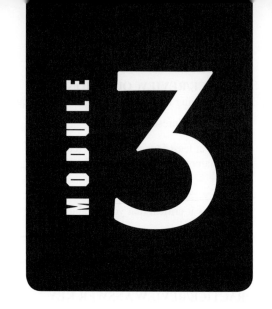

MODULE **3**

DIANE J. ANGELINI, E. JEAN MARTIN, AND DONNA J. RUTH

Skill Unit 1

Physical Examination of the Laboring Woman

Skill Unit 2

Testing for Ruptured Membranes
- Sterile Speculum Examination
- Nitrazine Paper Test

Skill Unit 3

Fern Testing for Ruptured Membranes

Skill Unit 4

Vaginal Examination

O b j e c t i v e s

As you complete this module, you will learn:

1. Key questions to ask the woman being admitted to the labor unit
2. To identify factors that make the laboring woman a high-risk patient
3. To recognize those characteristics that help to distinguish between true labor and false labor
4. Physical assessment skills used in admitting the laboring woman
5. How to use the Fern test, the Nitrazine paper test, and a sterile speculum examination to evaluate pooling of fluid in determining if membranes have ruptured
6. To evaluate cervical effacement, dilatation, station, and fetal presentation during labor.
7. The importance of preparing for and informing the expectant mother of examination and test procedures

K e y   T e r m s

When you have completed this module, you should be able to recall the meaning of the following terms. You should also be able to use the terms when consulting with other health professionals. The terms are defined in this module or in the glossary at the end of this book.

ABO incompatibility
abruptio placentae
amniotic fluid index (AFI)
arborization
bradycardia
chancroid
chorioamnionitis
cleft palate
clonus
Down syndrome
eclampsia
esophageal atresia
group B streptococcus (GBS)
herpes simplex virus (HSV) type 1, type 2
hydramnios (polyhydramnios)
macrosomia
meconium

meconium aspiration syndrome (MAS)
microcephaly
multipara
nullipara
oligohydramnios
perinatal
perinatal morbidity
perinatal mortality
postterm infant
pyloric stenosis
Rh incompatibility
spina bifida
tachycardia
term infant
thrombophlebitis
vertical transmission

Identifying Critical Information

- **What critical information must be identified for the woman being admitted to the labor unit?**

Certain information is needed immediately to evaluate the following:
- The extent of the woman's labor
- Her general physical condition
- Her risk status
- Her preparation for labor and delivery

This assessment must be carried out quickly to determine how active the labor is and to become alert to women with a history of rapid deliveries or those with problems denoting risk.

Questions	Information Needed
1. What made you come to the hospital?	1. Presenting complaint
2. When were you told the baby was due?	2. Expected date of delivery/confinement (EDD/EDC) and how it was determined: • by dates • by size • by ultrasound and during which trimester the ultrasound was performed Dating criteria by ACOG: Ultrasound confirmation of gestational age should be in agreement with menstrual dates within 4 days when performed at 6 to 9.6 weeks; within 7 days at 10 to 13.6 weeks or within 10 days when performed at 14 to 20 weeks. Dating after 20 weeks by ultrasound is not completely accurate.[1]
3. How many babies have you had?	3. Projection about possible rapid labor due to multiparity
4. When did your labor begin? How far apart are the contractions? Have they changed in intensity? Have you had any bleeding?	4. Stage of labor she is in: • Frequency, duration, and intensity of contractions • Amount and character of bloody show • Identification of abnormal bleeding versus bloody show
5. Has the bag of water (membranes) broken, and when did it occur? What color was the fluid?	5. Whether or not membranes have ruptured Risk of chorioamnionitis owing to prolonged rupture of membranes Presence or absence of meconium-stained or bloody amniotic fluid
6. How has your pregnancy been? Did you have any problems that required special treatment? Have you had any bleeding?	6. Any abnormalities in the pregnancy—specifically ask about problems with blood pressure (BP), bleeding, or infections
7. When did you last have anything to eat or drink? What were these foods?	7. Extent of gastric fullness
8. Are you allergic to any foods or drugs that you know of?	8. Any known allergies to drugs
9. Who has come with you? Will they be staying with you during labor?	9. Presence of a support system
10. Have you had any preparation for this labor and delivery?	10. Knowledge level regarding the birth experience
11. Is there anything special about your pregnancy that I should know?	11. To elicit information that could affect her labor/delivery or the newborn Opportunity for woman to share specific concerns regarding her care

Guidelines for History Taking

- Maintain eye contact.
- **Introduce yourself** and confirm the name by which the woman wishes to be called.
- Inform the woman that you need to ask several questions and that you will stop whenever a contraction begins.

- Ask open-ended questions when possible. For example, "Can you tell me about any problems you have had during this pregnancy?" instead of "Have you had an infection (or problem) during this pregnancy?" and "What preparation have you had for your labor and delivery?" instead of "Have you attended childbirth preparation classes?"

You might need to ask specific questions to follow up on the answers to your open-ended questions.

Identifying the High-Risk Mother and Fetus

• How can you identify a mother and fetus who are at risk?

Mothers with high-risk pregnancies tend to have high-risk infants. These patients need to be identified as early as possible on admittance to the labor unit. Women who begin pregnancy as a low-risk patient may develop complications that make them high risk during the labor and delivery process. Assessment on admission and throughout the labor process will help to identify these women in a timely manner.

Taking a good history and reviewing the prenatal record of the woman when she is admitted to the labor unit is necessary for identifying the high-risk intrapartal patient. Risk status may have changed in the period between the last prenatal visit and admission for delivery.

Risk Factors for Laboring Women

Extremes of age
Fifth or more pregnancy
Height 60 in or less
Little or no weight gain during pregnancy
Cigarette smoking
Rh incompatibility or ABO incompatibility
  problems
Previous premature deliveries
Previous birth to a large infant (>4,000 g/9 lb—
  macrosomia)
Previous perinatal loss
Less than a high school education or in the
  poverty-level income group
Single marital status
Unplanned pregnancy
Little or no antenatal care
History of a congenital anomaly or medi-
  cal disorder, such as anemia, diabetes,
  renal disease, cardiac problems, malignant
  tumors, or psychiatric disorders
Symptoms of oral (type 1) or genital (type 2)
  herpes simplex virus (HSV) or a current positive herpes culture; current symptoms, especially significant if the genital herpes infection
  present is the woman's first infection (primary
  infection) experienced during pregnancy
Lesions appear as blister-like vesicles, which
  progress to a crusted or ulcer-type appearance. HSV of either type 1 or 2 can be shed
  at the cervix in symptomatic and asymptomatic women. Women with prior HSV type 2
  infections who are asymptomatic have a low
  risk of shedding the virus during delivery

Maternal smoking is associated with preterm labor and delivery, growth restriction, birth defects, and other pregnancy complications.[2]

NOTE: Ulcerative genital complaints are symptomatic of many kinds of infections (e.g., chancroid, secondary infected syphilis, contact dermatitis).

Cesarean delivery is recommended when typical herpes lesions are present at labor, regardless of time since membrane rupture[3]
Risk factors for HSV include: (a) previous infant with invasive GBS disease; (b) GBS bacterium with this pregnancy; (c) delivery at less than 37 weeks' gestation; (d) unknown GBS status with amniotic membrane rupture >18 hours or intrapartum temperature ≥100.4°F

Vertical transmission of GBS during labor or delivery may result in newborn sepsis, pneumonia, or less frequently meningitis. All pregnant women should be screened at 35 to 37 weeks with a single culture swab from both the lower vagina and rectum[4,5]

Partner currently has or has a history of herpes

Active herpes in a partner can expose the sexually active mother and can unwittingly infect a newborn after birth. Parents need to be educated on the possible risk that HSV imposes on the newborn. Sources of risk include children, grandparents, and so on, who have oral lesions as well. Contact with the newborn should be avoided by anyone with a current infection

At risk for hepatitis B carrier status and no documentation of a negative screen

> The hepatitis B virus can be transmitted to the fetus during delivery and, perhaps, in rare cases, transplacentally.

At risk for HIV infection

History of previous obstetric complications, such as preeclampsia, multiple pregnancy, or hydramnios

Abnormal presentation (breech presentation or transverse lie)

Fetus has failed to grow normally or fetus does not reach the expected size for dates

> Any woman with an undocumented HIV status at the time of labor should be offered screening with a rapid HIV test.[6]

> A preterm birth is one that occurs before 37 completed weeks of gestation. *Gestational age is more important than weight in determining perinatal morbidity or mortality.*

• Can women who are clearly at risk for problems during labor be identified ahead of time?

The following factors are associated with the development of complications for either the mother or the baby both during and after labor and delivery.

Factors Identified From the Mother's History

- Diabetes
- Preeclampsia or eclampsia
- Rh sensitization
- Sickle cell disease
- Heart disease
- Sexually transmitted infections
- Chronic hypertension
- Previous perinatal loss
- Anemia
- Renal disease
- Carrier state for blood-borne infectious disease (e.g., hepatitis B, syphilis, or HIV)
- Group B streptococcus (GBS) carrier status

> Women who are partners of intravenous drug abusers, bisexual males, or those who have multiple partners exhibit high-risk behavior for sexually transmitted diseases, some of which could be life threatening to both the mother and the fetus. Screening for syphilis, hepatitis B, and HIV infection, and possibly Hepatitis C, is strongly recommended.

Factors That Develop During Pregnancy

- Preeclampsia
- Gestational hypertension
- Postterm pregnancy (more than 42 weeks' gestation)

- Hydramnios or oligohydramnios
- Third trimester bleeding of undetermined origin
- Abruptio placentae or placenta previa

Factors Related to the Fetus

- Irregularity in fetal heart rate (FHR) or nonreassuring FHR patterns
- Intrauterine growth restriction
- Prematurity
- Malpresentation
- Significant increase or decrease in current fetal activity
- Meconium-stained amniotic fluid

Factors Developing During Early Labor

- Chorioamnionitis
- Premature rupture of membranes (PROM) at term
- Fresh meconium-stained fluid
- Abnormal fetal heart tones or nonreassuring FHR patterns
- Suspected cephalopelvic disproportion

The presence of any high-risk factors requires that the mother and fetus be continually evaluated throughout labor.

Determining True Labor

• Is the woman in true labor?

The uterus undergoes intermittent contractions once pregnancy is established. These contractions are called Braxton–Hicks contractions, and they are often associated with false labor. After the 28th week of pregnancy, these contractions become definite and more noticeable by the woman.

As the 37th week of pregnancy approaches, contractions can be strong and are sometimes perceived by the expectant mother as a sign of true labor. Braxton–Hicks contractions usually stop or become highly irregular with a change of activity.

True Labor	**False Labor**
Show—is often present. Show is blood-tinged mucus released from the cervical canal as labor nears or begins. It is pink, red, or brownish.	*Show*—is absent or can be related to intercourse or to a recent vaginal examination. It is brownish when the bleeding occurs hours before discovery.
NOTE: *Bloody show without contractions indicates that the body is preparing for labor but labor is not present without regular contractions and cervical change.*	
Contractions—tend to occur at regular intervals. They start at the back and sweep around to the abdomen, increasing in intensity and duration over several hours. They often intensify with walking.	*Contractions*—are irregular. They may be felt only in the back or in the lower abdomen. They do not intensify with walking and gradually diminish over several hours.
NOTE: *Regular and intensifying contractions are the single most important indication that labor might have begun.*	
Fetal movement—no significant change is noted.	*Fetal movement*—can increase for a short time or remain the same.
Cervix—becomes effaced and dilated.	*Cervix*—no change is noted or very small changes in thinning out (effacement) occur. Contractions help to bring about effacement.
NOTE: *Progressive cervical dilatation is the hallmark of progress in labor.*	

True Labor	False Labor
Walking—increases the intensity of contractions.	*Walking*—does not change the intensity of contractions.
Sedation—does not stop true labor.	*Sedation*—tends to stop false labor or prodromal labor.
In addition, for some women:	
Bowel status—can have loose stools 1 or 2 days before the onset of labor.	*Bowel status*—is usually unchanged.
Nesting—women tend to experience a flurry of activity in housecleaning 1 or 2 days before the onset of labor.	*Nesting*—none is present.

When the mother is discharged home, instruct her to return if any of the following occur:
- Membranes rupture, even without contractions
- Contractions become more frequent
- Excessive bleeding
- Headache, visual complaints, epigastric pain
- Decrease fetal movement

Evaluating the Status of Membranes

• What is meant by "membranes"?

While developing inside the uterus, the fetus lives in a sac. The sac has two layers: the inner layer, called the *amnion,* and the outer covering, called the *chorion.* This sac is filled with fluid that is made up of water, various chemicals (e.g., salts), and particles that come from the fetus itself (e.g., body cells and hair).

• What is normal amniotic fluid like?

By the end of pregnancy, the uterus contains approximately 1 L of amniotic fluid. The fluid is clear or straw colored and has a characteristic (not foul) odor. When tested for its acid–base content, it ranges from neutral to slightly alkaline. A close relationship exists between the status of the fluid and the health of the fetus. By studying various components of amniotic fluid, one can learn much about the gender, health, and maturity of the baby.

• Does the fluid serve a special purpose?

The fetus derives many benefits from amniotic fluid, which does the following:
- **Protects** the fetus from a direct blow. Pressure from a blow spreads in all directions within the fluid-filled sac, so the fetus does not receive the full impact of the blow.
- **Provides** a fluid environment in which the fetus moves. This fluid continually changes in amount and consistency, promoting the growth and development of the fetus.
- **Prevents** loss of heat and permits the fetus to maintain a constant body temperature.
- **Provides** a source of oral intake. The fetus swallows amniotic fluid from approximately the fourth month until delivery.
- **Acts** as a collection system for the waste products of the fetus. The fetus urinates into the amniotic fluid from the fourth month until delivery.

• What can happen to the amniotic fluid and membranes that indicates a problem?

A. Premature Rupture of Membranes (PROM) Before Labor Begins With a Term Fetus at 37 Completed Weeks or More Gestational Age

Membranes ("bag of waters") can rupture before labor begins. The break in the membranes can be complete, with a large gushing of fluid from the birth canal, or a small tear with a slow leak.

Many women go into labor spontaneously within a few hours after membranes rupture.

B. Preterm Premature Rupture of Membranes (PPROM) Before Labor Begins With a Preterm Fetus Less than 37 Weeks' gestation

When rupture occurs before the fetus has reached the 37th completed week of gestation, perinatal morbidity and mortality increase. These women should be monitored for signs and symptoms of infection.

C. Meconium-Stained Amniotic Fluid

Fetal stool is referred to as *meconium*. It is largely made up of water, but also contains proteins, cholesterol, lipids, vernix, and other substances. Large concentrations of bile pigments give meconium its green color. Meconium present for more than 24 hours begins to turn yellow-green.

Almost all fetuses and newborn infants who pass meconium are at term or postterm gestation. From 20 to 34 weeks' gestation, fetal passage of meconium remains infrequent.[7] Although 12% to 22% of labors are complicated by meconium, only a few are linked to infant mortality.[2]

The significance of meconium-stained amniotic fluid as a predictor of fetal compromise may depend on the following:
- Concentration and type of meconium (e.g., thick or thin, color, amount)
- Gestational age
- Stage of labor when the meconium is passed (often not known)
- The presence of other fetal compromise markers such as FHR abnormalities or oligohydramnios

Birth of a depressed infant occurs in 20% to 33% of infants born through meconium-stained amniotic fluid. It is likely caused by pathologic intrauterine processes, primarily chronic asphyxia and infection.[7]

Meconium aspiration syndrome (MAS) is thought to be caused by an initial hypoxic event resulting in the release of meconium into the amniotic fluid. The normal fetal response to hypoxemia is to gasp, and thus in this instance, the meconium is aspirated and can be seen below the vocal cords on examination.

The pathophysiologic process set up in MAS often leads to a poor perinatal outcome.

NOTE: MAS is significantly associated with fetal acidemia at birth.[8]

Related Facts

Meconium is rarely passed before the 34th gestational week.

Clinical studies indicate an association between the passage of meconium and high-risk clinical situations, including the following:
- Acute chorioamnionitis
- PROM
- Abruptio placentae
- Cocaine use
- Postterm pregnancy

Meconium alone is not an indicator of fetal hypoxia. Look at other fetal assessment parameters.

Electronic fetal monitoring maybe recommended when meconium-stained amniotic fluid is present. Meconium-stained infants should not have suctioning on the perineum. They should be handed directly to pediatrics for evaluation.

Be prepared for the birth of a high-risk infant.

The presence of meconium is managed differently at different institutions. In most scenarios, neonatology is called for the birth to assess for meconium aspiration. In most situations, there is no suctioning of the fetus during the birth process and the infant is handed to neonatology for evaluation. If the infant is vigorous, no evaluation below the vocal cords is necessary.

Postterm pregnancies are defined as those lasting beyond 42 weeks' gestation. Most women are offered induction early in the 41st week.

In postterm laboring women, you should look for the following:
- The presence of meconium-stained fluid
- The absence of any amniotic fluid—This should alert you to the almost certain presence of meconium even though you cannot see it!

- Placental dysfunction—Watch for late decelerations
- Umbilical cord compression—Watch for variable decelerations
- Macrosomia

D. Infection

Amniotic membranes and fluid can become infected, especially after 24 hours of ruptured membranes. Infection can be detected by the presence of a foul odor, fundal tenderness, and an elevated temperature in the mother of 100.4 or greater.

E. Port Wine–Colored Amniotic Fluid–AN EMERGENCY

Port wine–colored amniotic fluid is an indicator of a premature separation of the placenta from the uterine wall, called *abruptio placentae or vasa previa.*

Signs of Abruptio Placentae

The following signs indicate that the placenta has partially or totally separated from the uterine wall:

- Tender abdomen
- Hard or rigid tone to abdomen
- Bradycardia or absence of fetal heart tones
- External bright red bleeding or concealed bleeding, shock

Vasa previa is noted when placental vessels overlie the cervix or portions of the cervix and are covered only with membrane. These vessels are vulnerable to compression which can lead to fetal anoxia and to laceration leading to fetal exsanguination. Vasa previa is relatively uncommon, 1 in 5,200 pregnancies.[9]

Abruptio placentae occurs in approximately 1 in 160 to 290 deliveries,[10,11] although most people consider it to be 1 in 200. Factors that may predispose a woman to developing abruptio placentae include the following:
- Hypertension
- Hydramnios
- Multiple pregnancies
- Trauma
- History of heavy smoking
- Cocaine use

F. Hydramnios/Oligohydramnios

There can be too much or too little fluid within the amniotic sac. Normally, the fluid volume is about 1 L toward the end of pregnancy. The presence of 2 L or more of amniotic fluid is considered excessive and called *polyhydramnios* or *hydramnios.* The mother's abdomen may look unusually large, tight, and glistening.

Amniotic fluid increases to about 1 L by 36 weeks and then begins to decrease. In postterm pregnancies, the amniotic fluid volume may be only 100 to 200 mL and hence the concern for oligohydramnios.

Ultrasonic techniques are used to measure amounts of amniotic volume. One method of evaluation involves adding the depth in centimeters of the largest vertical pocket of fluid in each of four equal uterine quadrants. The numerical value is called the *amniotic fluid index* (AFI).[12]

Ultrasound measurement of amniotic fluid is used during fetal surveillance by estimating amniotic fluid in a single vertical pocket (2×2) or the AFI. The AFI is the sum of the largest vertical fluid pocket in each of the four quadrants which does not contain umbilical cord.

Hydramnios, an AFI of greater than 20 to 25 cm, is commonly associated with fetal malformations and chromosomal abnormalities including:
- Hydrocephaly, microcephaly, and anencephaly
- Spina bifida

Common maternal antepartal conditions associated with polyhydramnios include:
- Idiopathic
- Multifetal pregnancies

- Cleft palate
- Esophageal atresia
- Pyloric stenosis
- Down syndrome
- Congenital heart disease

- Fetal anomalies
- Multiple pregnancy
- Diabetes
- Macrosomic
- Isoimmunization

Oligohydramnios, an AFI of ≤5 cm or the absence of a 2-cm vertical pocket and has been associated with fetal compromise. With oligo at term, evaluation for ruptured membranes should be considered. Women at term without ruptured membranes but with oligo are at risk for cord compression and sequelae and are often admitted for labor induction.[12,13]

Oligohydramnios may be associated with the following conditions:

- Chromosomal abnormalities
- Congenital anomalies
- Postterm pregnancies
- Ruptured membranes
- Maternal hypertension
- Preeclampsia
- Intrauterine growth restriction
- Defects of the fetal urinary tract

Oligohydramnios is primarily associated with the following:

- Cord compression
- Congenital defects of the fetal urinary tract
- Intrauterine growth restriction
- Postterm pregnancies

Cord compression during labor is common with oligohydramnios. Whenever women are diagnosed as having oligohydramnios or when there is no amniotic fluid on rupture of membranes, close surveillance is warranted.

PRACTICE/REVIEW QUESTIONS

After reviewing this part, answer the following questions.

1. List at least five types of information you need to elicit from a woman being admitted to the labor unit.

   a. _____

   b. _____

   c. _____

   d. _____

   e. _____

2. Which of the following factors predict a strong possibility of problems developing for the mother or infant during or after labor and delivery? Select all that apply.

   a. Maternal history of heavy smoking

   b. Fresh, meconium-stained fluid

   c. Induction of labor

   d. Fetal tachycardia

   e. Multiple pregnancies

   f. Mild anemia

   g. Prematurity

3. A birth occurring before _____ completed weeks' gestation is identified as preterm.

4. A fetus of more than _____ completed weeks' gestation (postterm) is considered high risk.

5. True labor includes regular contractions and _____.

6. What are the four risk factors for GBS?

   _____

   _____

7. Amniotic fluid generally peaks in volume by the _____ gestational week and then slowly _____ until the _____ week. It can _____ quickly after 40 weeks.

8. Which of the following descriptions are characteristic of normal amniotic fluid? Select all that apply.

   a. Clear or straw colored

   b. Neutral to slightly acid

   c. Composed of water, salts, and other particles from the fetus

   d. Alkaline

9. Which of the following situations indicates that you should prepare for the birth of a high-risk infant? Select all that apply.

    a. Rupture of membranes before labor begins with a 38-week gestational age fetus

    b. Rupture of membranes before labor begins with a fetus less than 37-week gestational age

    c. A laboring woman at a documented 43 weeks gestation

    d. Rupture of membranes with little fluid at 41 weeks' gestation

10. Which of the following can indicate that the fetus may possibly be in distress? Select all that apply.

    a. Greenish-brown meconium staining with a cephalic presentation

    b. Mother's temperature of 100.4°F or greater

    c. Tender abdomen

    d. Excessive amniotic fluid

    e. Port wine–colored amniotic fluid

    f. Absence of amniotic fluid

11. State the difference between PROM (premature rupture of membranes) and PPROM (preterm premature rupture of membranes).

    _____

    _____

12. Meconium passage at delivery in a term fetus is present in approximately _____% of labors.

13. When pregnancy is prolonged beyond 42 completed weeks of gestation, one should be prepared for a high-risk infant that is _____

14. In prolonged pregnancies, one should watch for placental dysfunction that can be reflected in an electronic fetal monitoring tracing with _____

15. The amniotic fluid index (AFI) is defined as

    _____

    _____

16. If a woman is diagnosed as having oligohydramnios, close surveillance is recommended.

    a. True

    b. False

17. Proteinuria is not necessary for the diagnosis of pre-eclampsia when other severe features present.

    a. True

    b. False

PRACTICE/REVIEW ANSWER KEY

1. Presenting complaint and symptoms, EDD/EDC, stage of labor, abnormalities in pregnancy, time of last snack or meal, known allergies to drugs, support system, review of patient's history (family and past history, current laboratory data, present obstetric status).
2. b, d, e, g
3. 37
4. 42
5. Cervical change
6. Four risk factors for GBS: previous infant with GBS disease, GBS bacteriuria, delivery <37 weeks gestation, and PPROM.
7. 36th, decreases, 40th, decrease
8. a, c, d
9. b, c, d
10. a, c, e, f
11. PROM pertains to rupture of membranes after the 37th completed gestational week, whereas PPROM signifies rupture of membranes before the 37th completed gestational week.
12. 12% to 22% (some say 30%)
13. Postmature/dysmature
14. Late decelerations
15. The sum of the largest vertical fluid pocket in each of the four quadrants which does not contain umbilical cord.
16. True
17. True

SKILL UNIT 1 | PHYSICAL EXAMINATION OF THE LABORING WOMAN

This section details how to perform a modified physical examination to screen for problems in the woman being admitted to labor and delivery. Study this section and then attend a skill practice and demonstration session scheduled with your preceptor. You will need to demonstrate the examination and correctly interpret the results. The steps of the examination are summarized at the end of this unit.

ACTIONS	REMARKS
What are the Techniques to Be Used in Performing the Physical Examination?	
1. *Inspection*—observing the general health and outstanding characteristics of the patient in a thorough, unhurried manner.	

skill unit continues on page 51

ACTIONS	REMARKS
2. *Palpation*–feeling or touching parts to be evaluated.	The physical examination of the laboring woman is not as extensive as that given at her first prenatal visit.
3. *Auscultation*–listening, usually with a stethoscope, for the sounds produced by the body.	

What Steps Should You Take to Prepare for the Examination?

1. Ask the woman to empty her bladder.	A full bladder can make examination of the abdomen or bladder uncomfortable.
2. Follow a logical order of assessment. Use all of your senses as the assessment is carried out.	In general, it is suggested that you begin at the head of the patient and work toward the toes. You are not likely to miss anything this way.
3. Explain to the woman what you are doing. 4. Warm your hands by rubbing them together or holding them under warm water. 5. Chart your findings in a logical order.	Unless you have a checklist, chart your findings in the same order in which you conduct the examination.

When Is the Best Time to Perform the Physical Examination?

The initial assessment is carried out immediately to evaluate the labor and any signs of problems.	The examination is conducted as quickly as possible. The woman can then assume a side-lying or upright sitting position. Cardiac output is better for the mother, and uteroplacental circulation for the fetus is optimized in these positions.
Assess the following: General appearance • Look for edema in face, hands, and feet (Fig. 3.1)	Early and careful assessment of the patient's physical status will provide clues to problems.

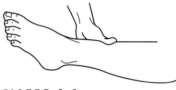

FIGURE 3.1

Vital signs Abdominal • Determine the frequency, duration, and intensity of contractions Fetal position Fetal heart tones Height of the fundus (top of uterus) Perform a vaginal examination to determine the following: Cervical effacement Cervical dilatation and station Amount of bloody show Whether membranes have ruptured Amount of amniotic fluid	For example, if the BP is elevated, evaluate for the following: • Edema in hands and feet • Protein in the urine • Presence of headache and blurred vision • Elevated preeclampsia laboratory indices • Epigastric pain In the presence of vaginal bleeding, the digital examination may be deferred until the location of the placenta can be verified and placenta previa ruled out.

NOTE: Women with preterm or term pregnancies who are not in labor and who present with ruptured membranes and no signs of fetal distress should not undergo a digital vaginal examination on arrival. Wait for the primary care provider to arrive.

Vaginal examination should not be performed on a nonlaboring woman who presents with ruptured membranes. A sterile speculum examination confirms rupture. If the woman is contracting and a baseline examination is needed, a digital examination can be performed after checking with provider.

skill unit continues on page 52

ACTIONS	REMARKS
	If the fetus is in a transverse or breech position and labor is active, you need to alert the primary care provider immediately. If the membranes are ruptured and there are signs of nonreassuring fetal status, you may need to perform a digital vaginal examination to assess the progress of the labor and to check for a prolapsed cord. Utilize ultrasound to confirm presenting part.

What Position Is Best for the Examination?

Ask the patient to lie on her back as you begin the examination. Elevate the head of the bed or the examining table enough to make the patient comfortable.	You need to ensure that the patient is not flat on her back to avoid supine hypotension syndrome.

Completing a General Assessment

Give *thoughtful attention* to the general appearance of the patient.
 Note the following:
  Signs of distress
  Skin color
  Movements
  Personal hygiene
  Odor
  Facial expression
  Speech
  Manner
  Mood
  State of awareness
	The woman who comes to the labor unit in active labor might appear stressed because contractions are strong and frequent. Note how she is coping with them—whether she is using a breathing technique or tensing up. You can reinforce her technique or teach her an effective one.
	 If she has come with a support person, find out whether she wishes the support person to remain with her during as much of the admission as possible. If she has no partner, you may need to assume a supporting role.

Vital Signs

1. Blood pressure: Be sure to assess BP between contractions.
   a. The cuff must fit snugly on the arm and be of appropriate size. The cuff should be approximately 20% wider than the width of the arm.
   b. Take BP measurements with the woman in a sitting position.
 	
 The patient may have a hypertensive disorder if the BP is:
   140/90 mm Hg or higher
   160/110 mm Hg or higher (severe features)
 You also need to do the following:
   New guidelines[14] have removed >5 g of proteinuria for severe disease and intrauterine growth restriction has also been removed in the severe category. It is now recommended to replace terminology of severe with severe features.
   Ask the mother if she is having headaches or blurred vision or epigastric pain.
   Notify the primary care provider if BP elevations approaching 140/90 mm Hg, hyperreflexia, and complaints of headaches or blurred vision or epigastric pain are noted.
	A cuff too small or too large can result in BP readings that are inaccurately high or low, respectively.
	
	 The method for taking BP readings (e.g., patient position and which Korotkoff sound to use) should be consistently used by all caretakers on the unit.
	 A woman with either of these BP changes can have gestational hypertension, chronic hypertension, preeclampsia or superimposed preeclampsia.
	 Assessment for HELLP syndrome which includes hemolysis, low platelets, and elevated liver enzymes can be seen often in preeclampsia and can be a life-threatening complication.

skill unit continues on page 53

ACTIONS	REMARKS
2. Pulse (normal range, 60–90 bpm)	Increased pulse rate can result from excitement, anxiety, dehydration, pain, and, in rare cases, cardiac problems.
3. Respirations	Avoid counting respirations during a uterine contraction because they can be abnormally high or low as a result of stress or because of the use of a breathing technique.
4. Temperature to 99.6°F (36.2–37.6°C)	Look for signs of infection, temperature ≥100.4°F or dehydration

Abdomen

1. Inspect for scars, striae (stretch marks), rashes, and symmetry of the abdomen.	Striae are shiny, reddish lines that appear on the breasts, abdomen, thighs, and buttocks of approximately half of pregnant women as a result of stretching of the skin and underlying tissue.
2. If you detect a scar that the woman tells you is the result of surgery done on the uterus and the woman is in active labor, notify the primary care provider immediately.	Vertical scars from previous classic cesarean births are much more likely to rupture than horizontal scars down low on the abdomen.

3. Assess the following:
  • Fundal height
  • Fetal position
  • Fetal heart tones
	An abnormal shape of the abdomen should alert you to fetal malposition (such as a transverse lie).
	See Skill Unit 1, Measuring Fundal Height, in Module 4.

Bladder

Gently palpate the lower abdominal area just above the symphysis pubis bone to determine bladder fullness or tenderness.	Suprapubic tenderness might suggest a bladder infection. Signs and symptoms of elevated temperature, burning on urination, and frequency of urination should be discussed.

Lower Extremities

1. Inspect for the presence of *varicosities.* If present, feel for warmth. Using both hands, palpate for *tenderness,* beginning behind the knee and working your way down the leg to the ankle (Fig. 3.2).	Warmth over a varicosity can indicate a *thrombophlebitis* (inflammation of a vein associated with a blood clot). The primary care provider should be alerted.

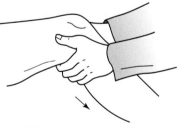

FIGURE 3.2

2. Evaluate for the following:
  • BP
  • Headaches or visual disturbances

Edema is not considered a reliable diagnostic criterion for preeclampsia.

skill unit continues on page 54

ACTIONS	REMARKS

3. To elicit a deep tendon reflex, the patient must be relaxed. Position the leg by supporting the knee with one hand or arm in a partially flexed position while asking the patient to relax that leg completely (Fig. 3.3). Briskly tap the patellar tendon just below the kneecap. This can also be done with the patient in a sitting position (Fig. 3.4). Watch for some degree of a brisk jerk.

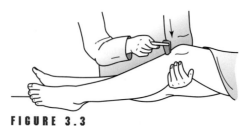

FIGURE 3.3

FIGURE 3.4

NOTE: Many women, including adolescents, have brisk reflexes. Do not consider this a major indication of a pathologic condition.

Reflexes are graded on a 0–4+ scale.

    4+ = extremely brisk (called hyperactive); often indicates a disease state of the central nervous system;

    3+ = brisker than average;

    2+ = average, normal;

    1+ = somewhat diminished, low normal;

    0 = flat, no response

Test for clonus if reflexes are 4+ (hyperactive). Support the knee in a partially flexed position. With your other hand, sharply dorsiflex the foot and maintain it in dorsiflexion (see Fig. 3.5). If clonus is present, you will see the foot moving back and forth in small rhythmic movements.

The presence of clonus indicates that the central nervous system is highly irritated, although in some patients it can simply be the result of anxiety. Clonus may be associated with moderate to severe preeclampsia.

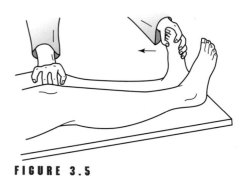

FIGURE 3.5

You will need to attend a skill session(s) to practice these skills with the help of your preceptor. Mastery of the skill is achieved when you can demonstrate techniques of physical assessment, including the following:

- Preparatory steps
- Logical order
- Appropriate positions for examining various areas of the body
- Accurate assessment of vital signs
- Abdomen (fundal height, fetal position, and fetal heart tones are demonstrated in Module 4)
- Bladder

SKILL UNIT 2 | TESTING FOR RUPTURED MEMBRANES

- *Sterile Speculum Examination*
- *Nitrazine Paper Test*

This section details accurate ways to test for the rupture of amniotic membranes. Study this section and then attend a skill practice and demonstration scheduled with your preceptor. You will need to demonstrate that you can perform and interpret the steps of this procedure. These steps are summarized at the end of this unit.

ACTIONS	REMARKS

Selecting the Speculum

1. The speculum is composed of two blades and a handle. A thumb piece attaches to the top blade; the bottom blade is fixed (Fig. 3.6).

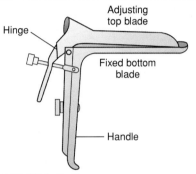

FIGURE 3.6

The top blade is hinged, and the thumb piece controls its motions (Fig. 3.7).

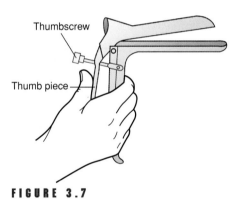

FIGURE 3.7

The thumbscrew, when turned, tightens and fixes the top blade in position (Fig. 3.8).

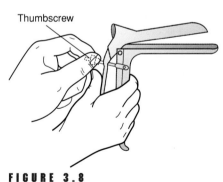

FIGURE 3.8

skill unit continues on page 56

| **ACTIONS** | **REMARKS** |

When the speculum is opened by using the thumb piece, a space is created between the blades, which, if placed in the vagina, permits a clear view of the vaginal walls and cervix (Fig. 3.9).

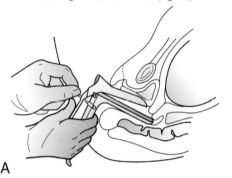
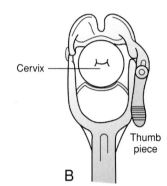

FIGURE 3.9

2. Two basic types of specula are as follows:
   a. The Graves speculum (Fig. 3.10A,B)
      • is the most common.
      • is used in the examination of the adult female.
      • comes in two sizes, standard and large, which vary in length from 3.5 to 5.0 in and in width from 0.75 to 1.50 in.

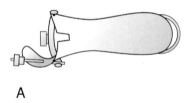
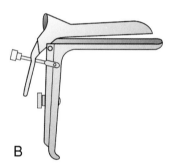

FIGURE 3.10 Graves speculum.

   b. The Pedersen speculum (Fig. 3.11A,B)
      • is as long as the Graves speculum but narrower and flatter.
      • is used more in women who have not had intercourse, women who have never had a baby, or women who are so tense that insertion of the Graves speculum is difficult.

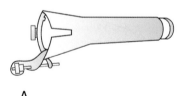
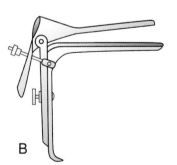

FIGURE 3.11 Pedersen speculum.

skill unit continues on page 57

ACTIONS	REMARKS
Preparing the Woman	
3. Tell the woman what you are going to be doing in terms she can understand.	An informed woman is more relaxed. She is more likely to cooperate with you throughout the examination.
4. Ask the woman to empty her bladder.	A full bladder can make the examination uncomfortable for the woman and more difficult to perform.
5. Have the woman remove her underclothing and lie on the examining table. Assist her to relax with her legs bent, feet resting flat on the table or in the stirrups. Place a pillow under her head and ask that she rest her hands across her abdomen or at her sides.	This increases comfort and relaxation. Sometimes women put their hands above their heads during a vaginal examination, which tightens abdominal muscles and makes the examination more difficult and uncomfortable.

What Should You Do Before Beginning the Examination?

6. Drape the mother's legs so that you cover her up to her knees. Make sure that you can see her face when you are sitting down.	
7. Position the light so that the perineum is well seen.	If the perineum appears wet and glistening, there is a good chance that the membranes have ruptured.
8. Position the stool on which you will sit for the examination so that you will not need to move it again.	
9. Select the appropriate speculum. The speculum must be *sterile*.	The appropriate speculum is the one that will cause the least amount of discomfort to the woman while providing a good view of the vagina and cervix.
10. Wash your hands.	
11. Put on sterile gloves.	
12. If you are alone, open the package containing the sterile speculum in such a way that you can grasp the handle for removal after you have put on a sterile glove.	It is a good idea to have someone assist you and support the woman throughout the examination.

Take care! Maintaining strict aseptic technique throughout the sterile speculum examination can reduce the risk of chorioamnionitis if membranes are ruptured.

Sterile gloves for question of ruptured membranes–otherwise gloves do not need to be sterile.

What Is the Best Way to Begin the Examination?

13. Sit down on the stool and ask the woman to separate or spread her legs. *Do not try to use force, or even to gently separate her legs.*	Because this examination is an intrusive procedure, it should be carried out when the woman is ready for it.
14. Tell the woman *how to relax.* If she knows a relaxation and breathing technique learned previously, have her use it. If not, have her do slow, deep, relaxed breathing. Ask her to let herself go limp, to think of herself as a rag doll.	
15. If the woman becomes upset or tense during the examination, *stop whatever you are doing.* Do not remove your fingers; simply hold your hand still. Find out what is bothering her. Try to distinguish among discomfort as a result of pressure, fear, and actual pain. Wait until she has regained control, helping her to relax.	
16. Often speculums are warmed. Often, additional lubricant is not needed because the vagina is moist from bloody show when the mother goes into labor. If a lubricant is needed, only *sterile* water should be used. No water or lubricant if you are confirming ruptured membranes.	If you use running tap water or a lubricant, you will lose the sterility of the speculum. This could introduce an infectious organism to the mother and to the fetus if membranes are ruptured. This accustoms her to your touch and prepares her for the more intrusive part of the examination.

skill unit continues on page 58

ACTIONS	REMARKS

17. Tell the woman what you are doing as you touch her inner thigh with the back of the gloved hand that is not holding the speculum.

18. Using this same hand, place two fingers just inside the introitus and gently press down on the base of the vagina.

19. With your other hand, introduce the *closed* speculum past your fingers at approximately a 45-degree angle downward (Fig. 3.12). Keep a moderate downward pressure on the blades to avoid upward pressure on the sensitive bladder and top vaginal wall.

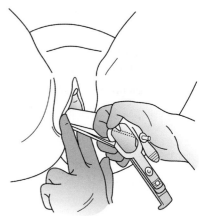

FIGURE 3.12

20. After the speculum is in the vagina, remove your fingers from the base of the vaginal opening. Turn the blades of the speculum into a horizontal position, all the while keeping a moderate downward pressure (Fig. 3.13).

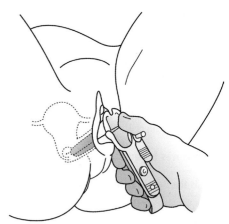

FIGURE 3.13

21. Tell the woman she might feel pressure. Move your thumb to the thumb piece and press to open the blades so that the cervix is in view (Fig. 3.14).

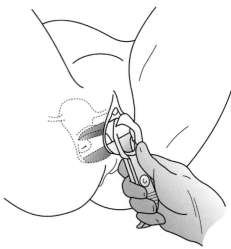

FIGURE 3.14

skill unit continues on page 59

ACTIONS	**REMARKS**

22. Sweep the blades slowly upward by gently pressing on the handle. If this does not bring the cervix into view, close the blades and withdraw the speculum a little. Warn the mother of the extra pressure she might feel. Then, while pressing down firmly, move the blades toward the back of the vagina again. Sometimes the tip of the blades needs to be directed more anteriorly or posteriorly, depending on the position of the cervix.
23. When the cervix is in view, tighten the thumbscrew to keep the blades open.

What Will You See If the Membranes are Ruptured?

24. Pooling fluid will be seen leaking from the cervical opening.
    - Pooling
    - Nitrazine
    - Ferning

Assessment for pooling, nitrazine and ferning compose the gold standard to confirm rupture of membranes.

> Viewing leaking fluid from the cervical opening is the best method for determining that the membranes have ruptured.

Note the color and odor.

- *Deep yellow, green, or brown color* indicates the presence of meconium.

Use this opportunity to screen for any signs of abnormalities, such as bleeding. Heavy bloody show can alert you to an advanced state of labor.

25. Obtain a specimen of the suspected leaking fluid by placing a *sterile* cotton-tipped applicator into the pool of fluid accumulating in the lower blade (Fig. 3.15).

Amniotic fluid is clear or straw colored. It does not have an unpleasant odor.

The presence of meconium should be noted. Check to confirm there is not a breech presentation.

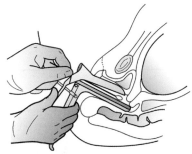

FIGURE 3.15

26. Touch the cotton-tipped applicator or cotton ball on a fresh strip of Nitrazine paper, moistening it well.

Nitrazine paper contains a dye that changes color when alkaline substances such as amniotic fluid moisten it.

How Do You Interpret the Color Change?

27. Compare the color that appears on the moistened paper against the standard color chart.

A standard color chart can be found on the box of Nitrazine paper, with a range of colors used to interpret the alkaline nature of substances. Because amniotic fluid is neutral (pH 7.0) or slightly alkaline (pH 7.25), it changes the yellow color of Nitrazine paper.

The pH values of blood, vaginal mucus, and certain secretions from vaginal infections are also alkaline. If the amount of amniotic fluid is small or absent but the above substances are present in large amounts, a false-positive test could result.

59

skill unit continues on page 60

ACTIONS	REMARKS

Findings on Nitrazine Paper

COLOR	pH	INTERPRETATION
Yellow	5.0	
Olive	5.5	Probably membranes are *not* ruptured
Olive-green	6.0	
Blue-green	6.5	Probably membranes are ruptured
Blue-gray	7.0	
Deep blue	7.5	May be caused by blood or cervical mucus

Be aware of the possibility of false-positive readings.	*The Nitrazine test is not considered a definitive test for diagnosing ruptured membranes. See the fern test for this.*

How Do You Remove the Speculum?

28. Release the thumbscrew on the thumb piece. Hold the blades apart by pressing on the thumb piece and begin withdrawing the speculum until the cervix is released from between the blades.	
29. Release your pressure on the thumb piece and allow the blades to close. Avoid pinching the vaginal tissue or pubic hair when the blades close. Rotate the blades to a sideways position and exert downward pressure. As the blades are eased out, hook your index finger over the top blade to control it.	This avoids pressure to the sensitive urethra and top vaginal wall.
30. Note the odor of any vaginal discharge pooled in the bottom blade.	Foul-smelling discharge might indicate amniotic fluid infection
31. Deposit the speculum in the proper container.	
32. Wipe any moisture or discharge from the perineal area.	

You will need to attend a skill session(s) to practice this skill with the help of your preceptor. Mastery of the skill is achieved when you can demonstrate the following:
- Selection and operation of an appropriately sized speculum for a variety of women
- Positioning and preparation of the woman for speculum examination
- The procedure for a sterile speculum examination
- How to obtain a specimen for Nitrazine paper testing
- Interpretation of color changes indicating that membranes have ruptured

SKILL UNIT 3 | FERN TESTING FOR RUPTURED MEMBRANES

This section details how to do the fern test to determine whether membranes have ruptured. Study this section and then attend a skill practice and demonstration section scheduled with your preceptor. You will need to demonstrate that you can perform the procedure and correctly interpret the results. These steps are summarized at the end of this unit.

ACTIONS	REMARKS
Preparing to Conduct the Test	
1. Who might need this test? • Any pregnant woman suspected of having ruptured membranes	Amniotic fluid contains a high amount of a salt called sodium chloride. If drops of the fluid are spread on a glass slide, allowed to dry, and examined through a microscope, a characteristic palm leaf pattern can be seen. This is why it is called *arborization* or the fern test.

2. What equipment is needed?
   • Sterile gloves
   • Sterile speculum
   • Two clean microscope slides
   • Two small, sterile cotton-tipped applicators
	No bacteria or other foreign material should be introduced into the vagina if ruptured membranes are suspected.

Performing the Test	
1. Assemble all the necessary equipment.	
2. Explain to the woman exactly what you will be doing.	
3. Help her assume the position for a speculum examination.	
4. Put on sterile gloves.	
5. Insert the sterile speculum.	
6. Locate the cervix.	
7. Insert a sterile cotton-tipped applicator and place it in the fluid accumulating in the lower blade. Be certain to use pooled fluid in the lower blade. Avoid touching the cervical opening.	If the membranes are ruptured, fluid can leak from the cervix if the woman is asked to cough or bear down.
8. Roll the cotton-tipped applicator on the first slide, spreading the specimen *thinly* over at least two thirds of the slide (Fig. 3.16).	

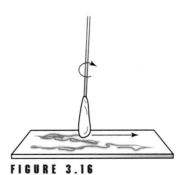

FIGURE 3.16

9. Repeat the procedure but place the second cotton-tipped applicator in the back of the vagina below the cervix.	
10. Roll the cotton-tipped applicator on the second slide.	Testing from two different areas offers a better chance of obtaining leaking fluid, which might otherwise be overlooked.
11. Allow the slide to dry for 5–7 min.	Some people remove the speculum and dip the cotton-tipped applicator in the fluid that has pooled in the lower blade.

skill unit continues on page 62

ACTIONS	REMARKS
	Drying permits the sodium chloride in the amniotic fluid to "arborize," or develop the typical "ferning" pattern (Fig. 3.17).

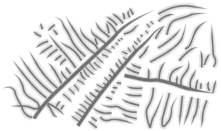

FIGURE 3.17

ACTIONS	REMARKS
12. Set the microscope on *low* power and examine all areas of each slide for the ferning pattern. If you have any doubt about the ferning pattern you see under low power, check again under high power.	The presence of the ferning pattern is a positive test result for ruptured membranes. Cervical and vaginal fluids per se do not fern. If you see ferning on the first slide, it is not necessary to check the second slide. However, you should always check the second slide if you do not see ferning on the first slide.

You will need to attend a skill session(s) to practice this skill with the help of your preceptor. Mastery of the skill is achieved when you can demonstrate the following:
- Collection of a specimen for testing
- Preparation of the slides for microscope viewing
- Use of low and high power on the microscope
- Interpretation of the ferning pattern seen under the microscope

SKILL UNIT 4 | VAGINAL EXAMINATION

This section details how to perform a vaginal examination to determine cervical effacement, dilatation, the status of membranes, and fetal presenting part and station. Study this section and then attend a skill practice and demonstration session scheduled with your preceptor. You will need to demonstrate that you can perform the procedure and correctly interpret the results. These steps are summarized at the end of this unit.

ACTIONS	REMARKS
Preparing the Woman for a Vaginal Examination	

Information you need before performing a vaginal examination:
- Gravidity
- Parity
- Gestational age
- History of any bleeding/spotting
- History of possible ruptured membranes

CAUTION: If membranes are ruptured and the mother is not contracting, do not perform a digital vaginal examination. Perform a sterile speculum exam. Check with provider if they want a baseline cervical examination. Confirm the presenting part.

skill unit continues on page 63

ACTIONS	**REMARKS**
1. Ask the woman to empty her bladder before the examination.	A full bladder makes the abdomen difficult to palpate thoroughly and is uncomfortable for the woman.
2. Tell the woman, in terms she can understand, what you will be doing and share your findings throughout the examination using her name.	An informed woman is more relaxed. She is more likely to cooperate with you throughout the examination. The woman has a right to know what is being done in regard to her body.
3. Warn the woman in advance if you are going to be exerting extra pressure or doing something that might be particularly uncomfortable.	
4. Help her to lie down on the examining table with legs bent so that her feet are resting on the table or in the stirrups. Place a pillow under her head and ask that she rest her hands across her abdomen or at her sides.	This increases her comfort and relaxation. Sometimes women put their hands over their heads during a vaginal examination, which tightens abdominal muscles and makes the examination more difficult or uncomfortable.
5. Drape the woman's legs to avoid unnecessary exposure. Make sure that you can see her face whether you are sitting or standing for any part of the examination.	The message given to the woman is that you respect her modesty and privacy. This will help her to relax. Making sure that you can see her face at all times might reassure her and enables you to note expressions of fear, discomfort, or embarrassment.
6. *Has the mother had any bleeding during the last part of her pregnancy?* *Do you see signs of bleeding that might be more than just bloody show? Blood running down her legs or bright red bleeding is abnormal.* *If you note any bleeding, do not proceed with the examination.*	**Vaginal examinations are never performed if there is a question of a placenta previa.** Sometimes the placenta grows partially or completely over the cervix. This condition is called *placenta previa* and is rare (Fig. 3.18).

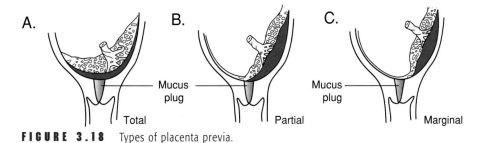

FIGURE 3.18 Types of placenta previa.

Getting Ready to Do a Vaginal Examination

7. Wash your hands and put on gloves. • If ruptured membranes are suspected, always use sterile gloves. • If membranes are intact, clean or sterile gloves can be used.	This procedure describes a two-gloved approach. One gloved hand is used to separate the labia (step 13) and the other gloved hand conducts the vaginal/cervical examination.
8. Ask the woman to separate or spread her legs. Do not try to use force or even gently separate her legs.	This examination is an intrusive procedure. It should be carried out when the woman is ready for it.
9. Tell the woman how to relax. If she knows a relaxation and breathing technique learned previously, have her use it. If not, have her do slow, deep, relaxed breathing. Ask her to let herself go limp, to think of herself as a rag doll.	

skill unit continues on page 64

ACTIONS	REMARKS
10. Ask the woman if you may proceed now. Watch your facial expression. Remain focused on the woman. Share your findings with her to the extent possible for the situation. Acknowledge the discomfort the examination may be causing her—even offer an apology.	This appropriately gives the woman some control, is empowering, and is humanizing in a difficult situation.

Performing the Examination

If the woman becomes upset or tense during the examination, *stop whatever you are doing.* Do not remove your fingers; simply hold your hand still. Find out what is bothering her. Try to distinguish between discomfort as a result of pressure, or fear, and actual pain. Wait until she has regained control, helping her to relax.

11. Generously lubricate the index and middle fingers of your examining hand with lubricating gel. As you squeeze the tube, let the lubricant drop onto your outstretched fingers. Do not wipe your fingers against the mouth of the tube to obtain the lubricant. The lubricant should be considered clean only—not sterile.
12. Be sure that you have good lighting.
13. Separate the labia with your gloved fingers (Fig. 3.19). Inspect the general area of the introitus (vaginal opening).

If it is uncertain whether the membranes have ruptured and a compelling reason exists for performing the examination, use only sterile water because some substances interfere with the Nitrazine paper color change.

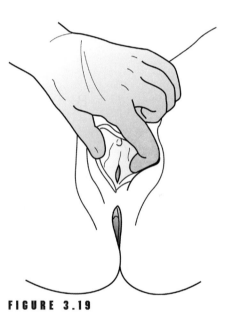

FIGURE 3.19

Look for the following:
- Amount of bloody show
- Wet, glistening perineum
- Malodorous discharge
- Deep yellow or greenish-brown discharge
- Ulceration of the labia
- Blisters or raised vesicles on the labia

Which might indicate the following:
Labor is advanced.
Membranes have ruptured.
Infection of the amniotic fluid and membranes is present.
Presence of greenish-brown fluid indicates fresh
   meconium or breech presentation.
Syphilis (chancre) or an HSV infection might be present.
HSV infection might be present.

skill unit continues on page 65

ACTIONS	**REMARKS**
Elicit signs and symptoms of current infection.	The appearance of a raised vesicle or a blistered area can mean that the mother has an active HSV infection. Mothers with herpes virus blisters on the cervix or genitalia can pass the disease on to a newborn delivered vaginally. In primary genital herpes infections, these babies experience high morbidity and mortality.

Newborns delivered through an infected birth canal should be isolated to protect other newborns in the nursery. The mucus membranes (e.g., eyes, nasopharynx) of the newborn should be cultured at 24–48 hrs after birth to avoid positive cultures resulting from contamination from the mother.

Current delivery recommendations for pregnant women with genital herpes infection include the following considerations:
- If there are no active lesions at term in a woman with intact membranes who has had active HSV lesions during pregnancy, vaginal delivery is acceptable.[5]
- If there are active lesions near or at term in a woman who is in labor or who has ruptured membranes, cesarean delivery is recommended.[5]

14. Insert the first finger of the other sterile gloved hand and then the second finger gently into the vagina. The hand should be turned sideways in this initial step. Continue to apply downward pressure as you insert the fingers to avoid pressing on the anterior vaginal wall or urethra. The thumb and forefinger on one hand separate the labia widely to expose the vaginal opening and prevent the examining fingers from touching the labia (Fig. 3.20).

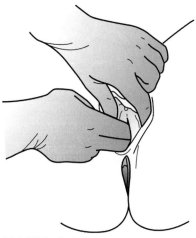

FIGURE 3.20

If you are doing a vaginal examination with one hand, avoid sweeping contaminants into the vagina by separating the labia with the thumb and little finger as you introduce the examining fingers.

The length of the vagina varies in women, but is usually 3–4 cm.

15. Move your fingers the full length of the woman's vagina. During the examination, the fourth and fifth fingers should not touch the rectal area. Keep the thumb straight up and stretched out. Keep the fourth and fifth fingers bent inward and touching the palm of your hand (Fig. 3.21).

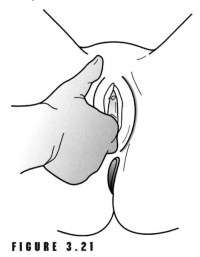

FIGURE 3.21

skill unit continues on page 66

ACTIONS	REMARKS

Assessing Progress in Labor

16. Are the membranes ruptured? Palpate for a soft, movable, bulging sac through the cervix (Fig. 3.22). Watch for running fluid during the examination.

If the membranes are not ruptured, they tend to bulge. If they are ruptured, amniotic fluid is likely to leak during the examination.

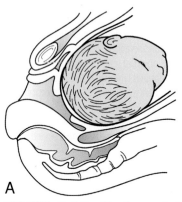

A   B

FIGURE 3.22 Membranes. **A.** Watchglass shape. **B.** Bulging into the cervix.

17. What is the degree of cervical dilatation?

Dilatation is measured in centimeters. One finger represents approximately 1-cm dilatation. Measurement of dilatation can be from 0 to 10 cm in diameter.

18. What is the degree of cervical effacement? Palpate the thickness of the cervix. Estimate the degree of thinness in percentages.

Effacement is measured in percentage. A cervix measuring approximately 1 cm (0.5 in) is 50% effaced. Transvaginal ultrasound is often used to measure cervical length in women suspected of cervical incompetency or at risk for preterm labor. The normal cervical length as measured by transvaginal ultrasound at midpregnancy is approximately 4 cm (1.6 in).

19. What is the presenting part of the fetus? (Figs. 3.23 and 3.24)

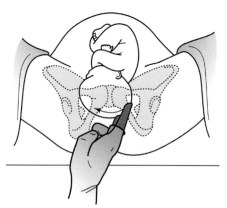

FIGURE 3.23 Identification of the posterior fontanelle.

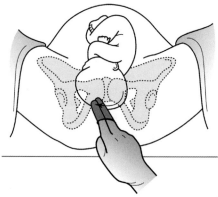

FIGURE 3.24 Identification of the anterior fontanelle.

skill unit continues on page 67

ACTIONS	**REMARKS**

Palpate for the presenting part. If you feel:
- The hard skull with the sagittal suture and follow it to the posterior or anterior fontanelle, it is a *cephalic presentation.*
- The softer buttocks, it is a *breech presentation.*
- Irregular, knobby parts like facial features, it is a *face presentation.*

20. What is the station? Has engagement occurred? Locate the lowest portion of the presenting part and then sweep the fingers deeply to one side of the pelvis to feel for the ischial spines (Fig. 3.25). Imagine a straight line from one spine to the other. To determine station, estimate how far (in centimeters) the tip of the presenting part is above or below the ischial spine (see Part 3 in Module 2). For example, if the fetal head is approximately 1–2 cm below the ischial spines, it is at +1 station.

Engagement occurs when the widest part of the fetal head has entered the inlet of the pelvis. Commonly, this occurs when the tip of the presenting part has reached the level of the ischial spines (i.e., station 0).

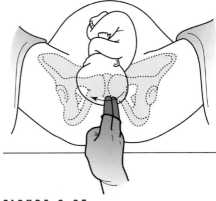

FIGURE 3.25

Station is +5 to −5 scale.

Station provides some information about the descent of the fetus through the pelvis. If the station is judged to be beyond 0, the pelvis is probably adequate for labor.

A vaginal examination can *begin* between contractions but should be *continued* throughout a contraction in the laboring woman.

Examination between contractions tells you about the degree of dilatation and effacement when the presenting part is not under the pressure of contraction. Examination during a contraction tells you the full extent of dilatation, effacement, and descent. It provides you with a clearer picture of how the laboring woman is doing.

21. Remove your fingers and discard the glove.

Informing the Mother

22. Tell the woman your findings and relate them to her progress in labor.

    Praise the woman for whatever you can at that point (e.g., working with you during the examination, achieving progress in labor to whatever degree, and recognizing the need to come in and be evaluated).

Information can be reassuring and supportive for the woman and for her support system.

Find some words of empowerment from the examination!

Labor consists of latent phase and active phase within the first stage of labor. Approximately 5% of women may experience a prolonged latent phase. 85% of women provided therapeutic rest will progress to active phase labor.[15,16]

You will need to attend a skill session(s) to practice this skill with the help of your preceptor. Mastery of the skill is achieved when you can demonstrate the following:
- Preparation and positioning of the woman for a vaginal examination
- Techniques used in a vaginal examination
- Accurate assessment of the status of membranes, cervical dilatation and effacement, fetal presentation, and station

REFERENCES

1. American College of Ob-Gyn. (2013). *ACOG Practice Bulletin #101: Ultrasonography in pregnancy* (pp. 1157–1167). Washington, DC: Compendium of ACOG Publications.

2. Cunningham, F. G., Leveno, K., Bloom, S., et al. (2010). *Williams obstetrics* (23rd ed., p. 329). New York, NY: Mcgraw Hill.

3. Creasy, R., Resnik, R. (2009). *Maternal-fetal medicine* (6th ed., pp. 769–770). New York: Elsevier.

4. American College of Ob-Gyn. (2013). *Committee Opinion #485: Prevention of early-onset group B streptococcal disease in newborns* (pp. 703–711). Washington, DC: Compendium of ACOG Publications.

5. Centers for Disease Control. (2010). Guidelines for Prevention on Perinatal Group B Strep tococcal (GBS) disease. *Morbidity and Mortality Weekly Report, 49*, 10. Atlanta, Ga: Author.

6. American College of Ob-Gyn. (2013). *Committee Opinion 418: Prenatal and perinatal human immunodeficiency virus testing: Expanded recommendations* (pp. 670–673). Washington, DC: Compendium of ACOG Publications.

7. Cleary, G., Wiswell, T. (1998). Meconium-stained amniotic fluid and the meconium aspiration syndrome: An update. *Pediatric Clinics of North America, 45*, 511–529.

8. Ramin, K., Leveno, K., Kelly, M., et al. (1996). Amniotic fluid meconium: A fetal environmental hazard. *Obstetrics and Gynecology, 87*, 181–184.

9. Lee, W., Lee, V. L., Kirk, J., et al. (2000). Vasa previa: Prenatal diagnosis, natural evolution and clinical outcome. *Obstetrics and Gynecology, 95*, 572–576.

10. Salihu, H., Bekan, B., Aliyu, M., et al. (2005). Perinatal mortality associated with abruptio placenta in singletons and multiples. *American Journal of Obstetrics and Gynecology, 193*, 198–203.

11. Martin, J., Hamilton, B., Sutton, P., et al. (2003). *Births: Final data for 2003. National Vital Statistics Report 2005; 54 #2.* Hyattsville, MD: National Center for Health Statistics.

12. Phelan, J., Smith, C., Broussard, P., et al. (1987). Amniotic fluid volume assessment with the four quadrant technique at 36–42 weeks' gestation. *Journal of Reproductive Medicine, 32*, 540–542.

13. Nabhan, A., Abdelmoula, Y. A. (2008). Amniotic fluid index versus single deepest vertical pocket as a screening test for preventing adverse pregnancy outcome. *Cochrane Database of Systematic Reviews, 3*, CD006593.

14. American College of Ob-Gyn. (2013). Hypertension in pregnancy. Executive summary. *Obstetrics and Gynecology, 122*, 1122–1131.

15. Howard, E. (2013). Labor evaluation. In Angelini D., LaFontaine D. (Eds.), *Obstetric triage and emergency care protocols* (pp. 159–167). New York: Springer Publishing.

16. Greulich, B., Tarrant, B. (2007). The latent phase of labor: Diagnosis and management. *Journal of Midwifery & Women's Health, 52*, 190–198.

Admission Assessment of the Fetus

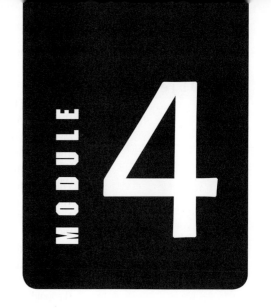

MODULE 4

SHARON L. HOLLEY

As you complete this module, you will learn:

1. Methods of fetal assessment
2. How to calculate fetal gestational age (GA)
3. Methods to obtain an accurate estimated date of delivery (EDD)
4. The relationship of fetal activity to fetal physiology and development
5. What fetal movement tells us about current fetal health
6. What to teach expectant women about fetal movement counting
7. The significance of the fetal alarm signal
8. Nursing implications for telephone triage when the expectant woman reports decreased fetal movement
9. Newer appreciations of the true capacities of the developing fetus and how to use this in humanizing the fetus for the woman and family during fetal assessment
10. An organized approach to evaluating fundal height and fetal lie, presentation, and position (Leopold's maneuvers), as well as how to estimate fetal weight and amniotic fluid in its extremes of low and high volumes
11. Clinical issues when findings for fundal height and fetal lie, presentation, and position vary from expected norms
12. What can and cannot be assessed with the auscultation method
13. How to apply an organized approach in locating and counting fetal heart rate (FHR) in intermittent auscultation (IA)
14. Definitions for and the significance of variations in FHR
15. Differentiation of sounds and rates when listening for fetal heart tones (FHTs)
16. Terminology to use when interpreting and charting FHRs heard by the auscultation method
17. Guidelines for fetal surveillance while caring for low- and high-risk laboring women

When you have completed this module, you should be able to recall the meaning of the following terms. You should also be able to use the terms when consulting with other health professionals. The terms are defined in this module or in the glossary at the end of this book.

acidosis	hypoxia
ballottement	oligohydramnios
fetal bradycardia	postterm
fetal tachycardia	

Assessing Fetal Health

• **How is fetal well-being assessed upon admission?**

When a woman in labor is admitted to the hospital, it is important to keep in mind that two patients are being admitted: the woman and the fetus. There are several important pieces of information that are gathered:

- Estimated gestational age (GA) of the fetus using the estimated date of delivery (EDD).
- Measure the fundal height of the uterus.
- Evaluate fetal position.
- Listen to fetal heart tones (FHTs).

There are important questions to ask the mother that have potential impact on the assessment of fetal well-being.

- Has she had any recent bleeding? Or is she bleeding now?
  - If so, how much?
  - Is it heavier than a period?
  - Is it bright red or brown in color?
  - Has she noticed any pain or other symptoms associated with the bleeding?
  - Has she recently taken any prescription or over-the-counter medications, herbal supplements, or street drugs?

- Has she noticed any recent of vaginal discharge consistent with leaking fluid?
  - If so, how much?
  - What color is it?
  - Has she noticed an odor with it?
  - Has she had any fever or chills recently?
- What is the woman's perception of recent fetal movement?

Gestational Age

• How is gestational age (GA) determined?

Predicting the EDD is another way of looking at GA. Determining the GA helps decision-making with regard to appropriate management of preterm labor, recommendations for timing of birth, as well as other fetal assessments that might be indicated. For example, knowing the GA, one can determine if the estimated fetal weight and maternal fundal height are consistent with expected measurements. Accurate GA determination decreases the incidence of the diagnosis of late-term and postterm pregnancies. Term pregnancy is considered between 37 0/7 weeks to 40 0/6 weeks, late-term pregnancy is defined as one that has been reached between 41 0/7 weeks and 41 6/7 weeks, and postterm pregnancy refers to a pregnancy that has reached or extended beyond 42 0/7 weeks.[1,2]

Obtaining an Accurate EDD

The estimated date of delivery, or EDD, represents a calculation based on 280 days (or 9 months and 7 days) from the onset of the last menstrual period (LMP), the approach used by most pregnancy wheels, or 266 days from the date of conception. Typically, ovulation is assumed to be approximately 14 days before the next 28-day menstrual cycle.[3] NOTE: You may also see the abbreviation last normal menstrual period (LNMP) is used.

Reliable criteria for accurately dating a pregnancy can be obtained in several ways. When assisted methods to achieve pregnancy are used, such as intrauterine insemination or embryo transfer, the conception/fertilization date is certain; therefore, that date should be used to calculate the EDD. Using an early first trimester ultrasound can facilitate obtaining an accurate EDD. Though the gestational sac is the first sonographic sign of an intrauterine pregnancy at 4.5 to 5 weeks, the crown-rump length (CRL) becomes visible at 5 to 10 weeks and is more accurate for dating and should be used to determine the EDD.[4] If the woman has been tracking her ovulation or knows her date of conception, these can be used to calculate her EDD as well. There are various methods used to track ovulation including over-the-counter ovulation kits, the use of basal body temperature chart with a coital record, as well as monitoring cervical mucus changes with coital record.

Often, the diagnosis of pregnancy begins when a woman presents with a positive home pregnancy test and cessation of menstrual periods. Only 4% of women give birth on the date predicted, which demonstrates that it is truly an estimate.[5] Though there are several methods to calculate an EDD, the ones most commonly used are Naegele's rule and ultrasound. The following questions help establish the EDD:

1. Use of the woman's first day of her last normal period (LMP). Use the following steps to help establish the LMP:
   - Explore with the woman whether her last menstrual period was normal in length, amount, color, and expected onset.
   - If the LMP was abnormal but the previous one was normal, use the first day of the last *normal* period.
2. If the pregnancy occurred during a time of amenorrhea for her, using the following techniques to help establish the EDD:
   - Ask the woman about her history of sexual intercourse. This helps establish a date of conception.
   - Question the woman about her use of birth control. For example, what type has she used recently, did she or her sexual partner use it consistently, or was this unprotected sexual intercourse?
   - Identify the date the woman first felt quickening, which is when the mother first feels the fetus moving. (This is generally around 18 to 20 weeks for nulliparous women and 16 to 18 gestational weeks for multiparous women.)

- Note when FHTs are first heard. When using a Doppler fetal monitor FHTs can first be heard between 10 and 12 weeks. When using a fetoscope, FHTs can be heard between 18 and 20 weeks.
3. Using the previous information one can use the following equation, known as Naegele's rule, to determine an EDD. Follow these simple steps:
    1. Determine the first day of the mother's LMP.
    2. Count back 3 months from the first day of the LMP and then add 7 days, adjusting the year if appropriate.

> **EXAMPLE:**
> LMP of August 18, 2014, the EDC is May 25, 2015.
> 8 − 3 = 5, or August − 3 months = May
> 18 + 7 = 25, or the 18th day of the month + 7 days = the 25th day of the month
> 2014 adjusted to 2015 to take into account the length of pregnancy.

NOTE: If there is a leap year this may alter the EDD by one day less.

> **EXAMPLE:** If LMP of August 18, 2015, the EDD is going to be May 24, 2016, because 2016 is a leap year making the month of February 29 days instead of 28 days, thus the extra day pushes the EDD back one day.

3. When using ultrasound to establish the EDD, remember that the earlier an ultrasound is done in pregnancy, the more accurate the information for estimating the GA. In general, ultrasound dating takes preference over LMP when the discrepancy is
    - >7 days in the first trimester;
    - >10 days in the second trimester;
    - ≥3 weeks in the third trimester.[4,6,7]

NOTE: Reassigning GA in the third trimester should be done with caution as there can be a 3 to 4 week range of accuracy. Using an accurate LMP for calculating the EDD is as reliable as using ultrasound in the second trimester. Ultrasound dating has a consistent margin of error of 8%.[7]

Factors That Influence the Accuracy of EDD Based on the LMP

Many women cannot remember the first day of their LMP.[2] Many also mistake implantation bleeding for an unusually short "period." Occasionally, a pregnancy is achieved during an amenorrheic period, when there is no menstruation. Amenorrhea, lack of menses, may occur in women experiencing certain conditions such as diabetes, thyroid problems, obesity, polycystic ovarian syndrome, or eating disorders. A woman who is exclusively breastfeeding will often have amenorrhea. Some women do not have regular 28-day cycles due to a longer follicular phase, thus affecting timing of ovulation earlier or later than day 14. Certain types of hormonal contraception may also lead to incorrect calculation of the date of ovulation.

Fetal Surveillance

Goals

Evaluation of fetal physical movements, FHR, and amniotic fluid production are currently used to predict fetal well-being at the time the testing is done. It is considered 99.8% predictive that fetal death is unlikely to occur within 1 week of a normal result.[8] For additional information regarding electronic fetal monitoring, see Module 7.

Fetal Physiology and Movement

Assessment of Fetal Movement Related to Fetal Health

Fetal activity requires oxygen consumption. When subjected to a hypoxic occurrence, one of the first fetal physiologic adjustments made is to economize movement. Compromise of fetal oxygenation elicits an adaptive response to decrease activity, thereby decreasing oxygen need.

TABLE 4.1 INDICATIONS FOR ANTEPARTUM TESTING	
MATERNAL INDICATIONS	**OBSTETRIC CONDITIONS**
Maternal age >40[14]	Assisted reproductive technology
Illicit substance use[15]	Cholestasis of pregnancy
Systemic lupus erythematosus	Decreased fetal movement
Cyanotic heart disease	Fetal growth restriction
Hypertensive disorders, including preeclampsia	Multiple gestation
Diabetes requiring insulin	Polyhydramnios
Hemoglobinopathies	Oligohydramnios
Hyperthyroidism	Postterm pregnancy (>41 wks)
Renal disease	Isoimmunization
Previous stillbirth	Gestational diabetes
Antiphospholipid syndrome	Preterm premature rupture of membranes
	Chronic abruption

From Fox, N. S., Rebarber, A., Silverstein, M., et al. (2013). The effectiveness of antepartum surveillance in reducing the risk of stillbirth in patients with advanced maternal age. *European Journal of Obstetrics & Gynecology and Reproductive Biology, 170*(2), 387–390; Izquierdo, L. A., & Yonke, N. (2014). Fetal surveillance in late pregnancy and during labor. *Obstetrics and Gynecology Clinics, 41*(2), 307–315.

This adaptive response can result from a physiologic or a pathophysiologic event. Fetal movements serve as an indirect measure of current central nervous system function. Maternal perception of fetal body movement has been used as a sign of fetal well-being. The goal of fetal movement counting is that when a woman identifies a decrease in her baby's normal movement pattern she can report this to her provider, and additional antepartum testing can be initiated with the goal of preventing fetal death.[9] Women who report decreased fetal movement have an incidence of stillbirth that is 60 times higher than women without this complaint. Various things can affect maternal perception of fetal movement such as fetal sleep cycles, maternal activity, and obesity.[10] Though there is fetal movement during the first trimester, this is generally only noted through the use of ultrasound. The term "quickening" is used to describe the woman's first fetal movement that is felt, usually like a small flutter.[11] Maternal perception of fetal movement generally starts in the second trimester. Primiparas typically begin to feel fetal movement between 18 and 22 weeks, while multiparous women often feel the fetus move earlier around 16 to 18 weeks.[11,12] Women who have an anterior placenta may begin to feel fetal movement later than those whose placenta has attached posteriorly. Fetal movement maximizes around 34 weeks GA, then decreases slightly due to the longer sleep cycles as the central nervous system matures.[13]

To date there is no specific level of fetal movement that can reliably identify a fetus at risk for fetal demise; there is generally a maternal awareness of what is normal movement for her own baby. There is no current evidence to support routine use of formal fetal kick count monitoring for women who are not at risk for chronic fetal hypoxia. Intrauterine fetal demise (IUFD), otherwise called stillbirth.[11] Formal fetal movement counting does not prevent all stillbirths, but there are those maternal or obstetric conditions that fall into a higher risk category, and these women may benefit by more formal fetal movement counts.[6] Table 4.1 outlines recommended fetal surveillance testing for women and fetal high-risk conditions.

Adequate functioning of the uteroplacental unit is necessary for the fetus to accomplish and maintain patterns of healthy behavior. There are both maternal and fetal factors that can affect fetal breathing and limb movements (see Table 4.2).

NOTE: *Women often report "less fetal movement" as term approaches. This change always requires careful evaluation, although what the mother perceives as "less movement" is often a result of less room in utero for the fetus to put "momentum" behind movements. The mother's perception of a significant change always requires further exploration.*

The normal fetus may move as many as 100 times per hour or as few as 4 times per hour. It is important to discuss with the woman the normal pattern of movement for her fetus. Attention should be given to any complaint of a decrease in the normal pattern of movement in the fetus. A period of decreased fetal movement commonly precedes fetal death, but the absence of perceived fetal movements does not necessarily indicate fetal death or compromise.

NOTE: *Any time an expectant woman calls reporting decreased fetal activity, it requires follow-up.*

TABLE 4.2 FACTORS AFFECTING FETAL MOVEMENT		
MATERNAL FACTORS	**FETAL FACTORS**	**OTHER FACTORS**
Timing of maternal meals	Gestational age	Time of day
Medication ingestion	Sleep cycles vs. wake cycles	Oligohydramnios
Diabetes	Intrauterine growth restriction (IUGR)	Rh disease
Hypertension disorders	Multiple gestation	History of previous IUGR
Systemic lupus erythematosus	Postterm pregnancy	Placental location
Tobacco, alcohol, or substance use		

Far too many expectant mothers avoid seeking care because they do not trust what they feel. Many have no prior frame of reference for what they are experiencing, but they also fear being seen as bothersome or a worrier. Anyone who might be a first-line contact for the expectant woman should demonstrate caring and concern.

If a mother calls reporting decreased fetal movement, explore her background for normalcy. Ask how today's fetal movements compare with those of the previous day and the days preceding. When movement is present but perceived as lessening, you might instruct the mother to do one of the various methods for fetal kick counts. If after doing the fetal kick counts the mother has not had a minimum number of perceived fetal movements, then she should be instructed to come into the office or hospital for further evaluation.

Most of the time, ultrasound or EFM reveals a normal FHR and activity pattern. Praise the mother for her vigilance, and as she leaves, offer professional assurance that you or the staff are there to help her in the weeks ahead.

Fetal Movement Counts ("Kick Counts")

Fetal movement counts have been utilized in the past as a simple, inexpensive, and noninvasive means of fetal surveillance for pregnant women. It can be done at home and has no contraindications. The rationale for fetal movement counting is the hope that fetal death can be prevented by acting immediately when there is a decrease in fetal movement. However, limitations of the test include the fact that the ideal number of movements or kicks has not been established, nor has the ideal duration for movement counting been clearly defined.[16] Additionally, the period between decreased fetal movement and fetal death may be too short for timely intervention in some clinical situations such as placental abruption or cord accidents.

Despite the fact that there is not enough evidence to recommend formal fetal movement counts for all expectant women, they are widely prescribed in both low- and high-risk women.[3] Fetal movement counts in high-risk women may begin as early as 28 weeks' gestation and in low-risk women at 32 to 36 weeks' gestation.

Many different methods have been devised to assess fetal movement. The intent of all methods is to have the expectant woman achieve a daily awareness of the patterns and level of activity exhibited by her baby in utero. One of the most popular is the "count to 10" method. This method requires that the mother dedicate 1 hour or less every day to tracking her baby's movements.[16]

To begin routine fetal movement counting, ask the woman to select a time of day when the baby is generally most active. Have the woman assume a comfortable position, but not flat on her back in order to avoid hypotension. Proceed to use one of the methods for fetal movement counting outlined in Table 4.3. If the appropriate fetal movements are noted, the counting is discontinued. However, if after 2 hours the woman has not felt the appropriate number of fetal movements she should notify her provider immediately. **Instruct the woman to not wait until the next day to notify the provider.**

Humanizing the Fetus for Parents

The Skill Units presented in this module not only offer methods to assess fetal health but involve a unique opportunity to help the woman and father/support person perceive the fetus as a developing human. While conducting any of the skills outlined, you can interact with the fetus through abdominal massaging, speaking to, and commenting about the fetus to the woman.

TABLE 4.3	METHODS TO ASSESS FETAL MOVEMENT		
NUMBER OF FETAL MOVEMENTS	**COUNTING TIMEFRAME**	**MATERNAL ACTIVITY LEVEL**	**GESTATIONAL AGE IN WEEKS**
10	12 hrs	Normal daily activity	28 or >
10	2 hrs	At rest and focused on counting	28 or >
4	1 hr	At rest and focused on counting	28 or >
10	25 min		22–36
10	25 min		37 or >

Research has shown the fetus responds to maternal voice and speech patterns.[17] Reactive movements or behaviors of the fetus include the following examples:

- Coughing or laughing in the mother brings about movement in nearly all fetuses between 10 and 15 weeks' gestation.
- Fetuses sometimes react to the needle during an amniocentesis by moving away from the needle or even attacking it.
- A bright light shining through the abdominal wall and fixed on the fetal head (vertex) increases the fetus' heartbeat.
- Some fetuses react to high-volume rock music and violent movies with vigorous movements that can even be painful to the mother.
- Variations in FHR and activity response to maternal voice.[17]

As you measure the fundus and palpate the maternal abdomen, talk to the baby and comment to the mother about any response you get. Educate and encourage the mother about fetal hearing and sensory perceptions. Newborns will thrive on nurturing attention after birth but what has become clear in the cited studies is that babies thrive with attention *before* birth.

PRACTICE/REVIEW QUESTIONS

After reviewing this module, answer the following questions.

1. State four pieces of information to gather when the woman is admitted to the labor unit.

   a. _____

   b. _____

   c. _____

   d. _____

2. If the LMP is June 6, 2015, when is the EDD? (2016 is a leap year)

   _____

3. Pregnancy can be achieved during an amenorrheic period if the woman has diabetes or thyroid problems.

   a. True

   b. False

4. An EDD represents a calculation of 280 days from a woman's LMP based on an average menstrual cycle of _____ days and assumed average ovulation day _____ of that menstrual cycle.

5. If the calculated EDD by a sure LMP is April 20, 2015, but the EDD based on a first trimester ultrasound is April 7, 2015, then the working EDD is April 20, 2015.

   a. True

   b. False

6. The woman can identify quickening around the 10th to 12th week of pregnancy.

   a. True

   b. False

7. A small amount of bleeding can occur with implantation.

   a. True

   b. False

8. List five reasons to begin antepartum fetal surveillance testing:

   a. _____

   b. _____

   c. _____

   d. _____

   e. _____

9. When the fetus is deprived of sufficient oxygen, a physiologic adaptive response is _____

_____

10. A *postterm pregnancy* is defined as one that has gone beyond which gestational week?

   a. 40

   b. 41

   c. 42

11. A significant overall decrease in fetal activity:

   a. Can be related to the awake/sleep state of the fetus

   b. Can signal a sign of maturity

   c. Can be a marker for fetal hypoxia

   d. Should be expected before the onset of labor

12. Name five factors that can affect fetal movement.

   a. _____

   b. _____

   c. _____

   d. _____

   e. _____

13. Name three evaluation methods used to predict fetal well-being.

14. Maternal intake of alcohol has an effect on fetal gross body movements.

   a. True

   b. False

15. A woman has called to tell you her baby has not moved much today. Her pregnancy has been uncomplicated, and she is 39 weeks today. She reports doing fetal movement counting for the last hour and has felt four movements. Your response is to:

   a. Offer reassurance this is normal, no further evaluation is needed

   b. Tell her to do aerobic exercise to wake up the baby

   c. Come in to the hospital now to obtain FHTs

   d. Schedule her for an induction of labor within 24 hours

16. Maternal perceptions of fetal activity:

   a. Are not reliable

   b. Are influenced by the time of day

   c. Are not influenced by the posterior implantation of the placenta

   d. Correlate poorly with actual fetal movement

17. A woman tells you her LMP is August 10, 2016. What is her EDD by Naegele's rule?

   a. November 17, 2017

   b. May 3, 2017

   c. November 17, 2016

   d. May 17, 2017

18. Select your response for question 16 if the mother had a history of stillbirth at 38 weeks' gestation with her last pregnancy and currently has gestational diabetes. You would choose response:

   a. "Come right in and let us evaluate what is going on."

   b. "Drink 1 or 2 glasses of fluids, go to bed this evening, but call your obstetric provider in the morning."

   c. "Take a walk and relax. Call tomorrow if you continue to have fewer than 10 movements in 1 hour."

   d. "Continue counting for 2 more hours, and call me back with your results. I'll want to talk with you then."

19. An insulin-dependent mother at 35 weeks' gestation calls to state that the baby has been moving a lot less over the past 2 days. When she is placed on the electronic fetal monitor, fetal activity with FHR accelerations is seen over 25 minutes. Subsequent to being reassured and sent home, she calls again 4 days later worried because, again, fetal movement appears significantly different. What will you recommend to her?

PRACTICE/REVIEW ANSWER KEY

1. Any four of the following:
   a. Estimate gestational age of fetus and EDD.
   b. Measure the fundal height of the uterus.
   c. Evaluate fetal position.
   d. Listen to FHTs.
   e. Ask about fetal movement.
2. March 12, 2016 (2016 is a leap year)
3. a. True
4. 28, 14
5. False
6. b. False
7. a. True
8. See Table 4.1
9. To decrease fetal movement
10. c. 42
11. c. Can be a marker for fetal hypoxia
12. See Table 4.2
13. a. Fetal movements
   b. FHR
   c. Amniotic fluid production
14. a. True
15. a. Offer reassurance this is normal, no further evaluation is needed
16. b. Are influenced by the time of day; and
   c. Are reliable
17. May 17, 2017 (2017 is not a leap year)
18. a. "Come right in and let us evaluate what is going on."
19. Tell her to come in for evaluation.

SKILL UNIT 1 | MEASURING FUNDAL HEIGHT

This section details how to measure the height of the uterine fundus to obtain information about fetal growth and body size. Study this section and then attend a skill practice and demonstration session scheduled with your preceptor. You will need to demonstrate the examination and correctly interpret the results. The steps of the examination are summarized at the end of this unit.

Key Points

- The fundus is the top of the uterus. Measuring fundal height in pregnancy is a way to evaluate fetal growth and screen for abnormal fetal growth. It is also used to screen for complications of amniotic fluid volume and can help detect for possible multiple gestation. If there is a discrepancy in the expected fundal height and what is found on examination, often an ultrasound is used to evaluate the discrepancy.
- Before the 20th week in pregnancy, fundal height is typically described as the uterine fundal height compared to the level of the symphysis pubis and umbilicus using fingerbreadth (fb) to note the measurement. For example, at 12 weeks GA, the fundal height for a singleton pregnancy is expected to be at the level of the symphysis pubis. If it is higher than expected it may be a sign of a multiple gestation or the estimated GA may be incorrect and an ultrasound would be ordered to determine the correct GA. However, at 16 weeks, the expected fundal height is halfway between the symphysis pubis and the umbilicus and would be recorded as 4 FB below the umbilicus. Following the 20th week, when the fundal height is at the level of the 1 to 2 FB below the umbilicus, a tape measure is used to measure from the symphysis pubis to the top of the fundus. The measurement between 20 weeks and term should be found to correlate within 2 to 3 cm with the tape measure to the number of weeks of GA. Factors that can affect the accuracy of fundal height are found in Table 4.4.
- If a contraction occurs, wait until the contraction has subsided before taking the measurement. Moving on to determining fetal lie, presentation, and position will then prepare you to know where to look for FHTs, the final assessment technique.

TABLE 4.4 FACTORS AFFECTING ACCURACY OF FUNDAL HEIGHT

FACTORS AFFECTING ACCURACY OF FUNDAL HEIGHT

MATERNAL	FETAL
Full bladder	Position, lie, attitude
Positioning	Multiple gestation
GA of pregnancy	Late third trimester
Incorrectly calculated GA	Factors affecting fetal growth
BMI ≥40	
Active labor	

ACTIONS	REMARKS
STEP 1: Measure the Fundal Height[18]	
1. Ask the woman to empty her bladder.	A full bladder gives a falsely high fundal height of as much as 2 to 3 cm.
2. Assist the woman to a supine position on the examination table. Avoid elevating the woman's trunk or flexing her knees, if possible. This may not be a comfortable position for her, so be prepared to move through the assessment without delay. When finished, elevate the examination table to her comfort. Ask her to expose her abdomen from below the breasts to the symphysis pubis.	Maternal position influences fundal height measurement.[20] No research data exist to support the use of a position other than supine for obtaining fundal height measurements. This helps improve accuracy of the fundal height measurement. Provide privacy and consider cultural needs.

skill unit continues on page 78

ACTIONS	**REMARKS**

3. Inspect the maternal abdomen before beginning fundal height measurements. Look at the abdominal shape. An elongated shape probably denotes a vertical lie; a triangular shape may indicate a transverse lie.

4. Facing the woman's head, place your hands on each side of the uterus approximately halfway between the symphysis and the fundus (Fig. 4.1). Feel along the sides of the uterus upward toward the fundus. As you near the top, your hands will begin to come together. They will meet at the top of the fundus.

This assists in identifying exactly where the fundus is located.

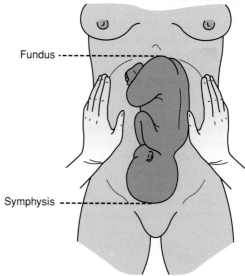

FIGURE 4.1 The fundal height is measured in centimeters.

5. Place the zero line of the tape measure on the anterior border of the symphysis pubis and stretch the tape upward in a straight line following the abdominal midline to the top of the fundus (Fig. 4.2).

The tape should be brought over the curve of the fundus. The measurement is read at the lowermost edge of the curved fundus.

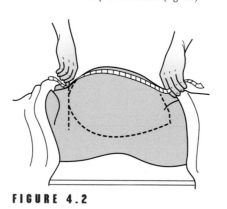

FIGURE 4.2

NOTE: *Slight variations in the way people measure the curve of the fundus result in discrepancies between examiners. There are several techniques for measuring fundal height; therefore, it is essential for clinicians to standardize their fundal height measurement technique so that all measurements are obtained in the same position and use the same anatomic landmarks.*[19]

skill unit continues on page 79

ACTIONS	REMARKS

Approximate Height of the Fundus During Pregnancy (Fig. 4.3)

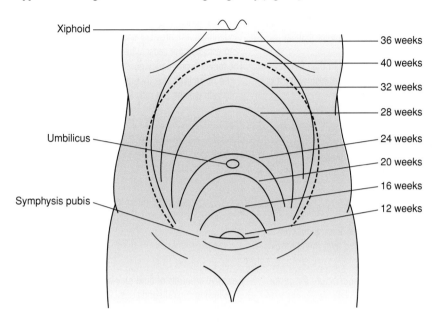

Xiphoid — 36 weeks
— 40 weeks
— 32 weeks
— 28 weeks
Umbilicus — 24 weeks
— 20 weeks
— 16 weeks
Symphysis pubis — 12 weeks

F I G U R E   4 . 3

WEEK	LOCATION OF THE UTERUS
1–11	The uterus is a pelvic organ for the first 3 mo of pregnancy, palpable on cervical examination.
12	The fundus is at the level of the symphysis pubis, approximately the size of a small grapefruit.
16	The fundus is halfway between the symphysis pubis and the umbilicus and is ovoid in shape.
20	The fundus is approximately 1–2 FB below the umbilicus.
24	The fundus is 1–2 FB above the umbilicus.
28	The fundus is halfway between the umbilicus and the xiphoid, approximately 3 FB above the umbilicus.
32	The fundus is three fourths the distance between the umbilicus and the xiphoid, or approximately 3 FB below the xiphoid process.
36–38	The fundus is at or 1 FB below the xiphoid process.
40	2–3 FB below the xiphoid process if lightening has occurred.[6]

NOTE: If the fetus is growing slowly or quickly, the fundal height will be too low or too high to give an accurate GA. Maternal BMI ≥40 also affects the accuracy of fundal height results; therefore, serial growth ultrasounds may be done to evaluate for fetal growth rather than rely on fundal height measurement screening.[20–22]

STEP 2: Evaluate the Fundal Height Measurement

Scenario A: What if you assess a lower fundal height than the woman's GA?

When you measure the mother's abdomen and find it is more than 2 cm less than what would be expected for her due date, it may indicate growth restriction in the fetus or oligohydramnios.

If this is the first time measuring fundal height, re-evaluate the calculated GA, and notify the obstetric provider.

The provider may choose to order an ultrasound for dating.

Consistently low fundal height can mean that the fetus is not growing appropriately for GA. This is called *intrauterine growth restriction* and can be a sign of placental insufficiency. Fetuses with IUGR require additional assessment and follow-up.

skill unit continues on page 80

79

ACTIONS	REMARKS
A lack of increase in fundal height over three consecutive weeks often indicates fetal growth restriction. Poor prenatal weight gain in a mother who is average size or smaller adds to the probability of this diagnosis.	Low fundal height can occur with a transverse lie. Careful abdominal palpation should be done.
When you have a lower fundal height than GA, review the woman's medical and prenatal history for the following:	There are multiple causes for IUGR. When IUGR is identified, the provider should be vigilant in trying to establish the cause when possible. The longer a pregnancy goes beyond the due date, the more likely it is that the fetus will not only fail to gain weight, but may lose weight.
• Heart disease • Elevated blood pressure and signs and symptoms of preeclampsia • Exposure to communicable diseases • An incidence of fever, chills, vomiting, or diarrhea during pregnancy • Smoking and drinking habits • Drug use • Fundal height measurements throughout pregnancy • Signs/symptoms of ruptured fetal membranes • Notify the provider	

Scenario B: What if a *high fundal height for gestational age* is found?
A high fundal height of more than 2 cm above the norm for GA can mean that the fetus is large for GA. However, you need to do the following:
• Palpate the woman's abdomen for the presence of an excessive amount of fluid (hydramnios).
• Palpate for the presence of more than one fetus.
• Review the woman's prenatal and medical history. Look for the following:
  ∘ The presence of a consistently high fundal height
  ∘ History of diabetes mellitus
  ∘ An ultrasound report noting a high amniotic fluid index.
	Excessive amounts of fluid may be present in the following clinical conditions:
	• Twin gestations
	• Fetuses with congenital anomalies
	• Women who have diabetes mellitus or syphilis
	• Women who have blood incompatibility—Rh isoimmunization

You will need to attend a skill lesson(s) to practice this skill with the help of your preceptor. Mastery of the skill is achieved when you can do the following:

- Identify the anterior border of the symphysis pubis bone as your starting point for measuring fundal height.
- Attain the same fundal height measurements as your coordinator or preceptor within 1 cm margin of error.
- Accurately interpret your measurements as normal, high, or low.
- Describe the implications for management of mothers with low and high fundal height measurements.

SKILL UNIT 2 | EVALUATING FETAL LIE, PRESENTATION, AND POSITION USING LEOPOLD'S MANEUVERS

This skill unit details how to use a systematic approach in abdominal palpation to determine fetal presentation and position. Study the section and then attend a skill practice and demonstration session scheduled by your preceptor. You will need to demonstrate that you can perform Leopold's maneuvers and correctly identify a variety of fetal lies, positions, and presentations. These steps are summarized at the end of this skill unit.

skill unit continues on page 81

ACTIONS	REMARKS

STEP 1: Prepare the Woman

Ask the woman to empty her bladder.

Assist the woman onto the examining table. She should lie on her back and expose her abdomen from below the breasts to the symphysis pubis.	Abdominal muscles are relaxed, and palpating for the fetal parts is generally easier. This allows for more accurate assessment of fetal lie, position, and presentation.
Facilitate relaxation of the abdominal muscles by putting a pillow under her head and upper shoulders, have her place her arms comfortably to the side, have her bend her knees so that the soles of her feet rest flat on the table (Fig. 4.4).	Moderately flexed knees decrease abdominal muscle tightening.
Carry out the examination between contractions if labor has begun.	A towel or small pillow may be placed on one side of the woman's hips and back to induce a lateral tilt. This is especially important if the woman is experiencing supine hypotension (faintness from diminished circulation to heart or brain while supine).

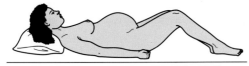

FIGURE 4.4

STEP 2: Determine the Presenting Part and Lie

Warm your hands by washing them under warm water or rubbing them together.	Cold hands cause abdominal muscles to contract and tighten.
Inspect the maternal abdomen before beginning palpation. Look for an elongated abdomen denoting a probable vertical lie or a triangular shaped abdomen indicating a possible transverse lie. Use gentle but firm motions. Start by lightly putting a hand on the woman's abdomen so she can adjust to the feeling of someone touching her. Use the flat palmar surface of the fingers for palpating, not the fingertips. Use smooth deep pressure as necessary to obtain accurate information, but avoid so much as to cause the woman discomfort or pain.[6]	Leopold's maneuvers should be done systematically to obtain the best results. This allows any muscle tightening of the abdomen time to relax and get used to the examiner's touch.
First maneuver: Face the woman's head. Place your hands up the sides of the abdomen and move them to the fundus (Fig. 4.5). Identify what is located in the fundus as being the fetal breech, fetal head, or unable to determine.	Typically the fetal breech, or buttocks, is found in the fundus and the fetal head is found near the maternal pelvis. A fetal breech typically feels less firm or as round as a fetal head. It is unable to move independently of the fetal body. The fetal head will feel firm and round as compared with the fetal breech. The head is movable and can be moved back and forth between the examiner's fingers (ballotable) or hands as the fetal head can move independently from the trunk. When the fetus is in a transverse lie, neither the head or breech will be felt in the fundus.

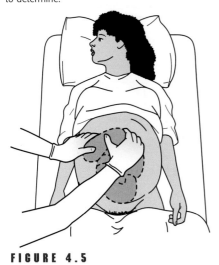

FIGURE 4.5

skill unit continues on page 82

ACTIONS	REMARKS

STEP 3: Locate the Back and Small Parts

Second maneuver: Continue to face the woman's head. Move your hands to the sides of the abdomen, about midway between the symphysis pubis and the fundus. Use one hand to apply steady pressure to the uterus and palpate with the other hand for the fetal back or small parts, such as hands and feet (Fig. 4.6). Keeping the fingers together, apply firm circular motions with the palmar surface of the hands. Move in a systematic fashion from mid-abdomen to the outer abdomen, and again from the symphysis pubis to the uterine fundus.

Applying pressure with one hand steadies the fetus/abdomen, so the other hand can palpate well for the fetal back or small part like arms and legs.

Using the palmar surface of the hands helps discriminate more accurately what you are feeling. Using only fingertips may cause maternal discomfort and will not elicit the information sought.

The side where the fetal back is located will feel firmer and smoother. The side where the fetal small parts are located, hands, elbows, knees, and feet, will feel softer and knobby and have more "give" as you palpate. When palpating the fetal small parts you may feel fetal movement. Fetal small parts should be opposite of the fetal back.

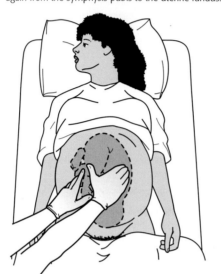

FIGURE 4.6

STEP 4: Examine the Fundus

Third maneuver: Face the woman's head. Use the palmar surface of one hand to steady the uterus by placing it on the fundus. Grasp the lower portion of the abdomen just above the symphysis pubis between the thumb and the fingers with the other hand (Fig. 4.7). Use gentle but firm pressure with the fundal hand while pressing deeply into the maternal abdomen just above the symphysis pubis with the other hand. Feel for the presenting part just above the symphysis pubis between the thumb and fingers of that hand. Gently move the presenting part back and forth between your thumb and fingers to determine if it is a fetal head or fetal breech.

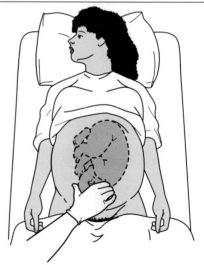

FIGURE 4.7

This maneuver can cause some discomfort and may be omitted if the woman finds it too uncomfortable. The fetal head will feel firm, hard, and more rounded than the fetal breech.

skill unit continues on page 83

ACTIONS	REMARKS

STEP 5: Locate the Cephalic Prominence and Fetal Attitude

Fourth maneuver: Turn and face the mother's feet. Move your hands to the sides of the maternal abdomen. Using your palmar surfaces, move your hands down toward the symphysis pubis and iliac crest with your fingers directed toward the symphysis pubis and into the pelvic inlet. Attempt to locate the cephalic prominence by moving your hands down the sides of the abdomen toward the symphysis pubis (Fig. 4.8). Note whether the head is:

• free and floating (ballotable)

OR

• flexed and approaching engagement.

The cephalic prominence, or brow, is located on the side where there is greatest resistance to the downward movement of the fingers. When the head is well flexed, it is found on the opposite side from the fetal back (Fig. 4.9). When the fetal head is not well flexed or is hyperextended, the cephalic prominence is found on the same side as the back.

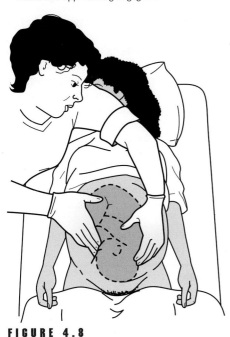

FIGURE 4.8

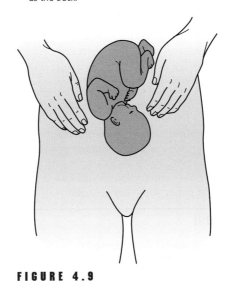

FIGURE 4.9

You will need to attend a skill session(s) to practice this skill with the help of your preceptor. Mastery of the skill is achieved when you can do the following:

• Prepare the woman and yourself for the examination.
• Systematically approach abdominal palpation using the first through fourth Leopold's maneuvers.
• Correctly identify fetal lie, presentation, and position on three different patients.

SKILL UNIT 3 | AUSCULTATION OF FETAL HEART TONES

This skill unit will teach you how to find and count the FHR and what to do if you hear a FHR that is not reassuring. Study this section and then attend a skill practice and demonstration session scheduled by your preceptor. You will need to demonstrate that you can perform the procedure and correctly interpret the findings. These steps are summarized at the end of this skill unit.

Key Points

• The information presented in this unit is limited to a discussion of auscultation of the FHR during admission assessment.
• Auscultation of the fetal heart is the practice of using a device to listen to the FHR, sometimes referred to as FHTs. Using any of the identified methods can be done intermittently; this is called intermittent auscultation (IA). Electronic fetal monitoring (EFM) is used for intermittent or continuous fetal monitoring

TABLE 4.5	RECOMMENDATIONS FOR INTERMITTENT FETAL MONITORING DURING LABOR		
ORGANIZATION	**PREGNANCY RISK STATUS**	**ACTIVE LABOR: FIRST STAGE**	**ACTIVE LABOR: SECOND STAGE**
AWHONN[a,23]	Low-risk status without oxytocin	Every 15–30 min	Passive fetal descent: Every 15 min Active pushing: Every 5–15 min
ACOG[b,24]	Low risk	Every 30 min	Every 15 min
	High risk	Every 15 min	Every 5 min
ACNM[c,25]	Low risk	Every 15–30 min	Every 5 min

[a]Association of Women's Health, Obstetric and Neonatal Nursing.
[b]American College of Obstetricians and Gynecologists.
[c]American College of Nurse-Midwives.

and has a readout that must be interpreted. Intermittent auscultation refers to the assessment of the FHT at selected intervals during labor, whereas continuous fetal monitoring is uninterrupted. Overall IA has been reported as equivalent to EFM in terms of neonatal morbidity and mortality outcomes based on randomized controlled trials (RTC).

- Decisions regarding the use of IA or EFM should, in the best practice approach, be a mutual one between each woman and her provider and should be determined by the woman's history, risk status, hospital policies and procedures, and the availability of personnel trained in IA (see Table 4.5).
- Evidence suggests a 1:1 nurse to patient ratio for IA. Therefore, staffing patterns may be a consideration when selecting IA or EFM as the primary method of fetal surveillance during labor.

NOTE: The frequency of intermittent auscultation should be individualized based upon the woman's wishes, risk status, assessment, unit staffing, and hospital policy. Listen to the FHR before, during, and after one full contraction. IA should be done at regular intervals, before and after cervical exams, rupture of membranes, the use of medications, or ambulation.[25]

NOTE: Every institution should have a policy on intermittent monitoring. Review your own hospital policy with your preceptor.

ACTIONS	REMARKS

STEP 1: Assemble the Equipment

The basic types of auscultation devices include:
A. A modified stethoscope worn on the head of the listener so that bone conduction from the skull increases hearing ability. Sounds associated with the actual opening and closing of fetal ventricular valves can be heard.

A. DeLee–Hillis fetoscope with headpiece (Fig. 4.10)

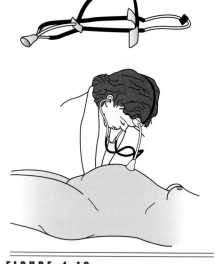

FIGURE 4.10

skill unit continues on page 85

ACTIONS	REMARKS
B. A large, heavy bell that magnifies fetal heart sounds.	B. Leff stethoscope (Fig. 4.11).

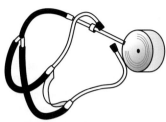

FIGURE 4.11

C. An electronic device that uses ultrasound technology to detect fetal heart motion such as the moving heart walls or valves and converts the ultrasound information into a sound that represents the cardiac activity. Some Doppler devices have been developed that can be submerged under water for use in women laboring in tubs.[11]

C. Doppler (Fig. 4.12)

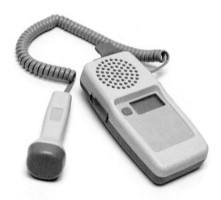

FIGURE 4.12

D. A Pinard is a handheld trumpet-shaped tool used to listen to the FHR. The wide end of the Pinard is held up against the maternal abdomen while the clinician listens through the flat end.

D. Pinard (Fig. 4.13)

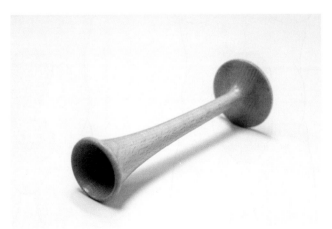

FIGURE 4.13

skill unit continues on page 86

ACTIONS	REMARKS

STEP 2: Obtaining FHR by Auscultation

Position the fetoscope, or other device, on the appropriate quadrant of the mother's abdomen. Use firm pressure.

In **right occipit anterior (ROA)** (Fig. 4.14), sounds are best heard in the right lower quadrant.

In posterior positions, such as **left occipit posterior (LOP)** (Fig. 4.15) or **right occipit anterior (ROP)** (Fig. 4.16), sounds are best heard at the woman's side.

In breech position (Fig. 4.17), sounds are best heard above the woman's umbilicus on her left side.

With a face presentation (Fig. 4.18), the fetal back becomes concave, and the best place to listen for the heart sounds is over the more convex chest.

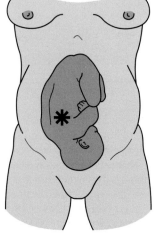

FIGURE 4.14   ROA.

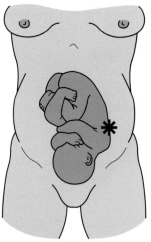

FIGURE 4.15   LOP.

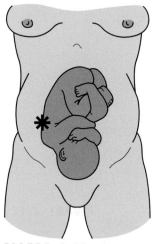

FIGURE 4.16   ROP.

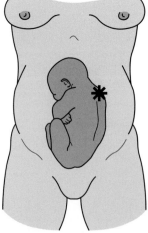

FIGURE 4.17   LSA.

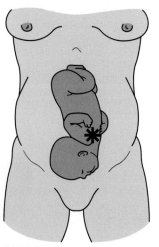

FIGURE 4.18   Face presentation.

skill unit continues on page 87

ACTIONS	REMARKS

STEP 3: Listening and Interpretation

Guidelines that can aid you in locating the fetal heart beat are as follows:

A. Between the *10th and 16th weeks of pregnancy,* use a Doppler. Apply a small amount of conduction gel to the contact portion of the Doppler. Begin listening at the upper border of the pubic hair. If you are unable to hear fetal tones, slowly move the instrument up toward the mother's umbilicus. Generally only light pressure is needed. You will need to apply more gel if the search is extensive.

B. Between the *16th and 24th weeks of pregnancy,* measure off 2 FB above the pubic hairline and listen along the midline of the abdomen.

C. After the *24th week of pregnancy,* search the abdomen in a methodical manner. Place the fetoscope or Doppler at position 1, as shown in Figure 4.19. If nothing is heard, move to position 2 in the lower left quadrant. Continue following the numbered positions.

D. If you do not detect FHRs at these eight positions, begin a systematic search of the abdomen. Place the fetoscope or Doppler at the umbilicus and move it centimeter-by-centimeter outward along the spoke-like pattern. Follow the sequence of numbers in Figure 4.20.

The ultrasound instrument is more sensitive than the fetoscope. It picks up FHTs about the 10th week of gestation. Conduction gel aids in the transmission of ultrasound waves.

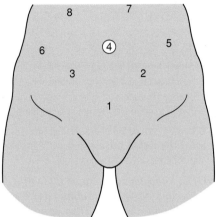

FIGURE 4.19 Methodical search pattern for FHTs. (Adapted with permission from Wheeler, L. A. [1979]. *Fetal assessment. Series 2: Prenatal care, Module 3* [p. 19]. White Plains, NY: The National Foundation—March of Dimes.)

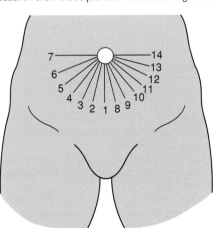

FIGURE 4.20 Systematic search pattern for FHTs. (Adapted with permission from Wheeler, L. A. [1979]. *Fetal assessment. Series 2: Prenatal care, Module 3* [p. 19]. White Plains, NY: The National Foundation—March of Dimes.)

STEP 4: Differentiating Sounds and Rates

A. Listen
- You may hear a soft "blowing" sound of maternal blood coursing through the uterine arteries; this is referred to as *the uterine soufflé.*
- A distinct "swishing" sound may be heard; this is synonymous with blood coursing through the umbilical artery and is referred to as the *funic soufflé.*

This is synonymous with the *maternal heart rate.*

This reflects the *FHR.*

NOTE: *Fetal heart valve opening and closing have very distinct cardiac sounds—not muffled or swishing sounds as in the uterine or funic soufflé.*

skill unit continues on page 88

ACTIONS	REMARKS
B. Check the woman's radial pulse while counting FHR. The goal in assessing FHR is to search for and count the fetal cardiac sound.	This distinguishes the maternal heart rate from the FHR.
C. Determine FHR by listening for a full 60 sec. If the rate is above 160 bpm or below 110 bpm, more frequent auscultation must be done.	The FHR must be counted long enough to determine changes in rate and rhythm. It is important to distinguish if the change is a brief, isolated increase or decrease (acceleration or deceleration) from the baseline or a change in the baseline rate.[11]
D. Determine the FHR rhythm. Rhythm is assessed for regularity and is described as regular or irregular. Irregular rhythms should be further assessed by ultrasound or cardiography to rule out artifact or to determine the type of dysrhythmia present.	An irregular rhythm should be reported to the provider.
E. Document each period of auscultation with a description of rate, rhythm, and the presence of gradual or abrupt decreases from the heart rate.	**EXAMPLE:** FHR 144 bpm by auscultation, regular rhythm, audible acceleration.

NOTE: Although auscultation allows the listener to hear gradual or abrupt changes from the baseline, baseline variability and the types of deceleration (late, variable, or early) cannot be identified with IA. There is no research to support that the expert listener can make these distinctions.[11]

REFERENCES

1. American College of Obstetricians and Gynecologists. (2014). Revitalize obstetric definitions. http://www.acog.org/About-ACOG/ACOG-Departments/Patient-Safety-and-Quality-Improvement/reVITALize-Obstetric-Data-Definitions. Accessed August 2, 2014.
2. American College of Obstetricians and Gynecologists. (2014). Management of late-term and postterm pregnancies. Practice Bulletin No. 146. *Obstetrics & Gynecology, 124*(2), 390–396.
3. Cole, L. A., Ladner, D. G., Byrn, F. W. (2009). The normal variabilities of the menstrual cycle. *Fertility and Sterility, 91*, 522–527.
4. American College of Obstetricians and Gynecologists. (2009). Ultrasonography in pregnancy. ACOG Practice Bulletin No. 101. *Obstetrics & Gynecology, 113*, 451–461.
5. Jukic, A. M., Baird, D. D., Weinberg, C. R., et al. (2013). Length of human pregnancy and contributors to its natural variation. *Human Reproduction, 28*(10), 2848–2855.
6. King, T. L., Brucker, M. C., Kriebs, J. M., et al. (2014). *Varney's midwifery* (5th ed.). Burlington, MA: Jones & Bartlett Learning.
7. Hunter, L. (2009). Issues in pregnancy dating: Revisiting the evidence. *Journal of Midwifery & Women's Health, 54*, 184–190.
8. Cunningham, F., Leveno, K. J., Bloom, S. L., et al. (2010). Antepartum assessment. In Cunningham, F., Leveno, K. J., Bloom, S. L., et al. (Eds.), *Williams obstetrics* (23rd ed.). New York, NY: McGraw-Hill.
9. Gilbert, E. S. (2011). *High risk pregnancy & delivery* (5th ed.). St. Louis, MI: Mosby Elsevier.
10. O'Neill, E., Thorp, J. (2012). Antepartum evaluation of the fetus and fetal well being. *Clinical Obstetrics and Gynecology, 55*(3), 722–730.
11. Raynes-Greenow, C. H., Gordon, A., Li, Q., et al. (2013). A cross-sectional study of maternal perception of fetal movements and antenatal advice in a general pregnant population, using a qualitative framework. *BMC Pregnancy & Childbirth, 13*, 32, 8.
12. Mangesi, L., Hofmeyr, G. J. (2007). Fetal movement counting for assessment of fetal wellbeing. *Cochrane Database of Systematic Reviews, (1)*, CD004909.
13. Hijazi, Z. R., East, C. E. (2009). Factors affecting maternal perception of fetal movement. *Obstetrical and Gynecological Survey, 64*, 489–494.
14. Fox, N. S., Rebarber, A., Silverstein, M., et al. (2013). The effectiveness of antepartum surveillance in reducing the risk of stillbirth in patients with advanced maternal age. *European Journal of Obstetrics & Gynecology and Reproductive Biology, 170*(2), 387–390.
15. Izquierdo, L. A., Yonke, N. (2014). Fetal surveillance in late pregnancy and during labor. *Obstetrics and Gynecology Clinics, 41*(2), 307–315.
16. American College of Obstetricians and Gynecologists. (2014). Antepartum fetal surveillance. Practice bulletin no. 145. *Obstetrics & Gynecology, 124*(1), 182–192.
17. Voegtline, K. M., Costigan, K. A., Pater, H. A., et al. (2013). Near-term fetal response to maternal spoken voice. *Infant Behavior and Development, 36*(4), 526–533.
18. Engstrom, J. L., Sittler, C. P. (1993). Fundal height measurement. Part 1: Techniques for measuring fundal height. *Journal of Nurse-Midwifery, 38*(1), 5–16.
19. Engstrom, J. L., Sittler, C. P., Swift, K. E. (1994). Fundal height measurement. Part 5: The effect of clinician bias on fundal height measures. *Journal of Nurse-Midwifery, 39*(1), 130–141.

20. Kither, H., Whitworth, M. K. (2012). The implications of obesity on pregnancy. *Obstetrics, Gynaecology & Reproductive Medicine, 22*(12), 362–367.

21. American College of Obstetricians and Gynecologists. (2013). Gestational diabetes mellitus. Practice Bulletin No. 137. *Obstetrics & Gynecology, 122*(2 p 1), 417–422.

22. Horton, A., Diaz, J., Mastrogiannis, D. (2014). Accuracy of estimated fetal weight by ultrasonography compared with the Leopold maneuver and effect of maternal obesity. *Obstetrics and Gynecology, 123*(suppl 1), 193S.

23. Association of Women's Health, Obstetric and Neonatal Nursing. (2008). Fetal heart monitoring. https://www.awhonn.org/awhonn/content.do?name=07_PressRoom/07_PositionStatements.htm. Accessed August 4, 2014.

24. American College of Obstetricians and Gynecologists. (2007). Intrapartum fetal heart rate monitoring: Nomenclature, interpretation, and general management principles. *Obstetrics & Gynecology, 114*(1), 192–202.

25. American College of Nurse-Midwives. (2010). Intermittent auscultation for intrapartum fetal heart rate surveillance. *Journal of Midwifery & Women's Health, 55*(4), 397–403.

Caring for the Laboring Woman

FRANCES C. KELLY, SUSAN C. SWART,
AND SUZANNE McMURTRY BAIRD

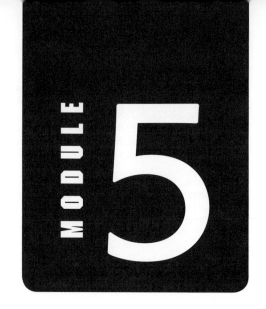

MODULE 5

Part 1
Intrapartum Nursing Care

Part 2
Patterns of Labor

Objectives

As you complete this module, you will learn:

1. Purpose and goals of intrapartum nursing care
2. Maternal and fetal assessments performed throughout first- and second-stage labor
3. Cultural influences on a woman's labor and birth experience
4. Incorporate cultural needs of the laboring woman
5. Expected patterns of labor for both nulliparous and multiparous women
6. How to differentiate expected from protracted or arrested labor progress through use of a partogram
7. Characteristics, causes, and interventions for abnormal labor progress
8. Characteristics, causes, and interventions for abnormal fetal descent
9. Physiologic care for woman in labor's second stage that optimizes progress and minimizes risk of maternal and fetal morbidity

Key Terms

When you have completed this module, you should be able to recall the meaning of the following terms. You should also be able to use the terms when consulting with other health professionals. The terms are defined in this module or in the glossary at the end of this book.

active-directed	labor down
active phase	latent phase
arrest of descent	lithotomy
arrest of dilation	molding
bloody show	multiparas
caput succedaneum	nulliparas
cephalopelvic disproportion	partogram
chorioamnionitis	physiologic care
engagement	primigravida
fetal station	second stage
first stage of labor	third stage
floating	

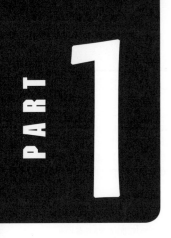

PART 1

Intrapartum Nursing Care

• What Is the Role of the Nurse during Labor and Birth?

Nurses are uniquely prepared to promote a safe and satisfying labor and birth experience, while partnering with perinatal healthcare providers to prevent the first cesarean birth or other complications.[1,2] The labor and delivery nurse is the nearly constant presence, who is likely to identify even subtle changes in the woman's or fetus' condition that require more intensive monitoring or intervention. By providing competent, caring, compassionate, and supportive care, the labor and delivery nurse can positively impact the outcomes of both the first and second stages of labor, which is essential to achieving safe passage for the mother and her newborn, and facilitating a positive birth experience.

The attributes of contemporary laboring women are different from those whom delivered five decades ago. Today, obstetric patients tend to be older, have a higher body mass index (BMI), and may experience one or more chronic illnesses.[3] Some of these women, who would otherwise not have survived to an age at which childbearing was feasible, are now getting pregnant. Many have chronic diseases such as diabetes mellitus or cystic fibrosis, or have surgically corrected heart defects with the associated long-term sequelae.[4]

The concepts that underpin this module are:
- labor and birth are natural processes;
- women do quite well if unnecessary interventions are avoided;
- the environment in which a woman labors and delivers should be supportive.[5,6]

***NOTE:** Labor practices such as non-medically indicated inductions of labor, admission to the hospital in false labor, and prematurely diagnosing arrest of cervical dilation or fetal descent may all contribute to an unplanned and potentially unnecessary cesarean birth.[6]*

• What Are the Goals of Intrapartum Nursing Care?

The goals of intrapartum nursing care include, and are not limited to, the following[1]:
- Promoting patient safety during labor and birth by performing thorough assessments and reassessments of maternal–fetal well-being, and speaking up to address any perceived safety concerns.[7]
- Understanding a laboring woman's expectations, and incorporating safe requests, and including her partner, significant other, or family.
- Advocating on her behalf.
- Educating laboring women and their partners or significant others about what to expect during labor and birth.
- Promoting physiologic labor and birth by implementing individualized interventions designed to promote effective coping and manage pain.
- Recognize and report complications, concerns, or changes in maternal or fetal condition.
- Organize the interprofessional team to achieve goals through effective coordination, communication, and collaboration.
- Promoting teamwork.

• What Are the Maternal and Fetal Assessments Completed during Labor and Birth?

Most pregnancies and the resultant labors and deliveries are low risk.[3] In order to achieve the goals of a safe and satisfying labor and birth experience, comprehensive assessments and

TABLE 5.1	MATERNAL VITAL SIGN PARAMETERS

VITAL SIGN	**NORMAL**	**CRITICAL THINKING**
Blood pressure (BP)	Systolic: 90–140 mm Hg Diastolic: 60–90 mm Hg	Increased BP may be related to unrelieved pain, fear, and/or anxiety. Increases may also be related to primary hypertension or the development of hypertensive disorders of pregnancy. Decreased BP may be related to hypotension, hypovolemia, or an infectious process.
Heart rate (HR)	60–100 beats per minute (bpm)	An increased heart rate may be associated with unrelieved pain, fear, and/or anxiety. Increases may also be associated with hypotension, hypovolemia, or administration of certain medications, such as betamimetics. Increased HR often precedes a rise in temperature.
Respiratory rate (RR)	12–20 breaths per minute	Increased RR may be related to unrelieved pain, fear, and/or anxiety. Increases may also be related to temperature >100.4°F/38°C, or complications such as pulmonary edema, pulmonary embolism, or amniotic fluid embolus (AFE). Decreases in RR may be related to certain medications, such as opioid analgesics or magnesium sulfate; or neuraxial anesthesia.
Oxygen saturation (SpO$_2$)	96% or greater	Decreases in SpO$_2$ may be related to chronic medical conditions, or complications such as pulmonary edema, pulmonary embolism, or AFE.
Temperature	Less than 100.4°F/38°C	Elevations in temperature may be sign of infection or medications (e.g., misoprostol). When membranes are ruptured, reassessments should occur at least every 2 hrs.

reassessments must be performed that include the physical, psychological, and sociocultural needs of the laboring woman. Module 3 provides a detailed review of the admission assessment of a laboring woman.

Maternal Vital Signs

Maternal vital signs are integral components of both admission and ongoing assessments during labor and birth. The results are compared to a woman's baseline or historical vital signs which are routinely documented in the prenatal record (if available). Obtain maternal vital signs regularly during labor and birth. It is important to interpret results within the context of the woman's history, her current status, and activities occurring during the labor and birth. Table 5.1 outlines individual components of maternal vital signs, expected findings, potential explanation of abnormal findings, and suggested nursing actions.

General Nursing Actions When Obtaining Vital Signs during Labor

- Avoid obtaining vital signs during uterine contractions.
- Be alert to any abnormal findings and consider possible causes. Is this an acute or chronic change? Is the change related to a procedure or medication administration?
- Do not assume an increase in BP, HR, or RR is due only to unrelieved pain, fear, or anxiety.
- Take action, such as assessing for obvious cause(s); discontinue any medication or therapy that may be related to the deviation; re-position the woman; or administer oxygen or intravenous fluids (according to provider and facility reviewed and approved orders and/or protocols).
- Repeat assessments if findings remain abnormal and alert the provider.
- Provide information, support, and feedback to the woman to decrease fear and anxiety, and increase feelings of control regarding assessments and actions.
- Document abnormal findings and assessments.

Cervical Examination

While a cervical examination provides important information, it is an invasive procedure for many if not all women. Performing a cervical examination requires a skillful, yet sensitive approach. The manner in which the caregiver approaches and conducts the examination must be respectful and patient-centered. The technical aspects of performing a cervical examination are outlined in Module 3.

When performing a cervical examination, the caregiver should review the maternal history for the following information:

- Gestational age, gravidity, and parity
- Presence or suspicion of placenta previa in current pregnancy
- Report or suspicion of ruptured membranes
- Report of vaginal bleeding or spotting
- Results of previous cervical examination, if applicable
- History of the present labor
  - when contractions began
  - contraction frequency and duration
  - when contractions became regular
- Fetal history (e.g., antenatal testing results, congenital or genetic abnormality)

There are several considerations in performing a sensitive cervical examination, including:

- Ask the woman's permission to perform the examination.
- Ensure privacy and draping prior to exam and consider the optimal position for you and the woman (experience in performing examinations while women are in alternative positions such as squatting or side-lying may optimize her tolerance of the examination).
- Establish an organized approach to performing a cervical examination.
- If possible, perform the examination between contractions.
- Use lubricant sparingly. Too much lubrication makes the area around the perineum wet and cold (if assessing for evidence of ruptured membranes by using pH paper or obtaining cultures, do so before using lubricants which may interfere with results).

The woman may have varying responses to cervical examination. Potential reactions to an exam may include the following:

- Inability to relax during the examination
- Tightening of vaginal muscles
- Body language that suggests fear and/or anxiety such as covering the eyes
- Crying

During the exam, visually inspect the perineum for evidence of:

- Amniotic fluid
- Bloody show
- Active bleeding
- Skin lesions

Perform cervical exam and note:

- Dilation from 0 cm (closed) to 10 cm (complete)
- Effacement from 0% (thick) to 100% (complete)
- Position (anterior, midline, posterior)
- Consistency (firm, soft)

Assess fetal membrane status:

- Intact
- Ruptured (color, odor, amount)

Assess presenting part:

- Degree of flexion
- Fetal station or degree of descent (−3 to +3 or −5 to +5 scale), where 0 is equal to the ischial spines
- Presence of molding of fetal cranial bones
- Presence of caput succedaneum (edema of fetal scalp)

NOTE: *There is no evidence to support or reject that routine cervical examinations in labor improve outcomes for women and/or newborns.[8] However, prudent judgment should be used when choosing to perform a cervical examination taking into consideration the woman's comfort, the indication for the procedure, and status of membranes. Indications to perform a cervical exam may include changes in fetal status (rupture of fetal membranes with fetal heart rate [FHR] decelerations), increase in bloody show (indicating possible cervical change), or evidence that the woman is making progress (e.g., spontaneous bearing-down efforts or urge to push).*

Fetal Heart Rate Assessment

The goals of monitoring the FHR during labor include establishing evidence of fetal well-being, and being able to detect signs of potential fetal compromise so that appropriate interventions may be initiated in a timely manner. Completing Module 7 will assist the labor and delivery nurse to differentiate normal from abnormal FHR tracings, as well as those tracings that require additional evaluation and/or intrauterine fetal resuscitation.[9,10]

During labor, assessment of the FHR may be accomplished by one of the following methods:
1. Intermittent auscultation with a stethoscope or a Doppler ultrasound device
2. Continuous electronic fetal monitoring

Although the early proponents of continuous electronic FHR monitoring asserted that using this monitoring method during labor would reduce the rate of cesarean births and may improve various birth outcomes, these assertions have not been supported in numerous published studies.[11] A recent Cochrane review, which included four studies representing more than 13,000 women, reported that while not statistically significant, the group of women assigned to receive continuous FHR tracing assessment an admission in labor was more likely to be delivered by cesarean, as opposed to those women who received intermittent FHR auscultation.[12] There is little evidence that continuous electronic FHR monitoring among **low-risk** laboring women is beneficial, and may potentially increase harm.

Both observation and technical skills are used to identify changes in maternal–fetal status; and fetal presentation, position, and descent. These skills, together with experience in FHR monitoring techniques, provide the caregiver with the ability to monitor maternal and fetal well-being. The laboring woman's risk status and birth plan should guide the care team in choosing the method of FHR monitoring. Regardless of the method chosen to assess for fetal well-being during labor, labor and delivery nurses must demonstrate current clinical knowledge and the ability to accurately interpret the findings. Because effective performance of intermittent auscultation of the FHR requires more hands-on time of the labor nurse, it requires one-to-one nursing care for the laboring woman.[13,14] Circumstances such as nurse staffing, as well as provider or patient preference, influence the method selected.

Uterine Activity

Assessing and reassessing uterine activity is an important aspect providing nursing care in the laboring woman. As labor progresses from early to active, uterine contraction frequency, strength, and duration increases due to release of prostaglandins and endogenous oxytocin.[15]

> • **What Is the Recommended Frequency of FHR and Uterine Activity Assessments during Labor and Birth?**

If, on admission the mother is in early labor, not receiving oxytocin, and has a Category I FHR pattern, fetal and uterine evaluation may be carried out less frequently than every 30 minutes, but should be done at least hourly. When active labor begins, evaluation intervals of 15 to 30 minutes are appropriate, depending on risk status. Many providers prefer a baseline strip with electronic FHR monitoring; however, there is no research to suggest a difference in outcome when this strategy is used. Table 5.2 summarizes frequency of assessment recommendations.

NOTE: If the woman or fetus has assessment parameters outside defined norms, assessments should increase until stabilization.

NOTE: When using electronic uterine and fetal monitoring, always palpate uterine contractions and auscultate maternal and fetal heart rates in the first few minutes of using the equipment and periodically throughout labor. This validates that the equipment is working properly.

TABLE 5.2 FREQUENCY OF UTERINE ACTIVITY ASSESSMENT[16]

	LOW RISK	**HIGH RISK**
Early labor	Every hour	Every 30 min
Active labor	Every 30 min	Every 15 min
Second-stage labor	Every 15 min	Every 5 min

From American Academy of Pediatrics and American Colleges of Obstetricians and Gynecologists. (2012). *Guidelines for perinatal care* (7th ed.). Elk Grove Village, IL: AAP.

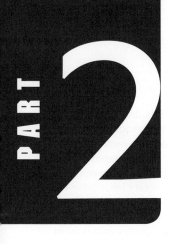

PART 2

Patterns of Labor

Early research conducted by Friedman to determine expected labor progress among "normal" nulliparous and multiparous women during the first stage of labor, found that cervical dilation progressed on average 1.2 and 1.5 cm per hour, respectively.[17] These rates of progress have served as benchmarks against which labor progress is evaluated, and care decisions made for countless numbers of laboring women since that time, even though these research findings were based on 100 "normal labors" that included women with multiple gestations and fetal malpresentations. In order to effectively promote physiologic labor and birth, an understanding of labor patterns of contemporary nulliparous and multiparous women is necessary.

- **What Are the General Characteristics and Patterns of the First Stage of Labor among Contemporary Laboring Women?**

The knowledge gleaned from the work of the Consortium on Safe Labor (CSL) study has informed perinatal healthcare providers about the characteristics of labor among contemporary women.[18] The purpose of the study was to identify labor curves according to parity. Based on these data, new definitions and criteria for labor management have been described.

Stage I labor is separated into two phases.
- The **early phase** (preparatory phase) extends from the onset of regular contractions that cause cervical change to the beginning of the active phase, when dilation occurs more rapidly. It usually extends over hours and appears as a nearly flat line on the labor curve.
- The **active phase** (dilational phase) of labor begins when the laboring woman reaches 6 cm of dilation, and ends when the cervix is 10 cm or completely dilated. Effective labor begins with the active phase.

Data included in the National Collaborative Perinatal Project (CPP) indicates that contemporary laboring women tend to[19]:
- be older;
- have a higher BMI;
- reach a maximum slope of cervical dilation not beginning until the laboring woman reaches 6 cms (as opposed to 4 cm as previously believed);
- have a slower than traditionally believed rate of dilation during the active phase of labor;
- have a longer first stage of labor even after accounting for maternal and pregnancy characteristics, by a median 2.6 and 2.0 hours in nulliparas and multiparas, respectively.

In another study of spontaneously laboring women with a single, vertex fetus and who experienced a vaginal birth with a normal newborn outcome, several key labor characteristics were described[18]:
- It may take more than 6 hours to progress from 4 to 5 cm of dilation.
- It may take more than 3 hours to progress from 5 to 6 cm of dilation.
- Before 6 cm, both nulliparous and multiparous laboring women progress at approximately the same rate (Fig. 5.1).
- After 6 cm, labor progress accelerates at a faster pace among multiparous laboring women (Fig. 5.1).
- Figure 5.2 depicts the 95th percentile for the cumulative duration of labor when admitted at various dilations. This partogram may serve as a useful guide to help identify when a nulliparous woman might be experiencing protracted labor.
- The 95th percentiles for the second stage of labor for nulliparous laboring women with and without a neuraxial anesthetic were 3.6 and 2.8 hours, respectively.

• How Should the Nurse Assess for Labor Progress?

Recall that contemporary laboring women tend to be older, have higher BMIs, and may have one or more comorbid conditions.[18] Along with these changes in their physical characteristics, contemporary laboring women tend to have their labors induced more often, undergo more obstetric-related interventions, and request neuraxial analgesia and anesthesia for pain management. As previously described in this module, the combination of the changes in physical characteristics coupled with more frequent obstetric interventions has altered the contemporary labor curve for both nulliparous and multiparous women (Fig. 5.1). Applying this knowledge to assess labor progress among contemporary laboring women is an essential competency of a labor nurse.

Plotting cervical dilation and fetal station on a graph in nulliparous and multiparous women has provided a norm for assessing and evaluating the adequacy of labor progress for many years. A partogram (sometimes referred to as a partograph) is a graphic illustration of labor progress, and was used originally in developing countries to identify women experiencing a deviation from expected progress. The partograph recommended by the World Health Organization

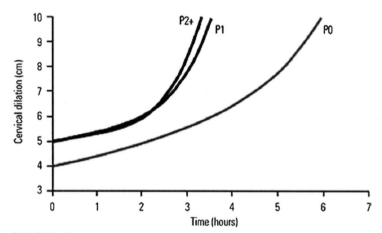

FIGURE 5.1 Labor curves by parity in singleton, term pregnancies with spontaneous onset of labor, vaginal delivery, and normal neonatal outcomes. (From Zhang, J., Landy, H. J., Branch, D. W., et al., for the Consortium on Safe Labor. (2010). Contemporary patterns of spontaneous labor with normal neonatal outcomes. *Obstetrics & Gynecology, 116*(6), 1281–1287.)

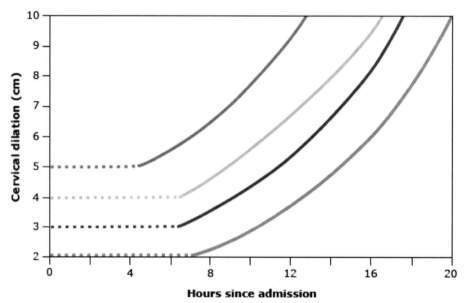

FIGURE 5.2 Contemporary estimates of labor duration by dilation at admission. (From Zhang, J., Landy, H. J., Branch, D. W., et al., for the Consortium on Safe Labor. (2010). Contemporary patterns of spontaneous labor with normal neonatal outcomes. *Obstetrics & Gynecology, 116*(6), 1281–1287.)

(WHO) is composed of alert and action lines (Fig. 5.3).[20] By plotting dilation, the alert line helped to identify progress that occurred slower than 1 cm an hour once a patient reached 4 cm. The action line, sequenced 4 hours to the right of an alert line, triggered notification of care providers, and facilitated a transfer from outlying birthing centers and hospitals to higher levels of care where a physician was available to perform a cesarean birth. Although available evidence varies, plotting labor progress on a partogram may reduce the risk of prolonged or obstructed labor and prevent a cesarean birth.[18,21]

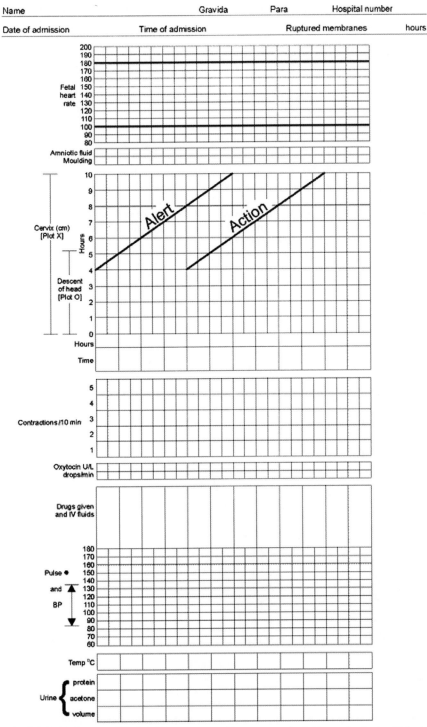

FIGURE 5.3 Modified WHO partogram. (From www.who.int/reproductivehealth/publications/maternal_perinatal_health/3_9241546662/en/)

• How Is the Descent of the Fetus Described and Assessed?

The degree of descent of the fetus through the maternal pelvis is determined by evaluating the fetal station. Fetal station may be assessed by palpating the gravid abdomen (Leopold's) or by performing a cervical examination, and described as the relationship of the presenting part of the fetus to an imaginary line drawn between the ischial spines of the maternal pelvis.

Fetal station is described utilizing either a −3 to +3, or a −5 to +5 scale. Each number represents the distance in centimeters of the fetal presenting part either above or below the maternal ischial spines (Figs. 5.4 and 5.7). The long axis of the birth canal is divided into thirds. The ischial spines are approximately halfway between the pelvic inlet and the pelvic outlet.

NOTE: *It is important that the same scale be understood and used consistently by all nursing and medical providers within the labor and delivery unit. For purposes of this module, the authors will use the −3 to +3 station scale.*

The following describes levels of fetal descent:
- If the presenting part is above the spines and at the level of the pelvic inlet, it is said to be at −3 station if using the −3 to +3 station range.
- ***Floating or Ballotable***—when the presenting part is entirely out of the pelvis and can be moved by the examiner abdominally just above the symphysis pubis bone or on cervical exam the fetal presenting part floats out of the pelvis (Fig. 5.5).
- If the fetal presenting part has descended one third the distance past the inlet, it is at −1 station.
- When the presenting fetal part (e.g., the head) is at the level of the ischial spines, the fetal station is 0 (the largest diameter of the fetal head enters into the smallest diameter of the maternal pelvis). This is fetal ***engagement*** (Fig. 5.6).

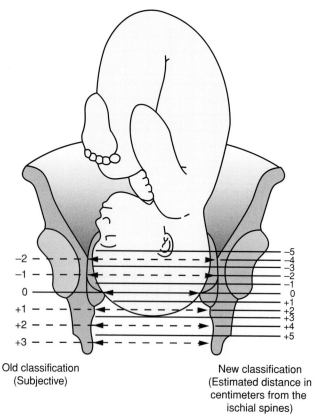

Old classification
(Subjective)

New classification
(Estimated distance in
centimeters from the
ischial spines)

FIGURE 5.4   Fetal station. (From Kilpatrick, S. & Garrison, E. [2012]. Normal labor. In Gabbe, S. G. Niebyl, J. R. Simpson, J. L. [Eds.], Obstetrics: Normal and problem pregnancies [5th ed., pp. 2267–286]. Philadelphia, PA: Elsevier Saunders.)

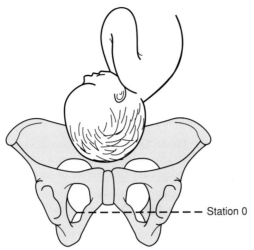

FIGURE 5.5   Floating. Fetal head is entirely out of the pelvis.

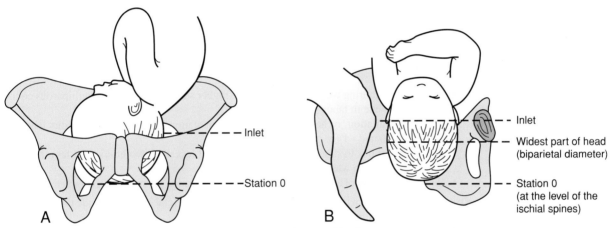

FIGURE 5.6   Engaged presenting fetal head. **A.** Front view. **B.** Side view.

- A similar division is assigned to the distances between the ischial spines and the pelvic outlet. If the level of the presenting part is one third or two thirds the distance between the spines and the outlet, it is said to be +1 or +2 station, respectively.
- When the presenting fetal part descends to the bony outlet, it is resting on the muscles of the vaginal opening and is at +3 station (Fig. 5.7).

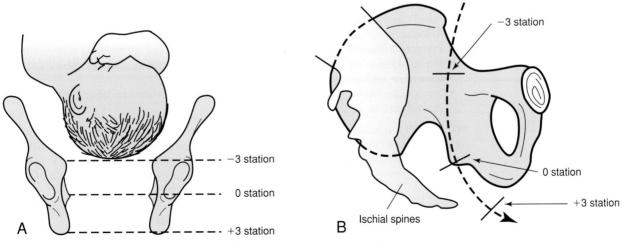

FIGURE 5.7   **A.** Descent of the presenting fetal part to station −3. Front view using a scale of −3 to +3. **B.** Descent pathway, side view.

- Sometimes the fetal scalp becomes edematous with the pressure of labor. This can be felt as a soft, swollen layer over the hard bony surface of the skull and is called caput succedaneum. Also, it is possible for molding of the fetal skull to occur, which can distort the examiner's evaluation of the fetal head descent.
- If the fetal head is severely molded, there is considerable caput succedaneum, or both, engagement might not have taken place even though the tip of the presenting part is at a 0 station.

NOTE: The presence of caput or molding is not an unusual finding in labor and is not an indication that the fetus will not descend.

For women pregnant for the first time (*primigravidas*), engagement usually occurs approximately 2 to 3 weeks before labor begins. For women who have had more than one pregnancy (*multiparas*), engagement occurs any time before or during labor.

Assessing and Promoting Fetal Descent

Assessing fetal descent is an important criteria to consider when evaluating the overall labor progress.[6] Similar to changes in patterns of cervical dilation among contemporary laboring women, there have also been changes in patterns of descent. In a study of more than 4,500 laboring women with term, singleton gestations, all of whom delivered vaginally, contemporary patterns of descent were identified using the −3 to +3 scale, including the following:[22]
- Faster descent can be expected among women in spontaneous labor as compared with those in whom labor is being augmented or induced.
- Multiparous laboring women experienced faster descent at all stations except at stations +2 to +3.
- Multiparous laboring women tended to have higher stations compared to nulliparous counterparts until late in labor's first stage.
- By 6 cm of dilation, or active labor, the median station for 95% of nulliparous laboring women was 0 and −1 for multiparous women.
- The median times to descend one station were all less than two hours, and less than one hour once 0 station was achieved.
- Ninety-five percent of all laboring women achieved 0 station or lower when completely dilated.

Risk factors associated with potential deviations in expected fetal descent include the following:
- Protracted dilation in the active phase
- Cephalopelvic disproportion (CPD) (a medical diagnosis made by the obstetric provider)
- Minor fetal malpositions, such as occiput posterior or mild asynclitic positions
- Neuraxial analgesia/anesthesia

NOTE: Cervical examination for assessment of descent must carefully distinguish between true descent and the occurrence of fetal scalp edema or molding of the cranial bones. If there is any question, the obstetric provider should come to the bedside and perform an assessment to determine the plan of care.

Nursing interventions which may promote physiologic fetal descent may include the following:
- Avoid factors which may delay or arrest descent (e.g., full bladder, position)
- Ambulation
- Position or frequent repositioning to maintain alignment and optimize the pelvic outlet
- Titrate oxytocin infusion (as ordered per provider) to facilitate adequate uterine contractions while maintaining uteroplacental perfusion.
- Provided the woman and fetus are tolerating labor well, advocate for labor to continue with vaginal birth as the goal

NOTE: CPD is a medical diagnosis and is not made by the labor nurse. The nurse's responsibility is to do a labor assessment and communicate progress with the obstetric provider. If the provider has a concern regarding labor progress, the provider should do an assessment to make a diagnosis, discuss options with the woman and labor nurse, and develop a plan of care.

• How Does the Nurse Assess for Deviations in Labor Progress?

Cervical dilation can progress too slowly (**protracted**) or stop completely (**arrest**).[23] Deviations from expected patterns of cervical dilation and fetal descent may occur in both the early and active phases of labor, as well as during labor's second stage. As previously described, the earlier a laboring woman is admitted to the hospital, the longer it may take to dilate between each successive centimeter (refer to Fig. 5.2). For example, 95% of women admitted to the hospital at 2 cm will take approximately 7 hours to progress to 3 cm. In contrast, 95% of women admitted at 5 cm will progress to 6 cm in approximately 4 ½ hours. Instead of using the mean duration of time to assess progress from 1 cm to the next, contemporary partograms use the more realistic 95th percentiles to help identify abnormal (protracted) or arrested dilation.[18] The 95th percentile in the contemporary partogram is equivalent to the action lines in traditional partograms, and are stair-like rather than straight lines because cervical dilation is not generally recorded as a continuous measure.[18] The contemporary partogram also does not have alert lines since most women in the United States give birth in a hospital setting.

Multiple factors should be considered when assessing labor progress, such as maternal BMI;[24] the phase and stage of labor; maternal position; maternal fear, anxiety and ability to cope; adequacy of uterine contractions; fetal size and position; the use of neuraxial analgesia/anesthesia; and the presence of an intrauterine infection. The following sections will describe how to assess for and identify these deviations, their risk factors, and the labor nurse's role in intervening and improving the odds of resolving them and promoting a vaginal birth. It is important to refrain from using these norms as rigid criteria for judging the adequacy of progress in every woman.

The diagnosis of protraction in the active phase is based on a deviation from the 95th percentile of the contemporary partograph. The United States National Institute of Child Health and Human Development (NICHD), Society of Maternal–Fetal Medicine (SMFM), and the American College of Obstetricians and Gynecologists (ACOG) have defined **arrest of cervical dilation** as a laboring woman who reaches 6 cm with ruptured membranes and has one of the following:[21]
- No cervical change for ≥4 hours despite adequate contractions (>200 Montevideo Units [MVUs])
- No cervical change for ≥6 hours with inadequate contractions.

Risk factors associated with protraction and arrest of labor in the active phase include the following:
- Hypocontractile uterine activity
- CPD
- Occiput posterior (OP) position
- Maternal obesity[23]
- Infection within the uterine cavity

NOTE: *The diagnosis of protracted or arrest of labor/descent is a medical diagnosis. The nurse's responsibility is to assess and notify the obstetric provider of the assessment findings.*

Nursing interventions to promote physiologic labor progress include, but may not be limited to the following:[25]
- Advocate for the woman in early labor by discouraging admission prior to cervical change in triage areas where nurses have primary responsibility for key clinical decisions, primary care, and communication to providers who are often offsite.[26]
- Provide continuous labor support.[1]
- Educate the laboring woman and her support person(s) about what to expect and set realistic expectations of progress,[1] explaining that progress will likely be slow but steady.
- Ensure adequate fluid and electrolyte intake, including oral if at low risk of complications.[27]
- Consider ambulation and upright positions as tolerated and appropriate for risk and maternal/fetal status or presence of complications.[28]
- Exhibit and model patience.
- Implement nursing interventions to manage pain and discomfort.
- Avoid routine or frequent cervical examinations, which may increase the risk of intrauterine infection.[8,29]
- Monitor for signs or symptoms of intrauterine infection such as maternal fever, maternal or fetal tachycardia, or complaint of abdominal pain or tenderness.

• What Is the Impact of Induction or Augmentation on the Labor Pattern and Mode of Delivery?

The percent of women who undergo induction of labor has increased over 100% since 1990.[30] According to a cohort of 208,695 electronic medical records from the CSL study,[18] 42.9% of nulliparas and 31.8% of multiparas underwent induction of labor.[19] Inducing or augmenting labor, with or without a medical indication, has the potential to impact both the length of labor and the mode of birth. In another study of over 5,388 women, the length of labor as well as the time it took to dilate each progressive centimeter, up until 6 cm, was longer among nulliparas and multiparas who underwent induction or augmentation, as compared to those whose labors were not induced or augmented.[31] For all indications, cesarean birth occurred more frequently among induced nulliparous women in the latent phase of labor, especially among those with complicated pregnancies.[19]

• What Is the Impact of Neuraxial Analgesia/Anesthesia on Labor Patterns?

Perinatal care providers have questioned if neuraxial analgesia/anesthesia (epidural, spinal, or combined spinal–epidural) impacted the length of labor or mode of birth.[32]

Similar to previously published data, the length of second-stage labor was at least 2 hours longer for both nulliparous and multiparous women who had neuraxial anesthesia/analgesia as compared to those who did not.[33] Several studies have shown there were no differences in rates of cesarean birth among women who received neuraxial analgesia/analgesia compared with those who did not.[34–36]

• How Does Maternal Positioning Affect Labor Progress?

Many, if not most, contemporary pregnant women receive labor and delivery care from a bed in a healthcare facility with potentially limited opportunities to move and ambulate. Low-risk laboring women should be encouraged to change positions based on their comfort.[37]

NOTE: Laboring women who are encouraged and allowed to assume upright positions and ambulate tend to experience:[28]
- *shorter labors;*
- *fewer neuraxial analgesia/anesthesia;*
- *fewer cesarean births;*
- *fewer admissions of their newborns to neonatal intensive care (NICU).*

Nurses are key members of the interprofessional team, influencing and advocating for positions that optimize labor progress and physiologic birth. Educating the low-risk laboring woman about the benefits of upright positions, ambulation, and encouraging her to assume a position that affords her the greatest comfort while considering her safety and needs for fetal monitoring are key.[28] When she is in bed, promote upright or lateral position. When a laboring woman assumes a lateral position, remember to facilitate alignment of hips. Proper alignment helps reduce pain and promote progress. Pillows or other aids (e.g., **Peanut ball**) may assist with optimal positioning of hips and avoidance of increased pressure on the vena cava. These actions help to optimize circulation to her heart, lungs, uterus, and placenta, and decrease her potential for developing supine hypotension (refer to Module 6 for further information on maternal positioning for labor).[38]

• Does Amniotomy Improve Labor Progress?

Performing an amniotomy has long been a traditional labor practice, the efficacy of which has rarely been questioned or supported by consistent published evidence.[39] The practice of amniotomy as an isolated intervention should be evaluated. While the results of published studies are mixed, one study demonstrated that intervening with amniotomy and administration of oxytocin resulted in a modest reduction in the rate of cesarean birth as compared to standard labor care.[40]

NOTE: Performing an amniotomy is outside the scope of nursing practice. Nurses should collaborate with providers about this practice when it is a part of a comprehensive management plan, the indications are clear, the woman's desires for labor have been considered, informed consent has been given and the plan agreed on, and risk status evaluated.

• How Does an Intrauterine Infection Affect Labor Progress?

There is some evidence that intrauterine infection inhibits effective uterine activity.[6] Although there has not been a causative link between chorioamnionitis and cesarean birth established, ineffective uterine activity may contribute to the diagnosis of dysfunctional labor. In addition, there is an increase in the utilization of oxytocin administration. The nurse's role includes the following:

* Prevention with limiting cervical exams with ruptured fetal membranes.
* Monitoring for signs and symptoms of infection which may include the following:
  * FHR tachycardia (may appear prior to an elevation in maternal temperature)
  * Maternal fever (≥100.4°F or 38°C)
  * Abdominal tenderness
  * Malodorous amniotic fluid
  * Maternal tachycardia

NOTE: *The diagnosis or suspicion of intra-amniotic infection in isolation and in the absence of other obstetric indications does not support the plan for cesarean birth.*

• How Does Maternal Obesity Affect Labor Progress?

The higher the woman's BMI, the longer it tends to take to progress from 1 cm to the next, even when accounting for induction of labor and gestational age.[23] In addition, laboring women with a BMI ≥40 take longer to reach 6-cm dilation as compared to women with a BMI of <25.[23] There is evidence that obese women are at higher risk for cesarean birth and other adverse outcomes. Therefore, BMI should be considered when evaluating the overall progress of labor and prior to a diagnosis of protraction or arrest of labor.[6,41] For a more in-depth discussion on obesity in pregnancy, refer to Module 14.

• How Does Hydration Affect Labor Progress?

If a laboring woman is restricted from oral intake, intravenous (IV) fluids are indicated to ensure adequate hydration and meet increased energy needs. Traditionally, 125 mL/hr of crystalloid fluid has been infused. However, this volume may be insufficient to meet the needs of laboring women and the resulting dehydration may negatively impact labor progress. Infusing 250 mL/hr may be more appropriate to maintain hydration, while taking care not to over hydrate.[42]

The components of IV solutions should also be considered. While somewhat controversial, IV solutions containing 5% dextrose in a balanced salt solution may help support energy needs as well as ensure hydration.[42] Uterine contractions require glucose for energy. Labor may deplete glucose stores resulting in lipolysis and ketone production, which may decrease fetal pH and impede optimal myometrial contractility.[43] To prevent maternal and fetal hyperglycemia and untoward impact, dextrose-containing IV fluids should not be bolused for neuraxial anesthesia/analgesia or with intrauterine resuscitation. Calculating intake and output is an important aspect of intrapartum nursing care.

Second Stage of Labor

The second stage of labor begins when the woman is completely dilated until the birth of the fetus. The second stage of labor may be characterized by numerous physical and emotional changes in the laboring woman. These changes may include the following:

* Increase in frequency and intensity of uterine contractions
* Increase in bloody show
* Complaining of perineal or rectal pressure
* Involuntary pushing with contractions
* Flattening of the perineum
* Bulging of rectum
* Uncontrolled shivering
* Nausea and vomiting
* Expressions of feeling out of control or an inability to copy
* Increased verbalizations or possibly crying out

• When Should a Laboring Woman Begin to Push?

The urge to push may not coincide exactly with reaching complete cervical dilation. Some women experience an involuntary urge to push prior to being completely dilated, while others may not experience this urge until sometime later. The urge to push is thought to be influenced more by the fetal station than by cervical dilation. When the woman's pelvic floor is distended by the descending and rotating fetal presenting part, stretch receptors are activated in the posterior vagina, which result in the release of endogenous oxytocin, resulting in the urge to push or bear down. This is called the "Ferguson reflex."

There is no clear evidence about the frequency that laboring women experience an urge to push before complete cervical dilation is achieved. There is also no clear plan to manage this in practice, though several recommendations have been suggested as potentially beneficial.[44] The recommendations that have been suggested include the following:

- Coaching the laboring woman to breathe through contractions with frequent, shallow breaths
- Changing positions (e.g., side-lying, hands and knees)
- Encourage and support the woman's vocalizations during the urge to push
- Considering use of water or bath (remember that the frequency of risk-based reassessments should be maintained)

"Laboring down" is a concept and clinical practice that promotes maternal rest once complete cervical dilation is achieved, when the laboring woman may feel no pelvic pressure or an urge to begin pushing. Instead of actively directing the woman to begin pushing immediately upon reaching 10 cm, she is encouraged to rest, allowing uterine contractions to facilitate further descent and rotation of the fetal presenting part. This period of rest or laboring down may continue until the urge to push is perceived by the woman, at which time spontaneous pushing should commence. Spontaneous maternal bearing-down efforts are found to be more effective and satisfying, resulting in less maternal fatigue.

Guidelines to Promote Physiologic Birth and Minimize Maternal–Fetal Complications[1]

- Provide 1:1 nursing care (one labor nurse to one laboring women).
- The woman in active and second-stage labor should not be left alone.
- Review and anticipate risks.
- Continue to support the woman's birth wishes, incorporating safe requests and preferences into the plan of care.
- If the woman is completely dilated and does not feel an urge to push, let her rest comfortably in a position that will facilitate fetal descent (e.g., side-lying). When no urge to push occurs after a rest period, the mother can be encouraged to move into an upright position in bed or sitting position. Use of a squat bar may also be useful for support during pushing efforts.
- Assess and respond to cues from the woman suggesting complete dilation and readiness to push. Suggestions like "push when you feel the urge" help women to begin stage II with minimal coaching.
- Avoid prolonged breath holding and bearing-down efforts (closed glottis) to decrease the likelihood of decreased fetal oxygen saturation. Studies show that when laboring women are supported to rely on their own bodies and are allowed and encouraged to push spontaneously and without rigid and active-directed coaching from the labor nurse or obstetric provider, they tend to push for less than 6 seconds, often taking several breaths between pushes and exhaling or releasing air while pushing (open glottis).[45,46]
- Position the woman to promote comfort and facilitate descent and rotation of the fetal presenting part. Positions that optimize the force of gravity may increase the pelvic diameter by as much as 30%, facilitating fetal descent and rotation, resulting in decreased use of vacuum and forceps, and possibly shortening the overall length of the second stage. Additionally, optimal positioning may minimize painful sensations, decrease the incidence of perineal trauma, and enhance maternal satisfaction with the birth experience.[28]

NOTE: *When the fetal position is posterior, it may be useful to position a mother in alternate positions, such as on hands and knees, to facilitate rotation. By doing so, she can do pelvic rocks during the contraction to provide additional pressure on the heaviest presenting part (the head) to rotate. Other positions such as the lateral position, squatting, or sitting may also assist with rotation. An exaggerated side-lying position may assist with rotation of the presenting part for mothers with regional anesthesia.*

- Continue to monitor and assess maternal vital signs, FHR, and uterine activity according to risk status.
- Maintain adequate hydration.
- Provide pericare, which remains an important comfort and hygiene measure.
- Warm compresses and perineal massage may decrease the potential for the third- and fourth-degree perineal lacerations.[47] However, warm compresses should not be placed on women with neuraxial anesthesia/analgesia.
- When neuraxial anesthesia/anesthesia is used, the urge to bear down can diminish. More active coaching may be needed.

NOTE: Using a mirror to view the perineum and encouraging the mother to touch the fetal head when it is visible at the perineum may promote effective pushing.

- Keep the woman and her support person(s) informed.
- Let her know when she is being effective in her efforts.
- Use terminology that she can understand (e.g., not all women understand "station +1").
- Avoid negative statements (e.g., "That baby's head is way up there!").
- Inform the mother when you are going to perform an examination and why.
- Maintain a calming, supportive environment (e.g., lighting, noise, temperature, room traffic).
- Be patient. Recall the impact of BMI, the presence of neuraxial anesthesia/analgesia, fatigue, and pain/discomfort.

• How Does the Nurse Assess for Progress in the Second Stage of Labor?

A number of factors should be considered when assessing the adequacy of maternal expulsive efforts during the second stage of labor. Such factors may include and are not necessarily limited to the woman's parity, BMI, emotional state and adequacy of support, fatigue, the presence of neuraxial anesthesia/analgesia, as well as fetal size, position, and in some cases, presentation. Progress in labor's second stage is primarily determined by noting rotation and/or descent of the fetal presenting part. Second stage arrest is a medical diagnosis made by the obstetric provider. The role of the labor nurse is to provide evidence-based physiologic support, and assist in identifying potential deviations as described by the time frames included in Table 5.3.[6,33]

TABLE 5.3	PROGRESS IN THE SECOND STAGE OF LABOR	
	WITH NEURAXIAL ANESTHESIA/ ANALGESIA	**WITHOUT NEURAXIAL ANESTHESIA/ANALGESIA**
Nulliparous	No progress after 4 or more hours	No progress after 3 or more hours
Multiparous	No progress after 3 or more hours	No progress after 2 hrs

From Spong, C. Y., Berghella, V., Wenstrom, K. D., et al. (2012). Preventing the first cesarean delivery: Summary of a Joint Eunice Kennedy Shriver National Institute of Child Health and Human Development, Society for Maternal–Fetal Medicine, and American College of Obstetricians and Gynecologists Workshop. *Obstetrics & Gynecology, 120*(5), 1181–1193; Cheng, Y. W., Shaffer, B. L., Nicholson, J. M., et al. (2014). Second stage of labor and epidural use: A larger effect than previously suggested. *Obstetrics & Gynecology, 123*(3), 527–535.

NOTE: As long as progress is being made, and signs of maternal and fetal well-being are present and reassuring, no absolutely rigid time limits or arbitrary rules related to the duration of the second stage are necessary.[6] Evidence supports the demonstration of patience and the practice of laboring down for women when there are no indications to expedite birth.

• What Should the Nurse Do to Prepare for Birth?

There are numerous processes and operations for the nurse to initiate in preparation for birth. Depending on how role delegation and tasks are assigned, the nurse may be responsible for the following:
- Setting up delivery table
- Checking neonatal resuscitation equipment
- Turning on neonatal warmer
- Maternal positioning
- Notification of appropriate team members
- Gathering appropriate medication and equipment

TABLE 5.4	EXAMPLE TRIGGERS
Maternal	Emergent maternal condition (e.g., hemorrhage, cardiac arrest)
	Abnormal placentation
	Suspected abruption
	Maternal fever >100.4°F from a suspected infectious etiology
	Prolapsed cord
	Operative vaginal birth
	Medications that may affect infant (e.g., magnesium sulfate, general anesthesia, insulin)
	Shoulder dystocia
	Emergent delivery outside of normal delivery areas
	Emergent cesarean birth
	Vaginal breech delivery
Fetal	Gestational age <36 wks
	Congenital anomalies with anticipated intervention at birth (respectful of birth plans), including, but not limited to:
	• congenital diaphragmatic hernia
	• congenital cardiac disease
	• other antenatal diagnoses requiring multidisciplinary care (e.g., omphalocele, gastroschisis, neural tube defects)
	Meconium-stained amniotic fluid with Category II/III FHR tracing
	Multiple gestation
	Intrauterine growth restriction (IUGR)
	Category III FHR tracing immediately prior to birth
	Consider calling for the following Category II conditions immediately prior to birth:
	• Bradycardia
	• Tachycardia
	• Absent baseline variability without recurrent decelerations
	• Recurrent variable decelerations with minimal baseline variability
	• Recurrent late decelerations with minimal baseline variability
	• Prolonged decelerations

In addition, approximately 8% of all labors are associated with an adverse neonatal outcome.[48] These adverse outcomes and obstetrical emergencies may increase the risk for neonatal morbidity and mortality.[16] Anticipating when a neonate may require resuscitation beyond that which is routinely provided is an important element of communication. Proactively calling the neonatal response team prior to birth during which they might be needed allows the neonatal response team members to proceed immediately to the delivery location, receive critically important information about either the maternal or fetal status, and prepare for resuscitation without being rushed. Anyone on the healthcare team, patient or family member, can request the neonatal team to attend a birth. Triggers that may initiate communication and attendance at birth are included (Table 5.4).

Episiotomy

Episiotomy is a surgical cut of the perineum to increase the diameter of the pelvic outlet. Doing an episiotomy is no longer recommended unless the provider determines an indication such as[49]:
- High risk for extensive vaginal or perineal tears;
- Expedited birth is needed for fetal compromise;
- Increased diameter to assist with shoulder dystocia.

NOTE: *There is very little evidence that performing an episiotomy decreases the risk of trauma to the perineum.*[49]

A median episiotomy (the most common type) is a vertical incision made from the vaginal opening toward the anus. If the provider cuts a mediolateral episiotomy, the incision extends either right or left at a 45-degree angle from the vaginal opening. A median episiotomy heals at a more rapid rate and results in less blood loss. However, it is more likely to extend during the birth process and result in a third- or fourth-degree laceration into the rectum.

Active Management of the Third Stage of Labor (AMTSL)

Previously, the third stage of labor (defined as the time period between the birth of the newborn and the expulsion of the placenta) was managed in an expectant manner with no interventions until spontaneous separation of the placenta occurred followed by administration of a uterotonic agent. As new research emerged, recommendations have changed to involve active management of the third stage (AMTSL), which includes the following:

1. Administration of a uterotonic agent (usually oxytocin)
2. Gentle cord traction
3. Fundal massage

Evidence has demonstrated that AMTSL:

1. decreases the duration of the third stage of labor;
2. reduces the risk of postpartum hemorrhage;
3. decreases the risk of anemia (maternal and newborn);
4. decreases the need for blood product administration; and
5. decreases the need for administration of additional uterotonic medications.

Women should be informed of risks and benefits of AMTSL versus expectant management. AMTSL is an interdisciplinary plan of care that should be standardized in each unit. The following AMTSL recommendations are based on current evidence and best practice.

Uterotonic Medication Administration

Prophylactic administration of oxytocin is recommended immediately after the delivery of the anterior shoulder of the newborn in all births.[50] Oxytocin is the first-line uterotonic medication and should be administered either by rapid IV drip or 10 units IM if the mother does not have IV access. Oxytocin should not be given IV push. The total dose or length of IV oxytocin administration should be determined by uterine tone, risk factors, and blood loss. All precautions related to oxytocin administration, as a high-alert medication should be taken. By adhering to these precautions, some hospitals may only have one premixed concentration of oxytocin solution. If this is the practice in the unit, set the pump to administer the desired amount per the obstetric provider's order. There are various guidelines supported for administration, but usually this is 10 to 40 units, with re-evaluation of uterine tone.[51,52]

***NOTE:** If the mother is low risk and chooses to not receive oxytocin administration, the risks should be explained, documented, and her decision supported.*[51]

Gentle Cord Traction

This component of AMTSL requires the obstetric provider to put gentle, continuous traction on the umbilical cord to facilitate placental expulsion. During traction, counter pressure should be applied to the fundus in order to support the uterus until the placenta is delivered. Cord traction decreases the amount of time for the third stage of labor, but does not significantly reduce blood loss. Cord traction may be considered as determined by the provider or patient, but is not a necessary intervention.[53]

Fundal Massage

Once the placenta has delivered, immediately assess uterine tone to ensure a contracted uterus. Continue to assess uterine tone every 15 minutes for 2 hours. If the uterus is boggy, perform fundal massage and monitor more frequently.[53] Nurses are in a key position to positively impact patient outcomes by performing thorough assessments before, during, and after birth; communicating abnormal assessment parameters; and anticipating the woman's needs (e.g., additional medications, equipment, or procedures). For additional information regarding management of the woman during the immediate postpartum period, refer to Module 17. Also, information on postpartum hemorrhage is discussed in Module 16.

Delayed Cord Clamping

In addition to the components of AMTSL, delayed cord clamping is now recommended. The umbilical cord should not be clamped for 1 to 3 minutes in order to allow physiologic transfer of blood volume to the newborn. Delaying the cord clamp has shown to decrease the risk of newborn anemia. Timing of cord clamping may be modified based on gestational age and resuscitation needs of the newborn. Gravity or placement of the newborn on the mother's abdomen does not influence the physiologic transfer.[53]

SKILL UNIT 1 | POSITIONING FOR THE SECOND STAGE OF LABOR

ACTIONS	REMARKS (PICTORIAL)

A woman may choose several positions during stage II, depending on the intensity of contractions, the urge to push, and the length of stage II. Stage II provides an opportunity for support person(s) to assist women as they move closer to birth and need reassurance and sensitivity.

1. Semi-sitting Positioning

Head and shoulders should be elevated at least 30–45 in. The head of the bed can be rolled up. If in the delivery room, use pillows to prop up the mother.

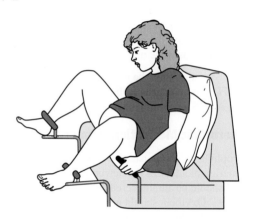

Mothers may grasp the legs with the hands behind or in front of the knees or have their partners sit behind them and hold their legs.

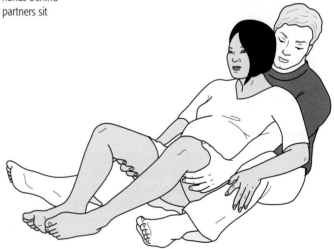

skill unit continues on page 109

ACTIONS	REMARKS (PICTORIAL)

Flex the thighs on the abdomen by grasping the legs behind the knees, in front of the knees, or at the ankles.

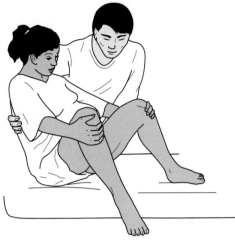

Variation: Permit the legs to relax in a frog-leg position with pillows under each knee.

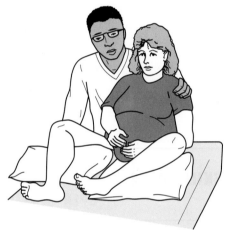

2. Squatting

The squatting position is extremely effective. Pushing efforts are maximized in this position, and the force of gravity assists the mother's efforts.

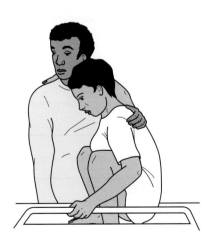

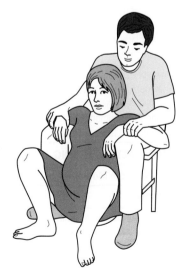

skill unit continues on page 110

109

ACTIONS	REMARKS (PICTORIAL)

3. Side-Lying

The side-lying position is useful for women who need to lie on their side for medical reasons or who are experiencing a rapid second stage and benefit from increased spacing of contractions that can occur in a lateral position.

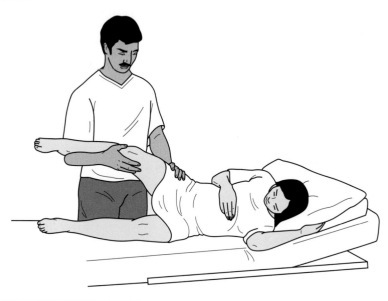

SKILL UNIT 2 | TECHNIQUE FOR PHYSIOLOGIC PUSHING (OPEN GLOTTIS)

SKILL 1: COUNTERACTING THE URGE TO PUSH

ACTION	REMARKS
This method can be used before the second stage for intensive pelvic/rectal pressure or during the second stage as the fetal head is crowning. Less intense pushing may facilitate a slow birth of the head and avoid lacerations.	Sometimes the urge to push is truly premature. If the cervix is not approaching 9 or 10 cm, pushing will only tire the mother. To push, the diaphragm is fixed and the breath held. Repeated blowing attempts help to counteract this tendency to push prematurely.
Blow out with short, forceful exhalations. An equal amount of air is taken in after each exhalation. Take caution that this is not done too rapidly, causing dizziness and numbness in fingers and lips from hyperventilation. This is sometimes called "feather blowing."	This technique is used only during that part of the contraction where the urge to push is felt.

SKILL 2: ACTIVE PUSHING

Encourage the Mother to do the Following:

ACTION	REMARKS
Assume the position of choice to enhance fetal descent. Take two cleansing breaths as the uterine contraction begins.	Examples: side-lying, hands/knees, squatting, sitting.
Take a slow, deep breath in and begin to expel the breath slowly through slightly pursed lips.	Breath-holding techniques should be discouraged.

skill unit continues on page 111

ACTION	REMARKS
Exhale slowly over 4–6 sec. Grunting may occur toward the end of the exhalation.	This is fine and provides effective effort in pushing. Remember to encourage the woman to keep the perineal muscles relaxed.
Take a cleansing breath at the end of the contraction and relax between contractions.	

Mastery of the skill is achieved when you can demonstrate the following:
- A variety of positions appropriate for pushing during stage II of labor
- The open glottis technique for pushing
- The technique for pushing using forceful exhalation
- Breathing to counteract the urge to push if not fully dilated

PRACTICE/REVIEW QUESTIONS

After reviewing this module, answer the following questions.

1. There are many goals in intrapartum care. List at least four.
   a. _____
   b. _____
   c. _____
   d. _____

2. List some ways the nurse might promote a woman's labor and birth goals.
   a. _____
   b. _____
   c. _____
   d. _____

3. Which of the following example vital sign data are considered abnormal for the laboring woman?
   a. BP 92/52 mm Hg
   b. HR 102
   c. RR 24
   d. SpO2 96%
   e. T 100.4°F

4. What are the causes of increased maternal heart rate during labor?
   a. _____
   b. _____
   c. _____
   d. _____
   e. _____

5. Name the two major techniques for monitoring fetal status during labor.
   a. _____
   b. _____

6. What is the appropriate nurse-to-patient ratio in active labor?
   _____

7. Prior to the initial cervical examination on a woman presenting to the birth setting, the nurse should evaluate for the following (list 5):
   a. _____
   b. _____
   c. _____
   d. _____
   e. _____

8. For the low-risk woman (a woman on oxytocin or with risk factors) in active labor who is dilated 8 to 10 cm, BP should be taken every _____ minutes; contractions should be monitored every _____ minutes; FHR, every _____ minutes.

9. Maintaining the supine position for a long time sometimes results in _____.

10. A cervical exam may provide the nurse what information?
    a. _____
    b. _____
    c. _____
    d. _____
    e. _____

11. Fill in the blanks. The goals of FHR assessment during labor are to establish evidence of _____, and being able to detect signs of potential _____ so that appropriate _____ may be initiated in a timely manner.

12. True or False. There is ample evidence that continuous electronic FHR monitoring among **low-risk** laboring women is beneficial.

13. Describe the two phases of stage I labor:

    a. _____

    b. _____

14. List possible reasons for recent changes in describing the labor curve.

    a. _____

    b. _____

    c. _____

15. When the presenting fetal part is at the pelvic inlet, it is said to be at _____ station.

16. When the presenting fetal part is at the level of the ischial spines, it is said to be at _____ station.

17. When the presenting fetal part is halfway between the ischial spines and the pelvic outlet, it is at _____ station.

18. When the widest part of the fetal head has passed through the pelvic inlet, _____ has occurred.

19. When engagement has taken place, the pelvis is thought to be _____.

20. What effect does molding have on assessment for the amount of descent?

    _____

21. Why is it important to assess the degree of descent?

    _____

22. You are caring for a G 1 woman with a BMI of 42. She is being induced for post dates pregnancy with an estimated fetal weight of 7 ½ pounds and is currently at 4 cm dilated with the fetal presenting part (cephalic) at +1 station. As the nurse caring for this woman, you understand that obesity may have what effect on cervical dilation?

    _____

    _____

23. As the nurse for a woman in active labor at 7 cm, you are planning for the second stage of labor. The woman has an epidural, but is able to change positions with assistance. Do best practice recommendations for nursing management may include the following actions: (Yes or No)

    a. Breath holding during pushing

    _____

    b. Open glottis pushing

    _____

    c. Lithotomy positioning

    _____

    d. Active coaching by counting to 10

    _____

    e. Laboring down until the woman feels the urge to push

    _____

    f. Side-lying positioning

    _____

    g. Turning off her epidural to assist with pushing

    _____

24. What are the three components of AMTSL?

    a. _____

    b. _____

    c. _____

25. You are the nurse caring for a woman in the second stage of labor. During labor, she had a fever (temperature maximum 101.2°F) and was treated with antibiotic therapy for chorioamnionitis. Is chorioamnionitis a trigger to notify the neonatal team to attend the birth?

    a. Yes

    b. No

PRACTICE/REVIEW ANSWER KEY

1. Any four of the following:
   a. Promote patient safety during labor and birth.
   b. Promote maternal coping behaviors.
   c. Support the mother and her family.
   d. Follow through on the mother's choices and desires whenever possible.
   e. Provide pain relief.
   f. Offer reassurance and information.
   g. Be an advocate for the woman and family
2. a. Create a quiet environment.
   b. Listen actively.
   c. Touch in a therapeutic manner.
   d. Integrate the support person.
3. a. abnormal
   b. abnormal
   c. abnormal
   d. normal
   e. abnormal
4. In any order:
   a. Hypovolemia
   b. Hypertension
   c. Medications
   d. Pain, fear, anxiety (don't assume it is attributable to these!)
   e. Infectious processes
5. Auscultation; continuous electronic fetal monitoring
6. 1:1

7. List in any order: gestational age, gravidity, parity; presence or suspicion of placenta previa in current pregnancy; report or suspicion of ruptured membranes; report of vaginal bleeding; results of previous cervical examination; history of the present labor; fetal history

8. 30; 30; 30

9. Supine hypotensive syndrome (i.e., lowered BP and hypotension)

10. Cervical dilation, effacement, position, consistency, membrane status, descent of presenting fetal part

11. Fetal well-being; fetal compromise; interventions

12. False

13. a. The early phase (preparatory phase) extends from the onset of regular contractions that cause cervical change to the beginning of the active phase, when dilation occurs more rapidly. It usually extends over hours and appears as a nearly flat line on the labor curve.

    b. The active phase (dilational phase) of labor begins when the laboring woman reaches 6 cm of dilation, and ends when the cervix is 10 cm or completely dilated. Effective labor begins with the active phase.

14. Any three of the following: older laboring women, higher BMIs, more comorbid conditions, increased use of neuraxial analgesia

15. −3

16. 0

17. Close to +2 station using the −3 to +3 scale; at +3 station using the −3 to +5 station

18. Engagement

19. Adequate

20. Sometimes, if severe molding of the fetal head has occurred, the examiner's assessment of the amount of descent can be distorted. That is, engagement might not have occurred even though the leading edge of the presenting part is at 0 station.

21. Assessment of the degree of descent is necessary to determine normal/abnormal progress in labor over time.

22. Cervical dilation may take longer. Also, reaching 6 cm may take longer.

23. a. No
    b. Yes
    c. No
    d. No
    e. Yes
    f. Yes
    g. No

24. Administration of a uterotonic agent (usually oxytocin); gentle cord traction; fundal massage

25. Yes

REFERENCES

1. Association of Women's Health, Obstetrics, and Neonatal Nursing. (2011). Nursing support of the laboring woman. *Journal of Obstetrics and Gynecologic Nursing, 40,* 665–666.

2. Committee for the Robert Wood Johnson Foundation Initiative on the Future of Nursing, at the Institute of Medicine. (2011). The future of nursing: Leading change, advancing health. Retrieved from http://thefutureofnursing.org/IOM-Report

3. Clark, S. L., Belfort, M. A., Herbst, M. A., et al. (2008). Maternal death in the 21st century: Causes, prevention, and relationship to cesarean delivery. *American Journal of Obstetrics & Gynecology, 199*(1), 36.e1–e5.

4. Callaghan, W. M., Creanga, A. A., Kuklina, E. V. (2012). Severe maternal morbidity among delivery and postpartum hospitalizations in the United States. *Obstetrics & Gynecology, 120,* 1029–1036.

5. American College of Nurse-Midwives. (2012). Supporting healthy and normal physiologic childbirth: A consensus statement by the American College of Nurse-Midwives, Midwives Alliance of North American, and the National Association of Certified Professional Midwives. *Journal of Midwifery & Women's Health, 57*(5), 529–532.

6. Spong, C. Y., Berghella, V., Wenstrom, K. D., et al. (2012). Preventing the first cesarean delivery: Summary of a Joint Eunice Kennedy Shriver National Institute of Child Health and Human Development, Society for Maternal–Fetal Medicine, and American College of Obstetricians and Gynecologists Workshop. *Obstetrics & Gynecology, 120*(5), 1181–1193.

7. Abbott, S., Rogers, M., Freeth, D. (2012). Underpinning safety: Communication habits and situation awareness. *British Journal of Midwifery, 20,* 279–284.

8. Downe, S., Gyte, G., Dahlen, H., et al. (2013). Routine vaginal examinations for assessing progress of labour to improve outcomes for woman and babies at term. The Cochrane Collaboration. John Wiley & Sons. DOI: 10.1002/14651858.CD010088.pub2.

9. Lyndon, A., Ali, L. (Eds.). (2015). *Fetal heart monitoring: Principles and practice* (5th ed.). Washington, DC: Association of Women's Health, Obstetric & Neonatal Nurses.

10. Clark, S. L., Nageotte, M. P., Garite, T. J., et al. (2013). Intrapartum management of category II fetal heart rate tracings: Towards standardization of care. *American Journal of Obstetrics & Gynecology, 209*(2), 89–97.

11. Grimes, D., Peipert, J. (2010). Electronic fetal monitoring as a public health screening program: The arithmetic of failure. *Obstetrics &Gynecology, 116*(6), 1397–1400.

12. Devane, D., Lalor, J., Daly, S., et al. (2012). Cardiotocography versus intermittent auscultation of fetal heart on admission to labour ward for assessment of fetal wellbeing. *Cochrane Database of Systematic Reviews Protocols,* CD005122. DOI: 10.1002/14651858.CD005122.pub4.

13. Association of Women's Health, Obstetrics, and Neonatal Nursing. (2010). *Guidelines for professional registered nurse staffing for perinatal units.* Washington, DC: Author.

14. Macones, G. A., Hankins, G. D., Spong, C. Y., et al. (2008). The 2008 National Institute of Child Health and Human Development workshop report on electronic fetal monitoring: Update on definitions, interpretation, and research guidelines. *Obstetrics & Gynecology, 112*(3), 661–666.

15. Simpson, K. R., O'Brien-Abel, N. (2014). Labor and birth. In Simpson, K. R., Creehan, P. A. (Eds.), *Perinatal nursing* (4th ed., pp. 343–425). Philadelphia, PA: Wolters Kluwer.

16. American Academy of Pediatrics and American Colleges of Obstetricians and Gynecologists. (2012). *Guidelines for perinatal care* (7th ed.). Elk Grove Village, IL: AAP.

17. Friedman, E. A. (1978). *Labor: Clinical evaluation of management* (2nd ed.). New York, NY: Appleton-Century-Crofts.

18. Zhang, J., Landy, H. J., Branch, D. W., et al., Consortium on Safe Labor. (2010). Contemporary patterns of spontaneous labor with normal neonatal outcomes. *Obstetrics & Gynecology, 116*(6), 1281–1287.

19. Laughon, S. K., Branch, D. W., Beaver, J., et al. (2012). Changes in labor patterns over 50 years. *American Journal of Obstetrics & Gynecology, 206*(5), 419.e1–e9.

20. World Health Organization. (2003). *Pregnancy, childbirth, postpartum and newborn care: A guide for essential practice.* Geneva: Author.

21. American College of Obstetricians and Gynecologists and Society for Maternal-Fetal Medicine. (2014). Safe prevention of the primary cesarean delivery. Obstetric Care Consensus Series. Retrieved from: http://www.acog.org/Resources-And-Publications/Obstetric-Care-Consensus-Series/Safe-Prevention-of-the-Primary-Cesarean-Delivery

22. Graseck, A., Tuuli, M., Roehl, K., et al. (2014). Fetal descent in labor. *Obstetrics & Gynecology, 123*(3), 521–526.

23. El-Sayed, Y. Y. (2012). Diagnosis and management of arrest disorders: Duration to wait. *Seminars in Perinatology, 36*(5), 374–378.

24. Kominiarek, M. A., Zhang, J., Vanveldhuisen, P., et al. (2011). Contemporary labor patterns: The impact of maternal body mass index. *American Journal of Obstetrics & Gynecology, 205*(3), 244.e1–e8.

25. Hodnett, E., Gates, S., Hofmeyr, G., et al. (2013). Continuous support for women during childbirth. *Cochrane Database of Systematic Reviews, 7*, CD003766. DOI: 10.1002/14651858. CD003766.pub5.

26. Simpson, K. R. (2014). Labor management evidence update: Potential to minimize risk of cesarean birth in healthy women. *Journal of Perinatal and Neonatal Nursing, 28*(2), 1080116.

27. Singata, M., Tranmer, J., Gyte, G. (2013). Restricting oral fluid and food intake during labour. *Cochrane Database of Systematic Reviews,* CD003930. DOI: 10.1002/14651858. CD003930.pub3.

28. Lawrence, A., Lewis, L., Hofmeyr, G., et al. (2013). Maternal positions and mobility during first stage labour. *Cochrane Database of Systematic Reviews, 8*, CD003934. DOI: 10.1002/14651858.CD003934.pub4.

29. Dixon, L., Foureur, M. (2010). The vaginal examination during labour: Is it of benefit or harm? *New Zealand College of Midwives Journal, 42*, 21–26.

30. Osterman, M. J. K., Martin, J. A. (2014). *Recent declines in induction of labor by gestational age.* NCHS data brief, no 155. Hyattsville, MD: National Center for Health Statistics.

31. Harper, L. M., Caughey, A. B., Odibo, A. O., et al. (2012). Normal progress of induced labor. *Obstetrics & Gynecology, 119*(6), 1113–1118.

32. Wong, C. A. (2012). Influence of analgesia on labor – is it related to primary cesarean rates? *Seminars in Perinatology, 36*(5), 353–356.

33. Cheng, Y. W., Shaffer, B. L., Nicholson, J. M., et al. (2014). Second stage of labor and epidural use: A larger effect than previously suggested. *Obstetrics & Gynecology, 123*(3), 527–535.

34. Anim-Somuah, M., Smyth, R., Jones, L. (2011). Epidural versus non-epidural or no analgesia in labour. *Cochrane Database of Systematic Reviews,* (12), CD000331. DOI: 10.1002/14651858. CD000331.pub3.

35. Wong, C. A., Scavone, B. M., Peaceman, A. M., et al. (2005). Risk of cesarean delivery with neuraxial analgesia given early versus late labor. *The New England Journal of Medicine, 352,* 655–665.

36. Wassen, M. M., Zuijlen, J., Roume, F. J., et al. (2011). Early versus late epidural analgesia and risk of instrumental delivery in nulliparous women: A systematic review. *British Journal of Obstetrics and Gynecology, 118*(6), 655–661.

37. Shilling, T. (2009). *Walk, move around, and change positions through- out labor. Healthy birth practices, #2.* Washington, DC: Lamaze International.

38. Hanson, L., & VandeVusse, L. (2014). Supporting labor progress toward physiologic birth. *The Journal of Perinatal & Neonatal Nursing, 28*(2), 101–107.

39. Jackson, S., Gregory, K. D. (2015). Management of the first stage of labor: Potential strategies to lower the cesarean delivery rate. *Clinical Obstetrics & Gynecology, 58*(2), 217–226.

40. Wei, S., Wo, B. L., Xu, H., et al. (2012). Early amniotomy and early oxytocin for prevention of, or therapy for, delay in first stage spontaneous labour compared with routine care. The Cochrane Collaboration. John Wiley & Sons.

41. Durie, D. E., Thornburg, L. L., Glantz, J. C. (2011). Effect of second-trimester and third-trimester rate of gestational weight gain on maternal and neonatal outcomes. *Obstetrics & Gynecology, 118*(3), 569–575.

42. Dawood, F., Dowswell, T., Quenby, S. (2013). Intravenous fluids for preventing prolonged labour in women giving birth to their first baby. *Cochrane Database Systematic Reviews, 6,* CD007715.

43. Shrivastava, V. K., Garite, T. J., Jenkins, S. M., et al. (2009). A randomized, double-blinded, controlled trial comparing parenteral normal saline with and without dextrose on the course of labor in nulliparas. *American Journal of Obstetrics and Gynecology, 200*(4), 379.e1–379.e6.

44. Borrelli, S. E., Locatelli, A., Newpoli, A. (2013). Early pushing urge in labour and midwifery practice: A prospective observational study at an Indian maternal hospital. *Midwifery, 29*(8), 871–875.

45. Hanson, L. (2009). Second-stage labor care: Challenges in spontaneous bearing down. *Journal of Perinatal and Neonatal Nursing, 23*(1), 31–39.

46. Osborne, K., Hanson, L. (2014). Labor down or bear down: A strategy to translate second-stage labor evidence to perinatal practice. *Journal of Perinatal and Neonatal Nursing, 28*(2), 117–126.

47. Aasheim, V., Nilsen, A. B., Lukasse, M., et al. (2011). Perineal techniques during the second stage of labour for reducing trauma. *Cochrane Database Systematic Review, 12,* CD006672.

48. Nielsen, P. E., Goldman, M. B., Mann, S., et al. (2007). Effects of teamwork training on adverse outcomes and process of care in labor and delivery: A randomized controlled trial. *Obstetrics & Gynecology, 109*(1), 48–55.

49. American Congress of Obstetricians and Gynecologists. (2006). ACOG recommends restricted use of episiotomy. Retrieved from: http://www.acog.org/About-ACOG/News-Room/News-Releases/2006/ACOG-Recommends-Restricted-Use-of-Episiotomies

50. California Maternal Quality Care Collaborative. (2015). *Improving health care response to obstetric hemorrhage, version 2.0: A California toolkit to transform maternity care.* Retrieved from: https://www.cmqcc.org/resources-tool-kits/toolkits/ob-hemorrhage-toolkit

51. Association of Women's Health, Obstetrics, and Neonatal Nursing. (2014). Quantification of blood loss: AWHONN practice brief number 1. *Journal of Obstetrics Gynecology and Neonatal Nursing, 3,* 1–3.

52. Association of Women's Health, Obstetric & Neonatal Nurses. (2015). Guidelines for oxytocin administration after birth: AWHONN Practice Brief Number 2. *Nursing for Women's Health, 19*(1), 99–101.

53. World Health Organization. (2012). *WHO recommendations for the prevention and treatment of postpartum hemorrhage.* Geneva: Author. Retrieved from: http://apps.who.int/iris/bitstream/10665/75411/1/9789241548502_eng.pdf

Nonpharmacologic and Pharmacologic Methods of Pain Relief for the Laboring Woman

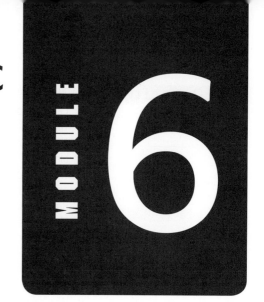

MODULE 6

Objectives

As you complete this module, you will learn:

1. Causes of pain in labor and nonpharmacologic therapies for pain control
2. The role of a professional doula in providing support to women giving birth
3. Those measures that need to be taken to safely use hydrotherapy for women in labor or giving birth
4. The technique for administering subcutaneous/intracutaneous injections of sterile water to treat severe back pain in labor
5. Breathing techniques to assist the woman in progressing through labor and birth
6. Pharmacologic interventions, rationale, and factors to consider when administering medications to laboring women for pain relief
7. Interventions and rationale for nursing care for women who choose neuraxial anesthesia to manage labor pain
8. Maternal and fetal effects of nitrous oxide when used as labor analgesia
9. Which peripartum patients and procedures are best suited for nitrous oxide use
10. Administration techniques for nitrous oxide delivery that support patient safety

Key Terms

When you have completed this module, you should be able to recall the meaning of the following terms. You should also be able to use the terms when consulting with other health professionals. The terms are defined in this module or in the glossary at the end of this book.

acupressure
acupuncture
anxiolytic
arachnoid space
catecholamines
conduction anesthesia
doula
effleurage
epinephrine
extradural space

homeopathy
hyperventilation
lithotomy
nonpharmacologic
neuraxial anesthesia
nitrous oxide
subdural space
transcutaneous electrical nerve
    stimulation (TENS)

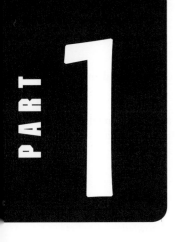

Pain in Labor and Nonpharmacologic Modes of Relief

MICHELLE R. COLLINS

The Experience of Pain in Childbirth

There are many characteristics universal to labor and birth, one of the most significant being the discomfort, or pain, that women experience. Though the physiologic cause of labor pain is universal for women, the experience of one's interpretation of that pain, as well as how it is dealt with, is certainly individualized. From the beginning of time, women have used various methods to cope with pain in labor and birth. Women in the Andes region of the world chewed coca leaves for pain (the same plant from which the modern cocaine is derived). According to ancient records, Greek women chewed willow bark during childbirth; willow bark being a predecessor to modern day aspirin.[1]

Pain, or rather one's experience with pain, is influenced by a multitude of factors, to include culture, age, personal experience with pain, parity, and physical/psychological and emotional support. Providers who are knowledgeable, clinically competent, caring, and skilled at providing both pharmacologic and nonpharmacologic methods of pain relief are needed in labor and delivery units and birth centers. Every laboring woman deserves kindness, compassion, and support as she navigates the process of giving birth. This aspect of your caregiving is really the art of nursing. Unfortunately, in today's fast-paced medical environment, nurses have limited time to spend providing supportive care.[2]

Studies indicate that the satisfaction a woman experiences during childbirth is related to either her ability to remain in control or to influence what happens to her.[3] For women, those factors which have great influence over the satisfaction with their birth experiences include their own personal expectations, the amount of support they felt was given by caregivers, the quality of the relationship between them and their caregiver, and their inclusion/involvement in decision-making.[4] Maternal perception of control is closely related to satisfaction, and the issue of control can be seen in terms of power. Both the birth setting and its participants powerfully influence the process of childbirth, shaping the role and amount of control held by a laboring woman, those who support her, and her caregivers. The birth experience belongs to the laboring woman and all efforts should be made to support, accommodate, and encourage both her and her support persons. Care providers should be committed to meeting the needs of the laboring women and their support persons and not committed to arbitrary and restrictive rules.

The goals of intrapartum care are to do the following:
- Promote maternal coping behaviors
- Provide a safe environment for mother and fetus
- Support the mother and her family throughout the labor and birth experience
- Follow through on the woman's desires and choices throughout labor, whenever possible
- Provide comfort measures and pain relief as needed
- Offer reassurance and information, doing so with attention to the mother's and family's cultural needs

The caregiver should do the following:
- Create an environment sensitive to the psychological, spiritual, and cultural needs of the woman and her family
- Monitor maternal and fetal well-being
- Listen actively
- Be vigilant in recognizing that body language, as well as spoken word, has a powerful influence over maternal perceptions of the birth experience

- Use language that is culturally appropriate, provides positive reinforcement, and empowers women and their families
- Touch so as to be therapeutic
- Use knowledge of both nonpharmacologic and pharmacologic therapies for pain relief
- Integrate the woman's support person(s) in all of these responsibilities so that he, she, or they become an essential and valued part of the profound experience of birth

Cultural Sensitivity

Diversity is the norm in our society, requiring healthcare providers to be aware of beliefs and cultural practices of the families for which they care. Quality of care in obstetrics can be measured by cultural competency or the ability of a provider to incorporate knowledge of beliefs and cultural norms as they relate to the birth experience.[5] Women give birth within the context of their cultural background and traditional norms, incorporating factors such as dietary practices and birth rituals. Other cultural norms surrounding birth, such as food intake, labor and birth positioning, support behaviors, and early infant caretaking need to be addressed by the caregiver.

Support for the Laboring Woman

Women tend to cope better, relax more readily, describe their babies more positively, have a more positive recall of the experience, and adjust more easily to parenthood when they receive kind and sensitive care during their labor. Women who are provided support in labor have shorter labors; use less medication; have less incidence of forceps-assisted, vacuum-assisted, or cesarean births; and have fewer babies with low Apgar scores.[6] An understanding of physiology shows us that undue fetal stress may occur if the laboring woman is anxious or frightened, as a result of increased catecholamine levels and subsequent vasoconstriction. This may contribute to a compromised fetal state in some cases.

Knowledge is empowering. Keeping women informed during labor about what to expect, interpreting the sensations they are experiencing, and explaining their progress in labor are important elements of care.

The following elements are essential to cover when providing supportive care:
- Helping the woman to feel that she can handle the sensations, intensity, and effort required of labor by giving constant feedback, explaining everything, being positive, and validating her efforts.
- Reviewing with her how to breathe and how to position herself, placing her hands on the fundus to feel the oncoming contraction, and showing her the baby's progress during pushing, in a mirror, if desired.
- Recognizing that some women may have an unrealistic, idealized view of labor and what is involved, and that they may need assistance navigating the reality of their labor versus the idealistic version they had envisioned. Conversely, respecting, and acknowledging, that women can very often accomplish what they set their minds to when it comes to labor and birth, despite what caregivers feel about their capability.
- Discussing potential barriers to labor progress such as fear, anxiety, or a history of sexual abuse or domestic violence.
- Being concrete and specific with descriptions of things such as findings on pelvic exams, and ongoing assessments and plans, always with an understanding that information might need to be repeated.

In addition, a significant other, whether family member or friend, should be encouraged to stay to support the mother. The support person needs nursing care and attention as well. Nursing personnel should show the partner how to offer support, and then praise the partner's efforts. Provision of snacks and fluids for the support person is an important component of supporting them as well. Additionally, being aware of any special needs of the support person assists nursing personnel in supporting them adequately.

Ambulation and Positioning

Healthy laboring women should be encouraged to change positions based on their comfort needs, as well as considering the position of the baby. Women who ambulate while in labor have shorter labors, less use of anesthesia, and report greater satisfaction with the birth process.[7] Additionally, the various pelvic diameters are different in various positions; moving about in labor may not

TABLE 6.1 MATERNAL POSITIONS FOR LABOR	
IN BED	**OUT OF BED**
Upright	Standing/walking/dancing
Semi-sitting	Sitting on a birth ball
	Sitting on a side chair or rocking chair
	Sitting on the toilet
	Sitting in a tub
Hands and knees	Hands and knees in the shower or tub
Lateral	Side-lying in a tub
Exaggerated lateral	
Squatting	Squatting in the shower or on the floor

From Simkin, P. (1995). Reducing pain and enhancing progress in labor: A guide to nonpharmacologic methods for maternity caregivers. *Birth*, 22(3), 161–170.

only facilitate pain relief, but enhance optimal fetal positioning and descent throughout labor.[8] Positions that women find helpful in labor include positions listed in Table 6.1 and Figure 6.1.

Positions that may provide comfort and help rotate a fetus from an occiput posterior position include the following[9]:

- Knee press
- Side or forward lunge
- Pelvic rock on hands and knees
- Exaggerated lateral position

Nurses should be advocates for promoting optimal positioning in labor and for birth. While important to consider such variables as fetal monitoring when positioning the woman, ease of monitoring should not be the main factor considered when position is chosen; very often women who do not require continuous electronic fetal monitoring have it applied and left on continuously, for the sake of nurse convenience. Women who are candidates for intermittent auscultation should be monitored that way. When she is in bed, promote right or left side-lying or sitting upright, to utilize gravity and facilitate descent.

Supine positions result in the heavy uterus resting on the major veins leading back to the heart, diminishing cardiac input. This may result in supine hypotension and fetal bradycardia. The risk is greatest when a lithotomy position is assumed.

Laboring women should be encouraged to avoid lying on their backs and to change position frequently.

It is unlikely that a supine position would be required to be maintained during labor for any reason. During a cesarean birth, however, the supine position cannot be avoided. To prevent supine hypotension, the woman's right hip is elevated with a pillow or wedge so that the uterus can be shifted to the left. Raising the right hip relieves pressure on the vena cava and may improve circulation to the maternal heart, lungs, uterus, and placenta, resulting in fewer low Apgar scores, though most recent research on maternal positioning is somewhat conflicting.[10]

Fluids and Food

The policy of NPO (nothing by mouth) during labor is, unfortunately, a well-established routine in many hospitals. This practice dates back to 1946 when it was suggested that aspiration of acidic gastric contents was a significant cause of maternal morbidity and mortality.[11] Although the risk of aspiration during childbirth has subsequently been proven to be extremely low, particularly because general anesthesia for childbirth is rarely used currently, and it is acknowledged that there is inherent risk in women being in a fasting state during labor and birth,[12]

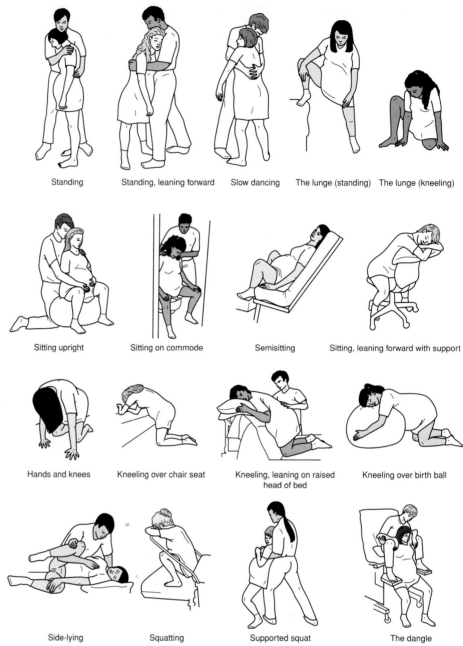

FIGURE 6.1 Maternal positions for labor and birth. **Top row:** Upright positions. **Second row:** Sitting positions. **Third row:** Kneeling positions. **Fourth row:** Second-stage positions. (Adapted with permission from Simkin, P. (1995). Reducing pain and enhancing progress in labor: A guide to nonpharmacologic methods for maternity caregivers. *Birth, 22*(3), 161–170.)

mandatory fasting for laboring women is a practice that continues in many hospitals today. Consider the following:

- Aspiration during general anesthesia in operative deliveries is directly related to difficult intubation, regardless of the patient's oral intake.
- Experts in anesthesiology agree that substandard management of anesthesia is a primary cause of pulmonary aspiration.
- Maintaining NPO status actually results in *increased* gastric acidity.
- Regional blocks have little effect on gastric emptying time and greatly reduce the risk of aspiration pneumonia.
- A regional block is appropriate for most emergency cesarean births, so general anesthesia is very rarely utilized.

- Routine intravenous (IV) fluid administration can induce fluid overload, hyperglycemia in the fetus, hypoglycemia in the newborn, and can alter plasma sodium levels.[13]
- Hydration and the energy needs of the laboring woman are akin to the needs of a competitive athlete. Deprivation of food and fluids can directly affect labor progress and outcome.[14]
- In 1999, the American Society of Anesthesiologists revised their recommendations regarding oral intake in labor. Clear liquids recommended for intake in labor include water, fruit juices without pulp, carbonated beverages, clear teas and coffee, flavored gelatin, fruit ices, popsicles, and broth. They recommend restrictions on a case-by-case basis only for those women who may be at increased risk for aspiration.[15] Again, the restriction of food intake during labor can have a negative effect on laboring women.[14]

Bladder Status

Provide the woman with the opportunity to empty her bladder every 2 hours. A full bladder can halt progress in labor, especially descent of the presenting part. If a woman goes into birth with a full bladder, it can impede her uterus from being able to contract, and thus involute successfully, after placental delivery, increasing her risk of hemorrhage.

Pain Management

As noted previously in this module, pain is a subjective experience, and is defined completely by the individual having the experience. Pain management is approached in various ways and usually varies according to the stage of labor; the rate of progress; the condition of the mother and fetus; the skill, experience, and attitude of members of the obstetric team; and the requests and attitudes of the mother and her family.

The methods of pain management include the following:
- Breathing and relaxation techniques
- Comfort measures
- Nonpharmacologic pain relief measures (e.g., hydrotherapy)
- Analgesia
- Anesthesia

Comfort Measures Nurses Can Use to Assist the Laboring Woman

- *Do not leave a woman in active labor alone;* merely the presence of another individual in the labor room can be calming to the laboring woman.
- Promptly change soiled and damp linen.
- For mothers who are NPO status, provide frequent mouth care, give ice chips, lubricate lips, and/or encourage frequent mouth rinses.
- Suggest ambulation, position change, or the use of a shower or tub, if available.
- Apply massage to abdomen, back, and legs as desired. Effleurage to the abdomen is particularly relaxing for some women.
- Ensure good ventilation in the room.
- Control the labor room environment according to the mother's wishes (e.g., lights, music, quiet, privacy).
- Promote the participation of a coach or significant family member.
- Offer support from a professional doula.

"*Doula* refers to a supportive companion professionally trained to provide labor support."[16] A doula's focus is to provide emotional and physical support; the doula is not trained as a clinical caregiver, and should not be asked to participate in, or perform independently, any clinical tasks. Doulas may provide support during labor, birth, and the postpartum period. Women who have a doula have been shown to have improved birth outcomes and more positive feelings about their birth experience.[17] Doulas may be particularly useful in busy birthing units where individualized care by a nurse or midwife is not possible.

• What Causes Pain in Labor?

Pain can be physiologic as well as psychological and is affected by a variety of factors, including level of anxiety, environment, support, and previous experience with painful stimuli.

The physiologic causes are thought to include the following:
- Hypoxia of the uterine muscle due to a diminished blood supply to the uterus during a contraction. While this is a normal, physiologic process, the hypoxia can cause muscle pain.
- Stretching of, and pressure on, the cervix, vagina, and perineal floor muscles.
- Distension of the lower uterine segment.
- Traction on reproductive structures, such as the fallopian tubes, ovaries, and uterine ligaments.
- Pressure on skeletal muscles.
- Pressure on the bladder, urethra, and rectum.
- Distension of the pelvic floor with laceration of the subcutaneous fascial tissue.

NOTE: Factors that undoubtedly influence the degree and character of pain include the following:
- *Nature of contractions (intensity, frequency and duration)*
- *Degree of cervical dilatation*
- *Degree of perineal distension*
- *Maternal age, parity, and general health*
- *Maternal position*
- *Fetal size and position (e.g., posterior positions are usually accompanied by intense back pain felt during contractions)*

Other factors that may influence a mother's response to pain include the following:
- Anxiety and fear
- History of abuse or previous traumatic birth or hospital experience[18]
- Cultural influences and upbringing
- Value system and education level
- Lack of knowledge or preparation
- Absence of supportive significant person

• Can Pain in Labor Have Harmful Effects on the Mother or Fetus?

Pain may have the following effects:
- *Hyperventilation,* or rapid breathing associated with pain, leads to oxygen and carbon dioxide imbalance in maternal blood and lungs. This results in decreased blood flow to the uterus and brain. Breathing changes may also lead to fetal acidosis.
- *Enhancement in physiologic decrease in blood flow to uterus and placenta.* With maternal stress, catecholamines, namely adrenaline, are released causing uterine blood vessel constriction, ultimately decreasing blood flow to the placenta and fetus.
- *Increase in maternal/fetal serum glucose levels.* Adrenaline also causes high serum maternal glucose levels, leading to an increase of glucose in fetal blood and, therefore, in brain tissue. Such high glucose levels decrease the fetal brain cells' ability to handle hypoxia and render those cells susceptible to damage.
- *Increase in maternal cardiac output and subsequently, blood pressure.* Severe pain can also change cardiac rhythms and decrease blood flow to the coronary arteries.
- *Perpetuation of the fear, tension, pain cycle.* Fear, tension, anxiety, and pain are intertwined; the greater the woman's fear, the more muscular tension she displays, which leads to greater anxiety and physical pain, which ultimately leads to more fear.[19]

• What Nonpharmacologic Pain Relief Measures Can Be Used with the Laboring Woman?

Many techniques and therapies can be used to provide nonpharmacologic pain relief during labor and birth. These can be used alone, or in combination with pharmacologic options, in an effort to delay, or completely forego, the use of pharmacotherapy.
The commonly used modalities include the following:
- Acupressure
- Acupuncture
- Hydrotherapy
- Massage, therapeutic touch, effleurage
- Intradermal injections of sterile water
- Heat and cold therapy
- Aromatherapy
- Music
- Meditation

- Hypnosis
- Transcutaneous electrical nerve stimulation (TENS)
- Herbal therapy
- Homeopathy

Nurses may use the following techniques, found to be useful for women in labor:

- Help mothers to identify the most comfortable position(s), as well as to encourage frequent position changes.
- Provide hot and cold therapy with hot packs/heating pads or ice packs.
- Utilize acupressure points.
- Encourage the use of a tub or shower.
- Provide or train a support person to use massage/effleurage techniques.
- Apply counter pressure to coccyx with tennis balls or other massage devices; particularly helpful for women who have a baby in occiput posterior position.
- Use the double hip squeeze to increase the outlet diameter and decrease pain. Hands are placed over the gluteus muscles with mothers assuming a position with hip joints flexed. Using the palms, pressure is given toward the center of the pelvis.[20]
- Use intradermal injections of sterile water for severe back pain.[21]
- Encourage support by a professional doula.

- **What Measures Should Be Taken to Safely Use Hydrotherapy for Women in Labor and/or for Birth? (Display 6.1)**

DISPLAY 6.1	SAFE USE OF HYDROTHERAPY FOR LABORING WOMEN
ACTIONS	**REMARKS**
Rule out any contraindications for hydrotherapy in labor.	Mothers requiring continuous electronic fetal monitoring are not appropriate candidates for water immersion, unless the facility has waterproof telemetric external monitoring available. Women who are appropriate for intermittent fetal monitoring may be auscultated while in the tub using a waterproof Doppler.
	Mothers should be able to get out of the tub or shower quickly if necessary. For this reason, it is important that there is always another person in the room with the woman while she is in the tub. That person does not need to be a nurse; a support person can fulfill this role.
	Maternal fever, defined as 38.0°C (100.4°F) is a contraindication. Presence of infectious disease is a contraindication. Women who are HIV positive, have active hepatitis, or infectious lesions (like herpes simplex) should not be placed in the tub. They may, however, use the shower for hydrotherapy.
	Prematurity is a contraindication. Mothers with gestations less than 37 wks may be restricted from water immersion, depending on individual unit policy.
	Women with epidural or spinal anesthesia are contraindicated to be immersed in the tub. The use of narcotic analgesia or nitrous oxide is not a contraindication to water immersion.
	Vaginal bleeding greater than a normal bloody show is a contraindication.
Use established protocols	Jets must be cleaned according to infectious disease protocols.
	Cleaning of tubs is to prevent bacterial growth and cross contamination between women.
Use of long gloves for vaginal examinations	Gloves that protect the caregivers from exposure to bodily fluids in the bathwater are necessary to use.

display continues on page 124

ACTIONS	REMARKS
Use water at normal body temperature, or at least in a range of 98–100°F.	Water temperatures much higher than body can result in elevated maternal temperatures, which in turn can cause fetal tachycardia. Water thermometers must be single use.
Determine baseline FHR and maternal vital signs before initiation of hydrotherapy.	
Cover IV lines or heparin locks with plastic.	
Provide a stool and/or pillow or a birth ball for maternal comfort.	Many women prefer to sit or lean in the shower.
Constant support must be available for women using hydrotherapy.	Neck pillows provide neck support for women using tubs. These must be single patient use items.
Discontinue hydrotherapy at any time if requested by the woman, or if conditions occur wherein the mother would be safer out of the water.	If water birth is anticipated, follow specific protocols established by a practice or institution.

Nursing Responsibilities in Performing Subcutaneous/Intracutaneous Injections of Sterile Water

Sterile water injections have long been used to relieve acute pain such as that associated with renal colic, as well as other types of musculoskeletal pain. Possible theories that explain the reason for its efficacy include the blocking of pain pathways via stimulation of large nerve fibers (gate theory). There may also be an accompanying release of endogenous endorphins.[22,23] This technique is particularly appropriate for women in labor who are experiencing acute back pain. A period of pain relief provided by this procedure gives an opportunity for rest and comfort and time for position changes to facilitate rotation of a posterior vertex to anterior (Display 6.2).[24]

Use of Acupressure and Acupuncture in Labor and Birth

Both acupuncture and acupressure have ancient origins in Chinese medicine. Acupuncture involves the strategic placement of specialized needles to stimulate particular points to produce analgesia. For labor pain, placement of needles depends on the degree and location of pain. Acupuncture has been used with some efficacy. How effective the acupuncture is depends on the degree of pain the woman is experiencing, as well as the stage of labor she is in, how fatigued she may be, as well as other mitigating forces like the woman's degree of anxiety and muscular tension.[25] Acupressure, or the application of touch at the same points used for acupuncture, stimulates the same points, but does not use needles. Research has indicated that women may experience good relief with the use of acupressure.[26]

DISPLAY 6.2 SUBCUTANEOUS/INTRACUTANEOUS STERILE WATER INJECTIONS	
ACTIONS	**REMARKS**
1. Secure informed consent.	
2. Explain steps in the procedure.	Emphasize to mothers that they will feel an acute "stinging" sensation associated with injection.
3. Assist the obstetric provider with injection.	Use 0.1 mL sterile water in four sites in the lumbar-sacral region area adjacent to the Michaelis rhomboid.[22–24] Some providers may prefer that all four injections are done simultaneously, with the nurse injecting at two sites, and the provider injecting at two sites.
4. Document the time of injection and pain relief.	Most women report relief soon after the injection, and for up to 60–90 min or longer. Use this time to reposition mothers to optimize rotation of the fetus to an anterior position. Figure 6.2 shows the location of the injection sites.

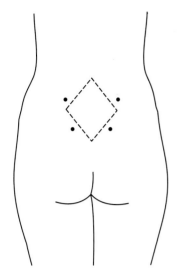

FIGURE 6.2 Location of injection sites in relation to the Michaelis rhomboid for intradermal injections of sterile water. (Adapted with permission from Martensson, L., & Wallin, G. (1999). Labor pain treated with cutaneous injections of sterile water: A randomized controlled trial. *British Journal of Obstetrics and Gynecology, 106*(7), 634.)

Massage and Therapeutic Touch in Labor and Birth

Human touch can convey such positive feedback from one person to another. The use of therapeutic touch does not require words; in fact, talk can be obtrusive for many laboring women, whereas the touch of another human being can convey exactly what is needed in the moment. Therapeutic touch in labor may be invited and welcomed by the woman in labor. Sometimes, another's touch may not be therapeutic, and in fact, may break the woman's concentration if she is using particular types of prepared childbirth methods. Caregivers should always ask permission before "assuming" that the laboring woman desires touch of any kind. Massage involves the specific manipulation of maternal tissue with the goal of relaxing certain areas of the body, or providing relief.[27] No harmful effects of either acupressure or acupuncture have been noted in studies specific to these modes.

Aromatherapy/Herbal Use for Labor and Birth

Aromatherapy involves the use of aromatic plant extracts, converted to essential oils, for topical use or inhalation. In labor, the essential oil may be applied to a handkerchief or washcloth, which the woman may then hold up to her nose at will. Sometimes essential oils are applied topically, but this practice requires that a professional trained in the use of essential oils be the provider to do so. As some oils can actually be harmful when applied to the skin, use of these requires knowledge as to the appropriate oils for use, contraindications, and side effects. Jasmine, geranium, rose, clary sage, neroli, ylang ylang, and lavender have been reported as having good relief when used in labor. Though effective, nurses need to remember that oils have medicinal properties, and as such, should be used in the smallest amount necessary for relief.[28]

Use of Heat and Cold Therapy for Labor and Birth

The application to the skin of either heat or cold may be soothing and pain relieving for the laboring woman. Though substantial scientific data on efficacy do not exist, anecdotally women report relief with this modality. Heat may be applied in the form of a heating pad, or warmed rice sock, water bottle, or even commercial heat packs. The most common places for heat application are the back, particularly the lower back/coccygeal area, the lower abdomen, and the groin. Typically during the second stage, the application of warm, moist compresses to the perineum provides relief from the burning sensation women often note with crowning of the fetal head. Nurses should be attentive to the temperature of anything applied to the woman's skin, to avoid burns.

Cold may be applied in the form of cold compresses or ice packs and is usually applied to the back, particularly the lower back/coccygeal area. If a woman notes she is very hot in labor, an ice pack, or washcloth soaked in ice water, may feel particularly good over her face, chest, or nape of her neck. Often times it is the alternating of cold and heat that brings relief; for example, application of heat to the coccyx for 20 minutes, then application of an ice pack to the area for 20 minutes, and then repeat. Particularly with ice packs, the cold may be too intense to be placed directly on the woman's skin; placing it over her gown may be much more tolerable. It should be understood that application of either heat or cold should only be done on a woman with intact sensation. A woman with an epidural in place, for example, will not have full sensation or perception of temperature and placing heat or cold on her skin could leave her vulnerable to skin damage.

Music for Labor and Birth

Music may be used by many women throughout labor to help relax, as well as to energize, them. The use of music to soothe patients postoperatively, or even while receiving chemotherapy, has been documented. Some women find it easier to use their rhythmic breathing patterns when they listen to music. Music, particularly music that holds special meaning for the woman, may result in the release of endorphins, which can alter the perception of pain. It is important to note that the selection of music that will be most efficacious is up to the individual woman, rather than the personnel in the room. While one woman may prefer classical music throughout labor, another may respond to a more lively jazz; it is not the type of music that is as important as is the woman's preference for, and response to, the style of music.

Use of Transcutaneous Electrical Nerve Stimulation for Labor Pain

TENS involves the transmission of electrical impulses from a hand-held device across the skin via electrodes applied to the woman's back.

TENS works basically on the same premise as the intradermal saline injections, which is the gate theory. By stimulating the large nerve fibers, the TENS causes a slight sensation that may ultimately block, or at least decrease, the woman's sensation of contractions. Though there is no strong research support that TENS is efficacious, when asked, most women who have used it report satisfaction, and a willingness to use it in a subsequent labor.[29] There is speculation as to why this may be the case, but some feel that because the woman maintains control of the TENS unit, the element of self-control adds to women's satisfaction with this mode.

Homeopathy for Labor and Birth

The practice of homeopathy has been around for approximately 200 years. Homeopathic remedies are derived from naturally occurring substances, be they plant, animal, or mineral. The original substance is diluted over and over again (via a particular process specific to the practice of homeopathy) until the resultant solution basically has only the essence of the original substance. Though somewhat contradictory to envision, the very substance that can cause particular symptoms is then used, in homeopathic form, to treat the condition. Chamomilla 200C, Sepia 200C, Aconitum Napellus 200C or 1M (1000C), and Nux Vomica 200C are homeopathic remedies that may be seen used for labor pain.[30]

UNIT 1 | TECHNIQUES FOR BREATHING AND EFFLEURAGE

This section details a breathing technique, and a massage technique called effleurage, which can be taught to the laboring woman and her coach if they have had no prior childbirth preparation. While in the past various childbirth education philosophies have ascribed to prescriptive methods of breathing, in the more recent past, there has been movement away from very prescribed techniques, and toward more physiologic patterns. The use of a breathing pattern during labor contractions has two objectives:

1. Helping the woman to relax by distracting her from the intense contraction sensations.
2. Ensuring a steady, adequate intake of oxygen.

ACTIONS	REMARKS
Begin the Breathing Technique	

This technique is done only during uterine contractions. Rest between contractions is important. Instruct the laboring woman to do the following:
• Assume a comfortable position.
• Try to maintain a relaxed state throughout the contraction.
• Concentrate on a focal point while doing the breathing (e.g., a picture of family, a button on someone's shirt).
• Begin and end each breathing technique with a cleansing breath. This is simply a very deep breath, like a big sigh. Inhalation is through the nose; exhalation is through slightly pursed lips. No counting is done through this breathing (Fig. 6.3).
	• Every woman enters labor with a different knowledge and skill of coping techniques. The nurse should assess the woman's ability to cope and provide simple instruction as indicated.
	• The use of a specific breathing pattern during labor contractions has two objectives:
	  1. Helping the woman to relax by distracting her from the contraction sensations.
	  2. Promote a steady, adequate intake of oxygen.
	• Concentrating on a focal point may provide relaxation or distraction for the woman.

Unit 1 continues on page 127

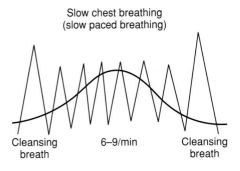

Slow chest breathing
(slow paced breathing)

Cleansing breath   6–9/min   Cleansing breath

FIGURE 6.3

ACTIONS	REMARKS
• After the cleansing breath, the woman should be urged to continue to breathe at her normal depth and rate, though she is inhaling through her nose, and exhaling through her mouth. For many women, the more intense the contraction becomes, the deeper they may want to inhale, so that their deepest breaths are over the peak of the contraction, with their normal depth and rate of breathing on either side of the peak. • Finish the contraction with a cleansing breath.	

Effleurage

This is a light massage over the abdomen with the fingertips. It can be done along with the breathing technique and/or during, or between, contractions. 1. Starting at the pubic bone, move the hands slowly up the sides of the abdomen in a wide circular sweep (Fig. 6.4). 2. During exhalation, move the fingertips down the center of the abdomen. 3. Effleurage can be done with one hand if a side-lying position is assumed.	Effleurage often has a soothing effect and provides a distraction for the mother when she concentrates on a stimulus that is not painful. Coaches can be encouraged to do this for the mother. This technique can be used to help mothers slow their breathing and match the rhythm of effleurage.

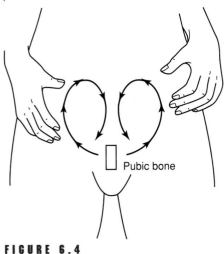

Pubic bone

FIGURE 6.4

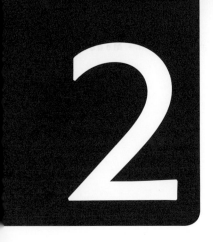

Pharmacologic Management of Labor Pain

SUSAN C. SWART AND FRANCES C. KELLY

The processes of labor and birth are intensely painful for most women. While labor pain is associated with normal, natural processes, many if not most laboring women require pain relief. Barring medical contraindications, a request from a laboring woman for pain medication, including neuraxial analgesia/anesthesia, should be honored in as timely a manner as one would respond to a nonobstetric patient in moderate-to-severe pain.[1–4]

Types of medications may include the following:

- Nonopioids
- Opioids
- Neuraxial analgesia/anesthesia
- Local anesthetic nerve blocks
- Nitrous oxide (inhaled analgesia)

• What Are the General Nursing Considerations during Administration of Pain Medications during Labor and Birth?

- Verify the laboring woman has given informed consent.
- Review and support her plan for pain relief. Remember that her plans may change as labor progresses related to unrelieved fear or anxiety, the severity of the pain, or a longer than expected labor.
- Review provider medication order.
- Assess for the presence of allergies.
- Review her medical and obstetric history, identifying any conditions or complications that could affect laboratory results, such as platelets in women with preeclampsia.
- Share pertinent history and all abnormal results with her obstetric and anesthesia providers.
- Obtain maternal vital signs prior to administration of medications.
- Evaluate FHR before and after administration of any medications.
- Assess progress of labor, the anticipated time of birth, and the gestational age of the fetus prior to administering medications. This is important because opioids cross the placenta and may cause dose-related respiratory depression in the neonate, as evidenced by:
  - reduced oxygen saturation;
  - increased carbon dioxide levels;
  - acidosis;
  - decreased suckling leading to impaired breastfeeding and diminished thermoregulation.[5]

Nonopioids

While providing better pain relief than either a placebo or no treatment, non-opioid medications are generally less effective than opioid medications in relieving labor pain.[6] Although there are few current studies, sedatives tend to improve a laboring woman's satisfaction with pain relief as compared to antihistamine. Among antihistamines, hydroxyzine may result in higher satisfaction with pain relief as compared to promethazine. There is insufficient evidence to support the administration of nonopioid medications to relieve labor pain.

Opioids

Parenteral opioids are often administered to laboring women to relieve pain. Compared with either no treatment or nonopioid medications, opioids result in higher levels of satisfaction with pain relief among laboring women. However, there is insufficient evidence to suggest that one opioid is superior to another.[4] Table 6.2 provides an overview of medications that may be administered to a laboring woman that includes common dosages; contraindications; side effects; as well as the onset, peak, and duration of action.[7]

Neuraxial Analgesia/Anesthesia

Neuraxial analgesia/anesthesia refers to administering a local anesthetic, an opioid, or more often, a combination of the two, a catheter in the epidural space, the spinal (intrathecal) space, or both.[8-10] These techniques are widely effective for managing labor pain and are increasingly requested by contemporary laboring women. Epidural analgesia/anesthesia involves threading a catheter into the epidural space to administer local anesthetics or opioids. Located between the dura mater and the enclosing vertebrae, the epidural space provides a passageway for nerve roots leaving the spinal cord. Medications administered into this space provide pain relief by blocking sensory and sympathetic nerves (Fig. 6.2). Spinal analgesia/anesthesia is the administration of medications directly into the spinal fluid in the subarachnoid space (Fig. 6.5). When administered together, local anesthetics and opioids act synergistically, allowing for lower doses of both. Neuraxial medications may be administered as a one-time bolus, as continuous infusions, as patient-controlled analgesia (PCA), or in modified dosages to promote pain relief while minimizing lower extremity motor nerve weakness and blockade.

• Are There Advantages of Neuraxial Analgesia/Anesthesia?[4]

- Superior pain relief compared to oral and parenteral medications during the first and second stages of labor
- Decreased maternal stress
- Decreased potential for maternal and fetal central nervous system (CNS) depression
- Effective pain relief for repairing perineal lacerations
- Dose may be increased to provide effective pain relief during cesarean deliveries
- Excellent alternative for women for whom general anesthesia poses an increased risk

---

• What Are the Contraindications to Neuraxial Analgesia/Anesthesia?[8-10]

- Allergy to local anesthetics (e.g., amino amide medications such as lidocaine)
- Localized infection at the proposed insertion site
- Maternal hemodynamic instability, hemorrhage, or shock
- Coagulopathy (increases risk of epidural hematoma)
- Anticoagulant, fibrinolytic, thrombolytic medication
- Indeterminate or abnormal FHR tracing requiring emergent delivery
- Maternal inability to cope
- Maternal increased intracranial pressure

• What Is the Nurse's Role in Preparing a Laboring Woman for Neuraxial Analgesia/Anesthesia?

Adequate nursing support is absolutely essential to the safe provision of neuraxial analgesia or anesthesia. The labor nurse's role in neuraxial analgesia and anesthesia is to collaborate with members of the interprofessional obstetric and anesthesia teams, organize care, monitor and document its effects, and initiate emergency care when indicated.[11] Institutional guidelines may vary regarding preparing a laboring woman for a neuraxial analgesia or anesthesia, but generally include the following:

- Reviewing her history for any contraindications, especially risk factors for hypotension.
- Initiating and maintaining IV access.

TABLE 6.2 MEDICATIONS ADMINISTERED DURING LABOR

DRUG NAME	TYPICAL DOSE	CONTRAINDICATIONS	SIDE EFFECTS	NOTES	ONSET OF ACTION (min)	PEAK EFFECT (min)	DURATION OF ACTION (hrs)
Morphine	1–2 mg IV over 4–5 min; may repeat at 5-min intervals—titrate to effect 5–10 mg IM	Altered level of consciousness (LOC), hypotension, depressed respiratory drive or rate	CNS and respiratory depression, hypotension, nausea and vomiting (N/V)		1–2 IV 10–20 IM	20 IV 60–90 IM	4–6 IV 4–6 IM
Fentanyl	10–25 mcg IV every 5–10 min 50–100 IM	Known intolerance to the drug	Dizziness, tachycardia, hypoventilation, respiratory depression, N/V		2–3 IV 7–15 IM	3–5 IV 20–30 IM	0.5–1 IV 1–2 IM
Butorphanol	1–2 mg IV, may repeat every 3–4 hrs 2–4 mg IM	Nasal form during labor or delivery	Depressed CNS, dizziness, headache (HA), N/V, hypotension, depression of fetus	Use with caution in myocardial infarction (MI) or cardiac disease. May precipitate withdrawal symptoms in narcotic-dependent patient	1–2 IV 10–30 IM	2–3 IV 30–60 IM	3–4 IV 3–4 IM
Nalbuphine	10–20 mg IV May be given every 3–6 hrs if IM	Head injury	CNS depression, crying, psychological reactions, cramps, dry mouth, bitter taste, dyspepsia, slurred speech	Caution: asthma, renal insufficiency	2–3 IV 15 IM	30 IV 60 IM	3–6 IV 3–6 IM
Remifentanil	0.2 mcg/kg and 0.8 mcg/kg	Not for intrathecal or epidural administration due to the presence of glycine in the formulation; hypersensitivity to remifentanil, fentanyl, fentanyl analogs, or any component of the formulation	Potent respiratory depressant, its use by PCA for labor has been associated with at least four case reports of respiratory and/or cardiac arrest	Remifentanil crosses the placenta; fetal and maternal concentrations may be similar	30–60 sec IV	2.5 IV	
Meperidine	25 mg IV slowly, 50–100 mg IM every 4 hrs prn	Altered LOC, patient receiving monoamine oxidase (MAO) inhibitors, hypotension, decreased respiratory rate	CNS and respiratory depression, hypotension, increased cranial pressure (ICP), N/V, tachycardia	Decreased use in clinical settings due to the neurobehavioral depression lasting for several days in the fetus	10 IV 50 IM	5–10 IV 40–50 IM	2–4 IV 2–4 IM

Table modified from: Lawrence, A., Lewis, L., Hofmeyr, G. J., et al. (2013). Maternal positions and mobility during first stage labour. *Cochrane Database System Review, 8*, CD003934.

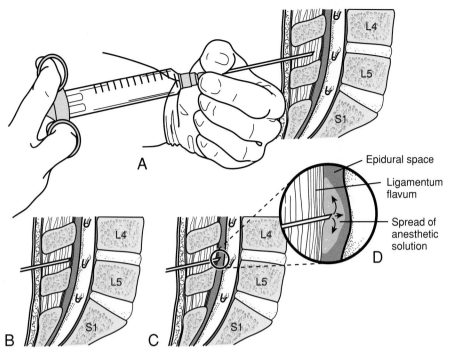

FIGURE 6.5 Technique of epidural block. **A.** Proper position of insertion. **B.** Needle in the ligamentum flavum. **C.** Tip of needle in epidural space. **D.** Force of injection pushing dura away from tip of needle. (Reprinted with permission from Taylor, T. (1993, March/April). Epidural anesthesia in the maternity patient. *Maternal-Child Nursing Journal, 18*(2), 86.)

- Hydrating patient with nondextrose containing IV fluids immediately before placement of neuraxial analgesia/anesthesia to reduce potential for hypotension. The volume of IV pre-hydration is often 500 to 1000 mL, but may vary according to the woman's condition.
- Avoiding neurotoxicity by helping to ensure that:
  - medications are sterile, preservative free, and formulated for neuraxial use; and
  - alcohol is not used on the catheter or infusion tubing.
- Avoiding initiation or changing of anticoagulation therapy prior to approval from licensed anesthesia care provider.
- Performing pre-procedure assessments of maternal–fetal well-being (e.g., maternal vital signs, interpretation of FHR tracing, etc.).

NOTE: Only a licensed anesthesia care provider may[9,11]:
- *obtain informed consent for the neuraxial analgesia/anesthesia;*
- *perform insertion and injection;*
- *bolus or re-bolus neuraxial medications;*
- *increase or decrease the rate of neuraxial analgesics/anesthetics.*

• What Is the Nurse's Role During and After Initiation of Neuraxial Analgesia/Anesthesia?

Blocking sympathetic nerves results in peripheral vasodilatation, which may decrease maternal blood pressure. Although neuraxial analgesia and anesthesia are generally considered safe for a laboring woman and her fetus, these effects may be exacerbated by the physiological and anatomic changes associated with pregnancy, resulting in adverse effects or complications.[4] The role of the registered nurse during the initiation of neuraxial analgesia/anesthesia to a laboring woman includes the following[11,12]:
- Augmenting information provided by the licensed anesthesia care provider about these pain relief techniques, and what she might experience such as feeling a warm tingling sensation down her legs after the initial bolus dose has been administered.
- Providing a calming, reassuring presence. Breathing techniques appropriate to the phase of labor may be encouraged to promote relaxation during the procedure.

- Assisting her to assume a side-lying or sitting position, with head flexed forward on chest and lower back bowed out (like a "mad" cat). If sitting, she can rest her elbows on her knees and place her feet on a chair. This promotes moderate spinal flexion to assist in locating the appropriate vertebrae.
- Monitoring the maternal and fetal status during and after the neuraxial analgesia/anesthesia procedure. Due to positioning of the mother, continuous electronic fetal monitoring may be difficult.
- The labor nurse remains present during the initial bolus or re-bolusing, and for at least 20 minutes after the administration of neuraxial analgesic or anesthetic medications and/or vital sign stabilization.
- Assess level of pain relief using facility-specific verbal or visual scales.

Table 6.3 outlines potential adverse effects and complications associated with neuraxial analgesia/anesthesia, common signs and symptoms, and the nurse's role in monitoring and helping to manage untoward effects.

Document the following per institutional policy:
- Maternal vital signs
- FHR rate or interpretation of tracing
- All position changes
- Time out as indicated by procedure
- Oxygen administration
- IV rate changes
- Maternal response to procedure
- Any complications
- Other supportive interventions, should they be necessary

Nitrous Oxide

Nitrous oxide inhalation has re-emerged as an alternative option for pain relief in laboring women in a growing number of birth facilities in the United States. Nitrous oxide (N_2O), familiarly known as "laughing gas," is a colorless, tasteless, odorless gas that may be inhaled to provide pain relief, decrease anxiety, and a feeling of euphoria within 30 to 60 seconds.[13] Benefits to the use of nitrous oxide include rapid onset of action, quick clearance through exhalation without accumulation in maternal or fetal tissues, maternal self-administration, the ability of the woman to remain awake and alert with complete functioning, and no effect on uterine activity.[13–19] Nitrous oxide may also be used in the intrapartum setting for vacuum- or forceps-assisted birth and perineal repair, or immediate postpartum procedures such as manual removal of the placenta, dilatation and curettage, or uterine exploration where local anesthesia may not meet all analgesic or anxiolytic needs.[13–15]

Contraindications for nitrous oxide use include the following[13–15,17–19]:
- Impaired consciousness
- Acute drug or alcohol intoxication
- Recent trauma
- Pneumothorax
- Increased intracranial pressure
- Increased intraocular pressure
- Intraocular surgery
- Bowel obstruction
- Middle ear surgery
- Emphysema
- Pulmonary hypertension
- Any medical history that includes the potential for physiologic spaces to form where gas could collect (recent bariatric surgery, collapsed lung as examples)
- Documented moderate to severe vitamin B_{12} deficiency
- *Inability of the woman to hold her own face mask*

NOTE: *Sedation from nitrous oxide administration is only possible if the woman continues to inhale the gas after she can no longer hold the mask tightly to her face or the tube tightly in her mouth.[17]*

TABLE 6.3	NURSE'S ROLE MONITORING FOR ADVERSE EFFECTS AND COMPLICATIONS OF NEURAXIAL ANALGESIA/ANESTHESIA

ADVERSE EFFECT OR COMPLICATION	ASSESS AND MONITOR FOR THESE SIGNS OR SYMPTOMS	NURSING CARE
Allergic or anaphylactic reaction to neuraxial medications	Swelling of face, tongue Difficulty breathing Progressive cardiopulmonary compromise or sudden arrest	Initiate emergency procedures (e.g., call for help, initiate cardiopulmonary resuscitation (CPR), promote left uterine displacement, prepare to support perimortem C/S if woman arrests and does not regain pulse or circulation within 5 min.
Intravascular injection of local anesthetic	Metallic taste in the mouth Tinnitus (ringing in the ears) Dizziness Tachycardia, bradycardia Possible hypertension Seizure Cardiopulmonary arrest	Note maternal BP and heart rate before and after test dose (often includes epinephrine). Obtain vital signs at least every 5 min during initiation of the anesthetic, and every 15 min thereafter. Initiate emergency procedures as indicated by patient condition.
Unintentional spinal (intrathecal) injection	Unexpected lower extremity motor blockade Sudden cardiopulmonary compromise or arrest	Stop neuraxial infusion. Notify anesthesia care provider. Initiate emergency procedures as indicated by patient condition.
Subdural puncture (the catheter may migrate into the subarachnoid space causing an overdose of opioid or local anesthetic)	Sudden or progressive increase in side effects such as sedation, loss of sensory and motor function leading to respiratory paralysis, and loss of consciousness	Stop neuraxial infusion. Notify anesthesia care provider. Initiate emergency procedures as indicated by patient condition.
Migration of catheter into epidural vessel that causes medications to be delivered systemically (occurs in approximately 5% of cases).	Blood in tubing Inadequate analgesia Local anesthetic toxicity such as dizziness, lightheadedness, hypotension, agitation, and seizures	Stop neuraxial infusion. Notify anesthesia care provider. Initiate emergency procedures as indicated by patient condition.
Maternal hypotension, related to peripheral vasodilation often resulting from sensory and sympathetic nerve blockade	Systolic BP <100 mm Hg or a 20% decrease from pre-procedure levels. Systolic pressure below 90 mm Hg is considered inadequate to maintain uterine blood flow necessary for fetal oxygenation. Nausea, vomiting Fetal responses such as changes in baseline rate and/or late decelerations	Pre-hydrate according to facility guidelines. Obtain vital signs at least every 5 min during initiation of the anesthetic and until patient is stable, and every 15 min thereafter. Promote semi-fowlers or lateral positioning. Avoid supine positioning. Administer additional IV fluid bolus according to facility guidelines (e.g., 500 mL). Oxygen 10 L by non-rebreather facemask. A vasopressor (e.g., ephedrine or phenylephrine) medication may be administered per anesthesia care provider order. Notify obstetric provider. Initiate emergency procedures as indicated by patient condition.

table continues on page 134

133

ADVERSE EFFECT OR COMPLICATION	ASSESS AND MONITOR FOR THESE SIGNS OR SYMPTOMS	NURSING CARE
Respiratory depression or sedation	Respiratory rate <12 breaths per minute. Difficult to arouse. Fetal responses such as fetal bradycardia and/or late decelerations.	No other opioid or CNS depressant should be administered. Stop neuraxial infusion. Oxygen 10 L by non-rebreather face mask. Naloxone may be administered by anesthesia care provider. Notify obstetric provider. Initiate emergency procedures as indicated by patient condition.
Urinary retention, which may impact physiologic labor progress and fetal descent. A full bladder may be traumatized during birth.	Diminished or absent bladder sensation. Bladder distention.	Encourage voiding before the procedure. Visually assess and palpate the area above the symphysis pubis for evidence of a full bladder. If unable to void on bedpan, perform intermittent urinary catheterization. There is no evidence to support routine insertion of urinary catheter to bedside drainage.
Impaired motor function (associated with administration of local anesthetic agents).	Inability to move legs. Unstable core strength when sitting up.	The woman should remain in bed when receiving epidural local anesthetic medications. Assist the woman to change position regularly, maintaining proper alignment, and protecting bony prominences.
Pruritus (associated with administration of opioids).	Complain of itching on face, arms, trunk, abdomen, or legs	Notify anesthesia care provider. Usually, the pruritus resolves within 1 hr of onset and fewer than 20% of women require medication. Diphenhydramine or naloxone may be effective.
Shivering	Uncontrollable shaking May not complain of feeling cold	Apply blankets for comfort and support. Assess maternal temperature at least every 4 hrs if membranes intact. Reassess maternal temperature every 2 hrs if membranes ruptured, or more often if ≥100.4°F.
Epidural hematoma	Changes in sensory or motor function, including progressive numbness, weakness, or bowel and bladder dysfunction	Avoid administering anticoagulants within 12 hrs before neuraxial analgesia or anesthesia. Notify anesthesia care provider.
Epidural abscess	Changes in sensory/motor function including: • Unexplained back pain • Bowel or bladder dysfunction • Fever • Neck stiffness.	Ensure site dressing intact while catheter in place, assessing site regularly. Assess maternal temperature. Notify anesthesia care provider.

From Centers for Disease Control and Prevention. (2014). *HIV transmission risk.* Atlanta, GA; Piot, P. (2006). AIDS: From crisis management to sustained strategic response. *Lancet, 368,* 526–530.

TABLE 6.4 GUIDELINES FOR ADMINISTRATION OF NITRUS OXIDE

Establish unit-specific criteria for use that represents consensus from obstetrical and obstetrical anesthesia, and neonatal providers (as well as institutional and risk management support) that addresses:
- role responsibilities;
- supervision of administration;
- equipment storage and set up;
- ongoing assessment parameters.

NOTE: *Nitrous oxide administration does not constitute anesthesia delivery because of the concentrations and intermittent use.*

Assessment and evaluation of the woman as a candidate for nitrous oxide may include the following:
- History
- Vital signs
- Fetal assessment
- Oxygen saturation

Ensure informed consent:
- may be verbal or written;
- possible benefits and side effects.

Proper equipment set up:
- Equipment attached to the tank of nitrous oxide and tank or wall O2 supply utilizing a blender designed for specific obstetric use
- Delivery up to a 50/50 nitrous oxide/oxygen delivery ratio in an intermittent, as opposed to continuous stream

Preparation of the woman and support persons:
- Instruction and reinforcement on self administration
  - Correct placement of facemask or mouthpiece to create a seal
  - Timing of breathing for maximum analgesic effects (to begin approximately 30 sec prior to the start of a contraction)
  - Woman is the ONLY one allowed to hold mask
  - Discontinue when the woman no longer desires or needs analgesia

Documentation:
- Note initial administration and duration of use in labor
- Nursing notes to include the woman's use of nitrous oxide, efficacy of use in providing pain relief, any side effects, or complications
- Ongoing assessment parameters
- Patient safety

From Centers for Disease Control and Prevention. (1987). Recommendations for prevention of HIV transmission in health-care settings. *Morbidity and Mortality Weekly Report, 36*(SU02), 1–19; Chin, J. (1994). The growing impact of HIV/AIDS pandemic on children born to HIV-infected women. *Clinics in Perinatology, 21*(1), 111–114; Barkowsky, W., Krasinski, K., Pollack, H., et al. (1992). Early diagnosis of human immunodeficiency virus infection in children less than 6 months of age: Comparison of polymerase chain reaction, culture, and plasma antigen captive techniques. *Journal of Infectious Diseases, 166*(3), 616–619; Centers for Disease Control and Prevention. (2006). *Revised recommendations for HIV testing of adults, adolescents and pregnant women in health-care settings.* Atlanta, GA.

Relative contraindications for use include women who experience intolerable side effects of the medication (nausea, vomiting, dizziness, dysphoria), hemodynamic instability or impaired oxygenation, and some category II or III EFM tracings.

Administration

Administration of nitrous oxide in the intrapartum setting requires a collaborative approach between the woman and her healthcare providers. Considerations for guidelines in administration of nitrous oxide are presented in Table 6.4.

As more institutions procure the necessary equipment and develop guidelines for use in the birth setting, nitrous oxide may become a more readily available pain relief alternative for all women in labor.

Local Anesthetic[20]

The primary care provider may inject local anesthetics into the perineum or vaginal wall during the second stage of labor to aid in pain management during labor/birth, application of vacuum or forceps, and/or perineal repair. Lidocaine hydrochloride or chloroprocaine hydrochloride may be used for a pudendal or paracervical block:

Pudendal Block

- Anesthetizes lower vagina, vulva, and perineum
- Used for assisted births and perineal repair
- Potential risks include hematoma, infection, nerve damage, local anesthetic toxicity, and extension of the nerve block

Paracervical Block

- Used for labor pain
- Newer superficial techniques along with lower concentrations of anesthetic have decreased the risk of fetal bradycardia historically associated with the technique.

PRACTICE/REVIEW QUESTIONS

After reviewing this module, answer the following questions.

1. There are many goals in intrapartum care. List at least four.

   a. _____

   b. _____

   c. _____

   d. _____

2. What steps can the caregiver take to promote achievement of the goals in question 1?

   a. _____

   b. _____

   c. _____

   d. _____

3. Discuss six ways that you, as a nurse, can help make the laboring woman more comfortable.

   a. _____

   b. _____

   c. _____

   d. _____

   e. _____

   f. _____

4. What activities do caregivers engage in that laboring women perceive as "supportive"?

   a. _____

   b. _____

   c. _____

   d. _____

5. List at least five theories and/or factors thought to be related to causes of pain in labor.

   a. _____

   b. _____

   c. _____

   d. _____

   e. _____

6. What are the three therapies commonly used for non-pharmacologic pain relief in labor?

   a. _____

   b. _____

   c. _____

7. What are the two reasons to provide sterile water injections in labor for women with a baby in an occiput posterior position?

   a. _____

   b. _____

8. Describe the technique for breathing through labor.

   a. _____

9. Describe the technique of effleurage.

   a. _____

10. Discuss the measures you should take when administering pain medication to the laboring woman.

    _____

    _____

    _____

    _____

11. Neuraxial anesthesia is intended to provide complete blockade of _____ nerves and minimal blockade of _____.

12. During the first stage of labor, the anesthetic dose is given so that the sensory block is limited to the lower _____ and the upper _____ segments. This allows _____ to be maintained to avoid interfering with internal rotation of the fetal head.

13. Who is responsible for explaining to the mother the essentials of the epidural procedure and possible complications?

    _____

14. State three contraindications to neuraxial anesthesia.

    a. _____

    b. _____

    c. _____

15. Why are IV glucose solutions not recommended for fluid loading before epidural administration?

    _____

16. Why is fluid loading done before neuraxial administration?

    _____

17. The mother's bladder status should be evaluated every.

    _____

18. The most common complication with an neuraxial is

    _____

19. List three steps to take in a maternal hypotensive episode with neuraxial anesthesia.

    a. _____

    b. _____

    c. _____

20. What are three signs associated with intravascular injection of local anesthetic?

    a. _____

    b. _____

    c. _____

21. The epidural catheter can be removed by a trained nurse if hospital policy and state practice act allow.

    a. True

    b. False

22. There are no known neonatal effects associated with maternal use of neuraxial during labor and delivery.

    a. True

    b. False

23. Nitrous oxide is most efficacious for laboring women when she begins inhaling:

    a. 2 minutes prior to a contraction

    b. 30 seconds prior to a contraction

    c. at the beginning of a contraction

PRACTICE/REVIEW ANSWER KEY

1. Any four of the following:
    a. Ensure a safe passage for mother and baby.
    b. Promote maternal coping behaviors.
    c. Support the mother and her family.
    d. Follow through on the mother's choices and desires whenever possible.
    e. Provide pain relief.
    f. Offer reassurance and information.
2. a. Create a quiet environment.
    b. Listen actively.
    c. Touch in a therapeutic manner.
    d. Integrate the support person.
    e. Explain your findings.
    f. Acknowledge that the examination might be painful.
    g. Pay attention to what the woman says about any pain.
    h. Apologize for causing her any pain.
3. a. Do not leave the mother alone while she is in active labor.
    b. Give frequent mouth care: give ice chips, lubricate lips, and encourage mouth rinses.
    c. Massage abdomen, back, and legs.
    d. Be sure the room is well ventilated.
    e. Control the environment so that quiet, privacy, and appropriate lighting are provided.
    f. Promote participation of a support person.
4. a. Helping the woman feel that she can handle her contractions
    b. Showing her how to breathe or position herself
    c. Anticipating her information needs
    d. Reinforcing information and being concrete
5. Any five of the following:
    a. Hypoxia of the uterine muscle because of diminished blood supply to the uterus during a contraction
    b. Stretching of and pressure on the cervix, vagina, and perineal floor muscles and perineum
    c. Traction on reproductive structures such as the fallopian tubes, ovaries, and uterine ligaments
    d. Pressure on the bladder, urethra, and rectum
    e. Nature of contractions (intensity and duration)
    f. Degree of cervical dilatation and perineal distension
    g. Maternal age, parity, and general health
    h. Fetal size and position (e.g., posterior positions are usually accompanied by intense back pain)
    i. Cultural influences and upbringing
    j. Value system and education level
    k. Anxiety and fear
    l. Lack of knowledge or preparation
    m. Absence of supportive significant person
    n. Lack of motivation

6. Any three of the following:
   a. Acupressure
   b. Heat and cold therapy
   c. Hydrotherapy
   d. Massage
   e. Intradermal injections of sterile water

7. a. Blocked pain pathways according to the gate theory
   b. Release of endogenous endorphins

8. a. The woman takes a cleansing breath at the beginning and end of every contraction, breathing at her usual rate and depth through the contraction. She may breathe more deeply over the peak of the contraction, as intensity builds.

9. a. Starting at the pubic bone, move the hands slowly up the sides of the abdomen in a wide circular sweep. During exhalation, move the fingertips down the center of the abdomen.

10. Know the mother's medical and obstetric history; check for allergies. Take vital signs, BP, and FHR readings before administering any medications. Know the status of labor and anticipated delivery at the time medication is given. Consider the mother's request. Be aware of the therapeutic effects, contraindications, and side effects of the drug being given. Use a large-bore (18-gauge) catheter when starting an IV infusion, which permits rapid fluid or blood administration if needed. Consider the mother's weight, the progress of labor, the maturity and size of the fetus, and the dosage of medicine being prepared. Give all IV medications at the beginning of a contraction, when the blood vessels of the uterus and placenta are somewhat constricted. If possible, inject the medicine over a few minutes. Because the medication is concentrated in bolus form, this technique enables a smaller amount of the drug to cross the placenta during the first few minutes of circulation so that the fetus does not receive a large amount of the drug all at once. Aspirate the syringe before giving any medication. Use filters with all IV medications and epidural catheters. Filters help to screen out glass particles and bacteria that are sometimes present in ampules after they have been broken open. Do not give any drug with which you are unfamiliar. Assess pain relief. Allow the mother to assume other optimal positions for fetal rotation.

11. Sensory; motor

12. T10 (thoracic); lumbar; perineal tone

13. The physician and anesthesiologist

14. Any three of the following:
    a. Refusal
    b. Maternal fear
    c. Coagulation defects
    d. Maternal hypotension

15. Because of possible fetal hyperglycemia with subsequent and rebound newborn hypoglycemia

16. The epidural induces vascular vasodilatation with resultant decreased BP. Adequate plasma volume helps offset hypotensive effects.

17. 30 minutes

18. Hypotension

19. a. Place mother in a full lateral position.
    b. Give oxygen.
    c. Give 250 to 500 mL IV bolus non–glucose-balanced saline solution.

20. Any three of the following:
    a. Change in maternal heart rate
    b. Metallic taste
    c. Loss of consciousness
    d. Seizures
    e. Tinnitus
    f. Maternal hypertension

21. a. True

22. b. False

23. c. at the beginning of a contraction

REFERENCES

Part 1

1. Cassidy, T. (2006). *Birth: The surprising history of how we are born.* New York, NY: Grove Press.
2. Simpson, K. R., Lyndon, A., Wilson, J., et al. (2012). Nurses' perceptions of critical issues requiring consideration in the development of guidelines for professional registered nurse staffing for perinatal units. *Journal of Obstetric, Gynecologic, & Neonatal Nursing, 41,* 474–482.
3. Nieuwenhuijze, M. J., de Jonge, A., Korstjens, I., et al. (2013). Influence on birthing positions affects women's sense of control in second stage of labour. *Midwifery, 29*(11), e107–e114.
4. Hodnett, E. D. (2002). Pain and women's satisfaction with the experience of childbirth: A systematic review. *American Journal of Obstetrics and Gynecology, 186*(5), S160–S172.
5. Fahey, J. O., Cohen, S. R., Holme, F., et al. (2012). Promoting cultural humility during labor and birth. Putting theory into action during PRONTO obstetric and neonatal emergency training. *Journal of Perinatal & Neonatal Nursing, 27*(1), 36–42.
6. Hodnett, E. D. (2000). Caregiver support for women during childbirth (Cochrane review). *The Cochrane Library,* (4). Oxford: Update Software.
7. Lawrence, A., Lewis, L., Hofmeyr, G. J., et al. (2013). Maternal positions and mobility during first stage labour. *Cochrane Database System Review, 8,* CD003934.
8. Michel, S. C., Rake, A., Treiber, K., et al. (2002). MR obstetric pelvimetry: Effect of birthing position on pelvic bony dimensions. *AJR American Journal Roentgenology, 179,* 1063–1067.
9. Niemczyk, N. A. (2014). Maternal positioning. *Journal of Midwifery & Women's Health, 59*(3), 362–363.
10. Fields, J. M., Catallo, K., Au, A. K., et al. (2012). Resuscitation of the pregnant patient: What is the effect of patient positioning on inferior vena cava diameter? *Resuscitation, 84*(3), 304–330.
11. Mendelson, C. L. (1946). Aspiration of stomach contents into the lungs during obstetric anesthesia. *American Journal of Obstetrics and Gynecology, 52,* 191–205.
12. Sharts-Hopko, N. (2010). Oral intake during labor: A review of the evidence. *The American Journal of Maternal/Child Nursing, 35*(4), 197–203.
13. James, D. (2011). Routine obstetrical interventions: Research agenda for the next decade. *Journal of Perinatal & Neonatal Nursing, 25*(2), 148–152.
14. Rahmani, R., Khakbazan, Z., Yavari, P., et al. (2012). Effect of oral carbohydrate intake on labor progress: Randomized controlled trial. *Iranian Journal of Public Health, 41*(11), 59–66.

15. American Society of Anesthesiologists. (1999). *Practice guidelines for obstetrical anesthesia care.* Park Ridge, IL.

16. Doulas of North America (DONA). What is a doula? Retrieved from: www.dona.org/faq.html

17. Kozhimannil, K. B., Attanasio, L. B., Jou, J., et al. (2014). Potential benefits of increased access to doula support during childbirth. *American Journal of Managed Care, 20*(6), e340–e352.

18. Veringa, I., Buitendijk, S., de Miranda, E., et al. (2011). Pain cognitions as predictors of the request for pain relief during the first stage of labor: A prospective study. *Journal of Psychosomatic Obstetrics & Gynecology, 32*(3), 119–125.

19. Curzik, D., Jokic-Begic, N. (2011). Anxiety sensitivity and anxiety as correlates of expected, experienced and recalled labor pain. *Journal of Psychosomatic Obstetrics & Gynecology, 32*(4), 198–203.

20. Simkin, P. (1995). Reducing pain and enhancing progress in labor: A guide to nonpharmacologic methods for maternity caregivers. *Birth, 22*(3), 161–170.

21. Simkin, P., O'hara, M. (2002). Nonpharmacologic relief of pain during labor: Systematic reviews of five methods. *American Journal of Obstetrics & Gynecology, 186*, S131–S159.

22. Reynolds, J. L. (1998). Practice tips. Intracutaneous sterile water injections for low back pain during labour. *Canadian Family Physician, 44*, 2391–2392.

23. Mårtensson, L., Nyberg, K., Wallin, G. (2000). Subcutaneous versus intracutaneous injections of sterile water for labour analgesia: A comparison of perceived pain during administration. *British Journal of Obstetrics & Gynecology, 107*, 1248–1251.

24. Hutton, E. K., Kasperink, M., Rutten, M., et al. (2009). Sterile water injection for labour pain: A systematic review and meta-analysis of randomised controlled trials. *British Journal of Obstetrics & Gynecology, 116*, 1158–1166.

25. Nesheim, B. I., Kinge, R., Berg, B., et al. (2003). Acupuncture during labor can reduce the use of meperidine: A controlled clinical study. *Clinical Journal of Pain, 19*, 187–191.

26. Hjelmstedt, A., Shenoy, S. T., Stener-Victorin, E., et al. (2010). Acupressure to reduce labor pain: A randomized controlled trial. *Acta Obstetricia et Gynecologica Scandinavica, 89*, 1453–1459.

27. Smith, C. A., Levett, K. M., Collins, C. T., et al. (2012). Massage, reflexology and other manual methods for pain management in labour. *Cochrane Database System Review, 2*, CD009290.

28. Tiran, D. (2000). Massage and aromatherapy. In Tiran, D., Mack, S. (Eds.), *Complementary therapies for pregnancy and childbirth* (2nd ed.). New York, NY: Balliere Tindall.

29. Dowswell, T., Bedwell, C., Lavender, T., et al. (2009). Transcutaneous electrical nerve stimulation (TENS) for pain relief in labour. *Cochrane Database System Review, 2*, CD007214.

30. McLeod, S. Homeopathy for natural childbirth: A simple guide for moms and birth professionals. http://prenatalcoach.com/homeopathy-natural-childbirth-guide/. Accessed November 14, 2014.

Part 2

1. American College of Obstetricians and Gynecologists. (2009). *Optimal goals for anesthesia in care in obstetrics* (Committee Opinion No. 433). Washington, DC: Author.

2. American College of Obstetricians and Gynecologists. (2004). *Pain relief during labor* (Committee Opinion No. 295). Washington, DC: Author.

3. American Society of Anesthesiologists. (2008). *Optimal goals for anesthesia care in obstetrics.* Park Ridge, IL: Author.

4. Jones, L., Othman, M., Dowswell, T., et al. (2012). Pain management for woman in labour: An overview of systematic reviews. *Cochrane Database Syst Rev, 2*, CD009234. Accessed July 29, 2015.

5. Reynolds, F. (2010). The effects of maternal labour analgesia on the fetus. *Best Practice & Research Clinical Obstetrics and Gynaecology, 24*(3), 289–302.

6. Othman, M., Jones, L., Neilson, J. (2012). Non-opioid drugs for pain management in labour. *Cohcrane Database Systematic Reviews, 7*, CD009223.

7. Burke, C. (2014). Pain in labor: Non-pharmacologic and pharmacologic management. In Simpson, K. R., Creehan, P. A. (Eds.), *Perinatal nursing* (pp. 488–529). Philadephia, PA: Wolters Kluwer.

8. Wong, C. (2009). Epidural and spinal analgesia for labor and vaginal delivery. In Chesnut, D. H., Polley, L. S., Tsen, L.C., et al. (Eds.), *Chesnut's obstetric anesthesia: Principles and practice* (4th ed., pp. 429–492). St. Louis, MO: Mosby.

9. Wahab, N., Robinson, N. (2011). Analgesia and anaesthesia in labour. *Obstetrics, Gynaecology & Reproductive Medicine, 21*, 137–141.

10. American Society of Anesthesiologsts. (2009). Statement on pain relief in labor. Approved by the House of Delegates on October 13, 1999, last amended October 21, 2009. Retrieved from: http://www. Asahq.org/publicationsAndServices/standards/47.pdf

11. Association of Women's Health, Obstetric & Neonatal Nurses. (2011). *Nursing care of the woman receiving regional analgesia/anesthesia in labor.* Washington, DC: Author.

12. Association of Women's Health, Obstetric & Neonatal Nurses. (2015). Role of the registered nurse in the care of the pregnant woman receiving analgesia and anesthesia by catheter techniques: Position statement. *Nursing for Women's Health, 19*(1), 89–92.

13. Starr, S. A., Collins, M., Baysinger, C. (2011). *Nitrous oxide use in the intrapartum/immediate postpartum period* (Labor and delivery, trans.) (pp. 1–10). Nashville, TN: Vanderbilt University Medical Center.

14. Stewart, L. S., Collins, M. (2012). Nitrous oxide as labor analgesia. *Nursing for Women's Health, 16*(5), 398–409.

15. Collins, M. R., Starr, S. A., Bishop, J. T., et al. (2012). Nitrous oxide for labor analgesia: Expanding analgesic options for women in the United States. *Reviews in Obstetrics and Gynecology, 5*(3–4), e126–e131.

16. Rosen, M. (2002) Nitrous oxide for relief of labor pain: A systematic review. *American Journal of Obstetrics and Gynecology, 186*(5), 110–127.

17. Rooks, J. P. (2011). Safety and risks of nitrous oxide labor analgesia: A review. *Journal of Midwifery & Women's Health, 56*(6), 557–565.

18. Likis, F. E., Andrews, J. C., Collins, M. R., et al. (2014). Nitrous oxide for the management of labor pain: A systematic review. *Anesthesia and Analgesia, 118*(1), 153–167.

19. Starr, S. A., Baysinger, C. L. (2013). Inhaled nitrous oxide for labor analgesia. *Anesthesiology Clinics, 31*(3), 623–634.

20. Volmanen, P., Palomaki, O., Ahonen, J. (2011). Alternatives to neuraxial analgesia for labor. *Current Opinion in Anesthesiology, 24*(3), 235–241.

Intrapartum Electronic Fetal Monitoring

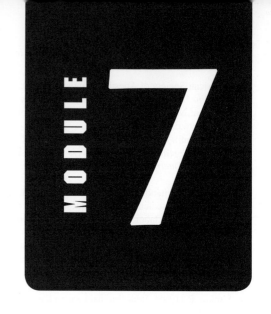

MODULE 7

LISA A. MILLER AND DONNA J. RUTH

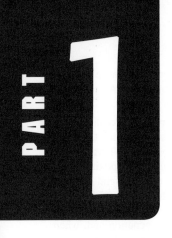

PART 1

Introduction and Overview

This module will provide clinicians with practical information on intrapartum fetal monitoring, with a primary focus on electronic fetal monitoring (EFM). The module is divided into six sections. Part 1 provides an overview of intrapartum fetal monitoring and includes information on the history of fetal monitoring, differences between intermittent auscultation (IA) and EFM, and the equipment and methods for both modalities. Parts 2 and 3 cover definitions, basic physiology, and offer a standardized approach to interpretation and management of EFM, while Part 4 provides information on umbilical cord gas analysis. Documentation is reviewed in Part 5, and Part 6 concludes this module with a self-assessment. The module has been written as a concise and practical guide to daily clinical practice, and is not meant to be an authoritative treatise on either EFM or IA. Clinicians are encouraged to obtain ongoing continuing education in fetal monitoring, and to regularly review the literature as part of the maintenance of professional practice.

Intrapartum Fetal Monitoring

Intrapartum fetal monitoring consists of the assessment and evaluation of fetal status during labor. During the intrapartum period, information related to both fetal heart rate (FHR) and uterine activity (UA) is obtained and interpreted to assist clinicians in three primary areas: (1) the evaluation of fetal oxygenation; (2) the application of conservative corrective measures; and (3) the ongoing management of labor and provision of appropriate labor support. Fetal monitoring may be done by IA, EFM, or a combination of both, but all laboring patients should have some type of ongoing evaluation over the course of labor.

Historically, monitoring of the FHR by auscultation has been in existence for over 200 years. The use of the electronic fetal monitor began in the late 1960s. Over the last several decades, the use of EFM has become ubiquitous in hospital labor and delivery settings.[1-3] But the routine use of EFM (especially continuous EFM throughout labor) is being questioned today, especially for low-risk patients. A systematic review of 13 randomized trials that included >37,000 women of varying risk status and compared continuous EFM to IA found no significant difference in the majority of outcomes including perinatal mortality, cerebral palsy, hypoxic ischemic encephalopathy (HIE), and neonatal intensive care unit (NICU) admission. While the review did demonstrate decreased incidence of neonatal seizures in the continuous EFM group, there were no differences in neurodevelopmental impairment at ≥12 months of age, and 661 women would need to be monitored in labor to prevent one neonatal seizure. The review also noted that continuous EFM is associated with significantly higher rates of cesarean and operative vaginal deliveries.[4]

Although it may seem that the results of systematic analysis would point to the complete abandonment of EFM for all patients, clinicians must understand some of the limitations of the current state of the science regarding EFM. These include the following:

- Only 2 of the 13 randomized trials in the systematic review were of high quality.
- None of the randomized trials utilized standardized nomenclature, interpretation, or management.
- Most of the trials did not include high-risk patients, so the safety of IA is not clear in the high-risk population, where continuous EFM continues to be recommended.[1]
- The vast majority of cases of cerebral palsy are related in whole or in part to antepartum events, not intrapartum events, and therefore the lack of a reduction in cerebral palsy related to EFM use is not an unexpected finding.[5]

- When used as a *diagnostic tool* for the development of cerebral palsy, the false-positive rate of EFM may be as high as 99.8%[5]; but no trials to date have compared IA to application of EFM as a *screening tool.*

While EFM has failed as a diagnostic tool, the value of EFM as a screening tool during the intrapartum period should not be lightly dismissed. There is wide consensus regarding the negative predictive value of two EFM components. The presence of either moderate FHR variability or an FHR acceleration provides reliable evidence to exclude the possibility of hypoxia-related central nervous system depression.[6,7] Combined with an understanding of basic fetal oxygenation, normal versus abnormal uterine activity, and the importance of clinical context, EFM used as a screening tool can assist clinicians in safe and effective labor support and assessment of fetal response to labor; intervening appropriately to correct interruption of oxygenation and, when necessary, proceeding with expedited delivery *prior* to the deterioration of fetal acid–base status. As Clark et al. correctly point out, "one important goal of intrapartum care is delivery of the fetus, when possible, prior to the development of damaging degrees of hypoxia/acidemia."[6]

Regardless of the ongoing debate regarding EFM versus IA, the use of EFM remains very common in many labor and delivery units. Clinicians need to be skilled in both EFM and IA to safely care for the variety of patients cared for in contemporary birth settings. Ultimately, the decision as to which monitoring method is used should be a joint decision between patients and healthcare providers. Factors that influence this decision may include clinical situation and risk status, availability of equipment, unit staffing patterns, and knowledge and skill level of staff (in the selected monitoring method). It has been suggested that informed consent be obtained before the initiation of any type of fetal monitoring[8,9]; however, clinicians should understand that when discussing options with patients, there are only two choices, IA and EFM, as no studies have been performed (nor are any likely) to compare monitoring versus no monitoring during labor. Regardless of which method of monitoring is chosen, each unit should have written policies and guidelines for *both* IA and EFM that are in accordance with guidelines endorsed by professional organizations such as the American Congress of Obstetrics and Gynecology (ACOG), the Association of Women's Health, Obstetric, and Neonatal Nurses (AWHONN), and the American College of Nurse-Midwives (ACNM). Unit guidelines should clearly list the procedures to be followed when using the chosen monitoring technique, define the standard terminology to be used for each method, and include the required frequency of assessments.[10] See Table 7.1 for the recommended frequency of assessment based on the phase and stage of labor. It is important to note that the recommended frequencies of assessments in latent phase of labor have not been established, and until further research is available, clinicians may be wise to comply with the standards set for active phase rather than choose an arbitrary standard.

TABLE 7.1 GUIDELINES FOR ASSESSMENT OF FETAL HEART RATE		
LOW RISK	**IA**	**EFM**
Active phase	q30min	q30min
Second stage	q15min	q15min
Risk Factors		
Active phase	q15min	q15min
Second stage	q5min	q5min

From American Academy of Pediatrics & American College of Obstetricians and Gynecologists. (2012). *Guidelines for perinatal care* (7th ed.). Washington, DC: Author.

Guidelines for Assessment of Fetal Heart Rate[10]

Intermittent Auscultation (IA)

While IA is not the primary focus of this module, it will be briefly reviewed here for two important reasons: (1) it may be the primary method of fetal assessment in labor for low-risk women following proper informed consent; and (2) it is the only alternative to EFM, making it an appropriate and necessary adjunct for situations where obtaining an interpretable EFM tracing is difficult. IA involves monitoring the FHR, through the use of either a fetoscope or Doppler, at specified intervals. IA allows for assessment of the FHR without belts, patches, or cables, and this means greater maternal mobility. Therefore, IA may be much more comfortable for the laboring woman, as well as promote a more natural, less technological environment for birth.

IA has been found to be a safe and reasonable option for monitoring low-risk women during uncomplicated labor when performed by a practitioner who:
- is experienced in the labor and delivery setting and competent in the use of IA;
- can discern, by auditory means, significant changes in the FHR;
- is practiced in palpating uterine contraction and relaxation;
- is capable of initiating appropriate interventions when indicated.[11]

Components Assessed with Intermittent Auscultation

In general, baseline rate and baseline rhythm can both be evaluated using IA. Baseline rate is assessed between contractions and during periods when the fetus is not active. In addition, baseline variations such as tachycardia (rate greater than 160 beats per minute [bpm]) and bradycardia (rate less than 110 bpm) can be readily identified. If tachycardia or bradycardia is suspected, then more frequent assessments may be warranted to determine if a baseline change has occurred or if the increase or decrease in rate was temporary. Auscultation can also be used to detect transient increases and decreases in the FHR, but adequacy of accelerations and types of decelerations based on current nomenclature cannot be confirmed without the visual assessment of an EFM tracing, as IA is a solely auditory assessment.

Baseline rhythm (regular or irregular) can also be evaluated with auscultation. Actual heart sounds can be heard using a stethoscope, fetoscope, or Pinard stethoscope. Doppler can be used to identify baseline rhythm, but the sound produced by the Doppler device is a representation of, not the actual, heart sounds. Auscultation may be used to verify the presence of a dysrhythmia.[11] If an irregular rhythm is heard, alternative methods of assessment, such as ultrasound or fetal echocardiogram, may be indicated to determine the type of dysrhythmia present. The majority of dysrhythmias discovered in the intrapartum period are benign and do not require intervention other than notification of the pediatric service for appropriate follow-up of the newborn.

Performance of Intermittent Auscultation

Follow these steps when performing IA:
1. Explain the procedure to the laboring woman.
2. Determine fetal position using Leopold's maneuvers.
3. Palpate the uterus to assess for contractions and resting tone. This helps the practitioner to assess the FHR response to uterine activity.
4. Apply the fetoscope or Doppler device on the maternal abdomen over where the fetal back is located (this is typically where fetal heart sounds will most audible).
5. Auscultate the FHR between contractions, beginning immediately after the end of the contraction and listening for at least 30- to 60-second intervals to determine the FHR and rhythm and response to uterine activity.
6. Count the maternal pulse to differentiate between fetal and maternal heart rates.
7. Document your assessments.
8. Share your findings with the laboring woman.

Assessment of fetal heart tones should be performed **before**:
- induction or augmentation of labor with oxytocin;
- initiation of anesthesia;
- administration of medications;
- ambulation;
- artificial rupture of membranes (amniotomy);
- transfer or discharge.

Assessment of the fetal heart tones should be performed **after**:
- rupture of membranes (either spontaneous or artificial);
- ambulation;
- vaginal examination;
- excessive uterine activity;
- change in oxytocin dosage;
- change in analgesia and anesthesia dosing;
- admission to the labor and delivery unit.

Advantages/Benefits of Intermittent Auscultation

Patient comfort—the woman may be up and about and may move easily in bed. Sometimes the abdominal area and the lower back of a laboring woman are extremely sensitive. Belts and other equipment can cause irritation and discomfort and interfere with her ability to concentrate and relax.

Facilitation of ambulation—ambulation often contributes to greater patient comfort and perhaps more rapid progress in labor. Freedom of movement (i.e., the ability to walk and stand) is supported by IA.

Requirement of caregiver to be at the bedside—this provides many benefits, such as comfort, support, and encouragement. The so-called doula effect, the presence of continuous labor support, has been shown to be of clear benefit to laboring women,[12] and is a critical component of intrapartum care for all patients, regardless of risk status. With IA, close, frequent contact between the patient and caregiver occurs routinely.

Less technology—women who desire an atmosphere in which birth is viewed as a normal, natural event might prefer this method of monitoring. The ACNM supports a judicious use of technology in labor, including avoidance of unnecessary use of technology, and specifically states that "use of technology may be influenced by a woman's preferences, and in the absence of clear evidence for use or avoidance of a certain intervention, a woman's choice should prevail."[9]

Neonatal outcomes—outcomes are comparable to those with EFM, at least in the low-risk population.

Lower cesarean birth rates—cesarean birth rates are lower in comparison with EFM as studied to date.

Equipment—equipment required for IA is less costly than that necessary for EFM.

Disadvantages/Limitations of Intermittent Auscultation

Practitioner skilled in auscultation—auscultation skills are required to perform assessments. Competency in the performance of auscultation should be demonstrated before the provision of care.

Nurse-to-patient ratio of 1:1—the nurse-to-patient ratio must be 1:1 and auscultation must occur on a regular basis for IA to be comparable to EFM. Nursing shortages and unit staffing patterns may sometimes preclude this capability.

Invasion of personal space—because very frequent, close personal contact is required to provide adequate assessment through IA, there may be some women who feel as if their personal space is being invaded.

Rapid heart rates (greater than 160 bpm)—heart rates greater than 160 bpm may be difficult to accurately count.

Inability to evaluate certain aspects of the FHR—examples include variability and the ability to discern the type of deceleration heard.

Physical limitations of equipment—maternal obesity, fetal position, and hydramnios may interfere with the practitioner's ability to adequately assess the FHR by IA.

Documentation of FHR Obtained by Intermittent Auscultation

Documentation of auscultation findings must be done with each assessment. Each entry should include baseline rate and rhythm, the presence or absence of changes (increases or decreases) in the baseline rate. Other information that should be documented includes any change in patient status, all nursing interventions and patient responses, and any communication that occurs with healthcare providers.

Electronic Fetal Monitoring

EFM is the primary focus of this module, specifically its use during the intrapartum period. EFM is an electronic method of providing a continuous visual record of the FHR and obtaining information about the laboring woman's uterine activity (Fig. 7.1). This information, which is recorded on *graph paper*, allows an ongoing minute-to-minute assessment of the FHR during labor. It also provides a permanent medical record, whether on paper or via electronic archiving.

NOTE: At the onset of EFM, validation of the equipment should be performed by auscultation of the FHR with a non mechanical means such as the fetoscope, and testing of the internal circuitry of the fetal monitor is accomplished by pushing the "test" button on the monitor and examining the test lines on the graph paper.

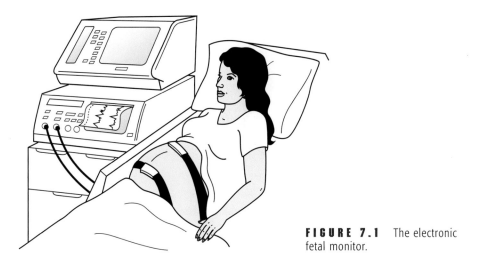

FIGURE 7.1   The electronic fetal monitor.

Indications for Electronic Fetal Monitoring

IA may not be appropriate for all labors.[1,9,10] Many factors can influence the decision to use EFM during labor, and whether EFM should be continuous or intermittent (alternated with IA). *Antepartum risk factors* are those that the woman either enters her pregnancy with (such as chronic hypertension) or develops during the antepartum period (such as gestational diabetes). Other indications for monitoring may not appear until the woman is already in labor; these factors are considered *intrapartum risk factors.*

Antepartum risk factors include the following:

Hypertension

Pregnancy-induced hypertension

Diabetes mellitus

Chronic renal disease

Congenital or rheumatic heart disease

Sickle cell disease

Rh isoimmunization

Preterm infants (37 weeks' gestation)

Age factors (younger than 15 years of age or older than 35)

Postterm infants (equal to or greater than 42 weeks' gestation)

Multiple gestations

Grand multiparity

Anemia

Intrauterine growth restriction (IUGR) or small for gestational age (SGA)

Genital tract disorders/anomalies

Poor obstetric history

Intrapartum risk factors include the following:

Prolonged rupture of membranes

Premature rupture of membranes

Failure to progress in labor or arrest disorders

Meconium-stained amniotic fluid

Abnormal FHR detected during auscultation

Abnormal presentations

Oxytocin augmentation/induction

Premature labor

Previous cesarean section in labor

Hypotensive episodes in labor

Bleeding disorders—abruptio placentae, placenta previa

EFM Equipment: External versus Internal

The electronic fetal monitor may be used in three different ways:

1. *External fetal monitoring,* also called *indirect fetal monitoring,* or *noninvasive fetal monitoring.* This method involves the use of an ultrasonic transducer to monitor the fetal heart while the contraction pattern is monitored with a tocodynamometer. Both are placed on the woman's abdomen and are secured in place by elastic belts (Fig. 7.2).

   The *ultrasonic transducer,* more commonly known as an *ultrasound* or *Doppler,* transmits high-frequency sound waves that detect movement within the fetal heart. The signal, which is similar to sonar used in submarines, is reflected back from moving structures and

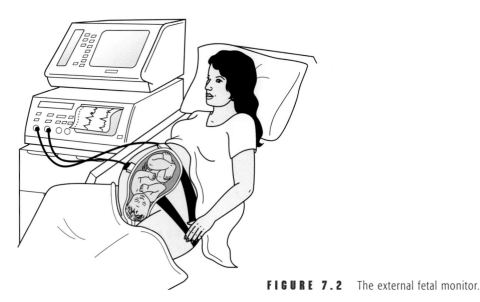

FIGURE 7.2   The external fetal monitor.

is recognized by the machine as a cardiac event. The movement detected is both ventricular contraction and the actual opening and closing of valves within the heart.

The *tocodynamometer,* more commonly known as a *toco,* provides information about the laboring woman's contraction pattern by detecting changes in the shape of the abdominal wall. It is usually placed directly over the uterine fundus. These changes in shape are the direct result of the effects of the uterine contraction on the contour of the maternal abdomen.

As a result of the manner in which the data are obtained, these methods are referred to as *indirect* or *external* monitoring because the techniques are performed external to the fetus and uterus. Because the vagina, cervix, and uterus are not invaded when applying an external monitor, the technique is also termed *noninvasive.*

External fetal monitoring may also be performed noninvasively by abdominal fetal electrocardiogram (fECG) (to capture FHR) and electromyogram (to capture uterine activity). This technology is not yet widely used, but may be superior to traditional external monitoring in patients with an elevated body mass index (BMI) where Doppler and tocotransducer use can be challenging.

2. *Internal fetal monitoring* is also called *direct fetal monitoring* or *invasive fetal monitoring.* With this method, the FHR is monitored by the use of a *fetal spiral electrode* (*FSE*), which is applied directly to the presenting part of the fetus, while the contraction pattern is monitored by the use of an *intrauterine pressure catheter* (IUPC) inserted vaginally into the intrauterine cavity through the cervix (Fig. 7.3). Note that a combination of internal and external monitoring may be used in some cases (Figs. 7.4 and 7.5).

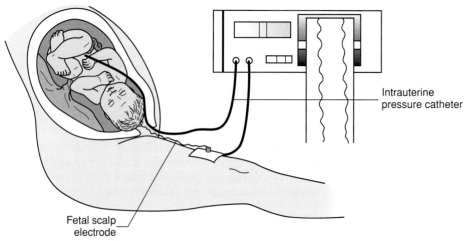

Intrauterine
pressure catheter

Fetal scalp
electrode

FIGURE 7.3   The internal fetal monitor.

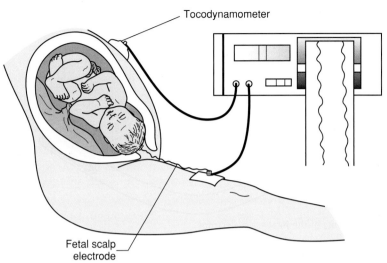

FIGURE 7.4 Combination of external and internal monitoring. The tocody-namometer and helix/fetal scalp electrode are used together.

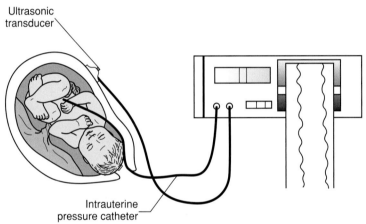

FIGURE 7.5 Combination of external and internal monitoring. The ultrasonic transducer and intrauterine pressure catheter are used together.

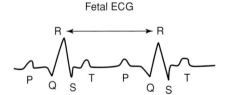

FIGURE 7.6 Determination of fetal heart rate with the use of a fetal scalp electrode.

The FSE tracks the FHR by picking up *R waves* on the fECG. The interval between each R wave is measured and processed by internal circuitry and calculated to a rate in bpm; the result is printed on graph paper (Fig. 7.6). During a vaginal examination, the examiner attaches the *spiral electrode* or *FSE*, directly to the presenting part of the fetus (Figs. 7.7 and 7.8). The FSE is then secured to a leg plate/pad that has been attached to the woman's thigh and connected to the monitor. FSE may be used when continuous information is required and a satisfactory tracing cannot be accomplished with external monitoring. *Use of the FSE should be avoided in women who are HIV positive, have chronic or active hepatitis, have herpes simplex virus, or have a known and untreated sexually transmitted disease.*[13]

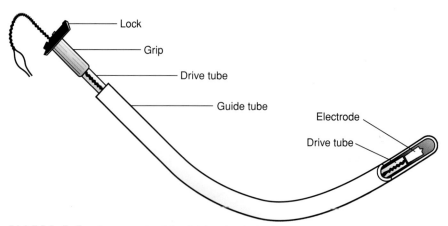

FIGURE 7.7 Components of the fetal scalp electrode.

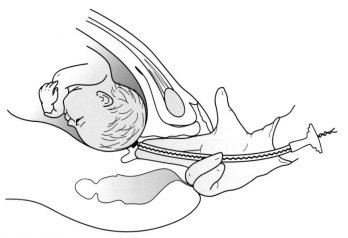

FIGURE 7.8 Application of a fetal scalp electrode to the presenting part of the fetus.

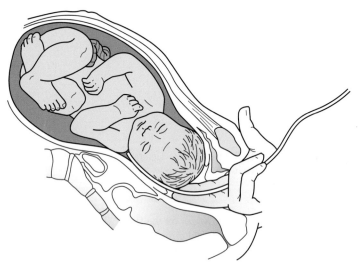

FIGURE 7.9 Insertion of intrauterine pressure catheter.

To monitor contractions internally, the IUPC is inserted through the cervix into the uterus beside the presenting part of the fetus (Fig. 7.9). The IUPC is used to determine the actual pressure inside the uterus during contractions, as well as the intrauterine pressure during relaxation time, which is called resting tone or *tonus* (Fig. 7.10). Changes in pressure at the tip of the

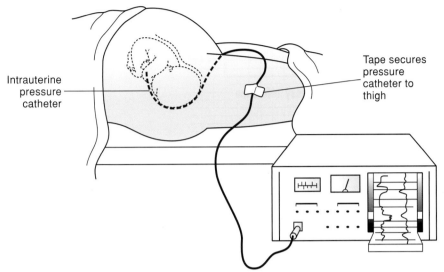

FIGURE 7.10 Intrauterine pressure catheter.

catheter (inside the uterus) are transmitted along the catheter. These pressure changes are caused by the force or intensity of the contractions and are translated into an electrical signal that is converted to a pressure reading expressed in mm Hg. This measurement is then displayed on the monitor. When clinical situations arise that require more precise measurements of uterine activity, an internal pressure catheter may be the preferred method of uterine monitoring.

Points to remember when using the IUPC include the following:

- When the IUPC is inserted, if resistance is met, the catheter must be slightly withdrawn and repositioned before insertion is attempted again.
- IUPCs must be "zeroed" to calibrate the instrumentation. (*Zeroing* means that the instrument is calibrated to air pressure so that pressure changes in the uterus can be compared against a baseline measurement.)

The Fetal Monitor Tracing

Figure 7.11 illustrates monitor paper. This graph is marked in specific time intervals of 3 minutes to allow easy readability (paper speed should be set at 3 cm/min, which is standard in the

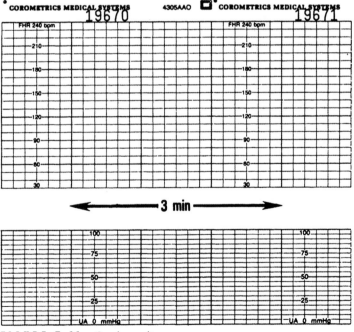

FIGURE 7.11 Graph monitor paper.

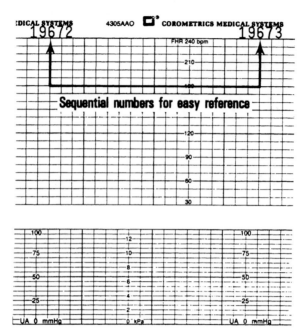

FIGURE 7.12 Sequential numbering of strip graph paper.

United States). Each small box represents 10 seconds. The numbers at the top of the strip in Figure 7.12 are reference numbers. They are sequential and appear at set intervals. On newer machines, these numbers may be located just above the uterine graph. These numbers assist in charting specific events by identifying their location on the strip. They also assist in chronologically reassembling a strip that has been separated for closer inspection.

The strip is divided into two sections: an upper section and a lower section (Fig. 7.13). The *upper* section is the portion of the graph on which the *FHR* appears. The *lower* section is the portion of the graph on which the *contractions,* or uterine activity, are recorded. The FHR (upper) section of the graph is divided vertically by dark lines, with five light, vertical lines between every two dark lines (Fig. 7.14). The time interval between any two dark lines is *1 minute;* therefore, the time interval between any two light lines is *10 seconds.* This section of the graph is also divided *horizontally* by dark lines, with two light, horizontal lines between

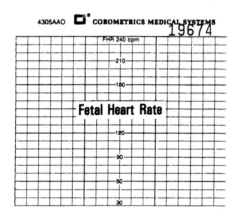

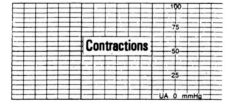

FIGURE 7.13 Strip graph monitor paper provides sections for tracing fetal heart rate and uterine activity.

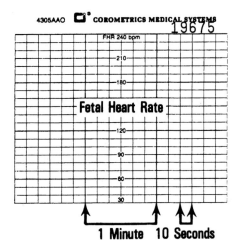

FIGURE 7.14 Division of fetal heart rate section into time intervals.

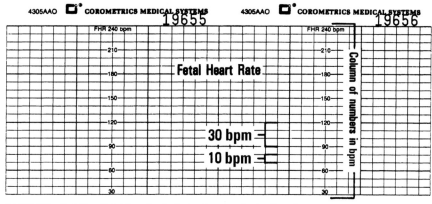

FIGURE 7.15 Fetal heart rate in beats per minute (bpm).

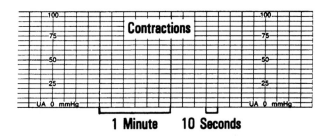

FIGURE 7.16 Division of uterine activity section into time intervals.

every two darker lines (Fig. 7.15). There is a horizontal column of numbers ranging from 30 to 240. These are reference numbers used in determining the FHR and are labeled *bpm*. The distance between any two darker lines is *30 bpm;* therefore, the distance between any two lighter lines is *10 bpm.*

The contraction or uterine activity (lower) section of the graph is divided *vertically* by dark lines, with five light, vertical lines between every two dark lines (Fig. 7.16). The time interval between any two dark lines is *1 minute;* therefore, the time interval between any two light lines is *10 seconds.* This portion of the graph is also divided *horizontally* by dark lines, with five light, horizontal lines between every two dark lines (Fig. 7.17). The numbers ranging from 0 to 100 in the horizontal column are reference numbers that are used to determine the intensity of contractions when a pressure catheter is used; they are labeled *mm Hg.* The abbreviation *UA* stands for "uterine activity."

Note that with the integration of electronic health records and perinatal data systems, many clinical systems no longer utilize paper tracings and clinicians read FHR tracings from a computer screen, tablet, or phone. The graphic representations still apply, and the parameters for

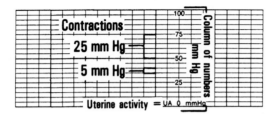

FIGURE 7.17 Uterine activity in millimeters of mercury (mm Hg).

evaluation horizontally (time, in seconds and minutes) and vertically (range, in bpm or mm Hg) are unchanged. All FHR tracings are interpreted based on visual assessment, whether on paper or electronic screen.

Summary

Intrapartum fetal monitoring may be accomplished by IA, EFM, or a combination of both. Data regarding which modality is superior for which patients is limited by a number of deficiencies with the research to date, including lack of standardization and sample size. IA is a reasonable choice for low-risk women having uncomplicated labors, while EFM is recommended for women with risk factors or those who develop intrapartum complications. All clinicians should be familiar with the benefits and disadvantages of both methods, as well as the equipment used for each and the parameters for the evaluation of the information obtained, which for IA is primarily auditory and for EFM is both auditory and visual. In the next section, clinicians will review standardized definitions for the evaluation of EFM findings and uterine activity.

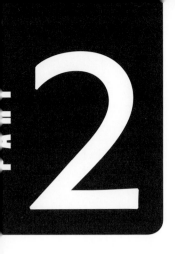

NICHD Definitions

In 1997, the National Institute of Child Health and Development (NICHD) of the National Institutes of Health gathered a panel of experts to look at some of the issues related to EFM. This group of experts proposed detailed, quantitative, and standardized definitions of FHR patterns.[14] These standardized definitions became known as the "NICHD definitions," and by 2006, all professional organizations had adopted or endorsed the use of the NICHD definitions. In 2008, a second panel of experts convened by the NICHD reaffirmed the 1997 terminology and provided additional information on uterine activity as well as a category system for classification of FHR tracings.[15] Part 2 of this module provides an overview of the current NICHD definitions and categories, as well as standardized definitions for uterine activity terminology.

Fetal Heart Rate Components

FHR Baseline

The FHR baseline has two components, the baseline rate and the variability of the baseline. The *baseline FHR* is defined as the approximate mean FHR rounded to increments of 5 bpm during a 10-minute segment, excluding:

1. Periodic and episodic changes, such as FHR accelerations or decelerations
2. Periods of marked variability
3. Any segments of the FHR tracing that differ 25 bpm or more

In the 10-minute segment, the minimum baseline duration must be at least 2 minutes (Fig. 7.18). The 2-minute minimum does not need to be contiguous. If there are less than 2 minutes of identifiable baseline, the baseline is considered *indeterminate.* In these cases, clinicians may need to assess additional portions of the FHR tracing to establish baseline rate. Baseline FHR is charted as a single number, not a range, and is always rounded to the nearest 5 bpm. Contrary to prior practices, the current definitions of FHR baseline *does not require* that baseline be read between contractions, rather it is assessed only by evaluation of the FHR portion of the monitor tracing.

Summary Terms for Baseline Fetal Heart Rate

- **Normal** FHR baseline ranges between 110 and 160 bpm, regardless of gestational age
- **Tachycardia** is an FHR baseline of greater than 160 bpm, regardless of gestational age
- **Bradycardia** is an FHR baseline of less than 100 bpm, regardless of gestational age

FHR Variability

The second component of FHR baseline is variability. *FHR variability* is defined as fluctuations in the baseline that are irregular in amplitude and frequency. Variability is quantified by the amplitude of peak to trough, in one of four ways:

- *Absent*—fluctuations are undetectable
- *Minimal*—fluctuations greater than undetectable but less than or equal to 5 bpm
- *Moderate*—fluctuations are in the range of 6 to 25 bpm
- *Marked*—fluctuations are greater than 25 bpm (Fig. 7.19)

It is important to note that variability is a component of baseline, as in the past some clinicians have mistakenly identified irregularity within the base of an FHR deceleration as variability.

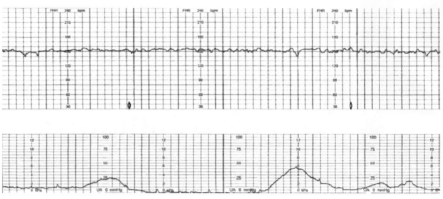

Baseline (highlighted) is identified over entire 10 minute window, exceeding the 2-minute minimum

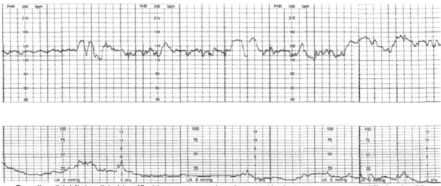

Baseline (highlighted) is identified between accelerations and/or between segments differing by 25 bpm or more, identifiable baseline is approximately 5 minutes total (note the 2-minute minimum is met)

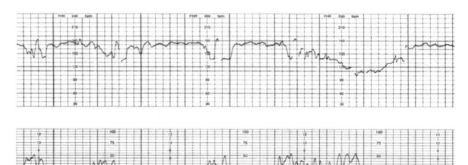

Baseline (highlighted) is identified between decelerations and/or between segments differing by 25 bpm or more, identifiable baseline is approximately 5 minutes total (note the 2-minute minimum is met)

FIGURE 7.18   Baseline fetal heart rate. (Courtesy PRMES, LLC.)

The NICHD makes it clear that secondary characteristics of variable decelerations, such as irregularity with a deceleration, have no known clinical significance based on the current evidence.[15] Research completed following the 2008 NICHD Workshop, evaluating atypical characteristics of decelerations, has confirmed that when evaluating FHR decelerations, atypical findings should not be considered clinically significant.[16] This means that *when clinicians evaluate FHR variability they must do so only in the context of variability as a component of the identifiable FHR baseline.*

Sinusoidal FHR Pattern

A sinusoidal FHR pattern is a *rare FHR pattern* that is defined by the NICHD as having the following visually apparent attributes[15]:
- Smooth, visually apparent, sine wave–like undulating pattern in FHR baseline
- Cycle frequency of 3 to 5 per minute
- Persistence for 20 minutes or more

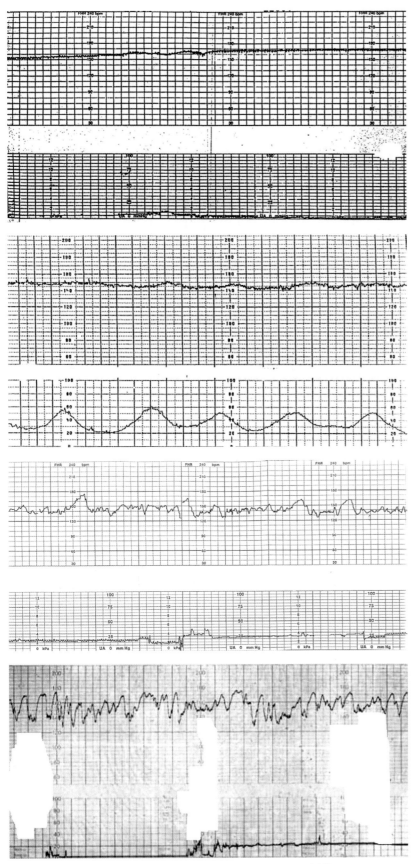

FIGURE 7.19 Absent, minimal, moderate, and marked variability. (Courtesy PRMES, LLC.)

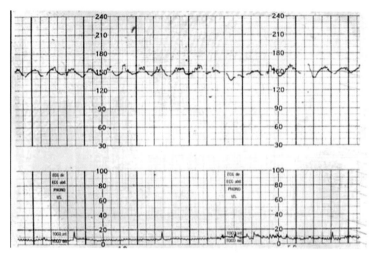

FIGURE 7.20   Sinusoidal pattern. (Courtesy PRMES, LLC.)

Sinusoidal patterns are characterized by smooth, sine waves that are regular in frequency and amplitude (Fig. 7.20). The sine waves should not be mistaken for variability. The pattern may be intermittent or continuous. Sinusoidal patterns have been seen in cases of fetal anemia, historically often related to Rh sensitization.[13] It has been suggested that intermittent sinusoidal baseline rate may be an early indicator of impending fetal compromise.[17] Because of both the rarity of the pattern and the correlation to potential fetal compromise, physician evaluation of the FHR tracing is recommended if a sinusoidal FHR tracing is suspected.

Medication Effect

A sinusoidal-like pattern may be seen following narcotic administration (Fig. 7.21). The appearance is similar to a true sinusoidal, but the amplitude is often less, and the pattern is transitory, resolving as the medication clears the maternal system. In the past, clinicians have used the term "pseudosinusoidal" to describe this medication effect on FHR, but this is not a term defined by the NICHD and is probably best avoided. Clinicians should use considerable clinical context and history of medication administration to determine whether an FHR pattern is related to medications administered to the mother or represents a true sinusoidal pattern.

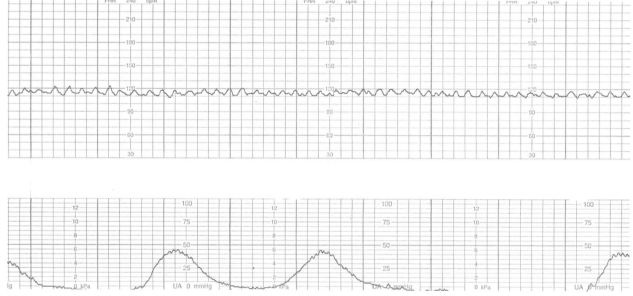

FIGURE 7.21   Medication effect, not to be confused with a sinusoidal baseline. (Courtesy PRMES, LLC.)

Periodic and Episodic Changes

FHR changes, which include both accelerations and decelerations, may be periodic or episodic in nature. Periodic changes are those that occur in association with a uterine contraction. Episodic patterns are those that occur randomly, unassociated with uterine contractions. By definition, late and early decelerations can only be periodic, as they require an association with a uterine contraction to be labeled as early or late. Accelerations, variable decelerations, and prolonged decelerations can be either episodic or periodic, as they can occur with or without an associated uterine contraction.

Accelerations

Accelerations are the most common type of periodic heart rate change. They are defined as a visually apparent abrupt increase in FHR (onset of acceleration to peak in less than 30 seconds) (Fig. 7.22). The peak of the acceleration is 15 bpm above the most recently determined baseline and the acceleration duration (onset to offset) is at least 15 seconds. Before 32 weeks' gestation, a peak of 10 bpm above the baseline and a duration of 10 seconds will satisfy the criteria for an acceleration.[15] Accelerations may occur spontaneously or in response to fetal movement, maternal movement, acoustic stimulation, fetal scalp stimulation, or contractions. *Prolonged accelerations* are those with a duration of 2 minutes or longer but less than 10 minutes. After a duration of 10 minutes, it is not considered an acceleration but rather a change in the baseline rate.

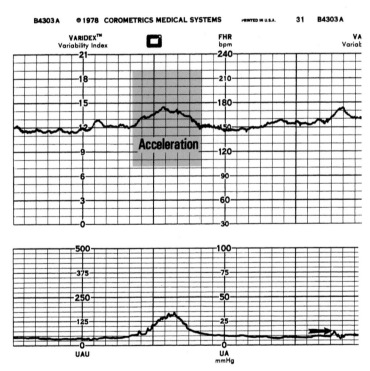

FIGURE 7.22 Fetal heart rate acceleration.

Early Deceleration

An *early deceleration* is defined as a visually apparent, *gradual* decrease (onset of deceleration to nadir greater than or equal to 30 seconds) and return to baseline associated with a contraction.[15] The onset, nadir, and return to baseline of an early deceleration correspond with the beginning, peak, and end of a uterine contraction (Fig. 7.23). Because the definition of an early deceleration is dependent upon the deceleration's relationship to an associated uterine contraction, early decelerations can only be periodic.

Late Deceleration

An *late deceleration* is defined as a visually apparent, *gradual* decrease (onset of deceleration to nadir greater than or equal to 30 seconds) and return to baseline associated with a contraction.[15]

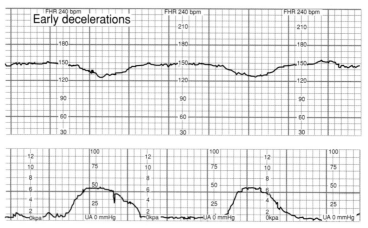

FIGURE 7.23 Early deceleration. (From Miller, L. A., Miller, D. A., & Tucker, S. M. (2013). *Pocket guide to fetal monitoring: A multidisciplinary approach* (7th ed.) St. Louis, MO: Mosby.)

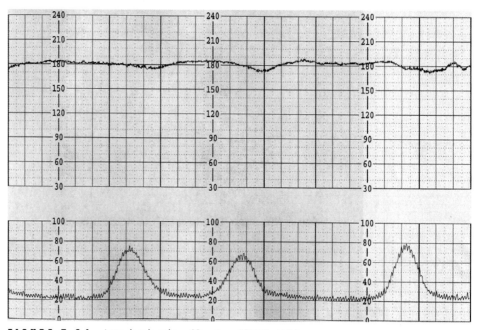

FIGURE 7.24 Late deceleration. (Courtesy PRMES, LLC.)

However, in contrast to the aforementioned early deceleration, the onset of the late deceleration is delayed, beginning after the onset of the contraction, with the nadir (lowest point) occurring after the peak of the contraction, and return to baseline generally following the offset of the contraction (Fig. 7.24). Because the definition of a late deceleration is dependent upon the deceleration's relationship to an associated uterine contraction, like early decelerations late decelerations can only be periodic.

Variable Deceleration

A variable deceleration is defined as a visually apparent, *abrupt* decrease (onset of deceleration to nadir less than 30 seconds) and return to baseline associated with a contraction.[15] The decrease in FHR from onset to nadir must be at least 15 bpm, and the duration (onset to offset) of the deceleration must be at least 15 seconds, but less than 2 minutes (Fig. 7.25). A variable deceleration may occur periodically (related to a contraction) or episodically (spontaneous, not associated with a contraction).

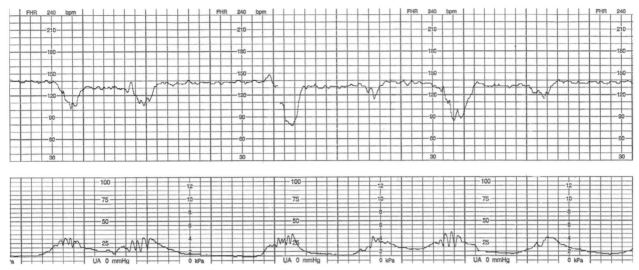

FIGURE 7.25 Variable deceleration. (Courtesy PRMES, LLC.)

Prolonged Deceleration

A prolonged deceleration is defined as a visually apparent deceleration from the FHR baseline that may be *abrupt* or *gradual* in onset.[15] The decrease in FHR from onset to nadir must be at least 15 bpm, and the duration (onset to offset) of the deceleration must be 2 minutes or longer, but less than 10 minutes (Fig. 7.26). Following a duration of 10 minutes, the prolonged deceleration would likely reflect a baseline change rather than a deceleration. A prolonged deceleration may occur periodically (related to a contraction) or episodically (spontaneous, not associated with a contraction). They are often seen immediately prior to delivery during the final expulsive efforts of the mother.

FHR Categories

The 2008 NICHD workshop report introduced a three-tiered system for the categorization of FHR tracings in the intrapartum period.[15] These summary terms have limited value in daily

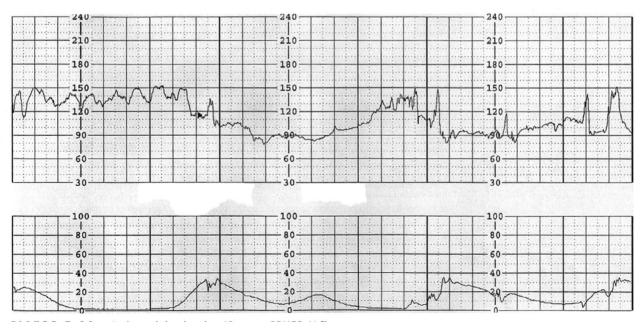

FIGURE 7.26 Prolonged deceleration (Courtesy PRMES, LLC).

clinical practice, but are important as an alternative to the vague and nonspecific terms (such as "reassuring" and nonreassuring") that many clinicians have utilized in the past when attempting to summarize FHR tracing characteristics. There are three categories:

Category I, or normal, requires a normal baseline rate, moderate variability of the FHR baseline, and may include early decelerations. A category I tracing is considered "strongly predictive of normal fetal acid-base status at the time of observation."[15]

Category II, or indeterminate, includes all FHR tracings that do not qualify as either category I or category III. These tracings represent the majority (80% or more) of FHR tracings that will be seen during labor.[6,18]

Category III, or abnormal, includes only four FHR tracings:
- Absent variability with recurrent late decelerations
- Absent variability with recurrent variable decelerations
- Absent variability with bradycardia
- Sinusoidal pattern

Category III tracings are considered predictive of abnormal fetal acid–base status at the time they are seen,[15] but the high false-positive rate of EFM means that even when delivered following a category III tracing, less than 50% will actually exhibit metabolic acidemia in umbilical cord blood, and even in those with abnormal cord gases at birth, not all will go on to develop any long-term morbidity.[7] Thus, "predictive of" is not equivalent to "diagnostic for" when discussing fetal acid–base status or neurologic outcome in relation to EFM tracings in category III. Nonetheless, as will be discussed in interpretation and management, category III tracings require prompt intervention and, if unresolved with conservative corrective measures, expeditious delivery with planned neonatal support.

Definitions for Uterine Activity

In addition to the reinforcement of previous FHR definitions and the implementation of a three-tiered category system for FHR tracings, the 2008 NICHD workshop report provided updated information on the components of uterine activity (UA), including summary terms for quantification of the frequency of uterine activity. Just as the rationale for standardized definitions of FHR components is to improve communication, standardized terminology related to uterine activity is paramount to appropriate and informative clinical discourse, especially during the intrapartum period, when management of uterine activity can be the key to fetal oxygenation. The NICHD specifically mentioned the importance of a *complete evaluation of uterine activity,* not simply evaluation of the frequency of contractions.[15] Clinicians should utilize standardized definitions for frequency, duration, strength/intensity, resting tone, and relaxation time. The following definitions and terms will be used in this module when the evaluation of uterine activity is being discussed:

Frequency: Uterine contractions are quantified as the number of contractions present in a 10-minute window, averaged over 30 minutes. Uterine contraction frequency is considered *normal* if there are five or less contractions in 10 minutes, averaged over a 30-minute window. If there are more than five contractions occurring in 10 minutes, averaged over a 30-minute window, this is called **tachysystole**. The term tachysystole applies to both stimulated and spontaneous labor, and when present, tachysystole should be qualified as to the presence or absence of FHR decelerations.[15] *It is important to note that the terms "normal" and "tachysystole" are summary terms that relate only to the frequency of contractions, and in clinical practice other parameters of uterine activity, such as contraction duration, strength or intensity, relaxation time, and resting tone must be included as part of a complete assessment.*

In daily clinical practice, contraction frequency is measured by the length of time from the beginning of one contraction to the beginning of the next contraction. In Figure 7.27, the contractions measured from start to start vary in occurrence from approximately every 1½ to 2½ minutes, or "q1½ to 2½ minutes." Contraction frequency is most often reported in a range, such as "q2 to 3 minutes" because contraction patterns are seldom uniform in frequency. *Note that as long as there is a contraction frequency of every 2 minutes or greater, tachysystole cannot be present,* as the average contraction frequency in a 10-minute window would be 5 or less.

Duration: Duration is the interval of time between the beginning (onset) and the end (offset) of the contraction. For contraction B on the FHR tracing in Figure 7.27, the duration is

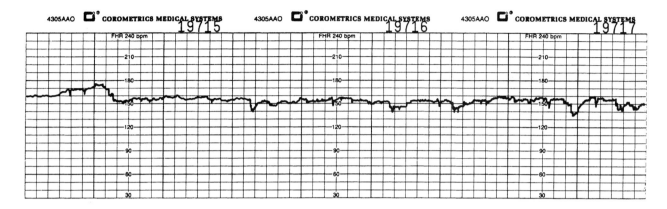

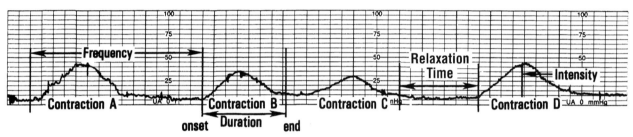

FIGURE 7.27 Components of the evaluation of uterine activity.

just over 70 seconds. Generally, contraction durations range from 45 to 90 seconds, with contractions in the first-stage labor typically having longer durations than contractions seen in the second stage. A contraction duration of 2 minutes or longer has been called a *tetanic* contraction, and can have a negative effect on fetal acid–base status if the pattern becomes recurrent; this is due to the lack of sufficient relaxation time for gas exchange. Contraction duration is usually recorded in a range because duration varies from one contraction to the next.

Strength/Intensity: Many institutions use these terms interchangeably, and this does not likely pose any clinical risk. Technically, strength was a term traditionally associated with palpation, while intensity was a specifically defined term used only when an IUPC was in place. It is important that clinicians understand the difference in assessing strength/intensity based upon the mode of monitoring (external vs. internal), and to facilitate that understanding, *strength* will be the term used in this module to discuss the evaluation of UA when palpation is being used (as with a tocodynamometer or with IA and palpation) and intensity will be the term used when discussing the assessment of UA in mm Hg with an IUPC.

When assessing using palpation (during IA or external monitoring) strength is determined by palpating uterine contraction with the fingertips, usually at the area of the uterine fundus. If the fundus is easily indented with the tips of the fingers, the contraction is considered "mild." If more pressure is needed to indent the fundus, the contraction is "moderate." The contraction is considered "strong" if the fundus cannot be indented at the contraction peak. In some patients, such as those with significant adipose tissue, the area where the contraction is most easily palpated may be below or to the side of the fundus.

When an IUPC is in place, the intensity of a contraction is commonly expressed in one of the two ways: (1) it may be expressed simply as the peak of the contraction in mm Hg, or (2) when using Montevideo units (MVUs) to assess UA over a 10-minute segment; intensity is defined as the peak of the uterine contraction in mm Hg less the baseline resting tone of UA in mm HG. Montevideo units may be used to evaluate the adequacy of uterine activity. The original formula from Caldeyro-Barcia was calculated by multiplying the average intensity in mm Hg by the frequency of uterine contractions in a 10-minute period.[19] For example, if there are three contractions in 10 minutes with an average intensity of 50 mm Hg, the MVUs for that period would be 3×50, or 150. An easier approach using simple arithmetic will provide essentially the same result, and it has become commonplace to calculate MVUs by simply adding the intensities (peak less resting tone) of each individual contraction in a 10-minute window. Thus, three contractions in 10 minutes where the intensities were 45, 50, and 55 mm Hg would result in an MVU total of 150 mm Hg. MVU assessments can be helpful in oxytocin management and in the evaluation of normal or adequate versus excessive UA.

Relaxation Time: Relaxation time is the time from the end of one contraction to the beginning of the next contraction and is often confused with resting tone. Resting tone is *assessed* during relaxation time, so the two components are related and interdependent, but are different assessments. This is extremely important for clinicians to grasp, as abnormalities of either relaxation time or resting tone, or both, can impinge upon fetal gas exchange and lead to hypoxemia. Normal relaxation times vary from the first to second stage of labor, with average relaxation times of 60 seconds being adequate to ensure sufficient oxygen/carbon dioxide exchange in the first stage, versus average times of 45 seconds in the second stage.[20]

Resting Tone: Resting tone (tone, tonus, baseline uterine tone) is the intrauterine pressure when the uterus is a contractile, and can be assessed by palpation or with an IUPC. When palpation is used to assess uterine resting tone it is often described as "soft" or "relaxed" when normal, or "firm" or "not relaxed" if abnormal. When an IUPC is in place, the resting tone is described in terms of mm Hg, normal resting tone in labor is usually between 8 and 10 mm Hg.[19] If resting tone exceeds 20 to 25 mm Hg with an IUPC, or palpates as firm or not relaxed when using external monitoring, the condition is called *hypertonus*. Hypertonus can negatively impact fetal oxygen uptake and carbon dioxide release, and should be promptly addressed if noted. Blood flow both from and to the placenta with hypertonus can be significantly decreased. Uterine resting tone can change between contractions, and is therefore often reported as a range when using an IUPC.

Summary

Standardization of terminology is crucial to ensuring clear communication between nurses, physicians, and midwives. In the United States, the use of the NICHD terminology for EFM is the standard of care. Clinicians should be comfortable with both the NICHD nomenclature as well as come to consensus regarding standardization of terminology for uterine activity, definitions for which are only partially addressed by the NICHD. Clarity when evaluating and discussing both FHR and UA findings is key to appropriate EFM interpretation and labor management, and will form the basis for interpretation and management approaches discussed in the following sections of this module.

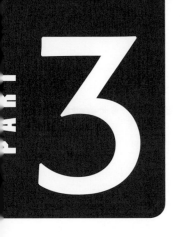

PART 3

Physiologic Approach to Interpretation and Management

Fetal Heart Rate Physiology

Overview of FHR regulation

The fetal heart is influenced by many factors, but it is primarily regulated by the autonomic nervous system, chemoreceptors, and baroreceptors. The two parts of the autonomic nervous system are the parasympathetic branch and the sympathetic branch. The parasympathetic branch exerts a tonal influence on the intrinsic rate for the fetal heart, and as it matures the intrinsic rate will decrease. The sympathetic branch primarily plays a role in stress response, and will cause an increase in FHR and/or peripheral vasoconstriction in response to oxygenation and blood pressure changes in the fetus. Both branches play a role in the variability of the FHR, along with the central nervous system. In addition to the parasympathetic and sympathetic influences, the FHR is regulated by baroreceptor and chemoreceptor activities. *Baroreceptors* are located in the carotid arch and the aortic sinus. Cells in these areas are sensitive to the stretching of surrounding tissue (changes in arterial wall diameter) caused by increased or decreased blood pressure. When fetal blood pressure changes, it is sensed by the baroreceptors, which transmit the message to the brainstem. Here the nervous system response will result in output to either slow the FHR (to decrease blood pressure) or increase the FHR (in an effort to return the low fetal blood pressure to normal).

Chemoreceptors also play a significant role in FHR regulation. They are sensitive to changes in oxygen, carbon dioxide, and pH of fetal blood. Reduction in blood oxygen and pH and/or increases in CO_2 are recognized by the chemoreceptors and may trigger a sympathetic response where FHR is increased in an effort to increase oxygenation or decrease CO_2. The sympathetic response may also (as seen in the mechanism of late decelerations) result in peripheral vasoconstriction in an attempt to move oxygenated blood from the periphery to the core organs (brain, heart, adrenals) in an effort to protect those organs from hypoxia.

Changes in FHR baseline rate resulting in tachycardia or bradycardia can have a variety of etiologies, not always related to hypoxemia or hypoxia. Tachycardia can be seen with infection, fetal activity or stimulation, and a wide variety of medications, including parasympatholytic drugs such as atropine or scopolamine, β-adrenergic drug such as terbutaline, and illicit drugs such as methamphetamine, cocaine, and Phencyclidine (PCP or angel dust). Other factors associated with tachycardia include elevated maternal heart rate, maternal fever, fetal anemia, fetal cardiac tachyarrhythmia such as supraventricular tachycardia (SVT) and atrial flutter, and maternal hyperthyroidism. Bradycardia may be the result of interrupted oxygenation, medications, and cardiac conduction abnormalities in the fetus (such as heart block), fetal heart failure, maternal hypoglycemia, and maternal hypothermia.[13,21]

Fetal Heart Dysrhythmias

Normally, the electrical impulse that governs heart rate and rhythm originates in the sinoatrial node located in the right atrium. Once initiated, the impulse then spreads downward to the atrioventricular (AV) node, the bundle of His, and Purkinje fibers. These impulses cause muscular contraction of the heart. Each part of this electrical system has the capacity for initiating cardiac contraction if the preceding mechanism fails. If abnormalities of the system exist, heart rate can be affected by dropped/skipped beats or premature contractions that can cause deviations in cardiac rhythm and rate. Deviations can also occur as a result of cardiac injury or are associated

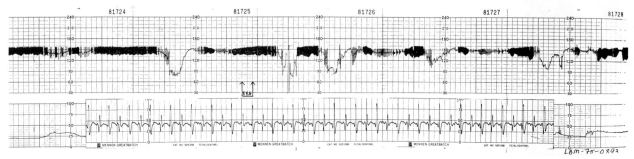

FIGURE 7.28 This tracing shows the fetal heart rate pattern above and fetal electrocardiograph below. (Reprinted with permission from Freeman, R. K., Garite, T. J., & Nageotte, M. P. [2003]. *Fetal heart rate monitoring* [3rd ed., p. 98]. Philadelphia, PA: Lippincott Williams & Wilkins.)

with maternal medical conditions. These deviations are called "dysrhythmias." The diagnosis of an FHR dysrhythmia is typically made in the antepartum period, and follow-up examinations with ultrasound and fetal echocardiograms are often the key to the diagnosis. The type of dysrhythmia can be identified only by its characteristics on an ECG (Fig. 7.28).

The appearance of the tracing with a dysrhythmia is unique. It may have an organized appearance that can help distinguish it from artifact, which tends to have a much more erratic and disorganized appearance. When a dysrhythmia is suspected, FHR auscultation should be done to audibly verify the dysrhythmia. The presence of a dysrhythmia can make assessment and interpretation of the fetal monitor tracing challenging, and clinicians may have difficulty assessing baseline rate and baseline variability.

Types of FHR Dysrhythmias

- **Premature atrial contractions (PACs) and premature ventricular contractions (PVCs)**—
  These are the most common sources of heart rate irregularity in the fetus. They are usually benign. They are not associated with hypoxemia or hypoxia and do not require intervention other than notification of the pediatric team for follow-up at birth. The majority of these will resolve when fetal circulation transitions to neonatal circulation at delivery (Fig. 7.29).
- **Supraventricular tachycardia (SVT)**—Although quite rare, this is the most commonly encountered tachydysrhythmia and should be evaluated carefully because this is associated with underlying cardiac disease. SVT is usually identified in the second trimester. The rate is often greater than 200 bpm but can exceed 250 bpm and can lead to fetal congestive heart failure, hydrops, and death. Management can include administration of medications such as digoxin, β-blocking agents, or calcium channel blockers to the mother to, hopefully, cause a conversion to a normal rhythm in utero. SVT will usually be managed by a

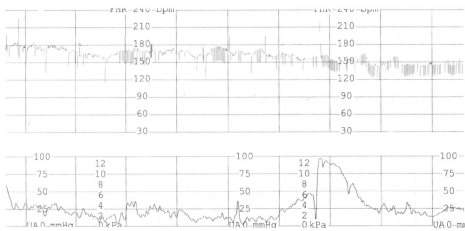

FIGURE 7.29 PACs during labor; normal outcome and no audible dysrhythmia at birth. (Courtesy PRMES, LLC.)

maternal–fetal medicine specialist once identified and is not often seen during the intrapartum period because it is usually diagnosed and managed prior to labor onset.[13,21]

- **Heart block**—Characterized by a bradycardic baseline rate, approximately 50% of fetuses with complete heart block have mothers who have evidence of connective tissue disease. In mothers who have systemic lupus erythematosus, the antibodies that damage the heart's conduction system can cross the placenta and attack cardiac tissue. When diagnosed prenatally, arrangements need to be made for care of the baby after delivery. This may include the need for a pacemaker. In the other 50%, congenital heart disease is usually the underlying case. In either case, consultation with a maternal–fetal medicine specialist is recommended to devise a plan of care that includes a recommendation regarding location and mode of delivery.[13,21]

The majority of clinically significant dysrhythmias will be diagnosed and managed in the antepartum period with maternal–fetal medicine specialists, and have little impact upon intrapartum EFM. Labor and delivery nurses will usually deal only with the more common PVC or PAC dysrhythmias, which simply require identification, observation, and review by the pediatric team at birth to assure that the dysrhythmia has resolved following transition to newborn life.

FHR Variability

Just as FHR baseline rate is the result of interplay between branches of the autonomic nervous system and other influences such as chemoreceptors and baroreceptors, FHR variability is also the result of sympathetic and parasympathetic signals from the medullary vasomotor center. The FHR changes in response to moment-to-moment changes in fetal PO_2, PCO_2, and blood pressure, as slight corrections in the heart rate result in optimal cardiac output and facilitate flow of oxygenated blood to the fetal tissues. These changes are seen in the FHR tracing as variability. The importance of moderate variability in FHR tracing interpretation and management cannot be overemphasized. In both the 2008 NICHD consensus report[15] and the more recent ACOG and AAP publication on neonatal encephalopathy,[7] it was noted that the presence of moderate variability and/or FHR accelerations reliably predict the absence of fetal metabolic acidemia (and related hypoxia-induced neurologic damage) at the time they are observed. These conclusions regarding fetal acid–base status are crucial components of informed clinical decision-making for FHR interpretation and management, and will be reinforced and reiterated later in this module. But if moderate variability is lacking, it is important to understand that minimal or absent variability does not mean that fetal metabolic acidemia or hypoxemia-related neurologic injury is present. There are many conditions that can be associated with minimal or absent variability, including fetal sleep cycles, medications administered to the mother, fetal tachycardia, prematurity, congenital anomalies, fetal anemia, cardiac arrhythmias, infection and pre-existing neurologic injury. Unfortunately, most of the literature reporting findings of "decreased" variability fails to distinguish between absent variability and minimal variability, making it impossible to ascertain the relative clinical significance of minimal versus absent, although some import may be given to the fact that three of the four category III FHR tracings require absent variability. On the other end of the variability spectrum, it should be noted that the clinical significance of marked variability is not known. Although it is most often seen in response to fetal stimulation or fetal movement, there is a plausible theoretical explanation that marked variability could at times be related to an exaggerated autonomic response to interruption of fetal oxygenation.[21]

FHR Accelerations

FHR accelerations frequently occur in with fetal movement or stimulation; the physiology is likely related to peripheral proprioceptor response, catecholamine release, and autonomic response. Umbilical venous compression, resulting in decreased fetal venous return and a subsequent rise in FHR due to triggering of baroreceptors is another possible mechanism. Like moderate variability, the presence of either a spontaneous or a stimulated FHR acceleration reliably predicts the absence of fetal metabolic acidemia at the time it is observed.[15] But the absence of an acceleration does not confirm the presence of fetal metabolic acidemia, and this is another important clinical point for interpretation and decision-making.

FHR Decelerations

Although most clinicians have been taught very simplistic explanations of the physiology of different FHR decelerations, such as "head compression" for early decelerations, "cord compression" for variable decelerations, and "uteroplacental insufficiency" for late decelerations, a deeper understanding of the mechanisms of FHR decelerations is not only available, it is likely beneficial to the evaluation of FHR tracings.

Early Deceleration

An early deceleration, commonly associated with the term "head compression," is thought to reflect a simple reflex fetal autonomic response to changes in intracranial pressure and/or cerebral blood flow caused by pressure exerted on the fetal head during a uterine contraction (Fig. 7.30). There is no correlation between early decelerations and systemic hypoxia or adverse neonatal outcomes, and early decelerations are considered clinically benign.[21] Early decelerations of the FHR are the only deceleration allowed in category I (normal) tracings.

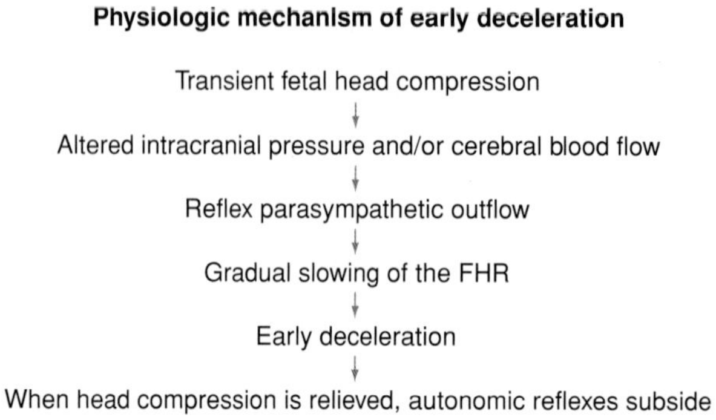

Physiologic mechanism of early deceleration

Transient fetal head compression
↓
Altered intracranial pressure and/or cerebral blood flow
↓
Reflex parasympathetic outflow
↓
Gradual slowing of the FHR
↓
Early deceleration
↓
When head compression is relieved, autonomic reflexes subside

FIGURE 7.30 Physiologic mechanism of early deceleration. (From Miller, L. A., Miller, D. A., & Tucker, S. M. (2013). *Pocket guide to fetal monitoring: A multidisciplinary approach* (7th ed.). St. Louis, MO: Mosby.)

Late Deceleration

The term "uteroplacental insufficiency" has long been associated with late decelerations and while not inaccurate, does little to further a clear understanding of the physiologic mechanism that results in a late deceleration. Figure 7.31 provides a schematic representation of the mechanism of late decelerations, most of which are combined chemoreceptor–baroreceptor-mediated reflex responses to transient fetal hypoxemia; the fetus will protect core organs such as the

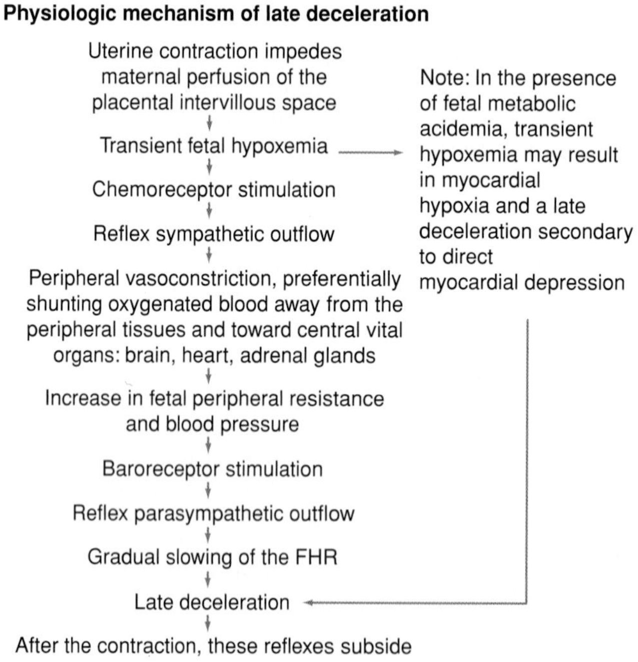

Physiologic mechanism of late deceleration

Uterine contraction impedes maternal perfusion of the placental intervillous space
↓
Transient fetal hypoxemia ────→
↓
Chemoreceptor stimulation
↓
Reflex sympathetic outflow
↓
Peripheral vasoconstriction, preferentially shunting oxygenated blood away from the peripheral tissues and toward central vital organs: brain, heart, adrenal glands
↓
Increase in fetal peripheral resistance and blood pressure
↓
Baroreceptor stimulation
↓
Reflex parasympathetic outflow
↓
Gradual slowing of the FHR
↓
Late deceleration ←────
↓
After the contraction, these reflexes subside

Note: In the presence of fetal metabolic acidemia, transient hypoxemia may result in myocardial hypoxia and a late deceleration secondary to direct myocardial depression

FIGURE 7.31 Physiologic mechanism of late deceleration. (From Miller, L. A., Miller, D. A., & Tucker, S. M. (2013). *Pocket guide to fetal monitoring: A multidisciplinary approach* (7th ed.). St. Louis, MO: Mosby.)

brain, heart, and adrenals during periods of transient hypoxemia by shunting blood from the periphery. If hypoxemia progresses and the fetus develops metabolic acidemia, late decelerations can be the result of direct myocardial depression, but these situations are rare and the late decelerations would be accompanied by other changes in the FHR tracing, such as loss of variability, lack of accelerations, and possibly changes in baseline rate.[21]

Variable Deceleration

Typically associated with the phrase "cord compression," variable decelerations are perhaps the most aptly named FHR deceleration regarding the underlying mechanism. Compression of the umbilical vein and two umbilical arteries results in baroreceptor response to changing fetal blood pressures, as seen in Figure 7.32. Although the degree of cord compression may always not be enough to result in changes in fetal PaO_2, the fact that the umbilical vein is being compressed means that the flow of oxygenated blood to the fetus is being interrupted to some degree.[21] This will be an important point for the interpretation of FHR tracings discussed later in this module.

Physiologic mechanism of variable deceleration

Umbilical cord compression
↓
Initial compression of umbilical vein
↓
Transient decreased fetal venous return
↓
Transient reduction in fetal cardiac output and blood pressure
↓
Baroreceptor stimulation
↓
Transient reflex rise in FHR
↓
Umbilical artery compression
↓
Abrupt rise in fetal peripheral resistance and blood pressure
↓
Baroreceptor stimulation
↓
Reflex parasympathetic outflow
↓
Abrupt slowing of the FHR
↓
Variable deceleration
↓
When umbilical cord compression is relieved, this process occurs in reverse

FIGURE 7.32 Physiologic mechanism of variable deceleration. (From Miller, L. A., Miller, D. A., & Tucker, S. M. (2013). *Pocket guide to fetal monitoring: A multidisciplinary approach* (7th ed.). St. Louis, MO: Mosby.)

Prolonged Deceleration

In the past, the word "prolonged" was used as an adjective and applied as a modifier to further describe late and variable decelerations. Since the publication of the 2008 NICHD Workshop Report, the term prolonged is a separately defined type of deceleration. The underlying physiology of prolonged decelerations may stem from the same mechanisms seen in late or variable decelerations, or may be a combination of multiple factors. Regardless of the presumed etiology(ies), prolonged decelerations should always be considered a reflection of an interruption of fetal oxygenation.[21]

Effects of Uterine Contractions on Maternal–Fetal Blood Flow

Normal uterine contractions produce repeated stress on the fetus by interfering with placental blood flow from the mother to the fetus. Before a contraction, blood flow is at its greatest, moving freely between the mother and fetus. As a contraction begins, *veins* in the myometrium are compressed. Compression of *arteries* in the myometrium occurs if the intensity of the contraction is greater than the mean arterial blood pressure of the mother. With the compression of the myometrial arteries, blood flow in the intervillous space ceases. The point at which blood flow stops is at approximately 40 to 50 mm Hg and has been referred to as *physiologic isolation*. In a normal contraction, this physiologic isolation is brief, and the fetus is fully able to maintain the heart rate. As the contraction subsides, the myometrial *arteries* open first, followed by an opening of the myometrial *veins*. Blood flow through the uterus to the placenta and fetus is restored. Thus, it is primarily during relaxation time with normal resting tone that the fetus is able to receive oxygen and release carbon dioxide, with the intervillous space of the placenta effectively serving as the fetal lungs would in an extra uterine environment. This may be one of the single most important physiologic concepts for clinical practice, as it follows that any periods of excessive uterine activity would negatively impinge on fetal O_2–CO_2 exchange. Additionally, every fetus will differ in the ability to tolerate excessive uterine activity, based primarily on the amount of stored glucose that can be used for anaerobic activity in times of diminished oxygenation.

It is important for clinicians to understand that tachysystole is a term that only describes the frequency of uterine contractions, and may or may not reflect excessive uterine activity. For example, a frequency of six contractions in 10 minutes, averaged over a 30-minute period, will *always* be tachysystole, but if the contraction duration is only 30 seconds on average, and the resting tone is normal, the fetus will have ample relaxation time to both receive oxygen and release carbon dioxide. On the other hand, a frequency of four contractions in 10 minutes, averaged over a 30-minute period will *never* be tachysystole, but if the contraction duration is 2 minutes, or the resting tone is elevated, the fetus may very well be compromised with respect to oxygenation. Clinicians must complete a full and thorough evaluation of uterine activity, not simply count the bumps, to ensure adequate opportunity for fetal O_2–CO_2 exchange. Excessive uterine activity may manifest as tachysystole, hypertonus, inadequate relaxation time, or any combination of these, and will require prompt attention and management. In Figure 7.33, baseline FHR is quickly affected by the contraction pattern. The first contraction lasts 130 seconds, and the second contraction lasts 230 seconds; both are tetanic contractions. There is insufficient relaxation time even if the uterine tonus is normal. Deterioration of fetal acid–base status could result if the contraction pattern is not corrected.

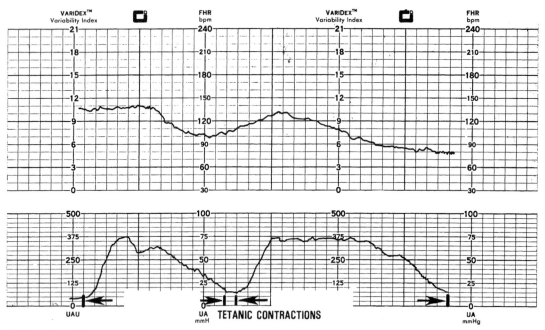

FIGURE 7.33 Excessive uterine activity (*but not tachysystole*).

Physiologic Principles of Interpretation

Every clinician, regardless of whether in the medical or nursing discipline, regardless of years of experience, must answer the same three questions when evaluating an FHR tracing. These questions, in simple terms, are the following:

1. What do I call it? (Definitions)
2. What does it mean? (Interpretation)
3. What do I do about it? (Management)

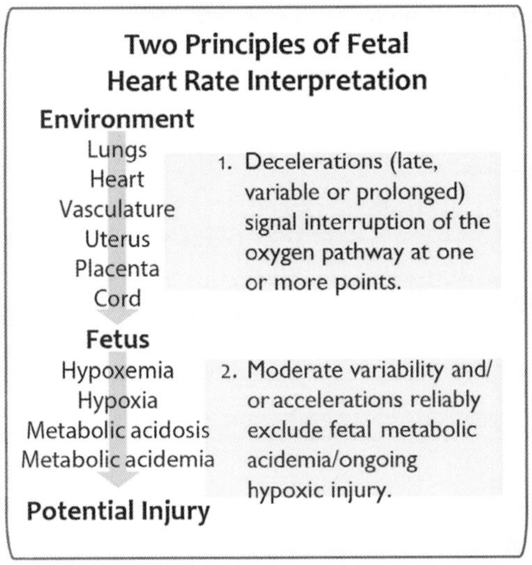

Two Principles of Fetal Heart Rate Interpretation

Environment

Lungs
Heart
Vasculature
Uterus
Placenta
Cord

1. Decelerations (late, variable or prolonged) signal interruption of the oxygen pathway at one or more points.

Fetus

Hypoxemia
Hypoxia
Metabolic acidosis
Metabolic acidemia

2. Moderate variability and/or accelerations reliably exclude fetal metabolic acidemia/ongoing hypoxic injury.

Potential Injury

FIGURE 7.34 Oxygen pathway and fetal response. (Courtesy David A. Miller, MD.)

In this module, the NICHD definitions, categories, and terminology for uterine activity evaluation that have already been presented will allow the clinician to effectively answer the first question (What do I call it?). In short, the FHR tracing is defined by its components (baseline rate, variability, accelerations, decelerations, uterine activity) and its category (I, II, or III).

It is now time to focus on the second two questions, which can be restated more simply as *interpretation* (What does this FHR tracing mean?) and *management* (What should be done about this FHR tracing by the clinical team?). To understand what an FHR tracing means, it is imperative that clinicians understand fetal oxygenation. Figure 7.34 shows both the fetal oxygenation pathway as well as the fetal response to interrupted oxygenation, should such interruption progress to hypoxemia and its eventual sequela, fetal metabolic acidemia (a precursor to potential hypoxic injury). The FHR tracing can provide information related to both parts of the pathway. As discussed earlier, variable, late, and prolonged decelerations can all be said to reflect interruption of the oxygen pathway at one or more points, which is the first principle of interpretation. Late decelerations reflect interrupted oxygenation because they are always triggered by hypoxemia; variable decelerations reflect interrupted oxygenation because they always reflect some decrease in umbilical venous flow (though not necessarily to the point of hypoxemia); and prolonged decelerations reflect interrupted oxygenation to some degree because they stem from the same mechanisms of late or variable decelerations, or in some cases perhaps a combination of these mechanisms.

The lower half of the oxygen pathway (Fig. 7.34) outlines the fetal response to interrupted oxygenation, which can progress from simple hypoxemia to metabolic acidemia if the interruption of oxygenation continues or worsens. The second principle of interpretations is based on the application of EFM as a screening tool, recognizing that the FHR tracing ***cannot reliably predict the development of fetal metabolic acidemia.*** In fact, FHR tracings with recurrent decelerations and minimal or absent variability have too high a false-positive rate to be considered diagnostic for fetal metabolic acidemia. Even category III tracings considered predictive of abnormal fetal acid–base status fail as *diagnostic* due to their high false-positive rate.

Where EFM fails as a diagnostic tool, it excels as a screening tool. The presence of either moderate variability or an FHR acceleration (spontaneous or stimulated) has already been described as reliable in excluding the presence of fetal metabolic acidemia and any ongoing hypoxic injury at the time it is seen, providing clinicians with the second principle of interpretation. Thus, while clinicians may not be able to use EFM tracings to diagnose impending hypoxic injury, they can effectively use the components seen in many EFM tracings to effectively rule out the possibility of clinically significant metabolic acidemia.[6,7,15]

When clinicians are working together in labor and delivery, understanding what an EFM tracing means related to fetal oxygenation will form the basis of any intervention or management, as well as the rationale for continued labor support versus an expedited delivery. The two principles of interpretation in EFM are:

1. Late, variable, or prolonged decelerations indicate interruption of oxygenation at one or more points.

2. Moderate variability or acceleration of the FHR precludes the presence of metabolic acidemia and ongoing hypoxic injury.

Application of these two simple principles to various FHR tracings is shown in Figures 7.35 to 7.38.

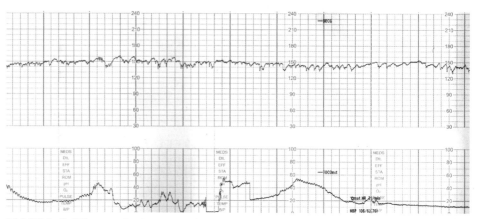

FIGURE 7.35 Application of standardized interpretation. In this tracing, the absence of any late, variable, or prolonged decelerations can be interpreted as an absence of interruption of the oxygen pathway. The presence of moderate variability excludes the possibility of ongoing hypoxic injury, by excluding fetal metabolic acidemia.

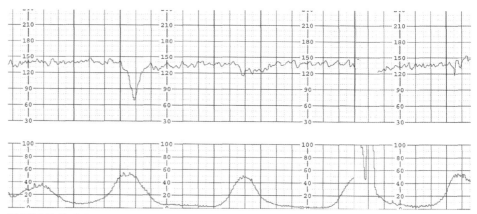

FIGURE 7.36 Application of standardized interpretation. In this tracing, the presence of variable decelerations can be interpreted as evidence of an interruption of the oxygen pathway. However, the presence of moderate variability excludes the possibility of ongoing hypoxic injury, by excluding fetal metabolic acidemia.

Standardized Intrapartum EFM Management

Standardization and incorporation of a shared mental model that promotes meaningful communication are the keys to patient safety.[22–24] The NICHD provides a standardized nomenclature, or terminology, which allows clinicians to answer the first question (What do I call it?) when reviewing EFM tracings. The second question (What does it mean?) can be answered by applying the two principles of interpretation related to (1) the presence or absence of interrupted oxygenation; and (2) the ability to rule out hypoxic injury through the presence of either moderate variability or an acceleration. That leaves the third and final question of management of EFM tracings, what do I do about it? The algorithm and supporting reference material shown in Figures 7.39 and 7.40 reflect an evidence- and consensus-based approach to the management of intrapartum EFM tracings that has been widely published and is based on the utilization of EFM as a screening tool.[13,21,25] *Using EFM as a screening tool relies not on the ability to diagnose impending hypoxic injury, but rather on the ability to screen for normal,* for example, the absence of impending hypoxic brain injury. Once the possibility of the development of hypoxic

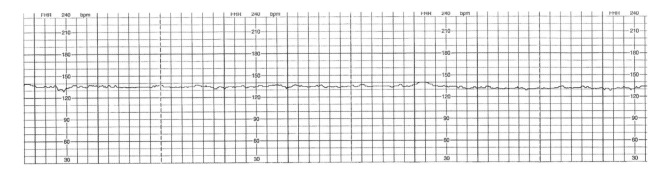

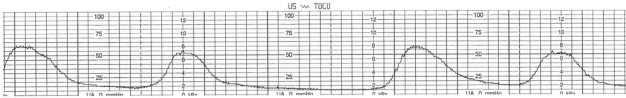

FIGURE 7.37 Application of standardized interpretation. In this tracing, the absence of any late, variable, or prolonged decelerations can be interpreted as an absence of interruption of the oxygen pathway. However, the absence of moderate variability or any acceleration prevents the clinician from excluding the possibility of ongoing hypoxic injury.

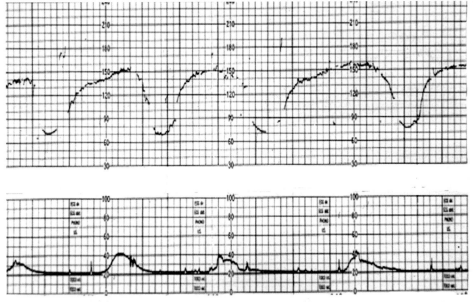

FIGURE 7.38 Application of standardized interpretation. In this tracing, the presence of late and/or variable decelerations can be interpreted as an interruption of the oxygen pathway, while the absence of moderate variability or any accelerations prevent the clinician from excluding the possibility of ongoing hypoxic injury.

injury can no longer be ruled out, the obstetric team must consider delivery. The model provided here (Fig. 7.39) can be divided into two sections, with management of category I tracings on the left (continued observation based on patient risk factors) and management of category II and III tracings on the right (application of the ABCD approach). The ABCD approach (Fig. 7.40) consists of four components:

A—Assess the oxygen pathway and review differentials[1]

B—Begin conservative corrective measures as indicated

---

[1]The term differentials here refers to other causes of FHR changes that may be unrelated to fetal oxygenation and can be either maternal or fetal in origin. In Figure 7.40, these are listed in a callout box on the left side.

Intrapartum FHR Monitoring Management Decision Model

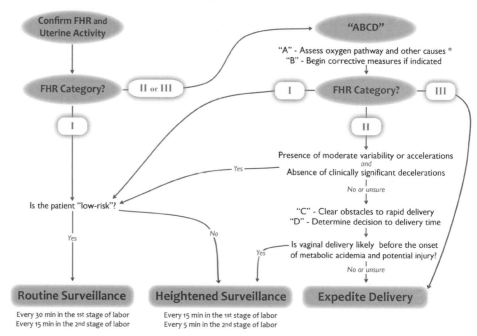

FIGURE 7.39 Intrapartum FHR management decision model. An algorithm for management of EFM tracings during the intrapartum period. (Courtesy of David A. Miller, MD.)

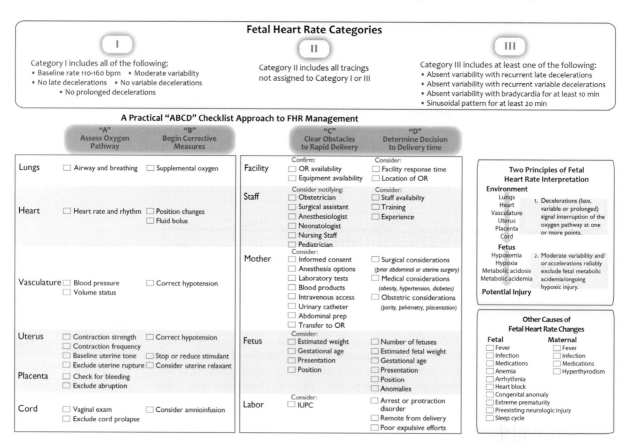

FIGURE 7.40 FHR categories, ABCD checklist, oxygen pathway with principles of interpretation, and other causes of FHR changes. These materials provide support for application of the management algorithm and critical thinking in the evaluation of EFM tracings in labor using a standardized approach. (Courtesy of David A. Miller, MD.)

C—Clear obstacles to rapid delivery

D—Determine a delivery plan (decision to delivery time)

Not all EFM tracings will require the implementation of steps A through D. In many cases, a review of the oxygen pathway and differentials will provide the clinician with sufficient information to simply continue observation, as in the case of minimal variability due to a fetal sleep cycle. In other cases, clinicians may decide to apply (B) conservative corrective measures (often called intrauterine resuscitation, discussed in the next section). If these corrective measures return the EFM tracing to a category I, the algorithm returns the patient to continued surveillance. If the EFM tracing worsens to a category III, or there is a category II tracing that does not resolve with corrective measures, expedited delivery is indicated.

But what if the EFM tracing remains a category II following corrective measures? This is where the C and D components of the algorithm come into play. If the EFM tracing has significant decelerations indicating interruption of the oxygen pathway, and/or the tracing does not allow clinicians to effectively rule out the possibility of the development of hypoxic injury (through moderate variability or an FHR acceleration), clinicians must work together to ensure that decisions are made regarding the timing of delivery. Ultimately, delivery decisions are made by the physician with surgical privileges, often an obstetrician, but in some cases a family practice physician trained in cesarean section.

NOTE: The only exception to this would be a setting where the only obstetric provider was a midwife, and cesarean delivery was performed by a general surgeon acting on the determination of the midwife.

To assist in this delivery decision process, Clark et al.[6] published an approach to persistent category II tracings that did not respond to conservative corrective measures (Fig. 7.41). In this algorithm, EFM tracings are separated into those with moderate variability or FHR acceleration (where metabolic acidemia and ongoing hypoxic injury can be effectively ruled out), and those

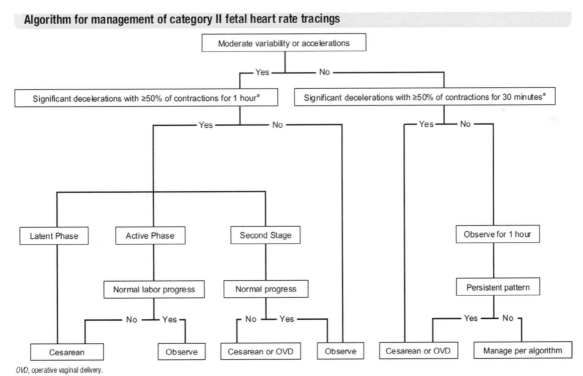

Algorithm for management of category II fetal heart rate tracings

OVD, operative vaginal delivery.

[a]That have not resolved with appropriate conservative corrective measures, which may include supplemental oxygen, maternal position changes, intravenous fluid administration, correction of hypotension, reduction or discontinuation of uterine stimulation, administration of uterine relaxant, amnioinfusion, and/or changes in second stage breathing and pushing techniques.

Clark. Category II FHRT. Am J Obstet Gynecol 2013.

FIGURE 7.41 Algorithm for management of category II fetal heart rate tracings. (From Clark, S. L., Nageotte, M. D., Garite, T. J., et al. (2013). Intrapartum management of Category II fetal heart rate tracings: Towards standardization of care. *American Journal of Obstetrics & Gynecology, 209*, 89–97.)

EFM tracings that lack either moderate variability or FHR acceleration (where the development of metabolic acidemia and ongoing hypoxic injury cannot be reliably excluded).

In the first case, where the EFM tracing demonstrates moderate variability or FHR acceleration, delivery timing decisions are based on several considerations:

1. The presence or absence of significant FHR decelerations
2. The pattern of recurrence of those decelerations over time
3. The stage and phase of labor
4. The determination of normal progress of labor (in either active phase of the first stage or the second stage)

In the second case, where the EFM tracing does not demonstrate either moderate variability or FHR acceleration, delivery timing decisions are based on the following:

1. The presence or absence of significant FHR decelerations
2. The pattern of recurrence of those decelerations over
3. The persistence of the lack of moderate variability or FHR acceleration even when recurrent, significant FHR decelerations are absent

It is extremely important to note that the consensus paper by Clark et al. represents expert opinion regarding delivery decisions made only in situations where the application of conservative corrective measures (intrauterine resuscitation) has failed to correct a category II tracing. In addition, Clark et al.[6] cite a number of very specific clarifications and exclusions, summarized in Table 7.2. Although the clarifications clearly state that the ultimate risk–benefit analysis regarding timing of delivery rests with the physician, all nurses and midwives should be aware of, and able to collaboratively discuss, the factors that go into the decision to continue labor with close observation versus expedite delivery through either operative vaginal delivery or cesarean section. Additionally, there are situations where the algorithm is not used (such as prolonged decelerations) but where the physician and obstetric team will still be faced with the

---

TABLE 7.2 MANAGEMENT OF CATEGORY II FETAL HEART RATE PATTERNS: CLARIFICATIONS FOR USE IN ALGORITHM

1. Variability refers to predominant baseline FHR pattern (marked, moderate, minimal, absent) during a 30-min evaluation period, as defined by NICHD.
2. Marked variability is considered same as moderate variability for purposes of this algorithm.
3. Significant decelerations are defined as any of the following:
   - Variable decelerations lasting longer than 60 sec and reaching a nadir more than 60 bpm below baseline.
   - Variable decelerations lasting longer than 60 sec and reaching a nadir less than 60 bpm regardless of the baseline.
   - Any late decelerations of any depth.
   - Any prolonged deceleration, as defined by the NICHD. Due to the broad heterogeneity inherent in this definition, identification of a prolonged deceleration should prompt discontinuation of the algorithm until the deceleration is resolved.
4. Application of algorithm may be initially delayed for up to 30 min while attempts are made to alleviate category II pattern with conservative therapeutic interventions (e.g., correction of hypotension, position change, amnioinfusion, tocolysis, reduction, or discontinuation of oxytocin).
5. Once a category II FHR pattern is identified, FHR is evaluated and algorithm applied every 30 min.
6. Any significant change in FHR parameters should result in reapplication of algorithm.
7. For category II FHR patterns in which algorithm suggests delivery is indicated, such delivery should ideally be initiated within 30 min of decision for cesarean.
8. If at any time tracing reverts to category I status or deteriorates for even a short time to category III status, the algorithm no longer applies. However, algorithm should be reinstituted if category I pattern again reverts to category II.
9. In fetus with extreme prematurity, neither significance of certain FHR patterns of concern in more mature fetus (e.g., minimal variability) or ability of such fetuses to tolerate intrapartum events leading to certain types of category II patterns are well defined. This algorithm is not intended as guide to management of fetus with extreme prematurity.
10. Algorithm may be overridden at any time if, after evaluation of patient, physician believes it is in the best interest of the fetus to intervene sooner.

FHR, fetal heart rate; NICHD, Eunice Kennedy Shriver National Institute of Child Health and Human Development.
From Clark, S. L., Nageotte, M. D., Garite, T. J., et al. (2013). Intrapartum management of Category II fetal heart rate tracings: Towards standardization of care. *American Journal of Obstetrics & Gynecology, 209,* 89–97.

decision regarding continued labor versus expedited delivery. In these cases, application of the previously discussed principles of interpretation, as well as consideration of clinical context as a whole, will be the key factors for consideration and decision-making. Regardless of the algorithms used or the decisions made, all EFM tracings being evaluated will require thoughtful assessment of the oxygen pathway and consideration of conservative corrective measures when managing changes in FHR related to oxygenation.

Conservative Corrective Measures

Conservative corrective measures, often referred to collectively as intrauterine resuscitation, are interventions applied as part of the previously described standardized management algorithm, under the "B-Begin corrective measures as indicated" portion of the ABCD checklist. The checklist lists seven conservative corrective measures at the level of the lungs, heart, vasculature, uterus, placenta, and cord. Two additional measures that may be more specific to the second stage are altered breathing and altered pushing. The institution of any of these measures follows the clinician's assessment of the oxygen pathway as well as clinical review of other causes of FHR changes unrelated to oxygenation. Types of conservative corrective measures and the basis for their inclusion in practice are listed alphabetically below.[6,7,13,21,25-29] All of the conservative corrective measures listed will provide improved oxygenation for any type of deceleration pattern, with the exception of amnioinfusion which would be primarily indicated for interruption of the oxygen pathway manifesting as variable decelerations. Patient context and clinical judgment will dictate which measure or combination of measures is warranted. It is important to note that clinical consideration of this group of interventions should be seen as the "standard of care" from a legal perspective. The implementation of any of these conservative corrective measures should be determined by assessment of the oxygen pathway as well as individual medical/ nursing judgment within the context of the patient's clinical condition, including risk factors and labor progress.

Alteration of Second-Stage Labor Pushing Efforts

1. Open glottis pushing (avoiding long Valsalva-style pushing)
2. Pushing with every other contraction

Recurrent variable, late, or prolonged decelerations as a response to maternal pushing efforts may prompt the clinician to alter those efforts. Open glottis pushing in the second stage has been shown to be an effective approach to improving fetal oxygenation. Altering the frequency of pushing efforts, such as pushing with every other or even every third contraction and/or pushing in a side-lying position, has also been effective. If these measures do not improve the FHR tracing, the clinician should consider discontinuation of all pushing efforts and repositioning the mother to her lateral side. Passive descent, which allows the contractions alone to move the fetus through the birth canal, may work best in such cases.

Consider Amnioinfusion

Amnioinfusion is an obstetric procedure in which normal saline or lactated Ringer's solution is placed transcervically into the uterus after adequate cervical dilation and rupture of membranes. Amnioinfusion can treat problems associated with decreased intra-amniotic volume, including oligohydramnios and variable decelerations during labor. The procedure requires an IUPC. The IUPC, also designed to accurately monitor uterine contractions, contains a port from which the saline or lactated Ringer's solution is infused. Amnioinfusion may reduce the number of variable decelerations that have not resolved with maternal position change or other corrective measures. The infusion usually begins with a bolus and is followed by a maintenance dose. The clinician should observe that the fluid is returning to avoid overdistention of the uterus. Overdistention of the uterus may cause pressure on the maternal diaphragm or even a placental abruption. Hospital policies and guidelines will dictate the use of this procedure.

Correction of Maternal Hypotension

A variety of factors can result in maternal hypotension, such as simple positioning causing supine hypotension, or as a result of a sympathetic blockade following regional anesthesia. Or the more serious situation which includes maternal hypovolemia is caused by hemorrhage. The resulting decrease in blood flow to the uterus may result in fetal bradycardia, prolonged or late decelerations. Infusion of intravenous (IV) fluids (500 to 1,000 cc) may improve maternal cardiac output which will in turn increase uterine perfusion. This should lead to improved oxygen delivery to the fetus, barring any interruption at the level of the uterus, placenta, or cord. Administration of medications such as phenylephrine and ephedrine may be used to correct hypotension following regional anesthesia. These medications are unlikely to reduce uterine blood flow and will often correct maternal hypotension when fluid bolus alone has failed to do so.

Intravenous Fluid Bolus

Appropriate maternal hydration is important for the optimal uterine perfusion, elimination of waste products of normal aerobic metabolism, and delivery of needed nutrients to the fetus. During labor a decrease in maternal fluid volume can lead to hypoperfusion of the uterus, and thus the intervillous space of the placenta, which could ultimately affect the fetus. Hypotension, regional anesthesia, and hypovolemia may also cause a reduction in blood flow. Fetal oxygenation may be improved by an administration of IV fluids to expand maternal intravascular volume. An IV fluid bolus generally consists of 500 of 1,000 mL of lactated Ringer's given over 20 to 30 minutes depending on the maternal clinical situation.

Maternal Repositioning

Compression of the maternal aorta by the contracting uterus during labor can be a factor resulting in changes in the FHR tracing. The combined weight of the uterus, fetus, amniotic fluid, and placenta may compress the vena cava and cause a reduction in uterine blood flow; this is especially an issue if the mother is in the supine position. Compression of the vena cava or aorta can also decrease blood return and lead to decreased maternal cardiac output, which can lower uterine perfusion. These changes in uterine blood flow may lead to clinically significant FHR decelerations. A maternal position change to the right or left lateral position may improve or resolve decelerations by improving maternal cardiac output and uterine blood flow. Maternal position change is often the first intervention chosen by the clinician, perhaps because of its simplicity and its ability to improve blood flow.

Oxygen Administration

Supplemental oxygen at 10 L/min by non rebreather mask increases the oxygen tension in maternal blood. This will increase the gradient across the uterine–placental interface and may result in increased oxygen transfer to the fetus. There is little evidence in the literature to determine how long oxygen therapy should be used or in what circumstances, and there is controversy in the literature regarding the safety and efficacy of supplemental oxygen.[30–35] Due to the number of other corrective measures available, as well as the paucity of evidence regarding appropriate oxygen administration in labor, oxygen should be used as a second-line response outside of emergency situations.

Reduction of Uterine Activity

1. Stop or reduce uterine stimulants
2. Administration of uterotonics

The NICHD defines uterine tachysystole as five or more contractions in a 10-minute window averaged over 30 minutes. But frequency of contractions provides only a partial assessment of uterine activity. Assessment of a contraction pattern also includes the duration, resting tone, and relaxation time. The clinician should not wait until there are changes in the FHR before responding to excessive uterine activity.[19,20] Uterine tachysystole may occur with or without uterine stimulants such as oxytocin or cervical ripening agents. Interventions for excessive uterine activity are dependent on the clinical context. Decreasing uterine contractions can increase uterine perfusion and allow the fetus appropriate relaxation time for oxygen and carbon dioxide exchange. Generally, the initial responses to decrease uterine activity are to change the maternal position and to discontinue or reduce the oxytocin infusion if it is being infused. Cervical ripening agents may need to be discontinued. A bolus of IV fluids may also be indicated. Tocolytics, such as terbutaline, may also be used to treat excessive uterine activity when other measures have failed; most hospitals require a provider order or midwife/physician involvement in the decision to administer tocolytics.

Summary

The interpretation and management of EFM tracings during labor is a responsibility shared by nurses, midwives, and physicians. Collaborative practice and communication is enhanced by the use of a standardized approach to EFM interpretation based on simple principles of interpretation related to whether or not fetal oxygenation has been interrupted and whether or not damaging degrees of acidemia can be easily excluded. Once the EFM tracing reveals issues with fetal oxygenation, a variety of conservative corrective measures (intrauterine resuscitation techniques) may be employed. Standardized management using an ABCD approach to EFM provides a template for a shared mental model that is both intra- and interdisciplinary. Should an EFM tracing remain in category II following the application of conservative corrective measures, expert consensus exists on how to proceed with decisions regarding continued observation versus expedited delivery.

But even algorithms culled from expert consensus will not provide guidance for every persistent category II tracing, and clinicians may need to individualize delivery and management decisions based on a wide variety of clinical considerations. There is no single, proven approach to EFM management that has proven to be superior, but application of the approach to standardized interpretation and management outlined herein provides nurses, midwives, and physicians with an opportunity to practice using a shared mental model that is consistent with evidence and consensus in the current literature. As Clark et al. state, "one important goal of intrapartum care is delivery of the fetus, when possible, prior to the development of damaging degrees of hypoxia/acidemia."[6]

The ability to understand acidemia, especially the difference between respiratory acidemia (which is essentially a normal finding at a birth that follows labor), as opposed to metabolic acidemia (which can be a precursor to hypoxic injury), is an important skill for all clinicians. The next section provides a simplified approach to understanding umbilical cord gases.

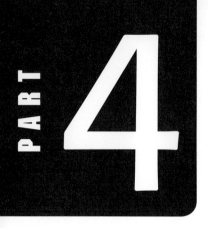

PART 4

Fetal Acid–Base and Umbilical Cord Gas Interpretation

The pH of the blood and tissues has an impact on all enzymes and proteins in the body, affecting organ function and infant status at birth. There are no FHR tracings that are reliably diagnostic for fetal metabolic acidemia, and even the majority of fetuses delivered with category III tracings will not exhibit metabolic acidemia in umbilical arterial cord blood; Category III tracings are deemed "predictive of abnormal fetal acid-base status at the time they are observed"[15] not because of a *majority finding,* but rather because of a *significant minority,*[7,36] which is why expedited delivery is recommended if the tracing does not promptly respond to conservative corrective measures. Regardless of the limitations in associating FHR changes with the presence of fetal metabolic acidemia, clinicians working with EFM can benefit from a basic understanding of cord blood gases and their analysis.

Terms Associated with Acid–Base Analysis

Acidemia—the buildup of acid (causing a reduced pH) in the *blood.* (The terms *acidosis* and *acidemia* are often used interchangeably. When blood values demonstrate a decreased pH, it can be assumed that the tissues are affected in the same manner.)
Acidosis—the buildup of acid (causing a reduced pH) in the *tissues.*
Base deficit (BD)—the amount of bases used by the body in an attempt to normalize a reduced pH (neutralize the acid); illustrates the degree of change in the bicarbonate concentration in the body; the more base used in attempting to normalize the pH, the larger the number becomes (the greater the deficit). Some laboratories report a *base excess* instead of a base deficit; in this case, the number will be expressed as a negative number (−4, −5, −6, etc.) to reflect the deficit (as there is no "excess"). Clinicians should not be confused by the math, but simply look at the number and compare it to the normal values.
Hypoxemia—reduction of oxygen in the *blood.*
Hypoxia—reduction of oxygen in the *tissues.*
pH—a representation of the hydrogen ion concentration.
PCO_2—the partial pressure of carbon dioxide (quantity of CO_2 in the blood).
PO_2—the partial pressure of oxygen (quantity of O_2 in the blood).

Understanding Cord Blood Gases

To understand acid–base evaluation in the fetus, it is helpful to have a brief review of fetal metabolism. In a healthy, well-oxygenated fetus, the primary mode of producing energy is via **aerobic metabolism** which is oxygen dependent. Oxygen and glucose are carried to the fetus via the oxygen pathway and then metabolized resulting in the production of heat and energy, with the byproducts of this metabolism being carbon dioxide and water (CO_2 and H_2O). The CO_2 and H_2O are returned to the placenta via the umbilical arteries. This is why the placenta is said to act as the fetal "lungs" until birth, it is the placental interface that provides oxygen and nutrients to the fetus via the umbilical vein, and then removes the waste products (CO_2 and H_2O) that are part of normal, aerobic metabolism.

When oxygen is not available for aerobic metabolism, the fetus will convert to *anaerobic* metabolism, which depends upon glucose and the conversion of glycogen stores (primarily from the fetal liver). The energy produced by anaerobic metabolism is much less than that produced by aerobic metabolism and is used to cover basal metabolic needs. The key byproduct of anaerobic metabolism is lactic acid, which must be buffered, or neutralized. Bicarbonate (HCO_3) is the base the fetus will use to buffer the lactic acid. Understanding these simple differences between aerobic and anaerobic metabolism is the key to a simplified understanding of cord gas results.

Respiratory versus Metabolic Acidosis

As just discussed, in normal aerobic metabolism, the end products are energy, heat, CO_2, and H_2O. When uterine, placental, and cord blood flows are all functioning properly, the byproducts CO_2 and H_2O are efficiently cleared. If the blood flow is decreased, CO_2 may not be effectively removed and will accumulate, quickly turning into hydrogen and bicarbonate ions. The bicarbonate ions shift into the tissue. But the accumulation of free hydrogen ions in the blood causes a decrease in pH. This results in a respiratory acidemia and is related to the accumulation of CO_2. Cord compression in the second stage and during active pushing can slow the clearance of CO_2 and H_2O, and that is why a respiratory acidemia at birth is common. A respiratory acidemia at birth is considered normal, as it is not caused by any lack of oxygen, rather it is due to the delayed clearance of CO_2. The first breath at birth usually resolves this issue, and *respiratory acidemia alone* at birth is not associated with neonatal morbidity or mortality.[7]

Should a decrease in blood flow or interruption of the oxygen pathway result in significant hypoxia, the peripheral tissues will shift into anaerobic metabolism, utilizing glucose as well as any stored glycogen. Lactic acid is the byproduct here and lactic acid must be buffered, or neutralized with a base, which is bicarbonate (HCO_3). When the amount of lactic acid exceeds fetal buffering capacity, metabolic acidemia is the end result. Should the hypoxia become severe enough (or prolonged enough), metabolic acidosis may occur not only in the peripheral tissues, but it may extend to the vital organs (brain, heart, adrenals) where blood flow was initially redistributed as a protective mechanism. Once metabolic acidosis reaches these vital tissues, the fetus is at risk for organ damage. The severity of metabolic acidemia is evidenced by the base deficit (reported as a positive number, known as base excess when reported as a negative number). The greater the base deficit, the more the fetus has "used up," or exceeded, its buffering capacity and, therefore, the more severe the metabolic acidemia.

Mixed acidemia is often confusing for clinicians, but it is simply the presence of both respiratory and metabolic acidemia in the cord gas result. Thus the sample will have a low pH and elevated base deficit consistent with metabolic acidemia, but the sample will also demonstrate and elevated CO_2, reflecting the "respiratory component" of a mixed acidemia.

Many clinicians use the terms acidosis and acidemia interchangeably, but this is not technically correct. Acidosis refers to tissue, while acidemia refers to blood. Neither respiratory nor metabolic acidosis can be measured directly as we do not sample tissue. Cord blood gases, specifically arterial cord blood samples, revealing either respiratory, metabolic, or mixed acidemia are what clinicians use to determine whether some type of acidosis has occurred in the fetus. The following tables provide information on approximate normal umbilical venous and arterial blood gases as well as respiratory versus metabolic acidemia. Remember, only an accurate arterial cord gas sample is diagnostic for respiratory, metabolic, or mixed acidemia. Clinicians must obtain both venous and arterial samples when drawing cord blood gases, as only comparison of the two will provide proof of an arterial sample (Tables 7.3 and 7.4).

TABLE 7.3	APPROXIMATE NORMAL VALUES FOR CORD BLOOD			
VESSEL	**pH**	**PCO$_2$**	**PO$_2$**	**BASE DEFICIT**
Artery	7.2–7.3	45–55	15–25	<12
Vein	7.3–7.4	35–45	25–35	<12

From Helwig, J. T., Parer, J. T., Kilpatrick, S. J., et al. (1996). Umbilical cord blood acid–base state: What is normal? *The American Journal of Obstetrics and Gynecology, 174*(6), 1807–1812; Victory, R., Penava, D., Da Silva, O., et al. (2004). Umbilical cord pH and base excess values in relation to adverse outcome events for infants delivering at term. *The American Journal of Obstetrics and Gynecology, 191*(6), 2021–2028; Nodwell, A., Carmichael, L., Ross, M., et al. (2005). Placental compared with umbilical cord blood to assess fetal blood gas and acid-base status. *Obstetrics and Gynecology, 105*(1), 129–138.

TABLE 7.4 GENERAL TRENDS FOR CORD GAS ANALYSIS			
VALUE	**RESPIRATORY**	**METABOLIC**	**MIXED**
pH	<7.20	<7.20	<7.20
PCO_2	>55	45–55	>55
Base deficit (mmol/L)	<12	≥12	≥12

Umbilical arterial cord gases represent the most objective measurements of fetal status at the time of delivery. ACOG recommends that umbilical cord gases be obtained in the following clinical situations[40]:

- Cesarean delivery for fetal compromise
- Low 5-minute Apgar score
- Fetus with IUGR
- Abnormal FHR tracings
- Intrapartum fever
- Multifetal gestations
- Maternal thyroid disease

Summary

Umbilical cord gases provide valuable information about the fetal status immediately preceding delivery. Understanding basic elements of umbilical cord gas interpretation is a useful and necessary skill for clinicians working in an intrapartum setting, and especially important is the need for clinicians to obtain both arterial and venous samples. Recognizing both key differences between respiratory and metabolic acidemia is key to recognizing the relationship between EFM findings and fetal acid–base status. ACOG has provided a simple list of recommended clinical situations that warrant the collection of umbilical cord blood gases and these recommendations can form the basis of a standardized protocol for cord blood gas collection in labor and delivery settings. Now that EFM history, mechanisms, interpretation, and management have been reviewed, including physiology and fetal acid–base status, the final section of this module will provide a brief overview of important documentation issues related to intrapartum EFM.

PART 5

Documentation

Documentation of the care provided in the intrapartum period is vitally important. The medical and nursing records should provide a complete, factual, and objective record of the care provided and include only clinically relevant data. These goals for documentation are much easier to discuss than to accomplish. Concerns related to inaccuracies and omission have forced providers to spend increasing amounts of time *documenting* care rather than *providing* care, which may be frustrating and unsatisfying for both patients and providers. The ideal documentation system should be easy to use, time and cost efficient, and comprehensive so that it accurately reflects the care provided.

Problems with Inaccurate and Incomplete Documentation

Despite the emphasis that many providers and institutions place on documentation, inaccuracies and omissions remain common. The results of these problems are many and include the following[41]:

- Decreased communication among members of the healthcare team, because an incomplete or inaccurate medical record may be used to plan care
- Lost information for both statistical purposes and outcome data for quality surveillance
- Denial of reimbursements by insurance carriers, resulting in lost revenue
- During litigation, difficulty for the defense to prove its case because of an incomplete or inaccurate record; additionally, omissions and inaccuracies may leave the impression of a provider who is careless and imprecise

Because litigation may occur several years following an event, the medical record is often the only source of information related to the event. Most providers may only have limited recall and have to rely on the information documented in the medical record. Even in litigation situations where the actions of the healthcare team were reasonable, or within the standard of care, poor documentation may lead to either settlement or a jury verdict favoring the plaintiff.[42]

Components of EFM Documentation

Several types of documentation systems may be used to chart care. These include flowsheets, clinical pathways, checklists, narrative notes, or plotted graphs such as labor progress curves. Clinicians may utilize these different forms electronically, on paper, or in some institutions a combination of both paper and electronic records are utilized. Each system may have benefits, but no one system has been proven to be superior. Regardless of the type of format or system, documentation elements that should be included in a complete evaluation of the EFM tracing during the intrapartum period are the following[15]:

- FHR baseline rate—usually documented as a single number, ending in a 5 or 0 because it is defined as a mean rounded to the nearest 5 beats
- FHR baseline variability—documented as absent, minimal, moderate, or marked
- Presence of FHR accelerations—on flowsheets, often noted with a check or plus sign
- Presence and type of FHR decelerations—documented as early, late, variable, prolonged, or may need to document multiple types of decelerations within an EFM tracing
- Uterine activity—documentation here should include at least contraction duration and frequency, along with resting tone; additional documentation of MVUs may also be included

- Changes or trend over time—demonstrated automatically with use of a flowsheet, but will require a narrative note if flowsheets are not used (as is the case with progress notes written by midwives and physicians)

There is no mandated requirement from the NICHD or any professional organization that summary terms such as categories (for EFM tracings) or the terms tachysystole and normal (referring to the frequency of contractions) be documented, although some institutions have protocols that dictate these summary terms be routinely recorded as part of the documentation process. From a risk management standpoint, to improve communication and enhance recall should litigation arise, it is preferable that the actual components of an assessment, rather than a summary term, be documented in the medical record.[43,44] Looking at a medical record during a deposition, often many years after the actual birth that prompted litigation, the clinician who can review the actual components of EFM and uterine activity evaluation will be better served than the clinician whose only record is one of summary terms.

Frequency of Documentation

The question "How often do I need to chart?" is frequently asked by nurses, midwives, and physicians, and there is really no absolute rule, or answer, from any of the professional organizations. ACOG recommends "health care providers should periodically document that they have reviewed the tracing."[1] AWHONN correctly differentiates between frequency of assessments versus frequency of documentation, and discusses the concept of regular summary documentation, but does not set any absolute timelines for documentation (providing instead "suggested guidelines").[45] Thus, most nursing policies on documentation with intrapartum EFM are determined by individual hospitals or hospital systems. Unfortunately, many policy writers may confuse guidelines on the frequency of assessment with guidelines for documentation.[44] For example, at-risk laboring women in the second stage require assessment of the FHR and uterine contraction pattern every 5 minutes.[10] Assessment is not documentation, yet many nursing managers who do not understand the difference (or perhaps believe the myth of "not charted, not done" myth) create policies requiring nursing documentation with every 5-minute assessment.[43] No nurse can concomitantly provide when trying to provide the second-stage labor support during active pushing and also chart a full evaluation of FHR and uterine activity every 5 minutes, even though nursing assessments are being made continuously during this time.

Rather than setting standards that no reasonable nurse can meet, management should draft protocols and guidelines that reflect nursing assessment expectations based on both patient acuity and phase or stage of labor, and outline reasonable *minimum* frequencies for documentation of these assessments. Should litigation arise, the hospital and nurse can rely on the use of the protocol or guideline coupled with testimony regarding routine or customary practice.

Summary

Documentation related to intrapartum EFM can be accomplished in a variety of approaches, using paper, electronic systems, or a combination of both. The NICHD provides requirements for EFM documentation that include FHR components, evaluation of uterine activity, and the inclusion of changes or trends over time. Summary terms such as categories for EFM tracings or terms such as tachysystole for uterine contraction frequency are unnecessary documentation burdens and can pose significant risk management issues if used in place of the actual FHR and UA components. Frequency of documentation will naturally vary by clinician and by institutional policies, but nursing guidelines should support recognition of the difference between assessment and documentation. Policies or guidelines that place unrealistic documentation burdens on nurses should be avoided.

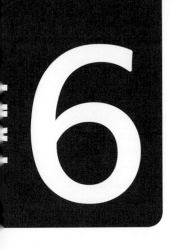

Self-Assessment

This self-assessment is divided into two parts. First, there are 24 questions that are either multiple choice or fill in the blank, followed by the answer key to those 24 questions. Second, there are 10 tracings with questions related to EFM definitions, interpretation, and management; these tracings are also followed by a corresponding answer key.

SELF-ASSESSMENT QUESTIONS

Part 1

1. Name two EFM components that cannot be assessed with IA.

   _____ and _____.

2. List three advantages of IA.

   a. _____

   b. _____

   c. _____

3. The FSE tracks the FHR by:

   a. assessing QT segment changes in the ECG

   b. tracking R to R intervals in the ECG

   c. calculating intervals between ventricular closure in the ECG

4. The shortest segment of time delineated on the graph paper used in EFM is:

   _____

Part 2

5. In a 10-minute segment, how much identifiable baseline is needed to establish a baseline rate?

   _____

6. Tachycardia is defined as an FHR baseline:

   a. >160 bpm

   b. >160 bpm in a term pregnancy

   c. >160 in a term pregnancy

7. A late deceleration requires all of the following, *except*:

   a. nadir that drops 15 bpm from baseline

   b. duration less than 2 minutes

   c. onset that is gradual

8. An EFM tracing reveals a baseline of 185 bpm with absent variability, no decelerations, or accelerations. This tracing should be considered:

   a. ominous

   b. category III, or abnormal

   c. category II, or indeterminate

9. Describe the difference between relaxation time and resting tone when assessing uterine activity.

   _____

   _____

   _____

   _____

10. A contraction duration of 2 minutes or greater is:

    a. considered hypertonus if persistent

    b. known as a tetanic contraction

    c. considered normal in latent phase of the first stage of labor

Part 3

11. Chemoreceptors are:

    a. located in the aortic arch and carotid sinus

    b. sensitive to changes in fetal blood pressure

    c. sensitive to changes in fetal oxygenation

    d. both a and c

    e. both a and b

12. The FHR dysrhythmia that can be associated with fetal hydrops is:

    a. SVT

    b. AV heart block

    c. persistent PVCs

183

13. Late deceleration of the FHR is associated most specifically with:

    a. transient fetal tissue metabolic acidosis during a uterine contraction

    b. transient fetal hypoxemia during a uterine contraction

    c. transient fetal asphyxia during a uterine contraction

14. A key point regarding the occurrence of tachysystole is that:

    a. it can occur in spontaneous or stimulated labor

    b. it requires FHR decelerations to be clinically significant

    c. it should be documented as only if oxytocin is being used

15. List, in order, the pathway that oxygen must follow to reach the fetus.

    _____

    _____

16. List the two principles of standardized interpretation of intrapartum EFM tracings.

    _____

    _____

17. According to the algorithm for delivery decision-making authored by Clark et al., the proper management of a patient with intermittent late decelerations and moderate variability in the second-stage labor with normal progress is:

    a. expedited delivery by operative vaginal delivery or cesarean section

    b. performance of fetal scalp stimulation to rule out acidemia

    c. continued observation

18. When an FHR tracing is category II, this means:

    a. it requires further evaluation

    b. it will progress to a category III if no intervention

    c. the fetus is at risk for acidemia

19. When applying the ABCD approach to a category II or III tracing, step B stands for:

    _____

    _____

20. Early decelerations are:

    a. the result of pressure on the fetal head

    b. gradual in onset

    c. unrelated to interruption of the oxygen pathway

    d. considered clinically benign

    e. all of the above

Part 4

21. Category III tracings are considered predictive of abnormal fetal acid–base status because:

    a. a majority of babies born following a category III tracing will have metabolic acidemia and are at risk for brain damage

    b. a significant number of babies born following a category III tracing will have metabolic acidemia

    c. at least 50% of babies born with a category III tracing will need neonatal resuscitation

    d. category III tracings are indicative of hypoxic ischemic encephalopathy

22. Respiratory acidemia at birth:

    a. is a common occurrence and generally unrelated to neonatal morbidity or mortality

    b. is the precursor to metabolic acidemia

    c. is caused by the buildup of excess lactic acid

    d. all of the above

23. For the following umbilical arterial cord blood gases, determine whether the values represent a normal blood gas, a metabolic acidemia, a respiratory acidemia, or a mixed acidemia.

    a. pH   7.02
       PCO_2 75   This is a _____
       Base deficit   16

    b. pH   7.22
       PCO_2 48   This is a _____
       Base deficit   6

    c. pH   7.16
       PCO_2 65   This is a _____
       Base deficit   11

    d. pH   7.01
       PCO_2 45   This is a _____
       Base deficit   14

    e. pH   6.98
       PCO_2 50   This is a _____
       Base deficit   20

    f. pH   7.24
       PCO_2 45   This is a _____
       Base deficit   5

    g. pH   7.11
       PCO_2 65   This is a _____
       Base deficit   15

    h. pH   7.06
       PCO_2 53   This is a _____
       Base deficit   18

Part 5

24. What must be included in the documentation of an EFM assessment per the NICHD?

    _____

    _____

25. Which of the following is true about EFM documentation?

    a. If something is not documented, it is legally considered not to have occurred

    b. Documentation frequency should be every 5 minutes in the second stage if a patient has risk factors

    c. Categories of the EFM tracing should be regularly documented

    d. None of the above

    e. All of the above

ANSWER KEY FOR SELF-ASSESSMENT QUESTIONS

Part 1

1. Variability of the FHR and the type of FHR deceleration (early, late, variable, or prolonged)
2. Any three of the following—patient comfort, facilitation of ambulation, doula effect, or requirement of caregiver to be at the bedside, less technology, no difference in neonatal outcomes, lower cesarean birth rates, less costly equipment.
3. b. tracking R to R intervals in the ECG
4. 10 seconds.

Part 2

5. 2 minutes, and the 2 minutes need not be contiguous.
6. a. >160 bpm. Gestational age does not alter criteria for baseline range, tachycardia, or bradycardia.
7. a. nadir that drops 15 bpm from baseline. There is no depth requirement with late or early decelerations, only with variable and prolonged.
8. c. category II, or indeterminate
9. Relaxation time is the time (measured in minutes and/or seconds) between the end of one contraction and the beginning of the next contraction. Resting tone is the uterine pressure when the uterus is a contractile (measured in mm Hg when an IUPC is in place, and by palpation when external monitoring or IA is being used). Thus, resting tone is evaluated during relaxation time,

and abnormalities of either can negatively affect fetal O_2/CO_2 exchange.

10. b. known as a tetanic contraction

Part 3

11. d. both a and c. Chemoreceptors are located in the aortic arch and carotid sinus and are sensitive to changes in oxygen, carbon dioxide, and pH of fetal blood.
12. a. Supraventricular tachycardia
13. b. transient fetal hypoxemia during a uterine contraction
14. a. it can occur in spontaneous or stimulated labor
15. The oxygen pathway consists of lungs—heart—vasculature—uterus—placenta—cord.
16. 1. Variable, late, and prolonged decelerations reflect interruption of the oxygen pathway at one or more points; 2. Moderate variability or FHR acceleration (spontaneous or stimulated) exclude the presence of fetal metabolic acidemia and any ongoing hypoxic injury at the time they are seen.
17. c. continued observation
18. a. it requires further evaluation
19. B stands for "begin conservative corrective measures, as indicated"
20. e. all of the above

Part 4

21. b. a significant number of babies born following a category III tracing will have metabolic acidemia
22. a. is a common occurrence and generally unrelated to neonatal morbidity or mortality
23. a. This is a mixed acidemia
    b. This is a normal blood gas
    c. This is a respiratory acidemia
    d. This is a metabolic acidemia
    e. This is a metabolic acidemia
    f. This is a normal blood gas
    g. This is a mixed acidemia
    h. This is a respiratory acidemia

Part 5

24. The NICHD lists six components to include in documentation. They are baseline rate, baseline variability, the presence of FHR accelerations, the presence and type of FHR decelerations, changes or trends over time, and uterine activity.
25. d. None of the above

Instructions for FHR Tracing Assessment

Please read carefully before proceeding to tracing review.

For the purposes of the FHR tracing review, *clinicians should assume that each tracing is reflective of what the clinician would continue to see over 30 minutes,* as this will allow for a clinical decision on whether tachysystole is present as well as assist in identifying some category III tracings where the recurrence of decelerations becomes a factor.

NICHD Terminology

For each tracing, please perform the following:
1. Identify the baseline rate
2. Identify the baseline variability
3. Circle any accelerations
4. Identify and label any decelerations as early, late, variable, or prolonged
5. Provide a description of the uterine activity
6. State the category of the FHR tracing (assume 30 minutes of similar tracing)

Standardized FHR Tracing Interpretation

For each FHR tracing, provide a standardized interpretation that answers the following two questions:
1. Is there evidence of interruption of the oxygen pathway?
2. Can fetal metabolic acidemia (and therefore ongoing hypoxic injury) be ruled out?

Please provide the interpretation of the tracing in sentence form, for example, "The late decelerations reflect interruption of the oxygen pathway, however, the moderate variability precludes (or rules out) the possibility of ongoing hypoxic injury."

"This tracings practicum is based on FHR tracings excerpted from The EFM Workbook, by Janice D. Gibbs and Lisa A. Miller, courtesy of the authors and PRMES, LLC."

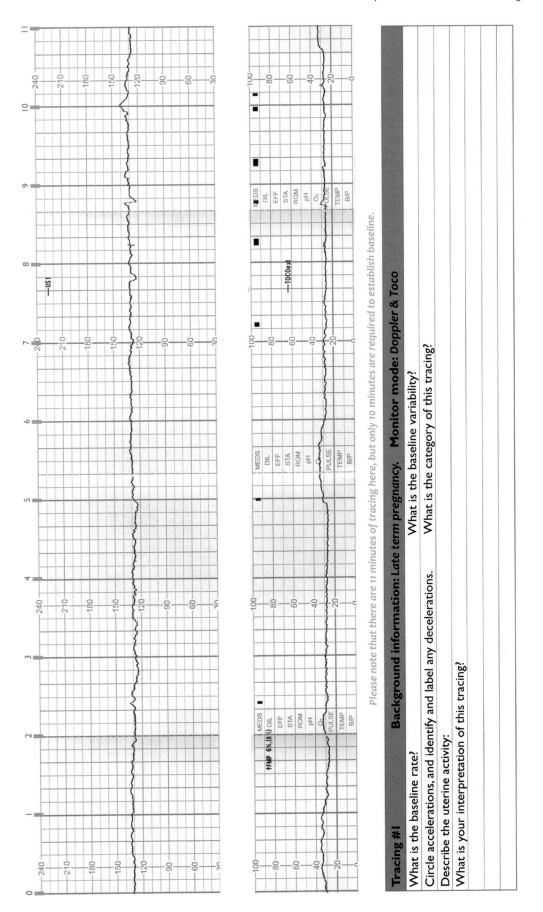

Please note that there are 11 minutes of tracing here, but only 10 minutes are required to establish baseline.

Tracing #1	Background information: *Late term pregnancy.*	Monitor mode: *Doppler & Toco*
What is the baseline rate?		What is the baseline variability?
Circle accelerations, and identify and label any decelerations.		What is the category of this tracing?
Describe the uterine activity:		
What is your interpretation of this tracing?		

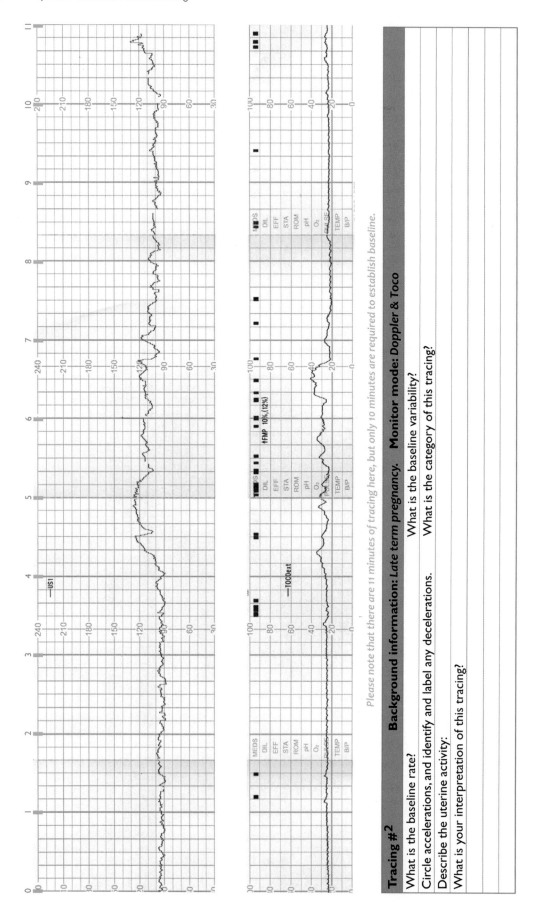

Please note that there are 11 minutes of tracing here, but only 10 minutes are required to establish baseline.

Tracing #2	**Background information:** *Late term pregnancy.*	**Monitor mode:** *Doppler & Toco*
What is the baseline rate?		What is the baseline variability?
Circle accelerations, and identify and label any decelerations.		What is the category of this tracing?
Describe the uterine activity:		
What is your interpretation of this tracing?		

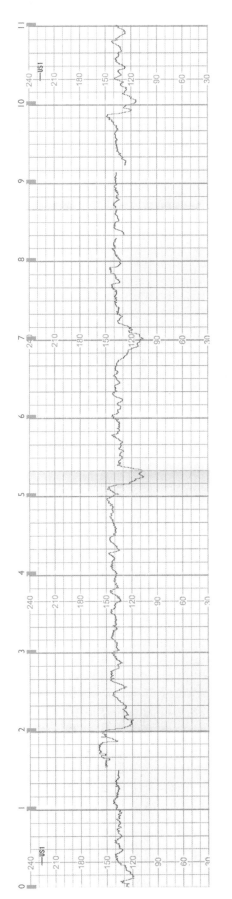

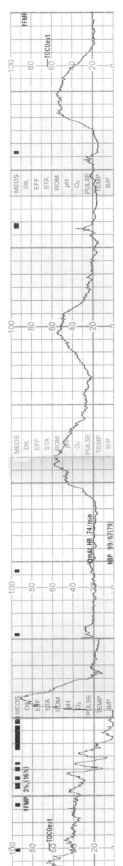

Please note that there are 11 minutes of tracing here, but only 10 minutes are required to establish baseline.

Tracing #3

Background information: Late term pregnancy.   Monitor mode: Doppler & Toco

What is the baseline rate?   What is the baseline variability?

Circle accelerations, and identify and label any decelerations.   What is the category of this tracing?

Describe the uterine activity:

What is your interpretation of this tracing?

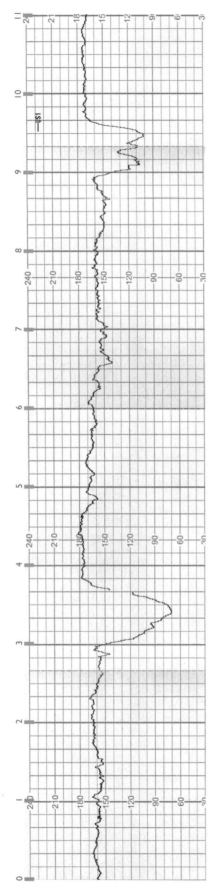

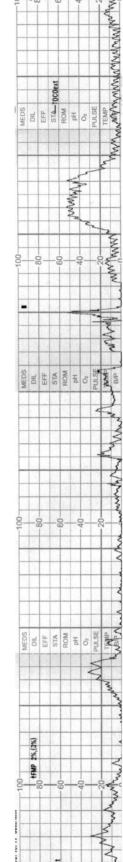

Please note that there are 11 minutes of tracing here, but only 10 minutes are required to establish baseline.

Tracing #4	**Background information: Late term pregnancy.** **Monitor mode: Doppler & Toco**
What is the baseline rate?	What is the baseline variability?
Circle accelerations, and identify and label any decelerations.	What is the category of this tracing?
Describe the uterine activity:	
What is your interpretation of this tracing?	

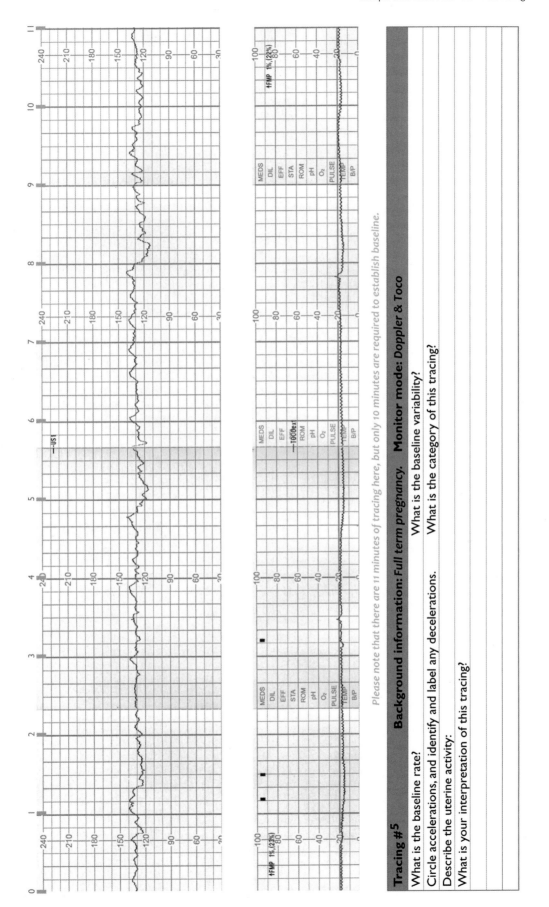

Please note that there are 11 minutes of tracing here, but only 10 minutes are required to establish baseline.

| Tracing #5 | Background information: *Full term pregnancy.* | Monitor mode: *Doppler & Toco* |

What is the baseline rate?

What is the baseline variability?

Circle accelerations, and identify and label any decelerations.   What is the category of this tracing?

Describe the uterine activity:

What is your interpretation of this tracing?

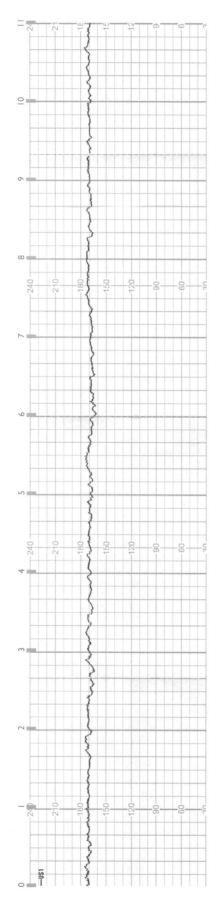

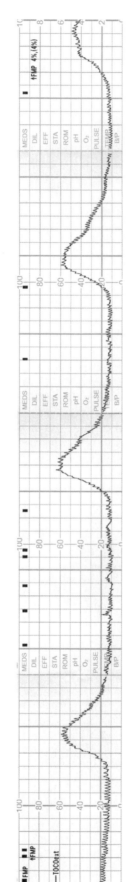

Please note that there are 11 minutes of tracing here, but only 10 minutes are required to establish baseline.

Tracing #6	**Background information:** *Preterm pregnancy at 35 weeks, SROM x 22 hours.* **Monitor mode:** *Doppler & Toco*
What is the baseline rate?	What is the baseline variability?
Circle accelerations, and identify and label any decelerations.	What is the category of this tracing?
Describe the uterine activity:	
What is your interpretation of this tracing?	

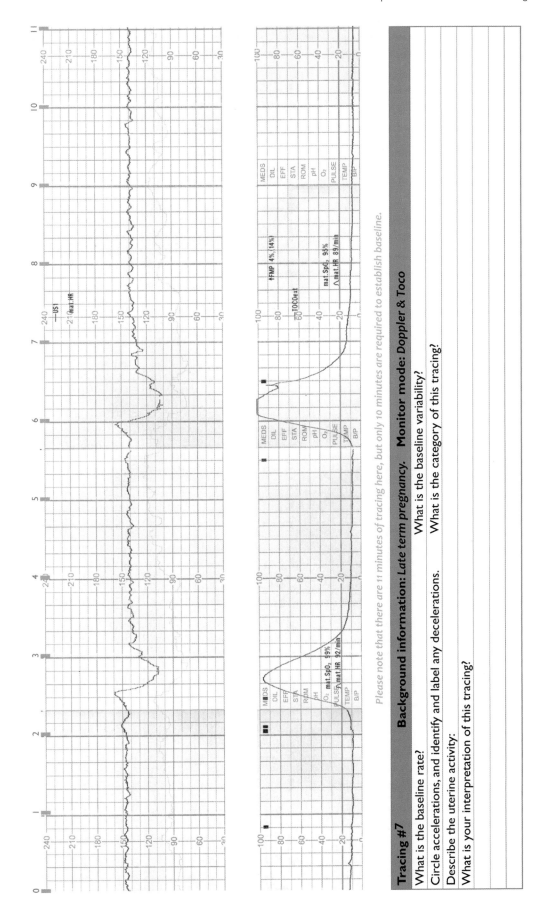

Please note that there are 11 minutes of tracing here, but only 10 minutes are required to establish baseline.

Tracing #7	Background information: *Late term pregnancy.*	Monitor mode: *Doppler & Toco*

What is the baseline rate?

What is the baseline variability?

Circle accelerations, and identify and label any decelerations.

What is the category of this tracing?

Describe the uterine activity:

What is your interpretation of this tracing?

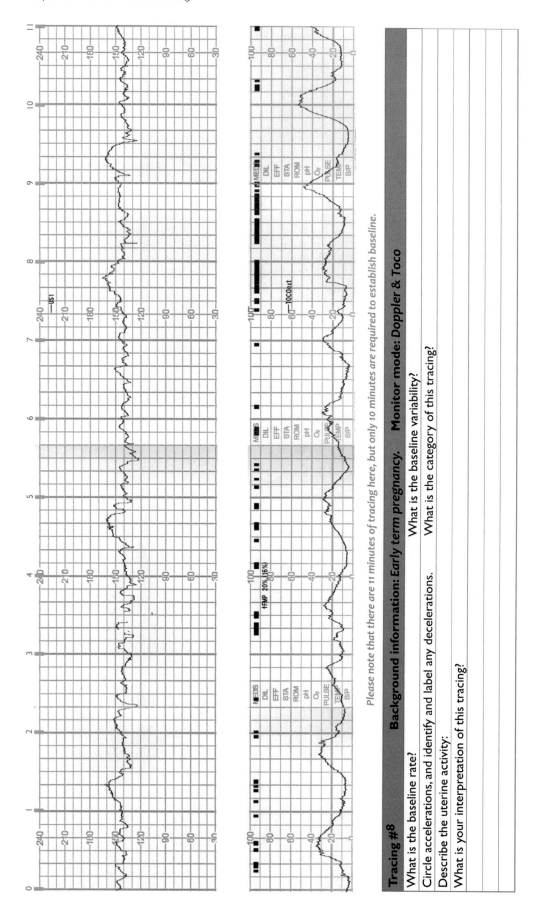

Please note that there are 11 minutes of tracing here, but only 10 minutes are required to establish baseline.

Tracing #8	Background information: *Early term pregnancy.*	Monitor mode: *Doppler & Toco*

What is the baseline rate?   What is the baseline variability?

Circle accelerations, and identify and label any decelerations.   What is the category of this tracing?

Describe the uterine activity:

What is your interpretation of this tracing?

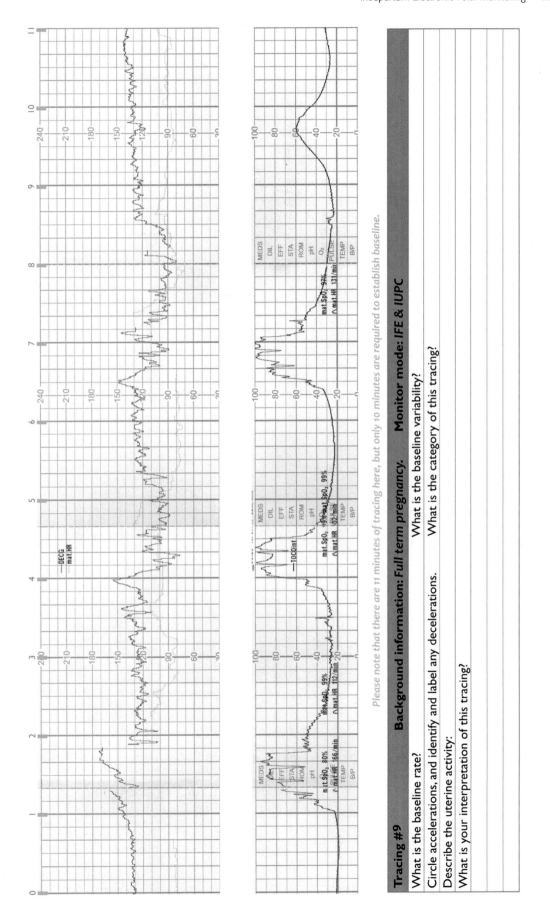

Please note that there are 11 minutes of tracing here, but only 10 minutes are required to establish baseline.

Tracing #9   Background information: Full term pregnancy.   Monitor mode: IFE & IUPC

What is the baseline rate?   What is the baseline variability?

Circle accelerations, and identify and label any decelerations.   What is the category of this tracing?

Describe the uterine activity:

What is your interpretation of this tracing?

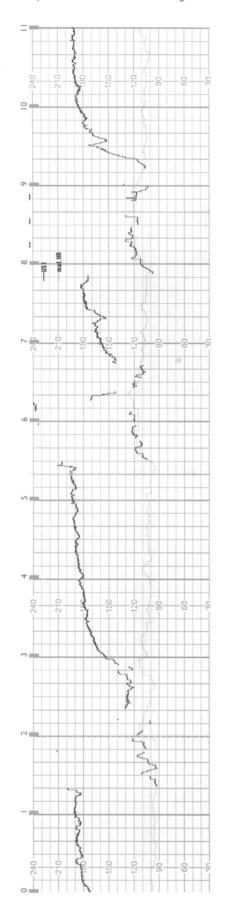

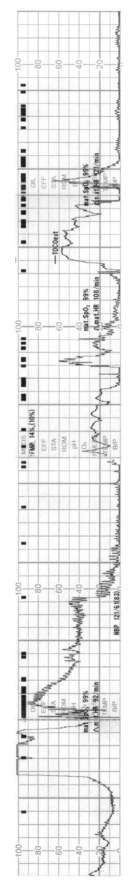

Please note that there are 11 minutes of tracing here, but only 10 minutes are required to establish baseline.

Tracing #10	Background information: *Late term pregnancy.*	Monitor mode: *Doppler & Toco*
What is the baseline rate?		
	What is the baseline variability?	
Circle accelerations, and identify and label any decelerations.		What is the category of this tracing?
Describe the uterine activity:		
What is your interpretation of this tracing?		

Instructions for Use of FHR Tracings Answer Key

The following FHR tracings provide answers to the questions posed by the practicum tracings review along with additional editorial comment that may be helpful in clinical practice. Both students and instructors will note that the authors have made every attempt to identify possible reasonable differences of opinion which can arise when visual interpretation of FHR tracings is occurring at the bedside; in such cases the clinical significance has been noted as well as an attempt to focus on the aspects of the FHR tracing components and interpretation where clinicians can agree. All too often in daily practice, nurses, physicians, and midwives get side-tracked and waste valuable time and energy by focusing on areas of disagreement. This workbook was specifically designed to refocus clinicians towards a shared mental model in EFM, and the answers provide to the tracings will reflect this underlying intention. *The authors realize that other experts in EFM (and individual clinicians) may differ in their analysis of the tracing, and welcome constructive discourse on any areas of disagreement.*

PLEASE NOTE: Due to the limitations of FHR tracing reviews in this format, discussion of the actual bedside management of these tracings is precluded for two reasons: 1) the application of the Intrapartum EFM Management Model requires clinical context; and 2) this type of exercise does not allow the clinician to view FHR tracing response to conservative corrective measures, making it impossible for clinicians to decide on expedited delivery vs. continued observation.

Guide to FHR tracing answer keys

Explanatory Text
The text portion found below each answer key tracing has been deliberately written in a conversational tone, to encourage clinicians to practice communication skills so vital to collaboration in EFM assessment and management. In addition to the discussion of each FHR tracing in text format, the tracings have been graphically illustrated to reflect correct answers related to FHR and UA tracing components.

Graphic Overlays for FHR Components & Uterine Contractions
Baseline Rate & Baseline Variability

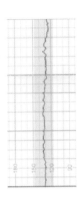

Areas of visually identifiable FHR baseline (which includes the two components, baseline rate and baseline variability) are demarcated by shaded rectangular overlays

FHR Accelerations

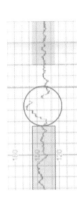

FHR accelerations are noted by a circle overlay surrounding the acceleration

FHR Decelerations

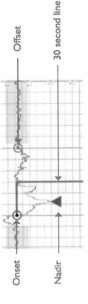

Decelerations are demarcated by an onset represented by the black dot outlined by a circle and connected to an inverted "L" shape that provides a 30-second marker. The nadir is represented by a blue triangle. If the peak of the blue triangle is located to the left of the line (as it is in the above example) the onset to nadir of the deceleration is "abrupt" per the NICHD guidelines. If the peak of the blue triangle is on the line or to the right of the line (as in the following example), the onset to nadir of the deceleration is "gradual" per the NICHD guidelines. The offset of the deceleration is noted as a red dot within a red circle.

Instructions for Use of FHR Tracings Answer Key

Graphic Overlays for FHR Components & Uterine Contractions

FHR Decelerations (continued)

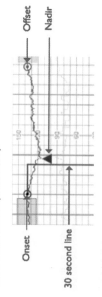

Onset

Offset

Nadir

30 second line

It is helpful to remind clinicians to measure the onset to nadir prior to evaluating any other facets of the deceleration, as decelerations with abrupt onsets by definition can only qualify as variable or prolonged, while decelerations with gradual onsets may be early, late, or prolonged.

Uterine Contractions

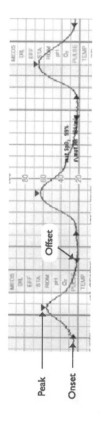

Peak

Offset

Onset

The onset, peak, and end, or offset, of a uterine contraction is identified with a small blue triangle (note that the onset triangle points to the right, the peak triangle points downward, and the end, or offset triangle points to the left).

Areas of FHR or Uterine Activity that are Questionable

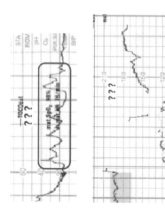

Any areas of either the FHR or UA that are questionable or deserve attention will be called out with a series of three question marks, and in some cases, a blue rectangular boundary box. These areas of the tracing will be discussed in the explanatory text.

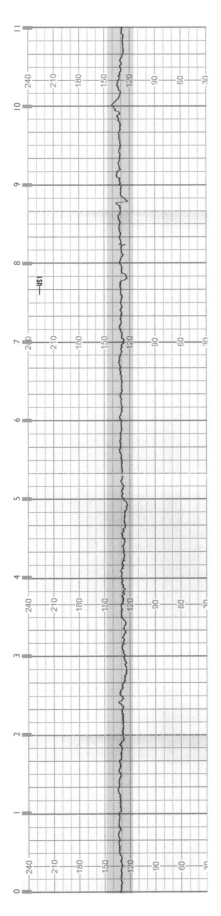

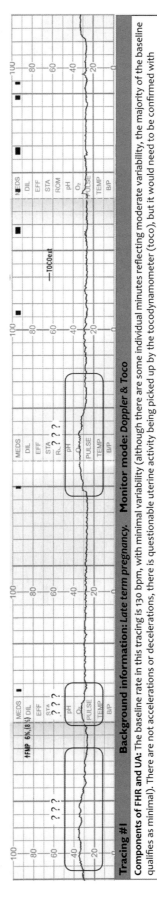

Tracing #1   Background information: *Late term pregnancy.*   Monitor mode: *Doppler & Toco*

Components of FHR and UA: The baseline rate in this tracing is 130 bpm, with minimal variability (although there are some individual minutes reflecting moderate variability, the majority of the baseline qualifies as minimal). There are not accelerations or decelerations. There is questionable uterine activity being picked up by the tocodynamometer (toco), but it would need to be confirmed with palpation.

Category: This tracing is Category 2, or indeterminate.

Interpretation: There is no evidence of interrupted oxygenation, but the possibility of metabolic acidemia cannot be ruled out due to the minimal variability and absence of accelerations. *Note for clinical practice:* decreased variability, when not preceded by evidence of interrupted oxygenation (late, variable, or prolonged) and occurring within the context of a normal baseline rate is usually due to factors unrelated to the oxygen pathway, such as fetal sleep cycles or analgesia.

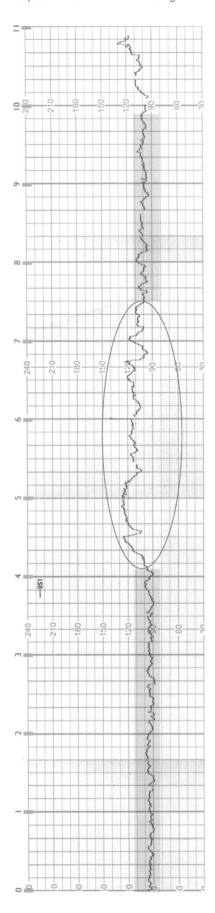

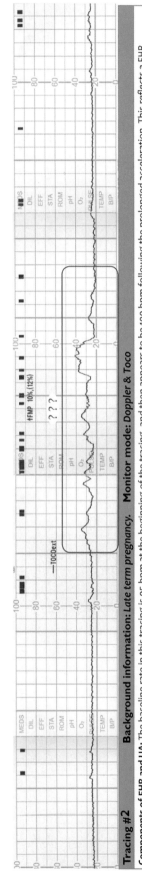

Tracing #2   Background information: Late term pregnancy.   Monitor mode: Doppler & Toco

Components of FHR and UA: The baseline rate in this tracing is 95 bpm at the beginning of the tracing, and then appears to be 100 bpm following the prolonged acceleration. This reflects a FHR bradycardia by definition, but this may be normal given the gestational age of late term (due to maturation of the parasympathetic system). It would be important for the bedside clinician to confirm that the tracing reflects fetal, and not maternal, heart rate. The variability is moderate. There are no decelerations. There is questionable uterine activity occurring at the time of the prolonged acceleration, it would require confirmation by palpation.

Category: This tracing is Category 2, or indeterminate (due to the bradycardic baseline).

Interpretation: There is no evidence of interruption of the oxygen pathway, and the presence of moderate variability and an acceleration rule out fetal metabolic acidemia. *Note for clinical practice:* As long as maternal heart rate/signal coincidence is ruled out, this tracing is an example of a situation where a bradycardia is a normal finding due to gestational age. It would warrant a note in the medical record to reflect the clinical team's understanding of this "bradycardia".

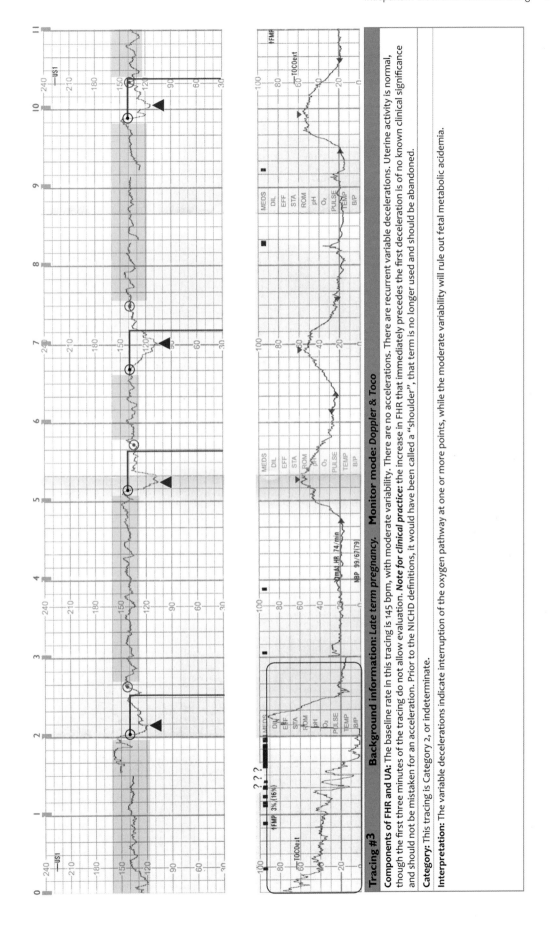

Tracing #3

Background information: *Late term pregnancy.*   **Monitor mode:** *Doppler & Toco*

Components of FHR and UA: The baseline rate in this tracing is 145 bpm, with moderate variability. There are recurrent variable decelerations. Uterine activity is normal, though the first three minutes of the tracing do not allow evaluation. *Note for clinical practice:* the increase in FHR that immediately precedes the first deceleration is of no known clinical significance and should not be mistaken for an acceleration. Prior to the NICHD definitions, it would have been called a "shoulder", that term is no longer used and should be abandoned.

Category: This tracing is Category 2, or indeterminate.

Interpretation: The variable decelerations indicate interruption of the oxygen pathway at one or more points, while the moderate variability will rule out fetal metabolic acidemia.

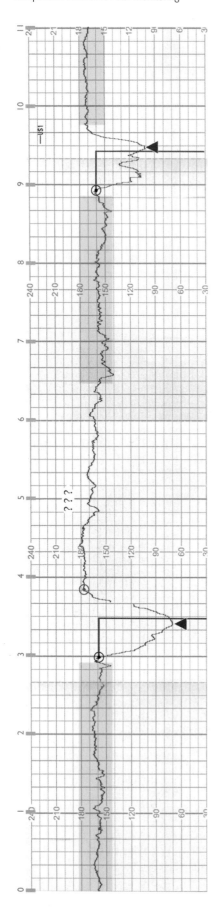

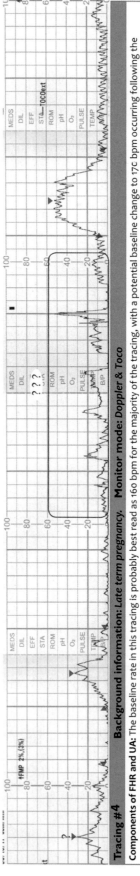

Tracing #4

Background information: _Late term pregnancy._   Monitor mode: _Doppler & Toco_

Components of FHR and UA: The baseline rate in this tracing is probably best read as 160 bpm for the majority of the tracing, with a potential baseline change to 170 bpm occurring following the second deceleration (although it could simply be an increase following the deceleration and may return to a baseline of 160 bpm as the tracing continues). The area of FHR between minute markers 4-7 may not actually reflect baseline, but rather a period of time where the fetus is returning to baseline, which means that baseline variability cannot be assessed again until closer to minute 7. Clinicians may therefore disagree as to whether the variability in this tracing is minimal or moderate, which will affect the interpretation of the tracing. But it will not affect the categorization of the tracing, and standardized management will "push" all Category 2 tracings towards an evaluation of the oxygen pathway as part of the ABCD approach, so clinicians will be doing the same things for the patient even when unable to agree on nomenclature or interpretation. There are two decelerations in this tracing, the first is a variable due to its abrupt onset, the second meets criteria for a late deceleration due to its gradual onset, duration of less than 2 minutes, and relationship to the contraction.

Category: This tracing is a Category 2, or indeterminate.

Interpretation: The decelerations indicate interruption of the oxygen pathway at one or more points, fetal metabolic acidemia cannot be ruled out (note that clinicians who determine baseline variability as moderate would be able to rule out fetal metabolic acidemia).

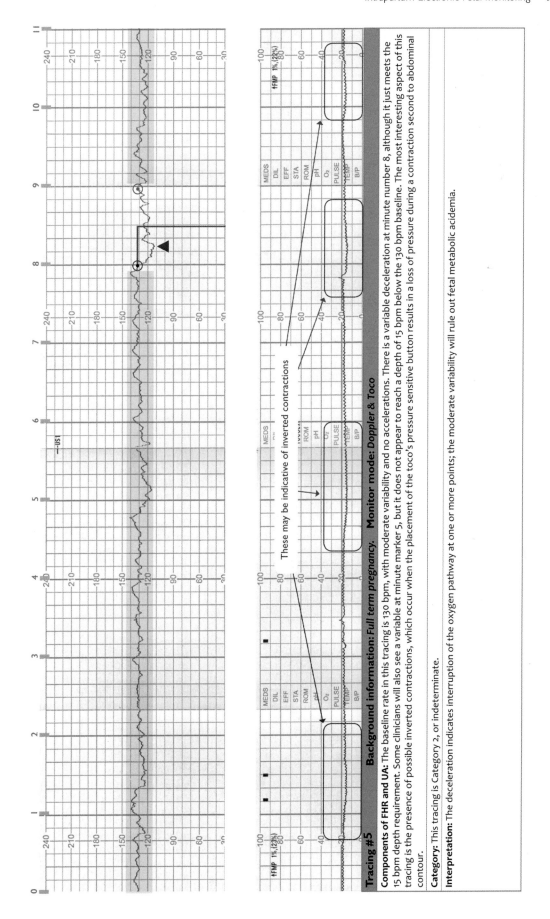

These may be indicative of inverted contractions

Tracing #5

Background information: Full term pregnancy.   Monitor mode: Doppler & Toco

Components of FHR and UA: The baseline rate in this tracing is 130 bpm, with moderate variability and no accelerations. There is a variable deceleration at minute number 8, although it just meets the 15 bpm depth requirement. Some clinicians will also see a variable at minute marker 5, but it does not appear to reach a depth of 15 bpm below the 130 bpm baseline. The most interesting aspect of this tracing is the presence of possible inverted contractions, which occur when the placement of the toco's pressure sensitive button results in a loss of pressure during a contraction second to abdominal contour.

Category: This tracing is Category 2, or indeterminate.

Interpretation: The deceleration indicates interruption of the oxygen pathway at one or more points; the moderate variability will rule out fetal metabolic acidemia.

203

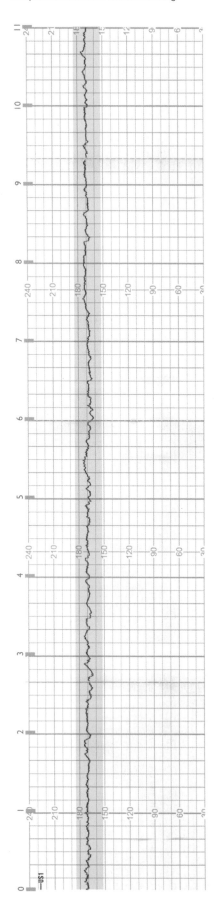

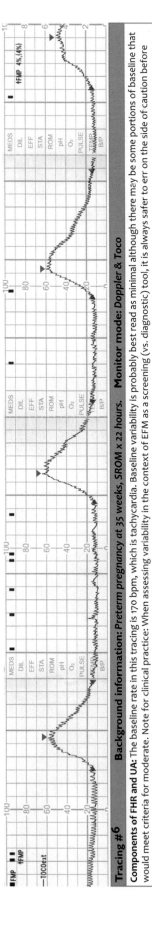

Tracing #6	Background information: *Preterm pregnancy at 35 weeks, SROM x 22 hours.* **Monitor mode: *Doppler & Toco***

Components of FHR and UA: The baseline rate in this tracing is 170 bpm, which is tachycardia. Baseline variability is probably best read as minimal although there may be some portions of baseline that would meet criteria for moderate. Note for clinical practice: When assessing variability in the context of EFM as a screening (vs. diagnostic) tool, it is always safer to err on the side of caution before calling baseline variability moderate, especially when there are no accelerations and the baseline is already complicated by tachycardia. There are no accelerations or decelerations. The uterine activity is normal.

Category: This tracing is Category 2, or indeterminate.

Interpretation: There is no evidence of interruption of the oxygen pathway, but the lack of consistently moderate variability or any accelerations prevents clinicians from ruling out fetal metabolic acidemia. ***Note for clinical practice:*** this type of tracing requires a very careful evaluation of both the oxygen pathway and the other factors that can affect FHR tracings. Prematurity and infection predispose the fetus to more rapid deterioration of fetal acid-base status, and cannot be overlooked as part of an integrated labor management plan. Delay in delivery has occurred (with resulting poor outcome) because clinicians "excused" lack of moderate variability, lack of accelerations, and tachycardia as being due to prematurity and infection. Once the obstetric team cannot rule out fetal metabolic acidemia in the setting of tachycardia and prematurity, decisions regarding continued labor versus expedited delivery must be carefully considered.

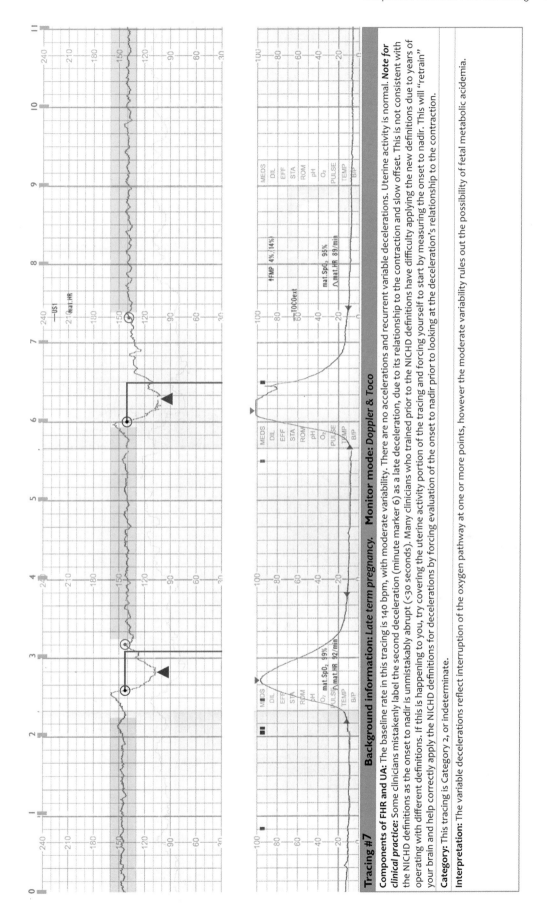

Tracing #7   Background information: *Late term pregnancy.*   Monitor mode: *Doppler & Toco*

Components of FHR and UA: The baseline rate in this tracing is 140 bpm, with moderate variability. There are no accelerations and recurrent variable decelerations. Uterine activity is normal. *Note for clinical practice:* Some clinicians mistakenly label the second deceleration (minute marker 6) as a late deceleration, due to its relationship to the contraction and slow offset. This is not consistent with the NICHD definitions as the onset to nadir is unmistakably abrupt (<30 seconds). Many clinicians who trained prior to the NICHD definitions have difficulty applying the new definitions due to years of operating with different definitions. If this is happening to you, try covering the uterine activity portion of the tracing and forcing yourself to start by measuring the onset to nadir. This will "retrain" your brain and help correctly apply the NICHD definitions for decelerations by forcing evaluation of the onset to nadir prior to looking at the deceleration's relationship to the contraction.

Category: This tracing is Category 2, or indeterminate.

Interpretation: The variable decelerations reflect interruption of the oxygen pathway at one or more points, however the moderate variability rules out the possibility of fetal metabolic acidemia.

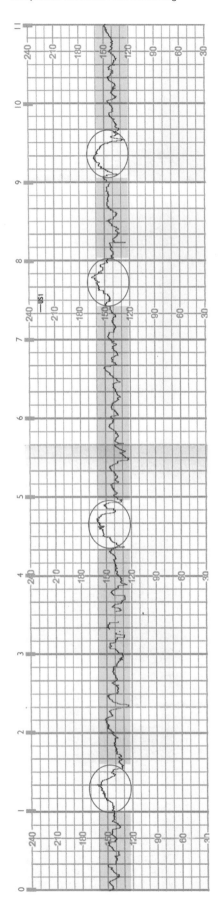

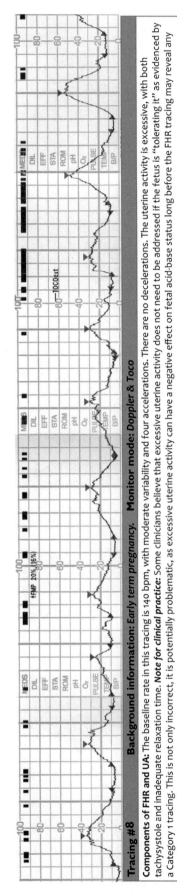

Tracing #8   Background information: *Early term pregnancy.*   Monitor mode: *Doppler & Toco*

Components of FHR and UA: The baseline rate in this tracing is 140 bpm, with moderate variability and four accelerations. There are no decelerations. The uterine activity is excessive, with both tachysystole and inadequate relaxation time. ***Note for clinical practice:*** Some clinicians believe that excessive uterine activity does not need to be addressed if the fetus is "tolerating it" as evidenced by a Category 1 tracing. This is not only incorrect, it is potentially problematic, as excessive uterine activity can have a negative effect on fetal acid-base status long before the FHR tracing may reveal any significant changes.

Category: This tracing is Category 1, or normal.

Interpretation: There is no evidence of interruption of the oxygen pathway and both the moderate variability and the accelerations rule out the possibility of fetal metabolic acidemia.

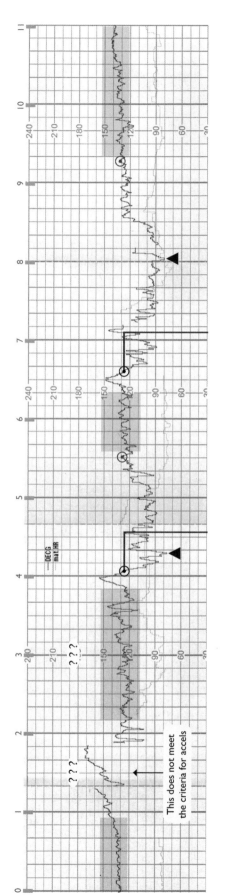

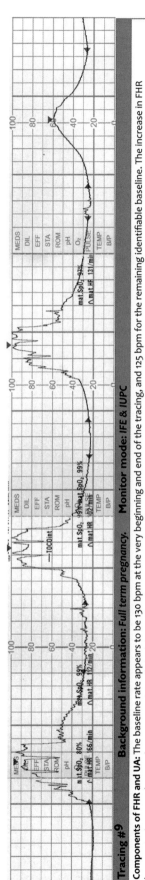

Tracing #9   Background information: *Full term pregnancy.*   Monitor mode: IFE & IUPC

Components of FHR and UA: The baseline rate appears to be 130 bpm at the very beginning and end of the tracing, and 125 bpm for the remaining identifiable baseline. The increase in FHR between minute marker 1 and 2 cannot technically be labeled an acceleration, as it has an onset to peak that is gradual (30 seconds or more) rather than abrupt (<30 seconds). This will not affect the interpretation of the FHR tracing as the baseline variability is moderate. There is one variable and one prolonged deceleration. The uterine activity is normal as to frequency (i.e., there is no tachysystole) but the relaxation time is inadequate following the second and third contractions and the resting tone seems to be increasing, which may result in hypertonus. It appears the patient may have been using closed glottis (long Valsalva) pushing during the first 3 contractions.

Category: This tracing is Category 2, or indeterminate.

Interpretation: The decelerations in this tracing reflect interruption of the oxygen pathway, however the moderate variability rules out the possibility of fetal metabolic acidemia.

207

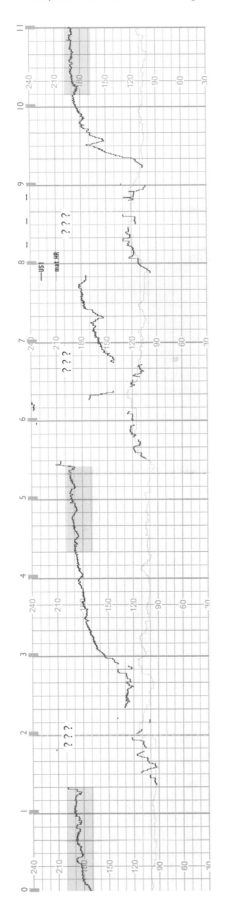

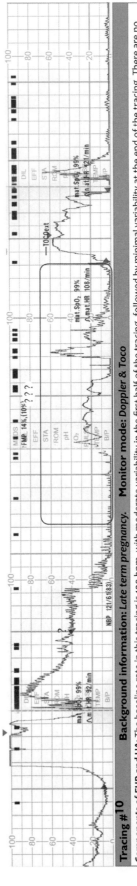

Tracing #10

Background information: *Late term pregnancy.*   **Monitor mode:** *Doppler & Toco*

Components of FHR and UA: The baseline rate in this tracing is 190 bpm, with moderate variability in the first half of the tracing, followed by minimal variability at the end of the tracing. There are no apparent accelerations. While much of the tracing between portions of identifiable baseline is missing, what little is present is indicative of probable prolonged decelerations and should be treated as such. The uterine activity is difficult to determine, and it appears the patient is utilizing closed glottis (long Valsalva) pushing maneuvers, which can have a deleterious effect on maternal (and therefore utero-placental) hemodynamics.

Category: This tracing is Category 2, or indeterminate.

Interpretation: The probable decelerations should be treated as indicative of interruption of the oxygen pathway and although the moderate variability at the beginning of this tracing rules out the possibility of fetal metabolic acidemia, this is not the case near the end of the tracing. **Note for clinical practice:** The tachycardia combined with the other features of the FHR tracing warrants an immediate response using conservative corrective measures (see the Intrapartum EFM Management model).

REFERENCES

1. American College of Obstetricians and Gynecologists. (2009). ACOG practice bulletin. Clinical management guidelines for obstetrician–gynecologists, number 106, July 2009; Intrapartum fetal heart rate monitoring: Nomenclature, interpretation, and general management principles. *Obstetrics & Gynecology, 114*, 192–202.

2. Resnik, R. (2013). Electronic fetal monitoring: The debate goes on . . . and on . . . and on. *Obstetrics & Gynecology, 121*(5), 917–918.

3. Stout, M. J., & Cahill, A. G. (2011). Electronic fetal monitoring: Past, present, and future. *Clinics in Perinatology, 38*(1), 127–142.

4. Alfirevic, Z., Devane, D., & Gyte, G. M. (2013). Continuous cardiotocography (CTG) as a form of electronic fetal monitoring (EFM) for fetal assessment during labour. *Cochrane Database of Systematic Reviews, 5*, CD006066.

5. Nelson, K. B., Dambrosia, J. M., Ting, T. Y., et al. (1996). Uncertain value of electronic fetal monitoring in predicting cerebral palsy. *The New England of Journal Medicine, 334*(10), 613–618.

6. Clark, S. L., Nageotte, M. D., Garite, T. J., et al. (2013). Intrapartum management of category II fetal heart rate tracings: Towards standardization of care. *American Journal of Obstetrics & Gynecology, 209*, 89–97.

7. American College of Obstetricians and Gynecologists & American Academy of Pediatrics. (2014). *Neonatal encephalopathy and neurologic outcome* (2nd ed.). Washington, DC: Author.

8. Wood, S. H. (2003). Should women be given a choice about fetal assessment in labor? *MCN, The American Journal of Maternal and Child Nursing, 28*(5), 292–298.

9. American College of Nurse Midwives (ACNM). *Position statement: Appropriate use of technology in childbirth.* http://www.midwife.org/ACNM/files/ACNMLibraryData/UPLOADFILENAME/000000000054/Appropriate-Use-of-Technology-in-Childbirth-May-2014.pdf. Accessed December 10, 2014.

10. American Academy of Pediatrics & American College of Obstetricians and Gynecologists. (2012). *Guidelines for perinatal care* (7th ed.). Washington, DC: Author.

11. Feinstein, N. F., Sprague, A., & Trepanier, M. J. (2009). *Fetal heart rate auscultation* (2nd ed.). Washington, DC: AWHONN.

12. Hodnett, E. D., Gates, S., Hofmeyr, G. J., et al. (2013). Continuous support for women during childbirth. *The Cochrane Database of Systematic Reviews, 7*, CD003766.

13. Freeman, R. K., Garite, T. J., Nageotte, M. P., et al. (2012). *Fetal heart rate monitoring* (4th ed.). Philadelphia, PA: Lippincott Williams & Wilkins, Wolters-Kluwer.

14. National Institute of Child Health and Human Development Research Planning Workshop. (1997). Electronic fetal heart rate monitoring: Research guidelines for interpretation. National Institute of Child Health and Human Development Research Planning Workshop. *The American Journal of Obstetrics and Gynecology, 177*(6), 1385–1390.

15. Macones, G. A., Hankins, G. D., Spong, C. Y., et al. (2008). The 2008 National Institute of Child Health and Human Development workshop report on electronic fetal monitoring: Update on definitions, interpretation, and research guidelines. *Journal of Obstetric, Gynecologic, and Neonatal Nursing, 37*, 510–515.

16. Cahill, A. G., Roehl, K. A., Odibo, A. O., et al. (2012). Association of atypical decelerations with acidemia. *Obstetrics and Gynecology, 120*, 1387–1393.

17. Kang, A. H., & Boehm, F. H. (1999). The clinical significance of intermittent sinusoidal fetal heart rate patterns. *The American Journal of Obstetrics and Gynecology, 180*(1), 151–153.

18. Jackson, M., Holmgren, C. M., Esplin, M. S., et al. (2011). Frequency of fetal heart rate categories and short-term neonatal outcome. *Obstetrics and Gynecology, 118*(4), 803–808.

19. Miller, L. A., Miller, D. A., & Tucker, S. M. (2013). Uterine activity evaluation and management. In *Pocket guide to fetal monitoring: A multidisciplinary approach* (7th ed., Chapter 4, pp. 75–97). St. Louis, MO: Mosby.

20. Bakker, P. C., Kurver, P. H., Kuik, D. J., et al. (2007). Elevated uterine activity increases the risk of fetal acidosis at birth. *The American Journal of Obstetrics and Gynecology, 196*(4), 313.e1–e6.

21. Miller, L. A., Miller, D. A., & Tucker, S. M. (2013). *Pocket guide to fetal monitoring: A multidisciplinary approach* (7th ed.). St. Louis, MO: Mosby.

22. American College of Obstetricians and Gynecologists. (2015). Committee Opinion No. 629: Clinical guidelines and standardization of practice to improve outcomes. *Obstetrics and Gynecology, 125*(4), 1027–1029.

23. Lyndon, A., Johnson, M. C., Bingham, D., et al. (2015). Transforming communication and safety culture in intrapartum care: A multi-organization blueprint. *Obstetrics and Gynecology, 125*(5), 1049–1055.

24. Miller, D. A. (2011). Intrapartum fetal heart rate definitions and interpretation: Evolving consensus. *Clinical Obstetrics and Gynecology, 54*, 16–21.

25. Miller, D. A., & Miller, L. A. (2012). Electronic fetal heart rate monitoring: Applying principles of patient safety. *The American Journal of Obstetrics and Gynecology, 206*(4), 278–283.

26. Simpson, K. R., & Creehan, P. A. (2014). *Perinatal nursing* (4th ed.). Washington, DC: AWHONN.

27. Garite, T., & Simpson, K. R. (2011). Intrauterine resuscitation during labor. *Clinical Obstetrics and Gynecology, 54*(1), 28–39.

28. Simpson, K. R. (2007). Intrauterine resuscitation during labor: Review of current methods and supportive evidence. *Journal of Midwifery Womens Health, 52*(3), 229–237.

29. American College of Obstetricians and Gynecologists. (2010). ACOG Practice Bulletin. Clinical management guidelines for obstetricians-gynecologists, number 116. Management of intrapartum fetal heart rate tracings. *Obstetrics and Gynecology, 116*, 1232–1240.

30. Fawole, B., & Hofmeyr, G. J. (2012). Maternal oxygen administration for fetal distress. *The Cochrane Database of Systematic Reviews, 12*, CD000136.

31. Hamel, M. S., Anderson, B. L., & Rouse, D. J. (2014). Oxygen for intrauterine resuscitation: Of unproved benefit and potentially harmful. *The American Journal of Obstetrics and Gynecology, 211*(2), 124–127.

32. Doyle, J. L., & Silber, A. C. (2015). Maternal oxygen administration for intrauterine resuscitation. *The American Journal of Obstetrics and Gynecology, 212*(3), 409.

33. Ross, M. G., & Amaya, K. E. (2015). Maternal oxygen use during labor. *The American Journal of Obstetrics and Gynecology, 212*(3), 410.

34. Garite, T. J., Nageotte, M. P., & Parer, J. T. (2015). Should we really avoid giving oxygen to mothers with concerning fetal heart rate patterns? *The American Journal of Obstetrics and Gynecology, 212*(4), 459.

35. Hamel, M. S., Hughes, B. L., & Rouse, D. J. (2015). Whither oxygen for intrauterine resuscitation? *The American Journal of Obstetrics and Gynecology, 212*(4), 461–462.

36. Parer, J. T., King, T., Flanders, S., et al. (2006). Fetal acidemia and electronic fetal heart rate patterns: Is there evidence of an association? *The Journal of Maternal–Fetal & Neonatal Medicine, 19*(5), 289–294.

37. Helwig, J. T., Parer, J. T., Kilpatrick, S. J., et al. (1996). Umbilical cord blood acid—base state: What is normal? *The American Journal of Obstetrics and Gynecology, 174*(6), 1807–1812.

38. Victory, R., Penava, D., Da Silva, O., et al. (2004). Umbilical cord pH and base excess values in relation to adverse outcome events for infants delivering at term. *The American Journal of Obstetrics and Gynecology, 191*(6), 2021–2028.

39. Nodwell, A., Carmichael, L., Ross, M., et al. (2005). Placental compared with umbilical cord blood to assess fetal blood gas and acid-base status. *Obstetrics and Gynecology, 105*(1), 129–138.

40. American College of Obstetricians and Gynecologists. (2006). *Umbilical cord blood gas and acid-base analysis.* Committee Opinion Number 348. Washington, DC: Author.

41. Simpson, K. R., & Chez, B. F. (2014). Perinatal patient safety and professional liability issues. In Simpson, K. R., & Creehan, P. A. (Eds.), *Perinatal nursing* (4th ed.). Philadelphia, PA: Lippincott William & Wilkins.

42. Clark, S. L., Belfort, M. A., & Dildy, G. A. (2008). Reducing obstetric litigation through alterations in practice patterns. *Obstetrics and Gynecology, 112*, 1279–1283.

43. Miller, L. (2011). Intrapartum fetal monitoring: Liability and documentation. *Clinical Obstetrics and Gynecology, 54*, 50–55.

44. Miller, L. A., Miller, D. A., & Tucker, S. M. (2013). Patient safety, risk management, and documentation. In *Pocket guide to fetal monitoring: A multidisciplinary approach* (7th ed., Chapter 10, pp. 216–251). St. Louis, MO: Mosby.

45. Lyndon, A., & Ali, L. U. (Eds.). (2009). *Fetal heart monitoring: Principles and practice* (4th ed.). Washington, DC: AWHONN.

Induction and Augmentation of Labor

VALERIE YATES HUWE

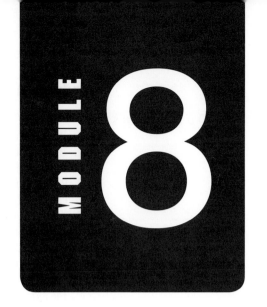

MODULE

8

Skill Unit 1

Oxytocin Labor Induction/Augmentation

Induction and Augmentation

As you complete this module, you will learn:

1. The indications for labor induction/augmentation
2. The current guidelines for cervical ripening, induction and augmentation of labor
3. The risks of induction and augmentation of labor
4. Principles of active management of labor
5. Contraindications for labor induction/augmentation
6. Conditions necessary for the safe administration of oxytocin
7. The state of the cervix as an important indicator of induction success
8. Prostaglandin preparations are hormonal medications used to promote cervical ripening and desired cervical change
9. To anticipate potential problems associated with the use of prostaglandins
10. The recommended method of oxytocin administration
11. To anticipate potential problems of oxytocin administration
12. The recommended nursing interventions when problems arise with the use of oxytocin or prostaglandins
13. The conditions necessary for safe administering of oxytocin including staffing ratios, assessment frequencies, and medical record documentation for inducing/augmenting labor

When you have completed this module, you should be able to recall the meaning of the following terms. You should also be able to use the terms when consulting with other health professionals. The terms are defined in this module or in the glossary at the end of this book.

active management of labor (AML)   oxytocin
amniotomy   cervical ripening
augmentation of labor   prostaglandins
Bishop score   uterine tachysystole
cephalopelvic disproportion (CPD)   dystocia
induction of labor

Induction and Augmentation of Labor

• What is induction of labor?

Induction of labor is the artificial stimulation of uterine contractions before spontaneous onset of labor for the purpose of accomplishing vaginal birth.[1] The goal of labor induction is to achieve vaginal delivery.[2]

• Why should labor be induced?

Before 41 0/7 weeks' induction of labor should generally be performed based on maternal or fetal indications. After 41 0/7 weeks' induction of labor should be performed to reduce the risk of cesarean and the risk of perinatal morbidity and mortality.[3]

• What is augmentation of labor?

Augmentation of labor is the stimulation of uterine contraction when spontaneous contractions have failed to result in progressive cervical dilatation or descent of the fetus.[4] Since uterine activity is characterized by frequency, intensity, and duration of contractions, it may be desirable to augment these forces in a patient who is in labor but not progressing adequately.

• What is oxytocin?

Oxytocin is a hormone, a peptide consisting of nine amino acids that is synthesized by the hypothalamus then transported to the posterior pituitary gland where it is released into the maternal circulation in a pulsatile fashion. Oxytocin is released in response to breast stimulation, cervical stretching, and stimulation of the lower genital tract. Oxytocin released in response to vaginal and cervical stretching results in uterine contractions.[5] Oxytocin is the most common pharmacologic agent used for both induction and augmentation of labor in the United States.[6] It is also the hormone responsible for the "let down" of milk from alveolar cells in the breast during the postpartum period.

• How does oxytocin function in labor?

Oxytocin increases free intracellular calcium, which is essential for smooth muscle activity. To exert its effect, oxytocin must bind with the oxytocin receptors. Oxytocin receptors in the uterus increase throughout gestation to reach their maximal levels at term.[7] In fact, oxytocin receptors at term are increased 300 times over nonpregnant level. Additionally, the increase of actual receptors is also accompanied by an increase in uterine responsiveness to oxytocin at term.[3,8] It is important to note that although oxytocin is an effective induction agent for women with a favorable cervix, it is not effective as a cervical ripening agent.[9]

• What is the half-life of oxytocin?

The pharmacokinetic half-life of oxytocin is generally accepted to be between 10 and 12 minutes.[10–13] Three to four half-lives of oxytocin are needed to reach steady-state plasma concentrations.[11] Uterine response to IV oxytocin administration occurs within 3 to 5 minutes of IV administration, and within 40 minutes a steady-state plasma concentration is achieved.[14] This information led Seitchik et al. to recommend at least a 40-minute interval between increases of oxytocin to allow time for the oxytocin to reach a steady state and exert its full effect on the uterus.[15] This dosing regime is intended to prevent women from receiving higher doses of oxytocin than are necessary.[15] Risks associated with oxytocin are generally dose related and the most common side effect is tachysystole. While oxytocin is the most common medication used for labor induction and augmentation, it is also the drug most commonly associated with preventable adverse events during childbirth.[16]

• What is tachysystole?

Tachysystole is now the preferred term to describe excessive uterine activity. Tachysystole is defined as:
  • More than five contraction in 10 minutes, averaged over 30 minutes
  • Contractions lasting 2 minutes or more
  • Contractions of normal duration occurring within 1 minute of each other
  • Insufficient return of uterine tone between contractions when palpated or >25 mm Hg between contractions when measured with an intrauterine pressure catheter (IUPC).[1,4,17,18]

*NOTE: Other terms like **hypertonus** and **hyperstimulation** are not well defined and should be avoided.*

Common Techniques for Induction and Augmentation of Labor

Common methods of inducing or augmenting labor include the following:
  • **Amniotomy**—is the artificial rupture of chorioamniotic membranes by a qualified provider using a plastic hook. It can be an effective method of labor induction in multiparous women with cervical dilation of 3 cm or more causing the uterus to begin contracting. For some women, this may be enough necessary stimulation for labor induction and no other medications are necessary. However, there is insufficient evidence on the safety and efficacy of amniotomy alone for labor induction.[1]

Amniotomy is done when the cervix is effaced and dilated. The head of the fetus should be against the lower uterine segment and at least dipping into the pelvis. It is essential to confirm the fetal vertex is the presenting part. Risks include umbilical cord prolapse, cesarean section, variable decelerations, intra-amniotic infection, fetal injury, bleeding from undiagnosed vasa previa, and commitment to labor with uncertain outcome, cesarean birth. Early amniotomy is contraindicated when there is maternal infection, such as HIV or viral hepatitis.

- **Nipple stimulation** is a nonmedical method of inducing labor. Some studies have shown that women with favorable cervices who had nipple stimulation were more likely to go into labor within 72 hours compared to similar women who did not receive nipple stimulation. Since oxytocin is released with nipple stimulation, theoretically tachysystole could result; therefore, uterine activity should be monitored. Nipple stimulation can be accomplished manually by the woman or by application of a warm compress to the breast.
- **Stripping membranes**—is the separation of the chorioamniotic membrane from the wall of the cervix and the lower uterine segment. This procedure is typically performed in an office visit at ≥39 weeks of gestation by inserting the examiner's finger beyond the internal cervical os and then rotating the finger 360 degrees along the lower uterine segment. This action causes a release of prostaglandins and may also stimulate oxytocin release.[19] Risks include discomfort during the procedure, prelabor rupture of membranes, vaginal bleeding, and irregular contractions.[9] Routine membrane stripping is not recommended, given there is no evidence of improved maternal and neonatal outcome.[20]
- **Use of oxytocin infusion**—Intravenous administration of oxytocin stimulates the smooth muscle of the myometrium of the uterus to contract. Oxytocin administration is covered in detail in Skill Unit 1.

Medical Indications for Induction/Augmentation of Labor

Indications for induction of labor are not absolute and should take into consideration maternal and fetal conditions, gestational age, cervical status, and other factors.[1] The following are examples of maternal and fetal conditions that may be indications for induction of labor:
- Abruptio placentae
- Chorioamnionitis
- Fetal demise
- Gestational hypertension
- Preeclampsia, eclampsia
- Premature rupture of membranes (PROMs)
- Postterm pregnancy
- Maternal medical conditions including but not limited to diabetes mellitus, renal disease, chronic pulmonary disease, chronic hypertension, and antiphospholipid syndrome
- Fetal compromise—including but not limited to severe fetal growth restriction, isoimmunization, and oligohydramnios

Prerequisites for Induction/Augmentation of Labor

- **What are some prerequisites for an induction/augmentation to be safe and effective?**

The woman should not have any of the contraindications for induction/augmentation. In addition it is recommended that the following occur[1,21]:
1. Gestational age, cervical status, pelvic adequacy, fetal size, and fetal presentation should be assessed before the administration of any cervical ripening agents or oxytocin.
2. Because of the known risks, the medical record should document that a discussion was held between the pregnant woman and her healthcare provider about the indications, the agents, and the methods of labor induction and cervical ripening, including the risks, benefits to the mother and the fetus, alternative approaches, and the possible need for repeat induction (if first attempt fails) or cesarean delivery.[1,9,23]

3. Nulliparous women undergoing induction of labor with unfavorable cervices should be counseled about a two-fold increased risk of cesarean delivery.[1,22-24]
4. A physician capable of performing a cesarean delivery should be readily available.[1]

Initiating an elective induction of labor for reasons of convenience, although very common, should not be encouraged by healthcare providers or hospitals. The pregnant woman should be at least 39 completed weeks' gestation to avoid the risk of iatrogenic prematurity.[1]

Healthcare providers should discuss the risks and benefits with the patient prior to admission. Perinatal nurses should confirm the woman has been fully informed of the risks, benefits, and alternatives.[25]

(See Fig. 8.1)

Patient Safety Checklist

SCHEDULING INDUCTION OF LABOR   Adapted from ACOG Safety Checklist No. 5, 3011.[26]

Date_____Patient_____Date of birth_____MR#_____
Physician /Certified Nurse Midwife_____ _____
Gravida/Parity_____EDD_____Gestational Age_____

Documented GA of 39 0/7 weeks or greater confirmed by either:

☐   Ultrasound measurement at less than 20 weeks or older of gestation that supports GA of 39 weeks or greater
☐   Fetal heart tones have been documented as present for 30 weeks of gestation by Doppler ultrasonography

Indication for induction: (choose one)

☐   Medical complication or condition: Diagnosis:_____
☐   Nonmedically indicated: Conditions/Circumstances_____

Patient has been counseled about risks, benefits, and alternatives to induction of labor
☐   Consent form signed as required by institution
Bishop Score (see below)

			Bishop Scoring System		
Score	Dilatation (cm)	Position of Cervix	Factor Effacement (1%)	Station*	Cervical Consistency
0	Closed	Posterior	0-30	-3	Firm
1	1-2	Midposition	40-50	-2	Medium
2	3-4	Anterior	60-70	-1, 0	Soft
3	5-6	---	80	+1, +2	---

*Station reflects a -3 to +3 scale.
Modified fro Bishop EH. Pelvic scoring for elective induction. Obstet Gynecol 1964;24:266-8.[30]

☐   Pertinent prenatal laboratory test results (eg, group B streptococci or hematocrit)
☐   Special concerns (eg, allergies, medical problems, and special needs):_____
To be completed by reviewer
☐   Approved induction after 39 0/7 weeks of gestation by aforementioned dating criteria
☐   Approved induction before 39 0/7 weeks of gestation (medical indication)
☐   **HARD STOP** – gestation age, indication, consent, or other issues prevent initiating induction without further information or consultation with department chair.

FIGURE 8.1   Induction of Labor Checklist. (Adapted from Patient Safety Checklist from ACOG No 5: Scheduling Induction of Labor.)

DISPLAY 8.1 CONTRAINDICATIONS TO INDUCTION/
AUGMENTATION

Vasa previa
Complete placenta previa
Transverse fetal lie
Umbilical cord prolapse
Previous classical cesarean delivery
Active genital herpes infection
Previous myomectomy entering the endometrial cavity

• Can every woman be safely induced/augmented?

No, although induction and augmentation have become a safer procedure for both women and their fetuses, there are some women for whom induction and augmentation carry an unacceptable risk.

Contraindications for Induction/Augmentation of Labor

Listed in Display 8.1 are clinical situations in which induction/augmentation should not be attempted.[15] This list is the same as the clinical situations contraindicated for spontaneous labor and vaginal birth.

- **Complete placenta previa** when the cervical os is completely covered by the placenta. This can be a life-threatening condition, therefore labor should be avoided and the fetus should be delivered by cesarean birth.
- **Vasa previa** when the umbilical arteries and veins cross the cervical os in front of the presenting part. It is a life-threatening condition for the fetus.
- **Transverse fetal lie**—fetus is not in the proper position for delivery and cannot be delivered vaginally.
- **Umbilical cord prolapse**—when the umbilical cord presents before the presenting part, blood flow to the fetus may be compromised. This is an emergency that requires immediate cesarean delivery.
- **Previous classical cesarean delivery** uterine contractions induced or augmented might be too powerful and may rupture the scar.
- **Active genital herpes infection**—in the presence of an active genital herpetic lesion, a cesarean birth is recommended to prevent transmission to the fetus.
- **Previous myomectomy** entering the endometrial cavity—contraction induced or augmented, might be too powerful and may rupture the scar.

> **KEEP IN MIND:** *For indeterminate fetal status (category II or category III FHR tracing) each contraction of the uterus, decreases blood circulation and oxygen supply to the placenta and the fetus. Because oxytocin increases the intensity and frequency of the contractions, there can be an even greater interruption of oxygen to the fetus. If the fetus shows signs of stress, it might not be able to tolerate the additional intensity of induced/augmented contractions.*

Conditions That Require Special Attention during Induction/Augmentation

There are some situations in which induction/augmentation of labor might present problems. These women require careful administration of a uterine stimulant and close monitoring (Display 8.2).

- **Trial of labor after a previous cesarean birth**—spontaneous labor appears to decrease the risk of uterine rupture in women desiring a trial of labor after cesarean (TOLAC). If induction of labor is done in this situation, a thorough discussion of the increased risk of uterine rupture must be documented by the provider in the medical record. Prostaglandin preparations for cervical ripening are contraindicated for these women.[27]

DISPLAY 8.2 RELATIVE CONTRAINDICATIONS TO
INDUCTION/AUGMENTATION

Trial of labor after a previous cesarean
Presenting part not engaged in pelvis
Severe maternal hypertension
Grand multiparity
Multiple gestations
Polyhydramnios
Abnormal or indeterminate fetal heart rate patterns (not requiring emergent intervention)
Maternal heart disease

- **Presenting part not engaged in pelvis**—there is space between the presenting part and the bony pelvis. With forceful contractions, the fetal membranes can rupture and increase the risk for umbilical cord prolapse. Also, if the presenting part is not engaged, it might indicate the fetus is too large for the pelvis.
- **Severe maternal hypertension**—control of maternal blood pressure should be the priority before induction of labor is initiated.
- **Grand multiparity**—in a woman who has had several children (five or more), the uterus is more likely to rupture with the powerful contractions caused by the induction/augmentation of labor.
- **Multiple gestations**—caution must be taken to prevent tachysystole of an overly distended uterus.
- **Polyhydramnios**—the uterus is overly distended and might not respond well. The possibility of an amniotic fluid embolus may be increased.
- **Abnormal or indeterminate fetal heart rate patterns** (not requiring emergent birth)—close monitoring of the fetal heart rate is necessary to rapidly identify any deterioration in fetal status.
- **Maternal heart disease**—these women may be induced, but require careful monitoring of maternal hemodynamic status throughout the labor and delivery process. Each clinical condition should be individually assessed. Some induction agents may worsen the patient's cardiac condition and have adverse effects.

- ## What is active management of labor?

Active management of labor (AML) is an augmentation protocol used in many institutions as a strategy to decrease cesarean births for labor dystocia. The goal is to establish effective contractions and accomplish a vaginal delivery within 12 hours of admission. Although active management is often considered a high-dose oxytocin protocol, it is really a labor management protocol and oxytocin administration is just one component of a whole program of labor.

The term *active management of labor* is interpreted differently from one institution to another. Many of the protocols are based on the belief that **once labor had been diagnosed, the rate of cervical dilatation should be 1 cm/hr.**[28] Two key management strategies are: if cervical dilatation does not progress at least 1 cm/hr, oxytocin augmentation is initiated, and if membranes have not spontaneously ruptured within 1 hour after labor has been diagnosed, amniotomy is performed.[28]

The original protocol was developed in Dublin, Ireland, to shorten labor and conserve resources in maternity hospitals.[29] All aspects of their protocol are not included in many U. S. hospitals. The following criteria are used for identification of patients for inclusion in AML protocols.
- Nulliparity
- Patient education
- More than 37 weeks' gestation
- Single fetus without compromise
- Spontaneous active labor
- Strict criteria to define labor and labor progress
- 1:1 nursing support

Cervical Ripening

Cervical ripening is the process of effecting physical softening and distensibility of the cervix leading to effacement and dilatation in preparation for labor and delivery.[6] A variety of different methods may be used to induce cervical ripening. These include mechanical devices and several different prostaglandin preparations. Before beginning any cervical ripening or induction, assessment of the cervix should be done and a Bishop score assigned. Since cervical status is the most important factor predicting the success of an induction, this score helps to identify those women who would benefit from cervical ripening before beginning an induction of labor.

• What is a Bishop score?

A Bishop score is a method of evaluating how ready or "ripe" the cervix is for induction.[30] A cervical examination is done to evaluate *dilatation, effacement, consistency* (i.e., softness or firmness), and *cervical position,* as well as *station* of the presenting part. The findings are scored on a scale that was developed based on studies of many women undergoing labor induction (Table 8.1). Inductions are more likely to be successful when a woman's cervix has undergone certain biochemical changes. Based on the assessment findings and using a scoring system for these changes, it identifies which women are good candidates for labor induction.

TABLE 8.1 BISHOP SCORE FOR ASSESSING READINESS FOR INDUCTION					
	SCORE				
	0	**1**	**2**	**3**	**SUBTOTALS**
Dilatation (cm)	0	1–2	3–4	5 or more	
Effacement (%)	0–30	40–50	60–70	80 or more	
Station (cm)	–3	–2	–1, 0	+1, +2	
Cervical consistency	Firm	Medium	Soft		
Cervical position	Posterior	Midposition	Anterior		
				Total	_____

A multiparous woman (has delivered a baby previously) can best be induced at a score of ≥5.
A nulliparous woman (has *not* delivered a baby previously) can best be induced at a score of ≥8.

From Bishop, E. H. (1964). Pelvic scoring for elective induction. *Obstetrics and Gynecology, 24,* 266.

Dr. Edward Bishop developed this scoring system based on observations of multiparous women in 1964. Over time, it was applied to nulliparous women. Best outcomes for multiparous women are seen with a score of 5 or higher. The nulliparous woman has a similar response to that of spontaneous labor with a score of 8 or greater.[1]

Mechanical Methods of Cervical Ripening

These methods should be limited to women who have a clear indication for induction and have little or no cervical effacement.[31] The devices used are placed in the endocervical canal by the healthcare provider. The most common methods include:

Laminaria—made from seaweed and absorbs fluid from the cervical tissues. They absorb fluid from the cervix and vagina, causing the seaweed to swell resulting in mechanical dilation of the cervix and prostaglandin release, which may stimulate contractions.

Synthetic osmotic dilators—made from polymer sponges and soaked in magnesium sulfate. They absorb fluid from the cervix and vagina causing the sponge to swell, resulting in mechanical dilation of the cervix and prostaglandin release.

TABLE 8.2 OXYTOCIN CONVERSIONS

SOLUTION CONCENTRATION
Premixed solution of (1 milliunit per minute [mU/min] = 1 milliliter per hour [mL/hr]) is preferred

RATE (mU/min)	10 U OXYTOCIN/1,000 mL (10 mU/mL) (mL/hr)	20 U OXYTOCIN/1,000 mL (0 mU/mL) (mL/hr)	15 U OXYTOCIN/250 mL (60 mU/mL) (mL/hr)
1	6	3	1
2	12	6	2
3	18	9	3
4	24	12	4
5	30	15	5
6	36	18	6
7	42	21	7
8	48	24	8
9	54	27	9
10	60	30	10
11	66	33	11
12	72	36	12
13	78	39	13
14	84	42	14
15	90	45	15
16	96	48	16
17	102	51	17
18	108	54	18
19	114	57	19
20	120	60	20

Adapted with permission from Poziac, S. (1999). Induction and augmentation of labor. In Mandeville, L. K, & Troiano, N. H. (Eds.), *High risk and critical care intrapartum nursing* (2nd ed., pp. 139–158). Philadelphia, PA: Lippincott Williams & Wilkins.

> **Transcervical balloon catheters**—a large-gauge (14 to 26) Foley catheter with a 30-mL balloon is inserted above the internal os. Once in position the balloon is inflated with sterile water or saline. The catheter is then loosely secured to the maternal leg. The inflated bulb puts direct pressure on the cervix and causes stretching of the lower uterine segment, resulting in prostaglandin release.

• What are the advantages and disadvantages when mechanical methods are used for cervical ripening?

There is a low risk of tachysystole with mechanical methods but there is a slight increased risk of maternal and neonatal infection. Some discomfort has been reported, and bleeding can occur if a low lying placenta is disrupted.

• If the cervix is not favorable but a woman otherwise meets the criteria for induction, can prostaglandin preparations be used to ripen the cervix?

There are a variety of prostaglandin preparations that may be used for cervical ripening before the induction of labor. These include both prostaglandin E_1 (PGE_1): misoprostol (Cytotec) and prostaglandin E2 (PGE_2) such as Cervidil vaginal insert and Prepidil gel. Healthcare providers should be aware that use of these preparations may lead to the onset of labor especially if the cervix is favorable. However, this result varies and is usually not a concern because the intent of the cervical ripening process is to prepare for labor.

> • **What are the potential concerns for the health of the mother and fetus when cervical ripening is achieved with prostaglandin preparations?**

According to the U. S. Food and Drug Administration (FDA) (2002), major adverse effects for the mother include the following:
- Uterine tachysystole that can progress to uterine tetany
- Marked decreased blood flow to the uterus, uterine rupture, or amniotic fluid embolism
- There have been reports of pelvic pain, retained placenta, severe genital bleeding, shock, and maternal death
- Increase chance of cesarean birth related to indeterminate or abnormal FHR pattern from tachysystole

Side effects include gastrointestinal upset (e.g., nausea, vomiting, and diarrhea)

Concerns for the fetus include the following:
- Indeterminate or abnormal fetal heart rate changes—which are usually related to uterine tachysystole
- Fetal bradycardia, and fetal death
- Commonly reported adverse effects are, umbilical artery pH less than 7.10, 5-minute Apgar score <7, and admission to NICU

Contraindications for Cervical Ripening Using Prostaglandin Preparations

Prostaglandins are not recommended in the following situations:
- Any time a vaginal delivery is not indicated (see clinical examples listed in Display 8.1).
- If there is an indeterminate or abnormal fetal heart rate tracing.
- If labor or oxytocin is contraindicated, prostaglandins for cervical ripening should be avoided.
- If tachysystole is present or there is an increase in uterine tone.
- Placenta previa or unexplained vaginal bleeding during the pregnancy.
- If there are not enough nurses to safely care for the patient. The current AWHONN 2010 recommendations are for 1:2 nurse-to-woman ratio for women undergoing cervical ripening with pharmacologic agents.[32]

Administration of Prostaglandins

> • **What is the ideal ripening agent?**

The ideal ripening agent should be easy to use, noninvasive, with timely effectiveness. It should not stimulate or induce labor during the ripening process, nor increase maternal, fetal, or neonatal morbidity. Unfortunately, the ideal agent or procedure for cervical ripening has not yet been identified.[6,33,34]

> • **What precautions should be taken to provide safe administration of vaginal PGE$_2$?**

Since all prostaglandin preparations used for cervical ripening tend to increase myometrial contractility and subsequently may intermittently impede blood flow to the placenta where oxygen exchange occurs, it is recommended that:
- The FHR pattern and uterine activity be monitored electronically for at least 20 to 30 minutes to establish baseline assessments before administration.
- The FHR pattern and uterine activity should be monitored continuously while insert is in place.
- After placement of the insert, the patient should remain supine for 2 hours and then may ambulate.
- Ambulation is encouraged if continuous EFM telemetry is available.[34]
- The vaginal insert should be removed with onset of active labor or 12 hours after placement.
- Maternal vital signs should be initially evaluated and then monitored every four hours, or as consistent with the patient's condition.

Prepidil gel must be placed by a physician or nurse midwife using a sterile speculum. Prepidil is less commonly used for cervical ripening, however, detailed information can be retrieved from: http://www.pfizer.com/files/products/uspi_prepidil.pdf

CERVIDIL VAGINAL INSERT (Fig. 8.2). Cervidil is approved by the FDA. It contains 10 mg of dinoprostone encased in a thin rectangular pouch of knitted Dacron. After placement, the pouch absorbs vaginal fluid, swells and slowly releases dinoprostone at a controlled rate of 0.3 mg/hr. Since Cervidil is relatively simple to insert it can be administered by a perinatal nurse that has demonstrated competence in insertion and the activity is within the scope of practice by the licensing state or provincial agency. Unlike transcervical gel preparations, proper placement of the vaginal insert does not require a speculum to visualize the cervix. Keep Cervidil frozen (–20°C) until immediate use. Remove the insert by tearing the aluminum package along the tear mark. Do not use scissors which could damage the knitted polyester pouch that contains the medication slab. Using sterile gloves apply a minimal amount of water soluble jelly to assist insertion. Avoid excess contact or coating of lubricant which could prevent optimal swelling and impede the release of dinoprostone from the insert. Place the insert transversely behind the cervix in the posterior fornix. The long axis of the insert should traverse the long axis of the vagina. To avoid accidental removal of the insert, tuck the end of the retrieval cord into lower vaginal space. Cervidil can be administered if membranes have ruptured.[35] The patient should remain recumbent for 2 hours following insertion.[9]

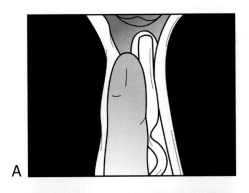

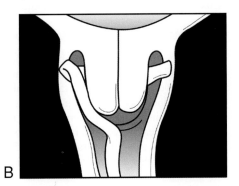

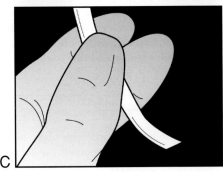

FIGURE 8.2 Cervidil vaginal insert. **A.** The Cervidil vaginal insert system is inserted into the vagina, up to the posterior fornix. **B.** The system is left in place, transverse to the posterior surface of the cervix. **C.** The Cervidil vaginal insert system can be easily grasped for gentle removal and discontinuation of drug administration.

• How does Cervidil work?

Dinoprostone directly softens the cervix, relaxes the cervical smooth muscle, and can stimulate uterine contractions. An added benefit of Cervidil is less oxytocin is needed postripening to produce coordinated uterine contractions.[36]

> • **If uterine tachysystole and/or category III FHR occur, what actions should the nurse take?**

Place the woman in either a left or right lateral position; administer an IV bolus of at least 500 mL lactated Ringer's solution. If improvement is not observed after 10 to 15 minutes, notify the patient's attending provider and remove the Cervidil vaginal insert. If maternal/fetal condition is not improved or worsens, consider tocolytic therapy, short-term oxygen at 10 L/min via nonrebreather face mask, and anticipate possible cesarean section. For some types of indeterminate (category II) FHR tracings, removal may also be indicated. Specific protocols regarding nursing management of prostaglandin-related uterine and fetal assessment should be developed by each hospital using prostaglandin ripening agents for induction of labor.[9]

> • **Can more than one dose of Cervidil vaginal insert be administered if inadequate ripening occurs?**

If after 12 hours the cervix has not ripened, the provider may consider alternative ripening methods. If a repeat dose of Cervidil is ordered, it is important to note that the safety and efficacy of a second Cervidil insert has not been published. The provider should document the assessment, plan, and rational for the repeat dose in the woman's medical record. The maximum vaginal duration should be 12 hours from insertion.[37]

> • **With adequate cervical ripening and no labor, how soon after prostaglandin administration can oxytocin be administered for labor induction?**

Oxytocin administration should be delayed until at least 30 to 60 minutes after the removal of the Cervidil insert.[9] Since previous exposure to PGE_2 potentiates the uterine contractile response to oxytocin, careful maternal–fetal monitoring is warranted.[36,38]

Use of Misoprostol (for Cervical Ripening)

In 2002, the FDA removed the contraindication for use in pregnancy because it was widely used for labor induction and cervical ripening. At that time, the FDA included warnings about potential adverse effects: uterine tachysystole that may progress to uterine tetany, marked impairment of uterine blood flow, uterine rupture, or amniotic fluid embolism. The FDA further noted that pelvic pain, retained placenta, severe genital bleeding, shock, fetal bradycardia, and fetal and maternal death have been reported. Misoprostol has been administered intravaginally in the posterior fornix using doses ranging from 50 micrograms (mcg) every 6 hours to 25 mcg every 3 hours. The higher dosage has been associated with increased incidence of uterine tachysystole and indeterminate or abnormal fetal heart patterns. When used for cervical ripening, 25 mcg placed in the posterior vaginal fornix should be considered for the initial dose.[9] Healthcare providers should be alert; even with 25 mcg intravaginally every 4 hours, uterine tachysystole may still occur.[1,6] Tachysystole with or without indeterminate or abnormal FHR changes is significantly higher with the use of misoprostol when compared with Cervidil, Prepidil, or oxytocin.[6,39] A 4- to 6-hour interval between doses has been associated with less uterine tachysystole than the 3-hour interval.[1,6,17,27]

> • **Are there additional restrictions or concerns for the use of misoprostol?**

It is recommended that the woman be admitted to the hospital labor and birth suites where continuous electronic monitoring is available. *Women with a history of prior uterine surgery, including a low transverse cesarean section, should not receive misoprostol.* Redosing is withheld if there are two or more contractions in 10 minutes, adequate cervical ripening is achieved, the woman enters active labor, or the fetal heart rate is abnormal. Tachysystole is more common with Misoprostol than Cervidil and oxytocin. Therefore, the healthcare provider should continuously monitor FHR and uterine activity. Brethine (terbutaline) 0.25 mg subcutaneously can be used in an attempt to correct uterine tachysystole.[9] Oxytocin should be delayed until at least 4 hours after the last dose. The medication is only available as a 100-mcg unscored tablet. Since the tablet must be cut into four equal pieces, the hospital pharmacist should prepare the 25-mcg tablets before administration.[9,40]

Recommendations for Safe Use of Misoprostol

To ensure the greatest safety for mother and fetus, it is recommended that *the following be true before administering misoprostol:*

- The perinatal nurse must demonstrate competence in insertion and the activity must be within the scope of practice as defined by state and provincial regulations
- The Bishop score is less than 6
- The fetal status should be normal before the drug is placed
- There is no history of uterine surgery
- The hospital pharmacist should use a pill cutter to prepare a 100-µg tablet in four equal parts to ensure a consistent dose of 25 mcg
- Tocolytic medications are available if needed to treat uterine tachysystole
- IV access is in place
- Continuous monitoring of FHR and uterine activity is indicated
- If membranes rupture after placement of misoprostol, the labor pattern and fetal response are observed for 2 hours before an additional dose is placed
- The facility has the capability of offering urgent/emergency cesarean delivery
- Protocols are developed by the department and include guidelines for misoprostol use, evaluation of outcomes, and documentation of adherence to guidelines

Oxytocin for Induction and Augmentation of Labor

Oxytocin remains the most commonly used induction agent in the United States and world-wide.[10] It is more fully discussed in Skill Unit 1.

PRACTICE/REVIEW QUESTIONS
After reviewing this module, answer the following questions.

1. Define *induction of labor.*

   _____

   _____

2. Define *augmentation of labor.*

   _____

   _____

3. Oxytocin is a _____ synthesized by the

   _____ then transported to the _____ gland.

   Oxytocin causes the uterus to _____.

4. What is the initial dose of misoprostol recommended by ACOG for cervical ripening?

   _____

5. List two reasons why the rate of oxytocin administration must be carefully controlled?

   a. _____

   b. _____

6. Describe the best way to administer oxytocin so that the rate of administration is controlled.

   _____

   _____

7. List at least five medical indications for the induction or augmentation of labor.

   a. _____

   b. _____

c. _____

d. _____

e. _____

8. What should be considered when a woman requests an induction for reasons of convenience?

   _____

   _____

9. List at least 5 induction of labor factors known to negatively impact the childbirth process?

10. List four criteria used to select women who might benefit from active labor management.

    a. _____

    b. _____

    c. _____

    d. _____

11. List at least five additional concerns of adverse effects for the mother who is experiencing induction/augmentation of labor.

    a. _____

    b. _____

    c. _____

    d. _____

    e. _____

12. List at least three concerns of adverse effects for the fetus during induction/augmentation.

    a. _____

    b. _____

    c. _____

13. List four situations that are absolute contraindications for induction of labor.

    a. _____

    b. _____

    c. _____

    d. _____

14. What are relative contraindications to induction of labor?

    _____

15. List four relative contraindications to the induction/augmentation of labor.

    a. _____

    b. _____

    c. _____

    d. _____

16. List at least three prerequisites for a safe and effective induction/augmentation.

    a. _____

    b. _____

    c. _____

17. The Bishop score is used to determine?

    _____

18. Mrs. J. is being assessed for induction of labor. Her cervix is dilated 1.5 cm and is 60% effaced. The vertex is at −1 station, cervical consistency is medium, and cervical position is midline. What is her Bishop score?

    _____

19. Match the definitions in Column B with the items in Column A.

    Column A

    1. _____ Labor
    2. _____ Complete placenta previa
    3. _____ Uterine tachysystole
    4. _____ Premature rupture of membranes
    5. _____ Used to evaluate cervical readiness

    Column B

    a. Bishop score
    b. Indication for induction
    c. Contraindications to induction
    d. Uterine contractions causing desired changes to cervix
    e. Relative contraindications to induction/augmentation

20. Oxytocin should always be administered using:

    _____

21. What evaluative/assessment technique is strongly recommended when using oxytocin?

    _____

22. List five items to be included in the written procedures for oxytocin administration?

    a. _____

    b. _____

    c. _____

    d. _____

    e. _____

23. List at least two concerns of effects for the fetus during preinduction cervical ripening.

    a. _____

    b. _____

24. Which one of the following dosages of misoprostol is recommended in the ACOG Committee Opinion?

    a. 50 μg every 6 hours in the posterior vaginal fornix

    b. An initial dose of 25 μg in the posterior vaginal fornix

    c. 50 μg every 6 hours by mouth

    d. 25 μg every 3 hours in the posterior vaginal fornix

25. The ACOG Committee Opinion on the use of misoprostol indicates that it is not recommended for women with a history of a low transverse cesarean section.

    a. True

    b. False

26. How often does tachysystole occur after insertion of Cervidil?

    _____

27. What is a major advantage of Cervidil versus Misoprostol?

    _____

• Can women who have had a prior cesarean section be induced?

Induction of labor for maternal or fetal indications remains an option for women undergoing TOLAC. However, the potential increased risk of uterine rupture exists with any induction, and the potential decreased possibility of achieving VBAC, should be discussed. Several studies have noted an increased risk of uterine rupture in the setting of induction of labor in women attempting TOLAC. Misoprostol should not be used for third trimester cervical ripening or labor induction in patients who have had a cesarean delivery or major uterine surgery.[41]

PRACTICE/REVIEW ANSWER KEY

1. The artificial stimulation of uterine contractions before spontaneous onset of labor for the purpose of accomplishing vaginal birth.
2. The stimulation of uterine contraction when spontaneous contractions have failed to result in progressive cervical dilatation or descent of the fetus.
3. Hormone; hypothalamus; pituitary; contract; where it is released into the maternal circulation in a pulsatile fashion.
4. 25 mcg.
5. a. Because it causes more powerful and frequent contractions than normal and can interrupt or decrease blood flow to the fetus.
   b. Oxytocin is a designated high-alert medication and requires careful titration and assessment of the maternal/fetal response.
6. Using an IV catheter in the arm, with a two-bottle system and the fluid flow rate controlled by an infusion control pump.
7. Any five of the following:
   a. Abruptio placentae
   b. Chorioamnionitis
   c Fetal demise
   d. Gestational hypertension
   e. Preeclampsia, eclampsia
   f. Premature rupture of membranes (PROMs)
   g. Postterm pregnancy
   h. Maternal medical condition disease state like diabetes mellitus, renal disease, chronic pulmonary disease, chronic hypertension, and antiphospholipid syndrome
   i. Fetal compromise such as severe fetal growth restriction, isoimmunization, or oligohydramnios
8. Women considering elective induction should have adequate information to make an informed decision. Common complications and potential risks associated with elective inductions should be discussed by the woman's provider in detail. ACOG advises against elective induction of labor between 39+0 and 41+0 weeks' gestation unless the cervix is favorable.
9. a. Intravenous line (IV line)
   b. bedrest
   c. continuous electronic fetal monitoring (EFM)
   d. amniotomy

e. significant discomfort
   f. analgesia/anesthesia
   g. prolonged hospital stay
10. a. Nulliparity
    b. More than 37 weeks' gestation
    c. Single fetus in no distress
    d. Spontaneous labor
11. Any five of the following:
    a. Hypertension or stroke
    b. Postpartum hemorrhage
    c. Embolism (amniotic fluid embolism)
    d. Too-rapid birth
    e. Lacerations to vagina, vulva, perineum, and rectum
    f. Water intoxication
    g. Increased fear
12. Any three of the following:
    a. Hypoxia
    b. Bradycardia
    c. Increased trauma
    d. Hyperbilirubinemia
    e. Less likely to breastfeed in the immediate postpartum period
13. Any four of the following:
    a. Previous transfundal surgical procedures: myomectomy, classical cesarean delivery
    b. Vasa previa or complete placenta previa
    c. Transverse fetal lie
    d. Umbilical cord prolapse
    e. Active genital herpes infection
14. Conditions that *might* or *might not* present severe problems for mother and baby
15. Any four of the following:
    a. Previous cesarean birth
    b. Presenting part not engaged in pelvis
    c. Severe maternal hypertension
    d. Multiple gestations
    e. Polyhydramnios
    f. Abnormal or Indeterminate fetal heart rate patterns not requiring emergent birth
    g. Maternal heart disease
    h. Trial of labor after cesarean (TOLAC) birth or history of uterine scar
16. a. The woman should not have any of the contraindications for induction/augmentation
    b. Gestational age of the fetus should be accurate
    c. The woman's healthcare provider should supervise the procedure
17. Whether the cervix is ripe or ready for induction
18. 7
19. 1. d
    2. c
    3. e
    4. b
    5. a
20. An infusion pump so that the lowest possible dose to achieve the desired therapeutic effect can be carefully titrated.
21. Continuous ongoing maternal–fetal assessment ideally utilizing a 1:1 nurse-to-patient ratio aimed to promptly

recognize and respond with corrective measures if tachysystole or indeterminate/abnormal FHR changes occur.

22. Any five of the following:
    a. Evaluation of cervical effacement and dilatation before administration
    b. Immediate availability, during administration, of a physician who has privileges to perform cesarean surgery
    c. Use of an IV catheter, infusion pump, two-bottle system
    d. The recommended waiting time when oxytocin is used after Cervidil or misoprostol
    e. A starting dose of 1 to 2 mU/min
    f. Gradually increasing the infusion by 1 to 2 mU/min every 30 to 40 minutes until adequate labor is established or contractions are 2 to 3 minutes apart
    g. Maximum concentration of solution and maximum rate of administration

    h. Evaluating the FHR pattern every 15 minutes or every 5 minutes during the pushing phase, or before the oxytocin infusion is increased
    i. Assessing uterine activity and the maternal response to labor
23. Any two of the following:
    a. Hypoxia
    b. Heart rate abnormality
    c. Sepsis
24. b. An initial dose of 25 µg in the posterior vaginal fornix
25. a. True
26. Tachysystole usually occurs 1 hour after placement, but can occur up to 9.5 hours after placement.[1]
27. One major advantage of Cervidil is that the system can be easily and quickly removed in the event of uterine tachysystole or other complications.

SKILL UNIT 1 | OXYTOCIN LABOR INDUCTION/AUGMENTATION

This skill unit instructs you on how to set up for an induction/augmentation of labor with oxytocin, how to identify the appropriate equipment needed, and how to regulate the infusion.

Remember, induction or augmentation with oxytocin is a procedure that stimulates regular uterine contractions. The procedure must *always* be ordered by the healthcare provider managing the woman's labor. There must be no absolute contraindications present for the induction/augmentation to proceed.

After you study this section, your preceptor should demonstrate the procedure and then give you an opportunity to demonstrate your skill.

Please remember that types of equipment and supplies vary from hospital to hospital, depending on the manufacturer and surgical supply houses used.

Administration of Oxytocin

• **What is the goal of oxytocin administration?**

In 2007, the Institute for Safe Medication Practices (ISMP) designated IV oxytocin as a high-alert medication. High-alert medication are drugs that carry a heightened risk of causing significant patient harm when they are used in error.[42] Each hospital should have a clinical protocol and unit policy for oxytocin administration. Key concepts for oxytocin administration are:
- Patient prioritization and proper documentation of provider.
- Staffing considerations that demonstrate nurse competency, availability and contingency plans such as on-call list.
- Frequent patient assessment that includes documentation of maternal/fetal well-being, documentation of fetal heart rate, resting uterine tone, frequency and characteristics of contractions, oxytocin dosage, maternal vital signs, and continuous electronic fetal monitoring (EFM) is recommended.
  - Use a standardized oxytocin protocol based on physiology that includes concentration and dosing regimen.
  - Carefully titrate oxytocin based on the maternal fetal response.
- Complication: define tachysystole, maternal interventions to resolve tachysystole and ensure fetal well-being, criteria to notify provider and obtain bedside evaluation.
- Immediate or urgent availability, during oxytocin administration, of a physician qualified to perform a cesarean delivery should problems arise.
- Chain of consultation for addressing clinical disagreements--algorithm flow chart. Oxytocin mismanagement has become a significant factor in perinatal liability.[16,43] AAP and ACOG recommend evaluation of the FHR and maternal condition every 15 minutes.[44,45] The lowest possible dose to achieve the desired therapeutic effect should be used.[42,46]

• What is the recommended method of oxytocin administration?

Oxytocin should always be piggybacked as a secondary infusion into the mainline solution in the port most proximal to the venous site. Since oxytocin is a high-alert medication, continuous administration must be controlled using an infusion pump. This IV set up allows the nurse to discontinue the oxytocin infusion while allowing the mainline infusion to continue.

INFUSION CONTROL PUMPS. Pumps provide a very carefully controlled flow of fluids. Many models are available on the market. It is critical to be aware of the manufacturer's guidelines for operation.

• What are the corrective measures nurses should know regarding oxytocin?

Oxytocin-Induced Tachysystole
(Normal FHR)
* Maternal repositioning (either left or right)
* IV fluid bolus of lactated Ringer's solution (~500 mL)
* If tachysystole persist after 10 minutes, decrease oxytocin rate by at least half
* If tachysystole persists after 10 more minutes, discontinue oxytocin until uterine activity is normal

Oxytocin-Induced Tachysystole
(Indeterminate/Abnormal FHR)
* Discontinue oxytocin
* Maternal repositioning (either left or right)
* IV fluid bolus of lactated Ringer's solution (~500 mL)
* Consider oxygen at 10 L/min via nonrebreather facemask if the above measure has not resolved. FHR pattern discontinues as soon as possible
* If still no response, consider 0.25-mg terbutaline SQ
* Notify primary provider of actions taken and maternal/fetal response

• When can oxytocin be resumed after Tachysystole?

If oxytocin has been discontinued less than 20 to 30 minutes, the FHR is normal, and the contraction frequency, intensity, and duration are normal, then oxytocin can be restarted no more than half the rate prior to tachysystole. If oxytocin has been discontinued for more than 30 to 40 minutes, resume oxytocin back at the initial dose ordered.[9]

NOTE: Multiple protocols for oxytocin administration exist. It is essential for each institution to have guidelines for induction, augmentation, or active management of labor that are specific for the institution.

NOTE: Comprehensive protocols that address nursing responsibility in oxytocin administration should include criteria for patient selection, responsibility for and information to be covered in the informed consent, drug preparation and administration, patient monitoring, potential side effects, and therapeutic goals.

ACTIONS	REMARKS
Assemble the Equipment	
Obtain premixed oxytocin solution in a 1:1 dilution.	Procedure is performed in labor and delivery 20 units of oxytocin in a 1,000-mL solution. 30 units of oxytocin in a 500-mL solution. 15 units of oxytocin in a 250-mL solution.
Infusion control pump (Fig. 8.3).	Need to be familiar with the operation of the infusion control pump.

skill unit continues on page 228

ACTIONS	REMARKS

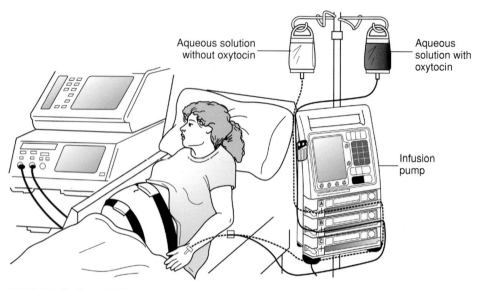

FIGURE 8.3   Infusion control pump: setup for oxytocin administration.

Prepare for IV Administration

Verify that the provider has obtained informed consent. Document the following: • Greater than 39 weeks' if elective. • If less than 39 weeks' indication is consistent with ACOG (2009) and TJC (2012) clinical indications.[47] Cervical readiness (Bishop score). Apply fetal and uterine monitor.	The woman must give permission with full awareness of the effects and side effects to herself and her baby.
Record baseline fetal heart rate and uterine contraction information for at least 20 minutes before administration of medication. Maternal temperature, pulse, respirations, and blood pressure should be assessed before the administration of medication.	**Do not start oxytocin in the presence of an abnormal FHR tracing.** Document all findings in the medical record. Follow-up with healthcare provider if there are any deviations from normal parameters. The fetal status is normal.

Start the Administration of Oxytocin

Connect the oxytocin infusion to the pump and start the piggyback infusion.	The woman's healthcare provider should order the initial dose. Maximum dose and interval of dose increases should be according to institutional guidelines (Table 8.2).
Adjust the dose until satisfactory contractions are established.	**Evaluate fetal and uterine response before all dose increases.** Steady-state plasma levels are reached only after 40 minutes.[15] Therefore, the full effect of an oxytocin increase will not be fully observed for 30–40 min.[48] As the uterus begins to contract and the cervix starts to dilate, the dose might need to be adjusted. The process of titrating oxytocin dosage is dynamic—assessment of the fetal heart rate, contraction pattern, maternal response, and labor progress should guide the titration of the medication.

skill unit continues on page 229

ACTIONS	REMARKS
Discontinuing Oxytocin Infusion	
Discontinue oxytocin in the presence of: • Tachysystole with indeterminate fetal heart rate changes. • Tachysystole—contractions that are more frequent than every 2 minutes (greater than 5 in 10 minutes over 30 minutes). • Contractions that last >90 seconds. • Uterine resting tone that is not relaxed to palpation.	Notify the provider of indeterminate or abnormal fetal status. Often these problems are related to uterine tachysystole and resolve with decreasing or discontinuing the oxytocin infusion.
Record the Procedure	
Documentation is required and should be according to institutional and unit guidelines.	Document in the medical record the following: • date and time for each entry • vital signs • fetal heart rate • resting uterine tone • frequency, duration, and intensity of contractions and response to contractions • vaginal findings: dilatation, effacement, station • oxytocin infusion rate • mainline IV infusion rate • fluid intake and output

Uterine Tachysystole

Uterine tachysystole is the most common complication of induction and augmentation of labor, yet much confusion exists regarding what defines excessive uterine activity. Uterine hyperstimulation, tachysystole, and hypertonus are all terms that may be used in reference to excessive uterine activity. Common themes emerge when reviewing definitions of uterine tachysystole such as hyperstimulation, the frequency of contractions, hypercontractility as the increased duration of contractions, and hypertonus as increased resting tone of the uterus between contractions. Some definitions of uterine tachysystole exist that require evidence of an adverse fetal response before uterine activity can be labeled as excessive. Such definitions may not be appropriate; it may encourage increases in oxytocin dosage **until** there is an adverse fetal response. Each institution should develop clinical guidelines that include a clear definition of uterine tachysystole and the expected interventions to be initiated when excessive uterine activity is noted.

You will need to attend a skill session(s) to practice this skill with the help of your preceptor. Mastery of the skill is achieved when you can do the following:
- Assemble all of the necessary equipment
- Prepare the IV solution administration setup including the mainline and piggyback infusions
- Regulate the oxytocin dose, using the infusion pump
- Apply the fetal and uterine monitor and interpret the findings
- Document findings and observations according to unit and hospital standards

• Should intrauterine pressure catheters (IUPCs) be routinely used?

Maternal fever is associated with IUPC usage but does not appear to impact neonatal outcomes negatively. Maternal fever is however associated with increased costs, antibiotic use, delay of breastfeeding, and increased length of stay. The use of an IUPC should be used in laboring patients with a clinical indication such as inability to monitor externally and fetal heart rate decelerations. The routine use of IUPC's in every laboring patient with ruptured membranes is not necessary, does not appear to reduce cesarean deliveries, and increases the risk of maternal fever.[49]

REFERENCES

1. American College of Obstetricians and Gynecologists. (2009a). *Induction of labor (Practice Bulletin No. 107)*. Washington, DC: Author. *Obstetrics & Gynecology, 114,* 386–397.

2. Spong, C. Y., Berghella, V., Wenstrom, K. D., et al. (2012). Preventing the first cesarean delivery: Summary of a joint Eunice Kennedy Shriver National Institute of Child Health and Human Development, Society for Maternal-Fetal Medicine, and American College of Obstetricians and Gynecologists Workshop. *Obstetrics and Gynecology, 120*(5), 1181–1193.

3. American College of Obstetricians and Gynecologists, Society for Maternal-Fetal Medicine. (2014). Obstetric care consensus no. 1: Safe prevention of the primary cesarean delivery. *Obstetrics and Gynecology, 123*(3), 693–711.

4. American College of Obstetricians and Gynecologists. (2003). *Dystocia and the augmentation of labor (Practice Bulletin No. 49)*. Washington, DC: Author; *Obstetrics and Gynecology, 102*(6), 1445–1454.

5. Association of Women's Health, Obstetric and Neonatal Nurses. (2002). *Cervical ripening and induction and augmentation of labor* (2nd ed.). Washington, DC: Author.

6. Wing, D. A., & Farinelli, C. K. (2012). Abnormal labor and induction of labor. In Gabbe, S. G., Niebyl, J. R., Simpson, J. L., et al. (Eds.), *Obstetrics:Normal and problem pregnancies* (5th ed., pp. 287–311). Philadelphia, PA: Elsevier Saunders.

7. Kimura, T., Takemura, M., & Nomura, S. (1996). Expression of oxytocin receptors in human pregnant myometrium. *Endocrinology, 137,* 780–785.

8. Fuchs, A. R., Periyasamy, S., & Alexandrova, M. (1983). Correlation between oxytocin receptor concentration and responsiveness to oxytocin in the pregnant rat myometrium. *Endocrinology, 113,* 743–749.

9. Simpson, K. R. (2013). *Cervical ripening. Labor induction and labor augmentation [AWHONN Practice Monograph]* (4th ed.). Washington, DC: Association of Women's Health, Obstetric and Neonatal Nurses.

10. Smith, J., & Merrill, D. (2006). Oxytocin for induction of labor. *Clinical Obstetrics and Gynecology, 49*(3), 594–608.

11. Dawood, M. Y. (1995a). Novel approach to oxytocin induction-augmentation of labor: Application of oxytocin physiology during pregnancy. *Advances in Experimental Medicine and Biology, 395,* 585–594.

12. Dawood, M. Y. (1995b). Pharmacologic stimulation of uterine contraction. *Seminars in Perinatology, 19,* 73–83.

13. Arias, F. (2000). Pharmacology of oxytocin and prostaglandins. *Clinical Obstetrics and Gynecology, 43,* 455–468.

14. Stringer, J. L. (1996). *Basic concepts in pharmacology.* St. Louis, MO: McGraw-Hill.

15. Seitchik, J., Amico, J., Robinson, A. G., et al. (1984). Oxytocin augmentation of dysfunctional labor. IV. Oxytocin pharmacokinetics. *American Journal of Obstetrics and Gynecology, 150,* 225–228.

16. Clark, S., Belfort, M. A., Dildy, G. A., et al. (2008). Reducing obstetric litigation through alterations in practice patterns. *Obstetrics and Gynecology, 112*(6), 1279–1283.

17. Simpson, K. R., & O'Brien-Abel, N. (2013). Labor and birth. In Simpson, K. R., & Creehan, P. A. (Eds.), *AWHONN's perinatal nursing* (4th ed., pp. 343–444). Philadelphia, PA: Lippincott Williams & Wilkins.

18. Macones, G. A., Hankins, G. D. V., Spong, C. Y., et al. (2008). The 2008 National Institute of Child Health and Human Development workshop report on electronic fetal monitoring: Update on definitions, interpretation, and research guidelines. *Journal of Obstetric, Gynecologic, and Neonatal Nursing, 37,* 510–515; *Obstetrics and Gynecology, 112*(3), 661–666.

19. Kilpatrock, S., & Garrison, E. (2012). Normal labor and delivery. In Gabbe, S. G., Niebyl, J., Simpson, L., et al. (Eds.), *Obstetrics: Normal and problem pregnancies* (6th ed., pp. 267–286). Philadelphia, PA: Elsevier Saunders.

20. Boulvain, M., Stan, C., & Irion, O. (2005). Membrane sweeping for induction of labour. *Cochrane Database of Systematic Reviews,* (1), CD000451.

21. American College of Obstetricians and Gynecologists. (1999). *Induction of labor (Practice Bulletin No. 10)*. Washington, DC: Author.

22. Moore, L. E., & Rayburn, W. F. (2006). Elective induction of labor. *Clinical Obstetrics and Gynecology, 49*(3), 698–704.

23. Luthy, D. A., Malmgren, J. A., & Zingheim, R. W. (2004). Cesarean delivery after elective induction in nulliparous women: The physician effect. *American Journal of Obstetrics and Gynecology, 191*(5), 1511–1155.

24. Vrouenraets, F. P., Roumen, F. J., Dehing, C. J., et al. (2005). Bishop score and risk of cesarean delivery after induction of labor in nulliparous women. *Obstetrics and Gynecology, 105*(4), 690–697.

25. American College of Obstetricians and Gynecologists. (2013). *Choosing wisely: Five things physician and patients should question.* Washington, DC: Author. Retrieved from: http://www.choosing wisely.org/doctor-patient-lists/delivering-your-baby/

26. American College of Obstetricians and Gynecologists. (2011). Patient safety checklist no. 5: Scheduling induction of labor. *Obstetrics and Gynecology, 118,* 1473–1474.

27. American College of Obstetricians and Gynecologists. (2010). ACOG practice bulletin no. 115: Vaginal birth after previous cesarean delivery. *Obstetrics and Gynecology, 116*(2 pt 1), 450–463.

28. Socol, M. L., & Peaceman, A. M. (1999). Active management of labor. *Obstetrics and Gynecology Clinics of North America, 26*(2), 287–294.

29. O'Driscoll, K., Jackson, R. J., & Gallagher, J. T. (1970). Active management of labour and cephalopelvic disproportion. *Journal of Obstetrics and Gynaecology of the British Commonwealth, 77,* 385–389.

30. Bishop, E. H. (1964). Pelvic scoring for elective induction. *Obstetrics and Gynecology, 24,* 266–268.

31. Ramsey, P. S., Ramin, K. D., & Ramin, S. M. (2000). Labor induction. *Current Opinions in Obstetrics and Gynecology, 12,* 463–473.

32. Association of Women's Health, Obstetric and Neonatal Nurses. (2010). Guidelines for professional registered nurse staffing for perinatal units. Washington, DC: Author.

33. Cromi, A., Ghezzi, F., Uccella, S., et al. (2012). A randomized trial of preinduction cervical ripening: Dinoprostone vaginal insert versus double-balloon catheter. *American Journal of Obstetrics and Gynecology, 207*(2), 125–127.

34. Fox, N. S., Saltzman, D. H., Roman, A. S., et al. (2011). Intravaginal misoprostol versus Foley catheter for labour induction: A meta-analysis. *BJOG: An International Journal of Obstetrics and Gynaecology, 118*(6), 647–654.

35. Zwelling, E. (2010). Overcoming the challenges: Maternal movement and positioning to facilitate labor progress. *MCN, The American Journal of Maternal Child Nursing, 35*(2), 72–78.

36. Keirse, M. J. (2006). Natural prostaglandins for induction of labor and preinduction cervical ripening. *Clinical Obstetrics and Gynecology, 49,* 609–626.

37. Forest Pharmaceuticals, Inc. (2010). *Cervidil prescribing information.* St. Louis, MO: Author. Retrieved from http://frx.com/pi/cervidil_pi.pdf

38. Maul, H., Mackay, L., & Garfiel, R. E. (2006). Cervical ripening: Biochemical, molecular, and clinical considerations. *Clinical Obstetrics and Gynecology, 49*, 551–563.
39. Hofmeyr, G. J., Gülmezoglu, A. M., & Pileggi, C. (2010). Vaginal misoprostol for cervical ripening and induction of labour. *Cochrane Database of Systematic Reviews,* (10), CD000941.
40. Wing, D. A., & Paul, R. H. (1999). Misoprostol for cervical ripening and labor induction: The clinician's perspective and guide to success. *Contemporary OB/GYN, 44*(4), 46–61.
41. American College of Obstetricians and Gynecologists. (2010b). *Vaginal birth after previous cesarean delivery (Practice Bulletin No. 115).* Washington, DC: Author; *Obstetrics and Gynecology, 116*(2 pt 1), 450–463.
42. Institute for Safe Medication Practices. (2007). *High-alert medications.* Huntingdon Valley, PA: Author.
43. Clark, S. L., Simpson, K. R., Knox, G. E., et al. (2009). Oxytocin: New perspectives on an old drug. *American Journal of Obstetrics and Gynecology, 200*(1), 35.e1–e6.
44. American Academy of Pediatrics, American College of Obstetricians and Gynecologists. (2012). *Guidelines for perinatal care* (7th ed.). Elk Grove, IL; Washington, DC: Authors.
45. American College of Obstetricians and Gynecologists. (2009c). *Intrapartum fetal heart rate monitoring: Nomenclature, interpretation, and general management principles (Practice Bulletin No. 106).* Washington, DC: Author; *Obstetrics and Gynecology, 114*(1), 192–202.
46. American Hospital Association, Institute for Safe Medication Practices. (2002). *Pathways to medication safety.* Chicago, IL: Authors.
47. Joint Commission. (2012). *Specifications manual for joint commission national quality core measures (version 2013A1).* Oakbrook Terrace, IL: Author.
48. Simpson, K. R., & Knox, G. E. (2009). Oxytocin as a high-alert medication: Implications for perinatal patient safety. *MCN. The American Journal of Maternal Child Nursing, 34*(1), 8–15.
49. Harper, L., Shanks, A., Tuuli, M., et al. (2013). The risks and benefits of internal monitors in laboring patients. *American Journal of Obstetrics and Gynecology, 209*(1), 38.e1–e6.

Unexpected or Precipitous Birth in the Absence of an Obstetric Provider

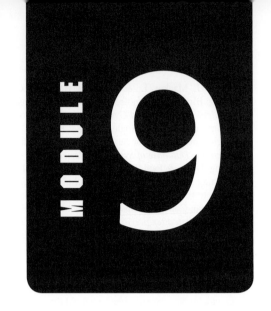

MODULE 9

JENNIFER G. HENSLEY AND
ELISABETH D. HOWARD

Objectives

After completion of this module, you will learn:

1. That remaining calm and attending to the woman is paramount, recognizing birth is a normal process and will occur whether or not you are anxious
2. Those situations that can result in an unexpected or precipitous birth before the obstetric provider arrives
3. Signs of an impending birth
4. What equipment should be ready and available (emergency birth pack)
5. How to deliver the baby, support natural birth, and help the newborn adapt to extrauterine life
6. What to do if another unexpected event occurs, that is, breech
7. What to do if there is meconium-stained amniotic fluid, difficulty delivering the baby's shoulders, excessive uterine bleeding, overt or occult bleeding from lacerations, or a newborn with difficulty breathing
8. What should alert you to the possibility of excessive uterine or birth laceration(s) bleeding
9. Dangers of an improperly conducted unexpected or precipitous birth
10. Immediate care of the newborn
11. Immediate care of the mother
12. Information that must be charted on the hospital record

Key Terms

Upon completion of this module, you will be able to recall the meaning of the following terms and use them when consulting with other health professionals. Terms are defined in this module or in the glossary at the end of this book.

hematoma	precipitous
"feather blow"	restitution
lochia	turtle sign
nasopharynx	shoulder dystocia
nuchal cord	thermoregulation
oropharynx	uterine atony

- **Why is it important for you to be able to deliver a baby in the absence of an obstetric provider?**

You, the maternity nurse have a responsibility to provide safe care for the mother and baby. If you make the assessment that a woman will give birth before her obstetric provider arrives, you must ask for help and be prepared to instruct and assist the woman while another nurse helps care for the newborn.

Comprehensive protocols addressing an unexpected or precipitous birth in the absence of the obstetric provider should be developed by each institution.

DO NOT WAIT TO PREPARE for the birth. **You should be ready:** *call for help*, **prepare the woman and her support person that birth is imminent, and prepare the place of delivery.**

- **Which women are at risk for delivery before the arrival of their obstetric provider?**

Women who are at risk include those who:
  - Have had at least one vaginal birth
  - Have preterm labor (smaller baby)
  - Have a history of a rapid labor or a previous precipitous birth
  - Have made rapid progress during the current labor
  - Are in active labor and have travelled a great distance to the hospital
  - Have an unexpectedly small baby

The Delivery Process

Signs and Symptoms of an Impending Delivery

- A woman having her second or subsequent baby who exclaims, "It's coming!," is probably correct. When the baby's head crowns and the woman experiences the maximal perineal stretch, or "ring of fire," you should stop what you are doing and attend to her. She needs you.
- New-onset early decelerations noted on the fetal monitor tracing of a laboring woman with an epidural may indicate descent of the head as the cervix fully dilates.
- A woman who has been comfortable with an epidural but suddenly feels pain or "pressure down there" may have rapidly progressed to the second stage.
- Involuntary shaking of the lower legs in a woman having an unmedicated birth (no epidural) may occur as the presenting part descends, putting pressure on nerves.
- Increased bloody show may be seen as the cervix completes dilation.
- A strong urge to "push" or to bear down (rectal pressure), or actual involuntary pushing with contractions may occur ("Ferguson's reflex").
- Separation or parting of the labia may be seen as the presenting part emerges (Fig. 9.1).

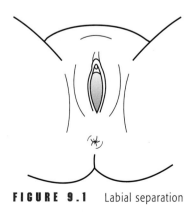

FIGURE 9.1 Labial separation

• Increased fullness and pressure against the perineum may be seen (bulging perineum) (Fig. 9.2).

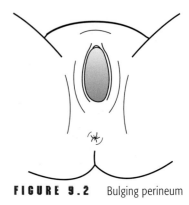

FIGURE 9.2   Bulging perineum

• Relaxation and bulging of the anus, with or without loss of stool, may also be seen (Fig. 9.3).

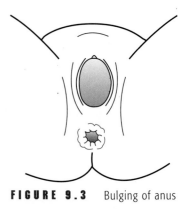

FIGURE 9.3   Bulging of anus

The Nurse's Role

> ### • What must you do to assist with the birth for consistency?

If the obstetric provider is not yet present, you should:

• Relax and stay calm. Help the mother and her support person prepare for the imminent birth. Remember, women have been birthing for centuries and birth is a natural process. It will happen whether or not you are in the room.
  • Birth is a clean, not a sterile event. Put on gloves, but do not waste time finding the correct size sterile gloves if they are not readily available.
  • It is not necessary to scrub the perineum with an antiseptic, this wastes time. Do wipe away stool with an x-ray detectable sponge.
  • Do not vigorously bulb suction the baby's oronasopharynx on the perineum. This can stimulate the vagus nerve and cause bradycardia. Wipe excess secretions away with an x-ray detectable sponge.
  • Allow the umbilical cord to stop pulsating before clamping and cutting. This allows the baby to receive extra blood.
  • Place the baby on the maternal chest/abdomen while drying him/her off. This should be sufficient stimulation to assist with spontaneous respirations. Cover both mother and baby with warm blankets.
  • It is not necessary to deliver the placenta immediately.
• Calmly call for assistance. Have another nurse in the room to help with the care of the mother and newborn.
• If chart information is not available, obtain pertinent information with a 30-second history:
  • Which baby is this for you?
  • When is your due date?
  • Did you have prenatal care?
  • Have you had any problems with the pregnancy?
  • Do you have any health problems?

- Inform the woman and her support person that the birth is about to take place.
- Reassure the woman that she will be assisted and will not be left unattended.
- DO NOT LEAVE THE ROOM. Send her support person for help if necessary.
- Instruct the woman to "feather blow" with each contraction, *unless* told to push.
- Open the emergency birth pack at the bedside or on the bed. It should contain the following items:
  - A package of x-ray detectable sponges
  - Absorbent towels
  - A soft bulb syringe (use only if necessary)
  - A small drape or sterile field barrier
  - Two clamps, such as Kelly or Rochester (use only if necessary)
  - A cord clamp or umbilical tape
  - Scissors
  - Baby blankets
  - Gloves
- Put on gloves (sterile preferred, but not essential), place the sterile barrier under the woman's hips, and prepare for birth of the baby. Do not take your eyes off the perineum.

Remember to observe universal precautions.

• Why should you instruct the woman to "feather blow" rather than push with some contractions?

When a woman pushes, she uses abdominal muscles and increases intra-abdominal pressure. This enhances the expulsive action of the contracting uterus. "Feather blowing" helps the woman to control the urge to push. To protect maternal tissue and the baby from trauma (facial bruising or subconjunctival hemorrhages), delivering the baby after gradual stretching of the perineal tissue is desired. The baby can also be delivered in between contractions.

• What aseptic techniques should be done in preparation before birth for consistency?

- Remember that birth is a "clean" (not a sterile) procedure. Instruments, however, should be sterile.
- If time, wash your hands and forearms thoroughly, then put on gloves (sterile or clean). Wipe away stool that appears as the woman pushes.

• Is control of the head important?

Research has shown the "hands-on" or "hands-off" approach to delivery of the head results in the same number of perineal lacerations.[1,2] The key is to talk to the mother, tell her when to "feather blow" and when to push. The mechanisms of labor can guide your hand maneuvers:
- Flexion
- Extension
- Restitution
- External rotation
- Lateral flexion
- Expulsion

Hand maneuvers include NEVER PULLING ON THE BABY'S HEAD!
- "*Hands-off*"
  - Allow the head to birth on its own
  - Support the body of the baby as it is born
- "*Hands-on*"
  - Maintain flexion of the fetal head with one hand by gently pushing downward
  - Allow slow, controlled extension of the head
  - With your other hand, gently ease the perineum over the baby's face
- Check for a nuchal cord by slipping one finger down the baby's neck as the head emerges
  - If possible, gently slide the cord over baby's head

- Deliver the anterior shoulder in a downward fashion and then the posterior shoulder in an upward fashion
- Support birth of the body by expulsion
- Place baby skin to skin on mother's chest or abdomen

• Why is it important *not* to hold back the delivery of the baby's head by pushing against it or crossing the mother's thighs?

Once it is clear that birth is about to occur, preparation must be made toward a safe and satisfying birth experience. Pushing back on the head to prevent birth can traumatize the baby and maternal tissues.

You can use "hands-off" or "hands-on" to assist with the birth: use the pads of the thumb, index, and middle fingers (Fig. 9.4) OR the cupped palm of the hand (Fig. 9.5) to maintain flexion of the head and to provide control as the head delivers. Talk to the mother.

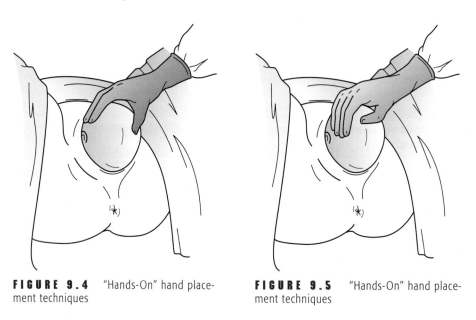

FIGURE 9.4 "Hands-On" hand placement techniques

FIGURE 9.5 "Hands-On" hand placement techniques

Never try to hold the head back from delivering!

• What other safety measures must you take to protect the mother during an unexpected or precipitous birth?

Position the mother comfortably so that the perineum, to which you must have access, can easily be viewed. Putting towels or pillows under the mother's hips can help provide downward traction when delivering the shoulders.

- Semi-Fowler's **in the labor bed:** on her back, with her head elevated to a 45-degree angle (Fig. 9.6).
- Side lying **in the labor bed:** have the support person elevate the mother's upper leg so the legs are separated.
- Squatting **in the labor bed or by the side of the bed:** after the head is born, support the body of the baby.

Maintain asepsis (clean technique). Careful handwashing, gloves, and use of the sterile emergency birth pack will help reduce the possibility of infection.

Allow delivery of the placenta without manipulation as it may take 30 to 60 minutes for this to occur. There is no need to tug on the cord. Observe for signs that the placenta is separating: the cord lengthens, a gush of blood comes from the vagina as the placenta detaches from the wall of the uterus, and the fundus changes from a discoid shape (flat) to a globular shape as the placenta drops into the lower uterine segment.

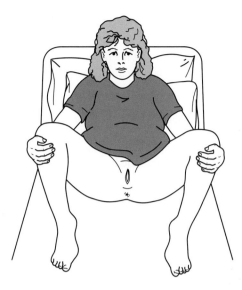

FIGURE 9.6 Position in the labor bed.

REMEMBER: If you are observing the progress of the mother's labor and watching closely for signs of an impending birth, the unexpected or precipitous birth can:
• Be planned and conducted in such a way as to eliminate last-minute rushing about
• Provide a safe and satisfying experience for the woman and her support

---

• What safety measures should be taken to protect the newborn?

In addition to "hands-on" or "hands-off" delivery of the head, you should:
• Inspect for a cord around the neck as the head emerges and gently slide it over the head.
  • If the cord is tight and will not slide over the head, try to gently push the cord over the anterior shoulder as it is born.
  • If the cord is twice wrapped around the neck and cannot be "reduced," allow the baby to birth and unwrap the cord as soon as possible.
  • If the cord is so tight the body of the baby cannot be born, place two clamps on the cord (1 inch apart from each other) and cut, unwrapping the cord as soon as possible.
• Wipe off the baby's face and head, gently sweeping away excess mucus from the nose and mouth if necessary.
• Gently (not vigorously) suction the oropharynx *then* nasopharynx with the bulb syringe *only* if the baby has excessive secretions and difficulty initiating respirations.
• Place the baby on the mother's chest or abdomen and allow the cord to stop pulsating.
• Prevent loss of body heat by drying the baby, then covering both mother and baby with warm blankets (**thermoregulation**).

Managing Problems

Meconium-Stained Amniotic Fluid

• Occurs more often in high-risk pregnancies[3]
• May be found in the presence of uterine tachysystole (precipitous labor; Pitocin drip)
• May be associated with maternal hypertension
• Is seen more often when the woman has a biophysical profile (BPP) of less than 6
• Occurs more often in postdate pregnancies
• May be associated with fetal hypoxic episodes
• May be found with decreased variability in the fetal heart rate baseline; late decelerations do not have to be present
• May be a physiologic indicator of a mature gastrointestinal tract
• Is not absolutely associated with fetal acidosis

Critical Interventions When Meconium-Stained Amniotic Fluid Is Noted

> Recent research has indicated that routine intrapartum suctioning of the oropharynx and nasopharynx does not always prevent meconium aspiration syndrome in infants.[4]

As for all impending births, a neonatal resuscitation program (NRP) trained nurse should be available to assist the baby with transition from intrauterine to extrauterine life. There is no need to suction the baby's oronasopharynx, even in the presence of meconium. If the baby is vigorously crying, he/she should be placed on the mother's abdomen and dried.

Shoulder Dystocia

For a detailed discussion of the nursing responsibilities in the event of a shoulder dystocia, refer to Module 16.[1] The following interventions relate specifically to delivery of the baby when an obstetric provider is *not* present.

A review of the woman's prenatal history may identify antepartum risk factors associated with a shoulder dystocia. Risk factors for shoulder dystocia are presented in Module 16.

• **What should you do in the presence of a "turtle sign," when baby's shoulders become "stuck" (*shoulder dystocia*)?**

Initial important steps to take include the following:
- Recognize the "turtle sign": when the baby's head retracts back against the perineum and does not attempt to externally rotate. This implies the shoulders are "stuck."
- Be prepared, remain calm, and have a nurse assistant in the room.
- If the mother's hips are not already on towels or pillows, do so now.
- After the head delivers, take advantage of the baby's rotating shoulders moving into the anteroposterior (AP) position. Do not allow the shoulders to rotate directly AP. Shoulders should be delivered in the oblique position.
- Have two nurses (or the woman and her support person) help the mother to sharply flex her knees and hips (McRobert's maneuver) backward by pulling back on her legs as far as they will go. This action flattens the lumbosacral spine and rotates the symphysis pubis anteriorly. In most cases, this will dislodge the fetal anterior shoulder (Fig. 9.7).

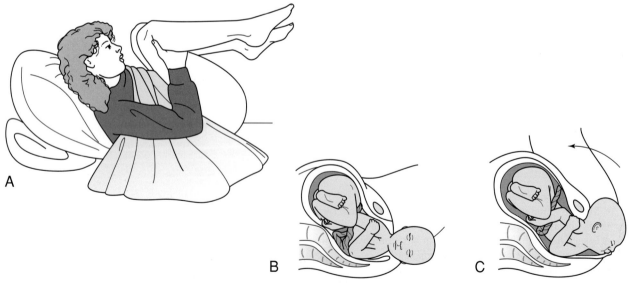

FIGURE 9.7 McRobert's maneuver. **A.** McRobert's maneuver position. **B.** Normal position of the symphysis pubis and the sacrum. **C.** The symphysis pubis rotates and the sacrum flattens. (Adapted with permission from Naef, R. W., & Martin, J. N. (1995). Emergent management of shoulder dystocia. *Obstetrics and Gynecology Clinics of North America*, 22(2), 252.)

• Have one of the nurses apply suprapubic pressure. This is best done while standing on a stool. Using the palmar surface of the hands placed above the pubic bone, apply reasonable pressure straight down (Fig. 9.8). This pressure causes flexion of the shoulder toward the fetal chest, decreasing the diameter of the shoulders. This may aid in delivery of the shoulder.

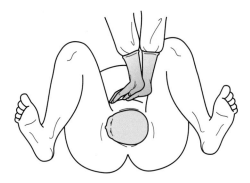

FIGURE 9.8   Pressure is applied by pushing down just above the pubic bone onto the fetal shoulder.

Additional maneuvers for the nurse assistant include:
• Identifying which maternal side the fetal back is facing.
• Positioning a stool on the side of the mother where the fetal back is lying and applying suprapubic pressure *away* from the fetal back, or toward the small parts.
• Lowering the maternal head (i.e., avoid a full Fowler's position) so there is room for the nurse(s) to do suprapubic pressure.

Suprapubic pressure is most effective when the person applying it is positioned higher than the maternal body. NEVER USE FUNDAL PRESSURE.

Bleeding

• **If the postpartum mother bleeds excessively, what should you do while waiting for the obstetric provider to arrive?**

Attempt to identify the source of the bleeding and perform the corresponding nursing interventions (Table 9.1). For a detailed discussion of postpartum hemorrhage, see Module 16. These actions are described for situations in which the obstetric provider is not present.

Hematoma (Hidden or Occult Bleeding)

It is possible for bleeding to occur under the surface of intact tissues (hematoma of the perineum or vagina). The woman may complain of increasing pelvic pain or rectal pressure out of proportion to the amount of lochia observed. Eventually a reddish-blue discoloration of the perineum might be seen, and a soft mass in the vagina might be palpated. This must be noted and observed over several hours. Occult bleeding can trap upward of 1,000 mL in hidden tissue planes not seen by the naked eye.
   Additional actions to take include the following:
• Notifying a physician or midwife
• Increasing administration of intravenous fluids to more than 125 mL per hour
• Taking and recording the woman's blood pressure and pulse
• Noting on the chart the amount, color, and type of blood loss

To treat a decreasing blood volume caused by excessive bleeding, lactated Ringer's solution should be administered for immediate fluid replacement and prevention of shock. Extreme caution should be used if a large volume of physiologic normal saline is used because it can increase the risk for electrolyte imbalance, coagulation problems, and renal failure.

TABLE 9.1 SIGNS AND SYMPTOMS OF AND INTERVENTIONS FOR ACTIVE MATERNAL BLEEDING

SOURCE	SIGNS AND SYMPTOMS	NURSING INTERVENTION
Uterine atony	1. Soft and poorly contracting uterus OR 2. Dark red vaginal bleeding	1. Massage the top of the uterus to stimulate a contraction and express clots, AND empty the bladder
Retained pieces of placenta	1. Clots	1. Give oxygen if needed 2. Increase rate of intravenous fluids 3. Take and record blood pressure and pulse
Laceration of cervix or vagina	1. Firm uterus 2. Bright red vaginal bleeding that is profuse	If orthostatic changes: 1. Place woman flat or in Trendelenburg position 2. Give oxygen if needed 3. Increase rate of administration of intravenous fluids 4. Start a second IV
Laceration of perineum or labia	1. Firm uterus 2. Obvious tear of tissue 3. Bright red bleeding from tear	1. Apply pressure using a sterile pad to tamponade bleeding 2. Place woman flat or in Trendelenburg position 3. Increase rate of administration of intravenous fluid

---

• **Which women are at greatest risk to bleed excessively after the birth?**

Women at greatest risk for excessive bleeding include those women who have had the following:
- A large baby, multiple pregnancy, or polyhydramnios
- A long labor
- A rapid or precipitous labor
- Oxytocin induction/augmentation
- A history of many pregnancies (grand multiparity)
- A history of excessive postpartum bleeding

Breech Delivery

• **If the unexpected birth is in a breech position, what should you do?**

- Stay calm and ask for assistance.
  - Elevate the mother's hips on towels or pillows.
  - Do not touch the breech until it has been born past the umbilicus. It will look funny as the breech dangles downward. This is good, especially if the back is facing you. It means the head is most likely flexed.
- If possible, prevent pressure on the umbilical cord by gently creating a loop of cord at the perineum *without tugging.* Tugging on the cord can create a vasospasm.
  - At this time, you can support the body by placing your thumbs on the sacral crests and your fingers on the pelvic brim and crests (not on the abdomen).
  - At this time, you can also take a "hands-off" approach and wait until you see the nape of the neck before supporting the body.
  - When the nape of the neck is seen, the assistant nurse should apply suprapubic pressure to keep the baby's head flexed.
- Support the baby in your hands (or with a towel that acts like a hammock on the abdomen) (Fig. 9.9).
  - After the baby is delivered, stimulate by drying with towels and place on the mother's chest or abdomen and cover with prewarmed blankets (thermoregulation).

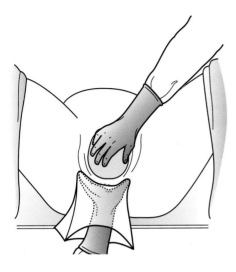

FIGURE 9.9 Use a warm towel and lift the body if available and there is time.

Immediate Care of the Newborn

Immediate care of the newborn involves the presence of an NRP nurse and the safety measures discussed previously:

- Maintain a clear airway
- Maintain body heat (*thermoregulation*)
- Assess general health status (i.e., inspect for any birth injuries or abnormalities)
- Observe vital signs
- Assess 1- and 5-minute Apgar scores

In addition, the following should be noted:

- Number of vessels in the cord (two arteries and one vein)
- Application of identification bands for mother and baby

Postpartum Care of the Mother

- Assess firmness and position of the uterus
- Note the color and quantity of the lochia
- Note any lacerations
- Observe and record vital signs every 15 minutes
- Assess the status of the bladder
- Assist woman to empty her bladder to help uterine contractions control bleeding
- Provide warmth, food, drink, rest, and initiate breastfeeding

The birth of a baby is a powerful emotional as well as physical experience. Studies indicate a most sensitive period exists immediately after the infant's birth. It is during this time that the parents are most likely to develop strong emotional ties ("bond") with their child. Touching, skin-to-skin contact, holding, nursing, and eye contact all help to develop this tie.

An unexpected or precipitous birth can often be so rushed and hectic that parents miss the opportunity to bond with their baby. The nurse's attitude toward every family's birth should be one of concern for health and safety and a commitment to promote family bonding.

Documentation

Information you should note in the legal record of the birth includes the following:

- Who was present at the birth
- Presentation and position of the baby
- Date and time of the birth
- Gender of the baby

- Apgar scores at 1 and 5 minutes
- Presence of cord around the baby's neck or body and the number of times the cord encircles that part
- Any lacerations to the maternal tissues
- The presence of birth injuries or abnormalities in the baby
- Time of delivery of the placenta
- Appearance of the placenta and membranes (intact, color, abnormalities)
- Appearance of the cord (number of vessels, abnormalities)
- Estimated blood loss
- Any drugs administered to the mother or baby
- Anything unusual about the birth
- First stooling or voiding by the baby
- Vital signs of the mother
- Vital signs of the baby
- Name of the person conducting the birth

PRACTICE/REVIEW QUESTIONS

After reviewing this module and those noted throughout, answer the following questions.

1. Which of the following situations could result in delivery of the baby before the arrival of the obstetric provider? Select all that apply.

    a. An unexpectedly small baby

    b. Rapid progress during labor

    c. Grand multiparous

    d. History of rapid labors

2. List six signs of an impending unexpected or precipitous birth.

    a. _____

    b. _____

    c. _____

    d. _____

    e. _____

    f. _____

3. List equipment that should be available in the sterile emergency birth pack.

    _____

    _____

    _____

4. "Feather blowing" may help the laboring woman control the urge to push.

    a. True

    b. False

5. A baby born with meconium-stained fluid requires vigorous suctioning to prevent meconium aspiration syndrome.

    a. True

    b. False

6. If the baby's head is delivering too fast, the nurse should hold it back.

    a. True

    b. False

7. List at least six actions you should do once the baby is delivered to ensure its safety.

    a. _____

    b. _____

    c. _____

    d. _____

    e. _____

    f. _____

8. Meconium-stained amniotic fluid may be associated with which of the following? Select all that apply.

    a. Tachysystole of uterine contractions

    b. Preterm pregnancies

    c. Postdated pregnancies

    d. Decreased variability in fetal heart rate baseline

9. What should you do for the baby if the amniotic fluid is stained with meconium?

    _____

    _____

10. Shoulder dystocia should be a concern when caring for a woman with which of the following? Select all that apply.

    a. History of shoulder dystocia

    b. Suspected macrosomia in current pregnancy

    c. You never know

    d. Slow labor progress

11. What should you do if the baby's shoulders become stuck?

_____

_____

_____

12. Match the signs and symptoms in Column B with the source in Column A.

Column A	**Column B**
_____ 1. Retained placenta	a. Uterus feels firm but bleeding easily seen from torn tissue
_____ 2. Lacerations of cervix or vagina	b. Bright red vaginal bleeding
_____ 3. Laceration of perineum or labia	c. Soft uterus and dark red bleeding and/or clots
	d. Watery discharge

13. If the source of excessive postpartum bleeding is retained pieces of placenta, what should you do?

a. _____

b. _____

c. _____

d. _____

14. Which of the following situations place the woman at risk for excessive bleeding after the birth?

a. Grand multiparity

b. Short, rapid labor

c. Small baby

d. Oxytocin induction/augmentation

15. What should you do to assist a breech delivery?

a. _____

b. _____

c. _____

d. _____

PRACTICE/REVIEW ANSWER KEY

1. a, b, c, and d
2. Any six of the following:
   a. Nausea and retching
   b. Increased bloody show
   c. Strong urge to push
   d. Separation of the labia
   e. Increased pressure against the perineum
   f. Bulging of the anus
   g. Early decelerations
   h. Epidural that "stops working"
   i. A statement from the mother such as, "It's coming!"
3. X-ray detectable gauze sponges, two absorbent towels, soft bulb syringe, small sterile drape, two clamps, scissors, baby blanket, gloves
4. a. True
5. b. False
6. b. False
7. Any six of the following:
   a. Do not hold the head back
   b. Inspect the baby's neck for a nuchal cord
   c. Place the baby on the maternal abdomen/chest
   d. Check the airway and wipe away excess secretions if the baby is having trouble establishing respirations
   e. Dry the baby
   f. Allow the umbilical cord to stop pulsating
   g. Prevent heat loss by covering mother and baby
8. c and d
9. Have an NRP nurse available.
   Do nothing if the baby is vigorously crying
   Double clamp and cut the cord and pass a depressed baby to the NRP provider for immediate resuscitation
10. a, b, c, and d
11. • Elevate the mother's hips on towels or pillows
    • Try and deliver the shoulders as the head is restituting, before they become lodged in the AP diameter
    • Have the mother sharply flex her knees and hips, bringing the thighs alongside her abdomen
    • Ask another staff member to apply suprapubic pressure
12. 1. c
    2. b
    3. a
13. a. Massage the top of the uterus
    b. Administer oxygen, if needed
    c. Increase the rate of administration of intravenous fluid
    d. Take and record blood pressure and pulse
14. a, b, and d
15. a. Elevate the mother's hips on towels or pillows
    b. Prevent stress on the cord by creating a loop at the perineum
    c. Allow the body to deliver on its own up to the umbilicus before placing hands on pelvic bones, OR, allow the body to deliver on its own up to the nape of the neck before supporting the body with a hand underneath
    d. Suprapubic pressure to maintain flexion of the head
    e. Lift the baby's body using two hands or a towel like a hammock to help deliver the shoulders and head
    f. Perform other safety measures, as with a normal delivery

SKILL UNIT 1 | MANAGING AN UNEXPECTED OR PRECIPITOUS BIRTH

The birth of a baby should be planned and conducted to ensure safety for the mother and baby and to promote bonding for the family. A birth conducted by the obstetric provider who has cared for the woman throughout her pregnancy is ideal. Sometimes, however, circumstances prevent this, and it is then the nurse in the labor and delivery unit who often assists the mother. The labor and delivery nurse must be prepared and have the necessary skills to provide the woman and her baby with the safest and most satisfying experience possible.

ACTIONS	REMARKS
Assemble Equipment	
Sterile emergency birth pack	Use universal precautions.
Prepare for the Delivery	
1. Call for assistance.	A second nurse who is NRP prepared can help care for the newborn, assist the nurse conducting the delivery, and help with any unexpected events.
2. Position the woman.	Position the woman on her back or side, whichever provides the most comfort for the woman and access to the perineum for the nurse. Elevate her hips on towels or pillows.
3. Wash hands.	
Control delivery of the baby's head with "hands-on" or "hands-off."	
4. Open the sterile emergency birth pack wherever the birth will take place.	You need to have the pack within easy reach. It is important to maintain sterile technique. This will help to decrease the chance of infection.
5. Put on (sterile) gloves. Place the sterile barrier under the buttocks.	

Be sure you know the presentation of the baby. If you are uncertain about the presentation, a vaginal examination should be done to see whether the baby is vertex or breech.

Conduct the Unexpected or Precipitous Birth	
6. If the head is crowning and the bags of water are still intact, focus on the birth.	The bags of water will usually rupture before birth. If not, rupture the bags with one of the clamps before (if there is time), or immediately after the birth. Birth with intact bags of water is known as "en caul."
7. Instruct the woman when to "feather blow" and when to push.	This helps to prevent uncontrolled, rapid delivery of the head.

Be clear when telling the woman what to do. Make your instructions short and easy to understand.

8. Slide your fingers down around the baby's neck to inspect for a nuchal cord as soon as the head has delivered (Fig. 9.10).	Need to determine whether or not a nuchal cord is present.

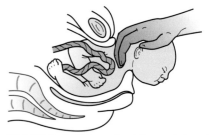

FIGURE 9.10 Check for nuchal cord

skill unit continues on page 245

ACTIONS	REMARKS

If the cord is loose, gently slip the loop of cord over the head (Fig. 9.11).

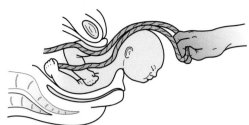

FIGURE 9.11   Gently slip loose nuchal cord over the head

If the cord is tight, try to slip the cord over baby's shoulders.

In the event a tight nuchal cord prevents birth of the body, place two clamps on the cord (approximately 1 inch apart) and cut between the clamps (Fig. 9.12). Quickly unwrap the cord from around the neck.

This baby may need stimulation after birth. The assisting nurse should be NRP prepared.

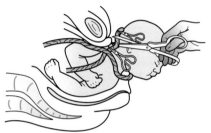

FIGURE 9.12   Clamp and cut tight nuchal cord

9. Wipe the head and face dry, paying special attention to mucus coming from the nose and mouth.

Mucus is forced out of the nose and mouth as the baby squeezes through the birth canal. *Only* if the baby has excessive secretions should a bulb syringe be used to suction the oronasopharynx.

10. Allow the head to **restitute**. You can place the hand palm-side up with the fingers toward the face, under the head for support (Fig. 9.13).

Head and shoulders are resuming normal alignment. The baby's head will turn slightly.

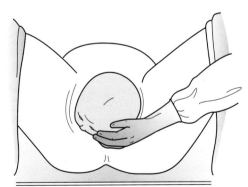

FIGURE 9.13   Support the head during restitution

skill unit continues on page 246

ACTIONS	REMARKS
Allow the shoulders to *externally* rotate (Fig. 9.14).	As the shoulders move into position for birth, you will observe another slight turn of the baby's head. The shoulders are now in the AP diameter of the maternal pelvis.

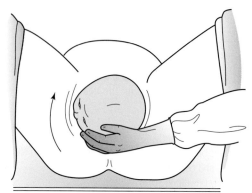

FIGURE 9.14 Continue support during shoulder rotation

11. Place the second hand on the other side of the baby's head and, with downward, outward traction on the head, deliver the anterior shoulder (Fig. 9.15).	Keep your fingers flat on the sides of the head. *Do not* grab the baby around the neck.

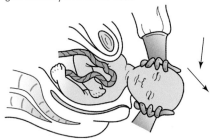

FIGURE 9.15 Downward and outward traction for delivery of anterior shoulder

12. As soon as the anterior shoulder delivers, provide upward, outward traction to the head to deliver the posterior shoulder (Fig. 9.16).	Keep fingers away from eyes and neck.

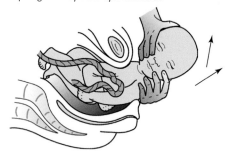

FIGURE 9.16 Upward and outward traction for delivery of posterior shoulder

13. As the shoulder clears the perineum, support the head with the heel of your hand and thumb. Using the fingers of this hand, grasp the baby's arm to the chest wall (Fig. 9.17). Support the baby in your lower hand.

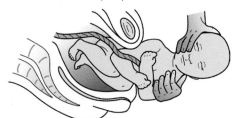

FIGURE 9.17 Support as shoulders clear the perineum

skill unit continues on page 247

ACTIONS	REMARKS
14. As the body delivers, slide the upper hand down the baby's back to grasp the feet (Fig. 9.18).	Holding the arm to the chest helps to prevent laceration of the perineum by the elbow.

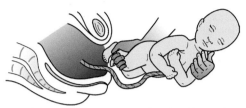

FIGURE 9.18 Support the shoulder and grasp the feet

15. Place the baby on the mother's abdomen or chest and dry. Cover both with blankets.	Skin to skin provides warmth, assisting with thermoregulation.
16. Allow the cord to stop pulsating on its own.	Delayed cord clamping allows the baby to receive extra blood.

Care of the Newborn (some repeated steps)

17. Place the baby directly on the mother's warm chest or abdomen.	This assists in maintaining the baby's body heat with skin-to-skin contact (or a heated crib).
18. Dry the baby thoroughly.	Wet babies lose a great deal of heat. It is important to replace wet towels immediately.
19. With skin-to-skin contact, cover the newborn and mother with warm towels or a blanket.	This helps to prevent heat loss in the newborn.
20. Double clamp the umbilical cord. Cut the cord between the two clamps (Fig. 9.19).	Take care to avoid wide spraying of the blood.

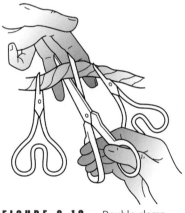

FIGURE 9.19 Double clamp and cut cord

21. Collect blood from the cord attached to the placenta.	Because the amount of cord blood drawn will depend on the tests needed, check the mother's chart and your hospital's guidelines.

Delivery of the Placenta

22. Check for uterine size, shape, and firmness.	The uterus must contract to expel the placenta and to control bleeding. Signs of placental separation are as follows: • A gush of blood • Lengthening of the cord • A change in the shape of the uterus from discoid (flat) to globular

skill unit continues on page 248

ACTIONS	REMARKS
23. Control the delivery of the placenta by keeping a gentle, steady, downward traction on the cord as the other hand supports the uterus with suprapubic pressure. The mother can assist by bearing down when she feels a contraction.	Tugging on the cord or vigorous rubbing of the uterus can cause problems and must not be done. Carefully inspect the placenta for signs of missing pieces or abnormalities. Count the number of vessels in the cord: there should be three (two arteries and one vein).
24. Observe the amount and color of the bleeding and the tone of the uterus.	If the uterus feels soft, it can be stimulated to contract by massaging the fundus (the top of the uterus) or by having the baby breastfeed.
25. Inspect for lacerations.	Gently inspect the perineum and labia for bleeding or tears in need of repair by the obstetric provider. An x-ray detectable sponge can be used to apply pressure to control bleeding of a perineal or labial laceration.
26. Facilitate bonding and initiate breastfeeding.	Families need time to inspect, hold, and "take in" the newborn. After birth, initiate breastfeeding and allow the family private time to begin to "attach."

You will need to attend a skill session(s) to practice these skills with the help of your preceptor. Mastery of the skill is achieved when you can demonstrate techniques of delivering a baby, including the following:

- Taking preparatory steps
- Positioning the woman for birth
- Using (sterile) gloves and drapes
- "Hands-off" and talking to the woman or "hands-on" with flexing and controlling delivery of the head
- Guiding the delivery of the baby's body
- Checking for a nuchal cord
- Cutting the umbilical cord or discussing the benefits of delayed cord clamping
- Delivering the placenta
- Inspecting the placenta and cord

REFERENCES

1. Albers, L. L., Greulich, B., & Peralta, P. (2006). Body mass index, midwifery intrapartum care, and childbirth lacerations. *Journal of Midwifery & Women's Health, 51*(4), 249–253.
2. Albers, L. L., Sedler, K., Bedrick, E., et al. (2006). Factors related to genital tract trauma in normal spontaneous vaginal births. *Birth, 33*(2), 94–100.
3. Kattwinkel, J., Perlman, J. M., Aziz, K., et al. (2010). Neonatal resuscitation: 2010 American Heart Association Guidelines for Cardiopulmonary Resuscitation and Emergency Cardiovascular Care. *Pediatrics, 126*, e1400–e1413.
4. American Heart Association, American Academy of Pediatrics. (2006). 2005 American Heart Association (AHA) guidelines for cardiopulmonary resuscitation (CPR) and emergency cardiovascular care (ECC) of pediatric and neonatal patients: Neonatal resuscitation guidelines. *Pediatrics, 117*, e1029–e1038.

FURTHER READINGS

Creasy, R. K., & Resnik, R. (2013). *Maternal-fetal medicine* (7th ed.). Philadelphia, PA: WB Saunders.
Cunningham, G., Leveno, K. J., Bloom, S. L., et al. (2014). *Williams obstetrics* (24th ed.). New York, NY: McGraw-Hill.
Gabbe, S. G., Niebyl, J. L., & Simpson, J. L. (2012). *Normal and problem pregnancies*. New York, NY: Churchill Livingstone.
King, T. L., Brucker, M. C., Kriebs, J. M., et al. (2015). *Varney's midwifery* (5th ed.). Burlington, MA: Jones & Bartlett Learning.
Perlman, J, M., Wyllie, J, Kattwinkel, J., et al.; on behalf of the Neonatal Resuscitation Chapter Collaborators. Part 7: neonatal resuscitation. International consensus on cardiopulmonary resuscitation and emergency cardiovascular care science with treatment recommendations. *Circulation, 132*(suppl 1), S204–S241.
Posner, G., & Black, A. (2013). *Oxorn-Foote human labor & birth* (6th ed.). New York, NY: Mc-Graw-Hill Companies.

Preterm Labor and Preterm Premature Rupture of Membranes

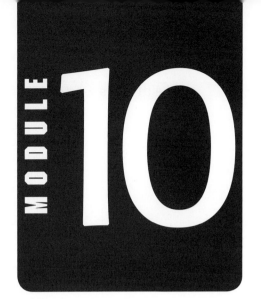

MODULE 10

DINEZ SWANSON AND
SUZANNE McMURTRY BAIRD

Part 1

Preterm Labor and Birth

Part 2

Preterm Premature Rupture of Membranes

As you complete this module, you will learn:

1. The definition of *preterm labor*
2. Strategies to identify women at risk for preterm labor
3. How to recognize and treat early symptoms of preterm labor
4. Management of preterm labor, including the following:
   a. Pharmacologic agents
   b. Nursing implications.
5. Appropriate education for women in preterm labor
6. The definition of *preterm premature rupture of membranes (PPROM)*
7. Risks to the mother and fetus associated with PPROM
8. Management methods when PPROM occurs in a preterm pregnancy, including the following:
   a. Chorioamnionitis
   b. Expectant management options
   c. The role of antibiotics for these patients
9. Priorities for nursing interventions in caring for the woman with PPROM
10. The role of steroid therapy in the prevention of neonatal complications
11. The use of magnesium sulfate for neuroprotection

Key Terms

When you have completed this module, you should be able to recall the meanings of the following terms. You should also be able to use the terms when consulting with other health professionals. The terms are defined in this module or in the glossary at the end of this book.

17-α-hydroxyprogesterone caproate (17P)
Bacterial vaginosis
β-Adrenergic agonist
β-Adrenergic receptor
Braxton Hicks contractions
Calcium channel blocker
Chorioamnionitis
Corticosteroid
Corticotropin-releasing hormone (CRH)

Fetal fibronectin (fFN)
Late preterm birth
Low birth weight
Neuroprotection
Preterm premature rupture of membranes (PPROM)
Preterm birth
Prostaglandins
Tocolytic therapy
Very preterm birth

This module reviews current information regarding spontaneous preterm labor (PTL) and preterm premature rupture of membranes (PPROM). Continuing research is constantly changing our understanding of the process leading to these events. There is very little evidence that any of the medical strategies or behavioral interventions that we use have had any significant impact on the prevention of PTL or reduction in the number of preterm births (PTBs). Nurses should stay informed of current evidence, understand recommended best practice, and provide diligent assessments in order for practice decisions to be based on proven strategies, optimize utilization of resources, and to avoid potentially harmful and unnecessary interventions.

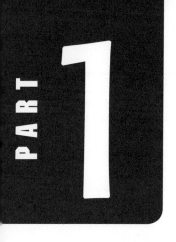

Preterm Labor and Birth

Epidemiology of Preterm Labor and Birth

A *PTB* is defined as the delivery of an infant at less than 37 weeks of gestation and account for 11.4% of live births in the United States.[1] PTB, although declining in rate, remains a significant issue with an estimated 450,000 babies are born too soon every year (US).[1,2] Improvements in the PTB rate since 2006 appear to be driven by reductions in late preterm births (LPTB), which increased rapidly between 1990 and 2006, peaking at 9.1% of live births.[2]

PTBs account for 85% of all perinatal morbidity and mortality.[2] A 2007 report from the Institute of Medicine estimated the annual cost of PTB in the United States to be $26.2 billion or more than $51,000 per premature infant.[3] Medical care services contributed $16.9 billion to the total cost and maternal delivery costs contributed another $1.9 billion.[3] In terms of longer-term expenditures, early intervention services cost an estimated $611 million, whereas special education services associated with a higher prevalence of four disabling conditions among premature infants added $1.1 billion.[3] It is estimated that lost household and labor market productivity associated with those disabilities contributed $5.7 billion.[3] Significant racial disparities persist in PTBs. In 2013, the PTB rate among African American women was 16%, 13.1% for American Indian or Alaska Native, 11.3% for Hispanic women, 10.2% for Asian or Pacific Islander, and 10.5% for Caucasian women.[1]

Complications of PTB arise from immature organ systems that are not yet prepared to support life in the extrauterine environment. In general, the more immature a preterm infant is at birth, the higher likelihood of required life-sustaining treatments, medications, and cost. Possible adverse outcomes for preterm infants are presented in Table 10.1.

PTBs are classified as **medically indicated** to optimize outcomes for maternal and/or fetal conditions, **spontaneous** due to PTL with intact membranes, **PPROM**, or **multiple gestations**.[5]

Preterm Definitions

Preterm: Birth that occurs between 20 0/7 and 36 6/7 weeks' gestation.[4]
Late Preterm: Birth that occurs between 34 0/7 and 36 6/7 weeks' gestation.
Low Birth Weight: Birth weight less than 2,500 g (5 lb, 8 oz).
Very Low Birth Weight: Birth weight less than 1,500 g (3 lb, 4 oz).
Extremely Low Birth Weight: Birth weight below 1,000 g.

NOTE: Low birth weight is not considered in the definition for PTL since it does not take into account the gestational age.

• What are the Risk Factors for PTL and Birth?[4–6]

The most common factors that increase the woman's risk of PTL and birth are:
- Prior PTB: Women who have had a previous PTB have approximately a 30% increased risk delivering prematurely in a subsequent pregnancy.
- Current multifetal pregnancy: Multiple gestations are associated with a high risk of PTL and birth. In general, the rate of PTL and birth is statistically higher in multifetal pregnancies. Contributing to the rate of prematurity among women with multifetal pregnancies is the use of assisted reproductive technologies (ART), such as in vitro fertilization, embryo

TABLE 10.1	NEWBORN COMPLICATIONS OF PRETERM BIRTH

Respiratory Distress Syndrome: The most common complication associated with PTB and low birth weight, primarily due to the premature newborn's immature respiratory system and lack of surfactant sufficient to maintain alveolar function.

Bronchopulmonary Dysplasia and Chronic Lung Disease: Chronic accumulation of fluid and scarring of the lungs, sometimes associated with medications used to facilitate mechanical ventilation.

Apnea: Periods of apnea and bradycardia are common among preterm neonates—premature and low birth weight babies also have a higher incidence of sudden infant death syndrome (SIDS).

Necrotizing enterocolitis (NEC): Disease of the gastrointestinal system that may be caused by immature immune system responses that predispose to infection or underdeveloped gastrointestinal flora.

Gastroesophageal reflux (GER): A back-up of acid or food from the stomach to the esophagus

Infection: Blood-borne infection

Interventricular hemorrhage (IVH): A brain hemorrhage, or bleeding within a premature infant's brain

Retinopathy of Prematurity (ROP): Abnormal proliferation of blood vessels in the eye, and occurs most frequently in neonates born before 32 wks.

White Matter Injury and Periventricular Leukomalacia: Occurs when the white matter of the brain is injured near the ventricles.

Hypothermia: Immature protective skin layer.

Hypoglycemia: Cold stress leads to utilization of glucose.

Feeding issues: Underdeveloped suck and swallowing reflexes that make feeding difficult.

Simhan, H., Iams, J., & Romero, R. (2012). Preterm labor. In Gabbe, S. G., Niebyl, J. R., Simpson, J. L., et al. (Eds.), *Obstetrics: Normal and problem pregnancies* (6th ed., pp. 627–658). Philadelphia, PA: Saunders Elsevier.

transfer, and donor transfer. There is also a higher rate of spontaneous multiple gestations in women over the age of 35.
- Fetal fibronectin (fFN) greater than 50 ng/mL between 22 and 34 weeks' gestation.
- Uterine/cervical abnormalities (which may be due to previous surgical procedures).
  - Cervical length less than 25 mm by transvaginal ultrasound (TVU) between 20 and 28 weeks' gestation
  - Previous pregnancy with cervical insufficiency
  - Abnormal placentation

Other factors that may *increase* risk for PTL and birth include:
- Interval between pregnancies
  - Less than 18 months
  - Greater than 59 months
- Vaginal bleeding not associated with previa or abruption
- Infection/inflammation
  - Bacterial vaginosis
  - Periodontal disease
- Ethnicity
  - African Americans and American Indians
- Age
  - Women younger than age 18
  - Women older than age 35 (more likely to have other conditions such as high blood pressure and diabetes that can cause complications requiring preterm delivery).
- Lifestyle factors
  - Substance abuse, including alcohol consumption
  - Smoking
  - Inadequate maternal weight gain
  - Domestic violence, including physical, sexual, or emotional abuse
  - Lack of social support
  - Depression, anxiety, stress
  - Long working hours with long periods of standing
  - Exposure to certain environmental pollutants

What Causes PTL

The initiation of labor involves two interdependent processes, that is, the triggering of rhythmic contractions that increase in amplitude and frequency, and the remodeling, effacement, and eventual dilatation of the cervix (with or without membrane rupture).[4–7] There are four pathways that lead to spontaneous PTL and birth, with the ultimate cause most likely some combination of these physiologic pathways (Fig. 10.1). Prostaglandins are key components to the labor process that:

- increase the number of contractions by stimulating the influx of calcium ions into smooth muscle cells.
- improve coordination of uterine muscle contraction by increasing the number of gap junctions between the individual myometrial (uterine muscle) cells.
- used in the production of proteases necessary for cervical ripening.

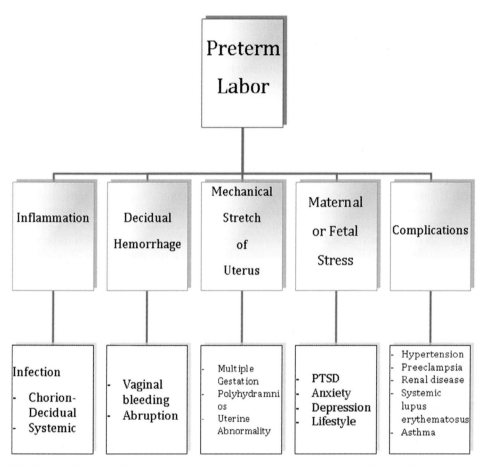

FIGURE 10.1 Pathways to preterm labor. PTSD, post traumatic stress disorde. (From Simhan, H., Iams, J., & Romero, R. (2012). Preterm labor. In Gabbe, S. G., Niebyl, J. R., Simpson, J. L., et al. (Eds.), *Obstetrics: Normal and problem pregnancies* (6th ed.,pp. 627–658). Philadelphia, PA: Saunders Elsevier; Cunningham, F., Leveno, K., Bloom, F., et al. (2013). Preterm labor. In *Williams obstetrics* (24th ed., pp. 829–861). New York, NY: McGraw Hill; American College of Obstetricians and Gynecologists, Committee on Practice Bulletins–Obstetrics. (2012). ACOG practice bulletin no. 127: Management of preterm labor. *Obstetrics & Gynecology, 119*(6), 1308–1317.)

Inflammation and Infection

Infection and inflammation are associated with the maternal or fetal cytokine response, which in turn produces prostaglandins and stimulates the production of matrix-degrading enzymes that cause breakdown of fetal membranes. Inflammation and infection may remain localized in a particular tissue or area of the body, pass into circulating blood, or ascend to the fetal membranes and fetus. Fetal inflammatory response syndrome (FIRS) is systemic inflammation and has been strongly linked to PTB, intracranial hemorrhage, periventricular leukomalacia, and cerebral palsy.[8] This fetal process is thought to be caused by the production of cytokines (tumor necrosis factor, interleukins 1, 6, and 8) which stimulate PTL. Blood vessels in the premature fetal brain are weak and susceptible to rupture and damage. In addition, the cytokines released due to inflammation have a damaging effect on oligodendrocytes and myelin, resulting in neuron death.[5]

Two micro-organisms that have been strongly linked to PTL and birth are *Ureaplasma urealyticum* and *Mycoplasma hominis.* Both organisms are thought to ascend from the lower genital tract. Bacterial vaginosis (BV) is associated with a twofold increase in PTL and a variety of other obstetric complications such as spontaneous abortion, chorioamnionitis, and low birth weight.[9] BV is a vaginal flora imbalance that occurs when the normal lactobacillus bacteria are replaced with anaerobic bacteria such as *Gardnerella vaginalis, Mobiluncus,* or *Mycoplasma hominis.* Women who are under chronic stress conditions, of certain ethnic groups, or who use vaginal douches have an increased risk of BV. Women with BV will have a watery and/or malodorous vaginal discharge. Screening and treatment have not been associated with a decreased risk of PTB. Routine screening is not recommend, but women who are symptomatic and diagnosed with an infection should be treated.[6]

Other infections, not associated with the genital tract, are also associated with PTL and birth. Urinary tract infections (cystitis, pyelonephritis), appendicitis, and periodontal disease increase risk. The pathophysiologic mechanisms are not well understood but are most likely linked to the maternal or fetal immune response. The woman's cervical length may also determine the effect of the infection and outcomes.[10]

Maternal or Fetal Stress

It has been suggested that stress stimulates the maternal–fetal hypothalamic–pituitary–adrenal axis. This in turn can cause increased production of corticotropin-releasing hormone (CRH). CRH is linked to cytokine release and prostaglandin production. Abnormal or early elevations of these hormone levels in maternal plasma have been documented in PTL. However, studies have not consistently shown the connection between stress, increased levels of CRH, and PTB.[5,11] A recent study indicated that pregnant women with posttraumatic stress disorder are at increased risk of PTB and should be treated as having high-risk pregnancies.[12] Further studies are needed to explain how stress may affect different women or why some women in very stressful situations deliver at term.

Decidual Hemorrhage or Abruption

Decidual hemorrhage or abruption initiates the coagulation cascade and production of thrombin. Thrombin has a uterotonic effect resulting in cervical ripening, uterine contractions, and a breakdown of the fetal membranes.[13] Any amount of vaginal bleeding between 6 and 13 weeks' gestation is associated with increased risk of pregnancy loss (before 24 weeks' gestation), abruption, and PTL.[14]

Mechanical Stretch of the Uterus

Another pathway of PTL is associated with overdistention of the uterus causing excessive uterine stretching in multifetal pregnancies, certain uterine malformations, macrosomia, or the development of polyhydramnios. The abnormal uterine stretching can stimulate prostaglandin production, thereby creating contractions. The mechanisms by which uterine overdistension might lead to PTL are not well understood. Uterine stretch induces the expression of gap junction proteins, as well as other contraction-associated proteins, such as oxytocin receptors. In multifetal pregnancies, a short cervical length (less than 25 mm) is the strongest risk factor for spontaneous PTB.[15,16]

• What are the Warning Signs of PTL?

The early warning signs of PTL are often subtle and can be difficult to differentiate from routine discomforts of pregnancy. These warning signs may go unrecognized until labor is advanced. The key to treating PTL and potentially preventing some of the morbidity associated with an early delivery is early recognition and treatment. Pregnant women should be educated to recognize the following symptoms[6]:
  • Change in type of vaginal discharge (watery, mucus, or bloody)
  • Increase in amount of discharge

- Pelvic or lower abdominal pressure
- Constant low, dull backache
- Mild abdominal cramps, with or without diarrhea
- Regular or frequent contractions or uterine tightening, often painless
- Ruptured membranes (your water breaks with a gush or a trickle of fluid)

NOTE: *A woman in PTL may have only one or all of these signs. The woman experiencing one or more of the signs of PTL should be examined and evaluated promptly.*

In addition to educating women and their families, all providers who might have contact with pregnant women should be knowledgeable about the early symptoms of PTL and the appropriate response. It is important to ensure the woman understands the terms used and can describe her symptoms. The importance of prompt reporting of these symptoms should be emphasized. The risks of delaying evaluation and treatment should be made clear, and women should be made to feel comfortable reporting symptoms or coming in for further evaluation, even when they are found not to be in labor.

NOTE: *Before giving instructions, the woman's knowledge level of PTL, her pregnancy history, and distance from the hospital should be ascertained.*

Assessment for Preterm Labor

Better identification of women in PTL not only provides timely and appropriate interventions but also promotes effective management to improve outcomes. Obstetric triage protocols should standardize assessment parameters according to best practice recommendations and prioritize the medical screening examination when a woman presents with PTL symptoms (Fig. 10.2). Units should establish a standardized clinical pathway for the assessment of women with suspected signs and symptoms of PTL, guidelines for management of asymptomatic women at risk of PTB, and management of women with confirmed PTL.[17] Early differentiation between "true" and "false" labor allows for timely decisions regarding management, which may include transport to a higher level of care, administration of antenatal corticosteroids and/or tocolytics, and assembly of the high-risk team. While it may not be possible to decrease the rate of PTB for these women, the outlined standardized interventions are well established to significantly improve neonatal outcomes.

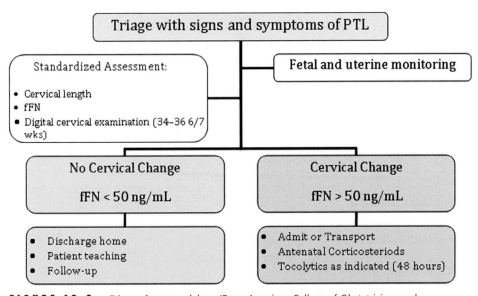

FIGURE 10.2 Triage of preterm labor. (From American College of Obstetricians and Gynecologists, Committee on Practice Bulletins–Obstetrics. (2012). ACOG practice bulletin no. 127: Management of preterm labor. *Obstetrics & Gynecology, 119*(6), 1308–1317; March of Dimes. (2012). *Preterm labor assessment toolkit.* White Plains, NY: Author. Retrieved from https://www.prematurityprevention.org/portal/server.pt; Howard, E. (2013). Labor evaluation. In Angelini, D., & LaFontaine, D. (Eds.), *Obstetric triage and emergency care protocols* (pp. 159–167). New York, NY: Springer Publishing.)

Spontaneous PTL, which accounts for approximately 50% of PTBs, is defined as regular uterine contractions occurring between 20 and 36 6/7 weeks' gestation accompanied by one or more of the following[2,6]:

- Change in cervical dilation **AND/OR** change in cervical effacement (assessment by digital examination or TVU).

OR

- Initial assessment of cervical dilation of 2 cm or more.

Timely and appropriate patient assessment by the nurse and provider is crucial to identify women at risk for PTB (Table 10.2). Preterm uterine contractions are not a reliable assessment parameter to determine if a woman is in PTL. Preterm contractions may be described as irregular or painless. A qualified medical provider should complete a thorough review of the woman's symptoms, prenatal record, and history soon after the woman presents and per Emergency Medical Treatment Labor Act (EMTALA) regulation.[6,17–19]

NOTE: If serial cervical examinations are indicated, ideally they should be done by the same examiner, when possible, to improve reliability of assessing early or subtle cervical change.

• What Tests are Used to Diagnose Preterm Labor?

Specific and objective diagnostic tools allow safe and cost-effective evaluation of women who present with uterine contractions without cervical change (a low-threshold sign and symptom of PTL). Current diagnostic tools include the fFN test and TVU for cervical length measurement. In combination with an fFN test result, cervical length more accurately predicts the likelihood of premature birth. However, either screen alone has also been found to distinguish between symptomatic patients at high and low risk for PTB.[18] Providers should use standardized criteria and protocols to identify those women at risk for having a PTB in order to reduce unnecessary hospitalizations and medical treatments, as well as the cost related to these interventions.

Fetal Fibronectin

fFN is a glycoprotein found in plasma produced by the fetus and that typically is present in maternal vaginal secretions.[17] During weeks 22 to 35 of a normal pregnancy, it is virtually undetectable in vaginal secretions. However, if disruption of the maternal–fetal interface occurs fibronectin is released into cervical/vaginal secretions and is an indicator of increased PTB risk. A positive fFN test is a value greater than 50 ng/mL. The positive predictive value of testing for fFN is low, meaning that many women who have fFN will not go into PTL. However, the negative predictive value is high. This means that when fFN is not detected in vaginal secretions, there is a very high likelihood that a woman will not experience PTL within 14 days of the test making this an important tool to determine whether a woman with preterm contractions should be admitted and treated for PTL.[20]

When the woman has signs and symptoms of PTL, samples should be collected using a sterile speculum with the following best practice recommendations[17]:

- between 24 and 34 weeks' gestation
- there is no evidence of vaginal bleeding
- the cervix is dilated less than 3 cm
- fetal membranes are intact and not bulging
- there are no open cervical and/or vaginal lesions present
- intercourse or digital cervical examination has not occurred during the 24 hours prior to specimen collection

NOTE: Use of a sterile speculum for collection of fFN is the only FDA-approved method. Vaginal swab collection is no longer recommended.[21]

Cervical Length Measurement

Cervical length obtained by TVU is superior to digital assessment due to subjectivity of the examiner.[17] The normal cervical length in the mid-trimester of pregnancy varies from 10 to 50 mm (median, 35 mm). When the cervix measures less than 25 mm in length by TVU, the woman has a greater than 95% risk for PTB before 32 gestational weeks. TVU should be done by an experienced provider in order to obtain accurate measurements. Contraindications and limitations of TVU for cervical length include[22]:

TABLE 10.2 SAMPLE TRIAGE AND INITIAL ASSESSMENT PLAN OF CARE

Triage	Chief complaint	
	Vital signs	Note any vital signs outside of normal parameters
	EDD and EGA	
	Fetal activity and heart tones	Fetal movement Fetal heart rate auscultation
	Pain	Per hospital policy

Notify Provider
Determine Priority for Medical Screening Exam

Initial Assessment	Review prenatal history	Note PTL risk factors Confirm EDD and EGA Note previous cervical exam (if applicable)
	Interview	Vaginal bleeding Leaking amniotic fluid Abdominal cramping or tightening Low back pain or pelvic pressure Onset, duration, and severity of symptoms What activities preceded the onset of symptoms? What relief measures have been attempted? Symptoms of infection (dysuria, uterine tenderness, fever, malaise)
	Physical assessment	Head-to-toe Palpate for uterine tenderness
	Fetal monitoring	Baseline rate Baseline variability Accelerations Decelerations Category
	Uterine monitoring	Frequency Duration Palpate intensity Palpate resting tone
	Psychosocial assessment	Interpersonal violence screening Substance use
Testing	Obtain urine specimen for analysis and culture	
	Sterile speculum exam for fFN (24–34 wks)	Observe for leaking of amniotic fluid through cervical os Obtain amniotic fluid or vaginal discharge for fern, microscopic examination, nitrazine
	Perform digital cervical exam	Position of cervix Dilation Effacement Presenting part Station of presenting part Consistency
	Transvaginal ultrasound for cervical length	As applicable Qualified provider

EDD, estimated date of delivery; EGA, estimated gestational age; PTL, preterm labor.

From American College of Obstetricians and Gynecologists, Committee on Practice Bulletins–Obstetrics. (2012). ACOG practice bulletin no. 127: Management of preterm labor. *Obstetrics & Gynecology, 119*(6), 1308–1317; March of Dimes. (2012). *Preterm labor assessment toolkit.* White Plains, NY: Author. Retrieved from https://www.prematurityprevention.org/portal/server.pt; Howard, E. (2013). Labor evaluation. In Angelini, D., & LaFontaine, D. (Eds.), *Obstetric triage and emergency care protocols* (pp. 159–167). New York, NY: Springer Publishing; American Academy of Pediatrics, The American College of Obstetricians and Gynecologists. (2012). *Guidelines for perinatal care* (7th ed.). *assessment toolkit.*

- Before 15 gestational weeks and after 28 gestational week measurements are considered invalid.
- Vaginal bleeding is present, the cause of bleeding should be investigated prior to conducting a TVU.
- Active bleeding from placenta previa. (If previa is not actively bleeding, an experienced operator who is aware of the woman's condition and mindful that the procedure may provoke bleeding may perform TVU.)
- A full bladder, as the cervix may be deviated in relation to the volume of fullness. A full bladder may also compress the cervix between the probe and the bladder, causing the cervix to appear closed or falsely long. Most women find it painful to undergo the procedure with a full bladder and, hence, should empty their bladders beforehand.

NOTE: *Not all institutions or birth settings have experienced providers and availability of ultrasound equipment to provide screening.*

Management of PTL

Management of women with PTL after triage and initial assessment is determined by the provider and based on gestational age, assessment findings, and hospital capabilities for care of preterm infants.

Gestational Age Between 34 0/7 and 36 6/7 Weeks of Pregnancy

There are many variables in management of the woman who presents in spontaneous PTL between 34 0/7 and 36 6/7 weeks' gestation. To determine cervical change, serial digital examinations are indicated since fFN and TVU are not objective assessment tools in this gestational age group. Tocolytics are not indicated during this gestational age unless administration is for stabilization and transport to a tertiary care hospital.

Tocolytic Therapy

Tocolytic medications are used to slow down or halt uterine contractions in order for **pregnancy** to proceed so that the fetus can gain size and maturity before birth. Unfortunately, studies comparing the effectiveness of tocolytics to placebos and to each other have only shown short-term efficacy with no direct neonatal benefit.[23] The focus of tocolytic therapy is to:
1. quiet uterine activity for 48 hours in order to administer antenatal corticosteroids.
2. provide an opportunity for transport to a regional medical center.[6]

There is no clear, first-line choice of tocolytic agent due to mixed efficacy and the potential for serious adverse effects with all agents. Due to the potential for maternal compromise, combination and prolonged tocolytic therapy is not recommended.[6,17]

- **What are the Contraindications to Tocolytic Therapy?**

NOTE: *Tocolytic therapy should not be initiated when the risks of labor suppression outweigh the risks of PTB.*

Factors that threaten maternal and fetal status are contraindications to labor suppression. Some examples include[5,6]:

Maternal Conditions

- Chorioamnionitis. Signs and symptoms include fever (temperature greater than or equal to 100.4°F), uterine tenderness, maternal and/or fetal tachycardia, elevated white blood cell count, purulent or foul smelling amniotic fluid
- Preeclampsia with severe features or eclampsia
- Maternal hemorrhage
- PPROM, except to facilitate transport or antenatal steroid administration
- Severe intrauterine growth restriction

- **What Medications are Currently Used for Tocolysis?**

NOTE: There are no recommendations on which tocolytic agent to use. The plan of care and management should be individualized.

β-Adrenergic Agonists

There are two types of β-adrenergic receptors in the body:

1. β_1-Adrenergic receptors are found in the heart, liver, pancreas, kidney, small intestine, and adipose tissue.
2. β_2-Adrenergic receptors are found in smooth muscle of the uterus, blood vessels diaphragm, and bronchioles.

By binding to these receptor sites, β-adrenergic agonists initiate a series of reactions resulting in reduced levels of calcium and reduced sensitivity of the actin–myosin contractile unit to calcium. With lowered intracellular calcium levels, smooth muscle contraction is less effective and uterine contractions may cease. However, continued exposure to these medications can lead to desensitization as the number of β-adrenergic receptors decrease.

NOTE: Injectable Brethine (Terbutaline) should not be used in pregnant women for prevention or prolonged treatment (beyond 48 to 72 hours) of PTL in either the hospital or outpatient setting because of the potential for serious maternal heart problems and death. In addition, oral Brethine should not be used for prevention or any treatment of PTL because it has not been shown to be effective and has similar safety concerns.[24]

Because β-adrenergic receptors are present in multiple sites, side effects can be seen in various organ systems and the probability of maternal risk is higher than with some of the other tocolytics. These effects are presented in Table 10.3.

TABLE 10.3 EFFECTS OF β-ADRENERGIC TOCOLYTICS	
Cardiovascular	Increases heart rate, systolic blood pressure, pulse pressure, stroke volume, and cardiac output.[6,25] Decreases diastolic pressure and peripheral vascular resistance. Cardiac dysrhythmias have been reported. Increased heart rate and myocardial contractility can predispose patients to myocardial ischemia.
Pulmonary	Increases plasma renin and arginine vasopressin, which is associated with sodium and water retention. This predisposes patients to pulmonary edema, especially in multiple gestations. Excessive intravenous fluids combined with the antidiuretic effect of high dosages of these medications can result in fluid overload.
Metabolic	Increases maternal blood glucose levels and insulin levels. This effect is enhanced by concomitant administration of corticosteroids. Lipolysis can also be included, which can lead to severe metabolic acidosis in diabetic women.

Reedy, N. (2014). Preterm labor and birth. In Simpson, K., & Creehan, P. (Eds.), *Perinatal nursing* (4th ed., pp. 166–202). Philadelphia, PA: Wolters Kluwer; American College of Obstetricians and Gynecologists, Committee on Practice Bulletins–Obstetrics. (2012). ACOGpractice bulletin no. 127: Management of preterm labor. *Obstetrics & Gynecology, 119*(6), 1308–1317.

Magnesium Sulfate

Magnesium sulfate is widely available and commonly used as the first-line tocolytic agent, even though randomized studies have not proven it to be effective for tocolysis.[6] The side effects of parenteral magnesium for the treatment of PTL appear to be less severe and less frequent than those of β-adrenergic therapy. Magnesium sulfate is also safer to use with insulin-dependent diabetic patients because it decreases the risk of uncontrolled hyperglycemia, which can occur with β-adrenergic medications. The mechanism by which magnesium sulfate inhibits uterine contractions is not fully understood, but is thought to be related to its ability to inhibit the reuptake of acetylcholine at the nerve synapse. In this way, magnesium sulfate blocks neuromuscular transmissions and uterine contraction.

Magnesium sulfate should not be administered to women with myasthenia gravis and used with caution in women with renal or cardiac conduction and function impairments. Administration of magnesium sulfate should follow a well-defined institutional procedure that includes best practice safety recommendations.[26,27] A sample procedure for magnesium sulfate administration is presented in Table 10.4.

TABLE 10.4 SAMPLE MAGNESIUM SULFATE PROCEDURE

Prior to magnesium sulfate administration	Review provider order.
	Educate woman/family concerning the indications for use and possible side effects and requirements of strict bed rest with side rails up while on magnesium sulfate.
	Initiate fall precautions per hospital policy/procedure.
	Obtain IV and begin mainline infusion if not previously started.
	Provide continuous electronic fetal monitoring. Assess fetal and uterine status according to hospital policy/procedure.
	Assess maternal status including vital signs, bilateral lung auscultation, oxygen saturation (SpO$_2$), level of consciousness (LOC), and deep tendon reflexes (DTRs) to establish a baseline.
Administration of magnesium sulfate loading dose	Obtain an infusion pump with two separate channels.
	Main line IV fluid infusion per order in first channel.
	Dose range is 4–6 g.
	Obtain prepared bolus infusion of magnesium sulfate, check expiration date, and prime tubing. (Premixed magnesium sulfate 4 g in 100 mL or 6 g in 150 mL of crystalloid solution 25cm^3 = 1 g).
	Place a "high alert" label on IV tubing above infusion pump channel, one just above insertion site, and one on magnesium sulfate IV bag.
	Load safety infusion pump and program for magnesium sulfate bolus infusion in second channel.
	Connect magnesium sulfate infusion into main line tubing at closest port to patient.
	A second licensed RN should perform a medication check prior to initiation of infusion. Independent medication confirmation should include verification of magnesium sulfate order, concentration of solution, dose, IV bag and tubing labeled appropriately, and pump set-up prior to initiation of infusion. The second licensed RN should document name, credentials, date and time in the medical record.
	Infuse as ordered. Dose range 4 or 6 g bolus over 20–30 min.
	RN should remain at the bedside during bolus administration assessing maternal and fetal status.
	Assess maternal status including blood pressure, respirations, heart rate, SpO$_2$, and tolerance to infusion bolus every 15 min.
Administration of magnesium sulfate maintenance dose	After receiving physician's order for maintenance infusion of magnesium sulfate, obtain the prepared premixed solution of 20 g in 500 mL crystalloid solution (1 g/25 mL). Check expiration date on bag.
	Once bolus dose is complete, reprogram the safety pump for magnesium sulfate maintenance dose infusion rate in g/hr as ordered.
	Perform second licensed RN medication check prior to initiation of infusion, IV bag change, rate change, and/or upon transfer to another unit (as outlined above).
	Begin infusion. Recommended dose is 2 g/hr.
	Assess maternal status and record magnesium sulfate assessment criteria every 15 min × 1 hr (includes bolus time), every 30 min for second hour, then hourly.
	Assess for signs and symptoms of magnesium sulfate toxicity including LOC, blood pressure, heart rate, respiratory rate, SpO$_2$, DTRs every hour.
	Assess and record hourly intake and output.
	Auscultate breath sounds every 2 hrs.

table continues on page 261

Discontinuation of magnesium sulfate	Stop magnesium sulfate infusion per provider order. Anticipate discontinuation of magnesium sulfate administration in 48 hrs. Remove magnesium line and discard bag and tubing. The woman should remain on bed rest × 1 hr, then up with assist upon first ambulation.
Notification of Provider	Vital signs that fall outside of normal values Significant changes in blood pressure from baseline values HR greater than 100 beats/min RR greater than 24 or less than 14 breaths/min SpO_2 less than or equal to 95% Adventitious breath sounds Changes in level of consciousness Absent DTRs Urinary output less than 30 mL/hr Category III EFM Vision changes (double vision or blurred vision)

EFM, electronic fetal monitoring; HR, heart rate; RR, respiratory rate.

Institute for Safe Medicine Practices, High Alert Medications in Acute Care Settings. Retrieved from: https://www.ismp.org/tools/institutionalhighAlert.asp; Simpson, K. R., & Knox, G. E. (2004). Obstetrical accidents involving intravenous magnesium sulfate. Recommendations to promote patient safety. *Maternal Child Nursing, 29*(30), 161–169.

Comprehensive nursing care during administration of magnesium sulfate is an essential component of patient safety with this "high alert" medication. Considerations for assessment during magnesium sulfate administration include:

- Magnesium toxicity is a potential complication of administration. Signs and symptoms of magnesium toxicity include loss of DTRs, respiratory, cardiac, and neurologic depression. Routine serum magnesium levels are costly and not necessary with routine assessment of these parameters. If magnesium sulfate toxicity is suspected, discontinue administration and notify the provider. The antidote to magnesium is calcium. Dosing is 1 g of calcium gluconate intravenously slowly over 3 minutes (each milliliter of 10 mL vial of 10% calcium gluconate solution contains 0.1 g of calcium gluconate). Trends in vital sign and DTR assessment data are clinical clues that magnesium levels are rising.
- Since magnesium sulfate is excreted by the kidneys, hourly I & O should be assessed. If urine output drops, magnesium levels rise.
- Pulmonary edema is also a potential complication of magnesium sulfate administration. Signs and symptoms of pulmonary edema include shortness of breath, increasing respiratory and heart rates, SpO_2 less than or equal to 95%, cough, and chest tightness.
- Lateral recumbent positioning optimizes maternal cardiac output and uterine perfusion. The woman should remain on bed rest during administration due to the neuromuscular blocking effects increasing the risk of falls.
- Continuous fetal and uterine monitoring is recommended during magnesium sulfate administration. However, this can be a challenge for the nurse and patient. Adjustments of the fetal ultrasound to obtain a continuous tracing may be difficult and disrupt sleep and comfort for the PTL patient.[28] Magnesium sulfate crosses the placenta and may decrease baseline variability and frequency of accelerations making it difficult to determine fetal well being.[29,30]
- Recommended staffing levels include 1:1 nurse to patient ratio during initiation of magnesium sulfate and continuous bedside nursing attendance during administration of the bolus. During maintenance administration and after assessments are recommended every hour, the nurse to patient ratio can increase to 1:2 to 1:3, depending on maternal and fetal status.[31]

NOTE: If the woman is transferred to an antepartum unit for maintenance magnesium sulfate administration, the same care recommendations apply.

Calcium Channel Blockers

Calcium channel blockers, such as nifedipine, have shown promise in inhibiting smooth muscle contractions, although the exact mechanisms are unknown.[32] They produce vasodilatation and decreased peripheral vascular resistance, resulting in flushing of the skin and a transient increase in maternal and fetal heart rates. Postural hypotension can occur with sudden position changes. However, in most women, the side effects of nifedipine are minimal. Nifedipine should not be used concurrently with magnesium sulfate due to increased risks of cardiovascular collapse.

Nonsteroidal Anti-Inflammatory (NSAID)

NSAIDs, such as indomethacin, decrease the synthesis of prostaglandin. As stated, prostaglandins play an important role in both preterm and term labors. Prostaglandins increase the frequency of contractions, help to coordinate contractions, and ripen the cervix. When used in appropriate pregnant patients at less than 32 weeks' gestation and for a short-term course (less than 72 hours (see Table 10.5 for a summary of all medications used in treatment of PTL), indomethacin can be very effective in delaying PTB with minimal side effects.[6]

TABLE 10.5 MEDICATIONS USED IN THE TREATMENT OF PRETERM LABOR		
MEDICATION	**COMMON DOSAGE**	**MATERNAL/FETAL CONSIDERATIONS**
β-Agonists Terbutaline	Typical initial dose is 0.25 mg subcutaneously every 20–30 min up to 4 doses until tocolysis is achieved, then 0.25 mg subcutaneously every 3 to 4 hrs for up to 48 hrs (hold for pulse >120 beats/min)	**Maternal** Cardiac arrhythmias Pulmonary edema Myocardial ischemia Hypotension Tachycardia **Fetal** Tachycardia Hyperglycemia Hypotension Intraventricular hemorrhage
Magnesium sulfate	4–6 g bolus for 20 min, then 2–3 g/hr	**Maternal** Flushing Diaphoresis Pulmonary edema Loss of deep tendon reflexes Cardiac arrest **Fetal** Hypotonia Respiratory depression Lethargy *Provides fetal neuroprotection*
Calcium channel blockers Nifedipine	30 mg loading dose, then 10–20 mg every 4–6 hrs	**Maternal** Dizziness Flushing Transient hypotension **Fetal** No fetal effects noted
Prostaglandin synthetase inhibitors Indomethacin	Loading dose of 50 mg rectally or 50–100 mg orally, then 25–50 mg orally every 6 hrs times 48 hrs	**Maternal** Esophageal reflux Nausea Gastritis **Fetal** Oligohydramnios Closure of the ductus arteriosus Pulmonary hypertension Intraventricular hemorrhage Hyperbilirubinemia Necrotizing enterocolitis Decreased renal function

table continues on page 263

MEDICATION	COMMON DOSAGE	MATERNAL/FETAL CONSIDERATIONS
Progesterone	Vaginal progesterone 200 mg supposi- tory or 90 mg gel daily to 36 wks 17P 250 mg intramuscularly every week starting at 10–20 wks until 36 wks	
Antenatal Steroids Betamethasone Dexamethasone	Women between 24 and 34 wks of pregnancy who are determined to be at risk for PTB within the next 7 d should receive either: Two doses of betamethasone 12 mg intramuscularly, 24 hrs apart OR Four doses of dexamethasone 6 mg intramuscularly, 12 hrs apart	

American College of Obstetricians and Gynecologists, Committee on Practice Bulletins–Obstetrics. (2012). ACOG practice bulletin no. 127: Management of preterm labor. *Obstetrics & Gynecology, 119*(6), 1308–1317; March of Dimes. (2012). *Preterm labor assessment toolkit*. White Plains, NY: Author. Retrieved from https://www.prematurityprevention.org/portal/server.pt; Reedy, N. (2014). Preterm labor and birth. In Simpson, K., & Creehan, P. (Eds.), *Perinatal nursing* (4th ed., pp. 166–202). Philadelphia, PA: Wolters Kluwer.

Progesterone

Recently, a lot of attention has been given to progesterone as another means of treating PTL. 17-α-*Hydroxyprogesterone caproate* (17P) is a naturally occurring metabolite of progesterone. Both 17P and progesterone itself are produced in large quantities during pregnancy. Administration of 17P has been shown to reduce the rate of a recurrent PTB, as compared with patients receiving placebo, in many women regardless of race. Women with a very PTB in a prior pregnancy demonstrated the greatest benefit. Despite the positive results, there are still many questions surrounding this treatment option. First, the mechanism of action of progesterone in preventing PTB is not clearly understood. In addition, these studies have focused on a specific population of women, those at risk owing to a previous PTB, and who also had singleton pregnancies. Further studies are being done on women with multiple gestations, with preliminary data suggesting that progesterone may not prolong those pregnancies. At this time, ACOG recommends that 17P be considered only for the treatment of women who have experienced a previous PTB.[6]

• How Effective are Tocolytics for the Treatment of Preterm Labor?

Although tocolytic therapy often temporarily stops contractions, none of the agents have been proven effective at preventing PTB. *Use of tocolytics in a maintenance capacity following an episode of acute tocolysis has not been shown to be effective. Also, the repeated use of tocolytics in women with a recurrence of PTL is usually not recommended except for maternal transport.*[6] **Tocolytics are only recommended for short-term use to provide time for steroid administration and, if necessary, maternal transport to a facility with appropriate neonatal care.**

NOTE: There is no evidence that outpatient use of tocolytics prolongs gestation.[6]

• In addition to tocolytic therapy, are there other recommendations for management of PTL?

Antenatal Corticosteroids

Appropriate use of corticosteroids to accelerate lung maturation in the fetus is one of the most effective ways to improve the outcomes of PTBs.[6,17] Evidence from clinical trials since the 1970s has proven antenatal corticosteroid administration effective in reducing infant mortality by 30% and neonatal respiratory distress by 50%. **All women at risk for preterm delivery between 24 and 34 weeks' gestation are candidates for corticosteroid therapy** in order to:
- Decrease the risk and severity of respiratory distress syndrome
- Decrease the risk of intraventricular hemorrhage
- Decrease mortality in the neonate.

The decrease in complications also lowers the cost and duration of neonatal care. The optimal benefit of antenatal corticosteroid therapy is greatest more than 24 hours after starting therapy. Repeated courses of antenatal corticosteroids given to women at risk for preterm delivery have not reduced neonatal morbidity when compared with a single course.

NOTE: Antenatal corticosteroid therapy is one of the most effective strategies in the prevention of mortality and disability in preterm infants. A single course of corticosteroids should be given to all pregnant women between 24 and 34 weeks' gestation if at risk for PTB.[6,17,33]

Group B Streptococcus Cultures

Group B streptococcus (GBS) disease is the leading cause of early-onset neonatal sepsis in the United States, and the leading cause of newborn infectious morbidity and mortality, with case fatality rates as high as 20% to 30% in premature newborns.[34] On admission, cervical–vaginal cultures are obtained for GBS and other infections as indicated by patient symptoms and/or state law. See Table 10.6 and Figure 10.3 for indications and an algorithm for GBS management.

At less than 37 weeks' and 0 days' gestation EGA:
- If the woman has undergone vaginal–rectal GBS culture within the preceding 5 weeks' the results of that culture should guide management.
- GBS-colonized women should receive intrapartum antibiotic prophylaxis.
- No antibiotics are indicated for GBS prophylaxis if a vaginal–rectal screen within 5 weeks was negative.

TABLE 10.6 INDICATIONS AND NONINDICATIONS FOR INTRAPARTUM ANTIBIOTIC PROPHYLAXIS TO PREVENT EARLY-ONSET GROUP B STREPTOCOCCAL (GBS) DISEASE

INTRAPARTUM GBS PROPHYLAXIS INDICATED	INTRAPARTUM GBS PROPHYLAXIS NOT INDICATED
Previous infant with invasive GBS disease	Colonization with GBS during a previous pregnancy (unless an indication for GBS prophylaxis is present for current pregnancy)
GBS bacteriuria during any trimester of the current pregnancy	GBS bacteriuria during previous pregnancy (unless an indication for GBS prophylaxis is present for current pregnancy)
Positive GBS vaginal–rectal screening culture in late gestation during current pregnancy	Negative vaginal and rectal GBS screening culture in late gestation during the current pregnancy, regardless of intrapartum risk factors
Unknown GBS status at the onset of labor (culture not done, incomplete, or results unknown) and any of the following: Delivery at <37 wks' gestation Amniotic membrane rupture ≥18 hrs Intrapartum temperature ≥100.4°F (≥38.0°C) Intrapartum nucleic acid amplification test (NAAT) positive for GBS	Cesarean birth performed before onset of labor on a woman with intact amniotic membranes, regardless of GBS colonization status or gestational age

Intrapartum antibiotic prophylaxis is not indicated in this circumstance if a cesarean birth is performed before onset of labor on a woman with intact amniotic membranes.
Optimal timing for prenatal GBS screening is at 35–37 wks' gestation.
If amnionitis is suspected, broad-spectrum antibiotic therapy that includes an agent known to be active against GBS should replace GBS prophylaxis.

Verani, J. R., McGee, L., & Schrag, S. J., Division of Bacterial Diseases, National Center for Immunization and Respiratory Diseases, Centers for Disease Control and Prevention (CDC). (2010). Prevention of perinatal group B streptococcal disease. *Morbidity and Mortality Weekly Report, 59*(RR–10), 1–36.

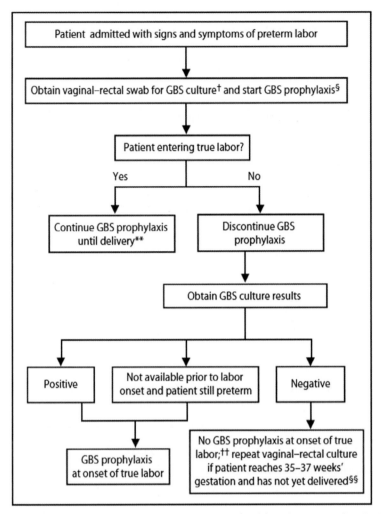

FIGURE 10.3 Preterm GBS management algorithm. (From Verani, J. R., McGee, L., & Schrag, S. J., Division of Bacterial Diseases, National Center for Immunization and Respiratory Diseases, Centers for Disease Control and Prevention (CDC). (2010). Prevention of perinatal group B streptococcal disease. *Morbidity Mortality Weekly Report, 59*(RR–10), 1–36.)

- The woman should be regularly assessed for progression to true labor; if the woman is considered not to be in true labor, discontinue GBS prophylaxis.
- If GBS culture results become available prior to delivery and are negative, then discontinue GBS prophylaxis, unless subsequent GBS culture prior to delivery is positive.

NOTE: A negative GBS screen is considered valid for 5 weeks. If a woman with a history of PTL is readmitted for PTL and had a negative GBS screen >5 weeks prior, she should be rescreened and managed according to the algorithm at that time.

Antibiotics

Although inflammation and infection have been linked to both PTL and PPROM, the benefit of antibiotics has been frequently debated. Because infection of the upper genital tract has been associated with preterm deliveries, there has been speculation that treatment with antibiotics could perhaps prevent delivery. For women experiencing PTL, without rupture of membranes, treatment with antibiotics has not been proven successful in preventing a preterm delivery. Therefore, antibiotics are not recommended in women with PTL, except for GBS prophylaxis before delivery.[35]

In women with PPROM, antibiotics have been shown to delay delivery and reduce neonatal morbidity.[35] Treatment with antibiotics is able to delay delivery for 7 days to up to 3 weeks' and newborns have a reduced need for oxygen, incidence of respiratory distress syndrome, necrotizing enterocolitis (NEC), and sepsis.[2] Ampicillin and erythromycin IV are recommended for 48 hours, followed by amoxicillin and erythromycin orally for 5 days during expectant management.[35]

Magnesium Sulfate for Neuroprotection

Cerebral palsy refers to a group of related disorders that are caused by nonprogressive damage to, or dysfunction of, the developing fetal or infant brain.[35–38] The hallmark of cerebral palsy is abnormal control of movement or posture that results in limitation of activity. Cerebral palsy is a leading cause of chronic childhood disability, affecting more than 200,000 American children between the ages of 3 and 13. PTB is a major risk factor for cerebral palsy, with infants born at the threshold of viability being 70 times more likely to be diagnosed with the disease than those born at term. In fact, almost half of all children with cerebral palsy were born preterm.

Magnesium sulfate is effective for neuroprotection with reduction in cerebral palsy with no increase in major maternal complications. While magnesium sulfate for neuroprotection is not presently a standard of care, many experts recommend this treatment for women at high risk for birth before 32 weeks' gestation.

Candidates for neuroprotection therapy:
- 23–0/7 to 31–6/7 weeks and
- PTL with high likelihood of birth within 12 hours (cervix greater than or equal to 4 cm)
- PPROM
- Planned birth for maternal/fetal complications

Delivery should not be delayed in order to administer magnesium sulfate for neuroprotection if there are maternal and/or fetal indications for emergent birth. A sample neuroprotection protocol in presented in Table 10.7.

TABLE 10.7 SAMPLE NEUROPROTECTION PROTOCOL

Bolus Dose: Magnesium sulfate 6 g loading dose IV over 20–30 min
Maintenance Dose: Magnesium sulfate maintenance infusion 2 g/hr until birth or for 12 hrs, whichever occurs first.
Repeated Dosing:
If a woman returns less than 6 hrs after receiving magnesium for neuroprotection, restart magnesium sulfate at
   2 g/hr without an additional loading dose.
If greater than 6 hrs has elapsed, begin with loading dose.

American College of Obstetricians and Gynecologists. (2012). Magnesium sulfate before anticipated preterm birth for neuroprotection. Patient safety checklist no. 7. *Obstetrics & Gynecology, 120*, 432–433; Constantine, M. M., & Weiner, S. J. (2009). Effects of antenatal exposure to magnesium sulfate on neuroprotection and mortality in preterm infants: A meta-analysis. *Obstetrics and Gynecology, 114*(2 pt 1), 354; Reeves, S. A., Gibbs, R. S., & Clark, S. L. (2011). Magnesium for fetal neuroprotection. *American Journal of Obstetrics and Gynecology, 204*(3), 202.e1–e4; Rouse, D., Hirtz, D., Thom, E., et al., Eunice Kennedy Shriver NICHD Maternal-Fetal Medicine Units Network. (2008). A randomized controlled trial of magnesium sulfate for the prevention of cerebral palsy. *New England Journal of Medicine, 359*(9), 895–905.

• What about Bed Rest, Hydration and Pelvic Rest?

Bed rest, hydration protocols, and/or pelvic rest have not been shown to be effective for the prevention of PTB and should not be routinely recommended. In fact, bed rest and excessive hydration have potentially harmful maternal complications.[6] There is no data indicating that activity restriction is of benefit for any obstetric condition. Disorders of pregnancy associated with elevated blood pressure, PPROM, multiple gestation, and inadequate growth of the baby are among the most common reasons for hospital admissions during pregnancy and often trigger a recommendation of activity restriction. Bed rest in pregnancy can be associated with these complications[6]:
- Venous thrombosis and embolism
- Muscle atrophy
- Bone loss
- Weight loss
- Cardiovascular deconditioning (decreased plasma volume, total blood volume, cardiac output, and red cell mass)
- Endocrine system changes

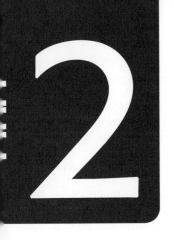

Preterm Premature Rupture of Membranes

Preterm Premature Rupture of Membranes (PPROM) is the rupture of membranes *before term* (i.e., before the completion of 37 weeks' gestation), with or without the onset of labor. PPROM complicates approximately 1% to 5% of all births, but remains a major cause of spontaneous PTB. African American women have a twofold increase in occurrence.[39]

- ## What are the causes of PPROM?

Although risk factors that appear to be related to PPROM have been identified, the exact cause is unknown and probably results from a variety of factors. Intra-amniotic infection has been found in anywhere from 13% to 60% of women with PPROM.[39] However, PPROM often occurs in women without recognized risk factors (Table 10.8).

- ## How is PPROM diagnosed?

TABLE 10.8 RISK FACTORS ASSOCIATED WITH PPROM

RISK FACTORS ASSOCIATED WITH PPROM

Maternal Factors
Prior preterm birth due to PPROM
Prior PTB due to preterm labor
Maternal medical complications (collagen vascular disorders, pulmonary disease)
Nutritional deficiencies in copper and/or ascorbic acid
Bacterial vaginosis (relationship unclear)
Cocaine use
Low body mass index (less than 19.8 kg/m^2)
Recent symptomatic uterine contractions and/or vaginal bleeding
Low socioeconomic status
Positive fetal fibronectin
Smoking during pregnancy
Infections of the urogenital tract
Abdominal trauma—direct, blunt
Chronic steroid use

Uteroplacental Factors
Placental abruption
Uterine anomalies
Advanced cervical dilation
Short cervical length (less than 25 mm)
Cerclage or cervical procedures
Intra-amniotic infection

Fetal Factors
Uterine overdistension (multiple gestation, polyhydramnios)

Cunningham, F., Leveno, K., Bloom, F., et al. (2013). Preterm labor. In *Williams obstetrics* (24th ed., pp. 829–861). New York, NY: McGraw Hill; Mercer, B. M. (2012). Premature rupture of the membranes. In Gabbe, S. G., Niebyl, J. R., Simpson, J. L., et al. (Eds.), *Obstetrics: Normal and problem pregnancies* (6th ed., pp. 659–672). Philadelphia, PA: Saunders.

Symptoms suggestive of PPROM should be evaluated promptly. An accurate diagnosis is essential for the appropriate management of suspected PPROM.

- When confirming PPROM diagnosis, a sterile speculum examination should be performed rather than a digital examination. A sterile speculum examination minimizes the risk of infection and allows the provider to inspect for cervicitis, umbilical cord prolapse, cervical dilation and effacement, and to obtain cervical cultures.
- When the sterile speculum examination is performed, observation of amniotic fluid coming through the cervix is the best method to confirm the diagnosis.
- If the diagnosis is still in question, Nitrazine paper can be used to test the pH of the fluid. The pH of vaginal fluids is usually 4.5 to 6.0. Amniotic fluid has a higher pH of 7.1 to 7.3 and therefore turns Nitrazine paper blue—a positive result. False positives may occur if blood, semen, or infection such as BV is present.
- Fluid from the posterior vaginal vault may also be placed on a glass slide and allowed to dry. Under microscopic examination, the presence of a *ferning* pattern is suggestive of amniotic fluid.
- The measuring of amniotic fluid volume by ultrasound may also be of value, but should not be the only method used to diagnose PPROM.
- If unable to determine PPROM with sterile speculum examination, the provider may do an amniocentesis to instill a dye to the amniotic fluid, or to obtain cultures if infection is suspected.

- ## What are the risks for PPROM complications in the woman, fetus, and newborn?[39]

Risks associated with PPROM are as follows:

- Intrauterine infection (chorioamnionitis): *Note: Risk of infection increases with duration of rupture.*
- Sepsis (maternal and newborn)
- Maternal death
- Retained placenta and hemorrhage requiring D&C (12%)
- Fetal malpresentation
- Umbilical cord compression and/or prolapse
- Placental abruption (4% to 12% of PPROM pregnancies)
- Complications of prematurity (respiratory distress syndrome [RDS], necrotizing enterocolitis [NEC], intraventricular hemorrhage [IVH], infection)
- Pulmonary hypoplasia (associated with rupture in the second trimester)
- Cesarean delivery for fetal status

Infection is inevitable in many women with PPROM, especially those with very early gestational age. The incidence of infection rises with the number of cervical examinations performed. Most women with PPROM deliver within 1 week regardless of management, leading to significant neonatal complications of prematurity.[39]

- ## What are the recommendations for management of PPROM?

There is no standardized approach to the management of PPROM. The plan of care is individualized for each woman based on examination of risks and benefits, and the following factors:

- Gestational age
- Presence or absence of labor
- Presence or absence of maternal infection
- Presence or absence of fetal reassurance
- Fetal presentation
- Cervical examination
- Availability of neonatal intensive care
- Patient/family desires

Gestational age and fetal well-being play important roles in the decision about how to best care for women with PPROM. Potential complications associated with prematurity are weighed against the risk of maternal and neonatal complications.

PPROM >34 weeks' EGA

Women with PPROM, who are at 34 weeks' gestation or more and who are hospitalized where neonatal intensive care is available may be best managed by induction of labor.

PPROM 32 to 33 weeks' EGA

Labor may be induced in women at gestational ages of 32 to 33 weeks only with documented fetal lung maturity.[32] At these gestational ages, the risks of prematurity are usually considerably less than the risks of infection with PPROM for the woman and fetus. However, in the absence of fetal lung maturity, corticosteroids are recommended.[39] Prophylactic tocolysis is not recommended, but may be used in the short term to administer corticosteroids.[40]

PPROM 23 to 31 weeks' EGA

Due to the increased risk for perinatal morbidity and mortality, prolonging pregnancy after PPROM between 23 and 31 weeks' gestation, the woman is usually managed conservatively unless there is clinical evidence of intra-amniotic infection, placental abruption, advanced labor, or there is a changes in fetal status.[39]

PPROM prior to 23 weeks' EGA

Previable PPROM is associated with significant risks including neonatal pulmonary hypoplasia due to oligohydramnios, stillbirth, as well as the complications of extreme prematurity, and complications of prolonged maternal bedrest. There is currently no consensus about management of these women as inpatient or outpatient, but should be hospitalized once viability the fetus reaches viability. The woman and family should be counseled about realistic outcomes and expectations.

NOTE: If the woman is being managed expectantly and not in active labor, she should be in a facility capable of performing an emergent cesarean birth, with 24-hour neonatal support for resuscitation and intensive care.[39]

*See Module 19 for more information on Maternal Transport.

Nursing care guidelines for expectant management may include the following:
- Review prenatal records
- Determine current gestational age and due date
- Determine if the woman has previously received corticosteroids during the pregnancy
- Obtain a complete history and note time of rupture and onset of labor, color, and odor of amniotic fluid
- Perform a complete physical examination; note abdominal tenderness
- Avoid digital cervical examination unless an emergent situation presents (e.g., suspected prolapsed cord) or if birth is inevitable
- Monitor trends in maternal vital signs

NOTE: Maternal tachycardia usually precedes a rise in maternal temperature and subsequent fetal tachycardia.

- Assess for intra-amniotic infection (chorioamnionitis)
  - Maternal (greater than 100 beats/min) and/or fetal tachycardia (greater than 160 beats/min baseline)
  - Temperature of 100.4°F or higher
  - Uterine tenderness noted with palpation
  - Foul-smelling, purulent amniotic fluid
  - Leukocytosis

NOTE: Elevated white blood cell counts are not a reliable indicator of infection in women with PPROM, especially if corticosteroids have been administered. During labor, even in the absence of infection, white blood counts can become elevated to levels of 25,000/mm³ or more.[39]

- Assess fetal well-being per provider order
  - Nonstress test or fetal monitoring
  - Ultrasound
  - Biophysical profile
  - Fetal movement counts

NOTE: Fetal assessments for hospitalized women with PPROM are typically done at least daily due to the potential for cord compression and fetal compromise.[39]

- Assess for signs/symptoms of abruption
- Administer prophylactic antibiotics per provider order

- Administer corticosteroids per provider order
- Administer course of tocolytics if necessary per provider order
- Assess positioning and limit activity according to due to fetal presentation, dilation, station, and medication administration (e.g., magnesium sulfate)
- Assess the woman's understanding of the implications of PPROM and management options
- Communicate with the neonatal team. If possible, provide early contact with the neonatal team in order to allow the patient and family to have anticipatory planning
- Provide psychosocial support

- **When PTL is advanced or is unresponsive to tocolysis, what preparations should be made for birth?**

- If possible, women who are at less than 34 weeks' gestation should be transported to a tertiary care center *before delivery* so that neonatal intensive care facilities will be immediately available for the infant. This intervention in itself has been proven to decrease perinatal morbidity and mortality. (See Module 19 regarding maternal transport.)
- Assess the family's understanding of the rationale for starting or stopping tocolytic therapy and their expectations for the preterm infant's appearance, needs, and care.
- Provide contact information for the neonatal care unit to facilitate communication.
- Provide 1:1 ratio due to high risk status.
- Apply continuous EFM.
- Limit cervical examinations.
- Delayed cord clamping (refer to Module 5 for active management of the third stage of labor)
- Notify neonatal resuscitation team members to be present for birth. Ensure neonatal resuscitation equipment in working order and readily available.
- Anticipate placenta to be sent to pathology for examination.

EFM in the Preterm Fetus

For a complete understanding of EFM concepts, refer to Module 7. Gestational age determines how the EFM strip should be interpreted. EFM definitions and assessment parameters are the same with the following significant differences:

- Accelerations are defined as abrupt increases in FHR (onset of acceleration to peak in less than 30 seconds). Prior to 32 weeks' gestation, accelerations are defined as having an acme greater than or equal to 10 bpm above baseline, with a duration of 10 seconds or more.[6,39,41]
- The preterm fetus is more likely to have variable decelerations, with or without association of uterine contractions. During labor, variable decelerations occur in 70% to 75% of preterm patients.[41]
- A more rapid decrease in baseline variability may occur during labor.
- With the combination of decreased variability and variable decelerations, Apgar scores and cord blood gases are more likely to be depressed at birth in the preterm neonate.[39]

Family Teaching

Education of the woman and family is essential as this can be a time of uncertainty, stress, and worry. Presence with the family, individualized teaching, and anticipatory guidance are important components of nursing care. Teaching should include, but is not limited to, the following:

- Signs and symptoms of PTL and PPROM and when to seek care if signs/symptoms of PTL or PPROM occur
- Technique for palpating and timing uterine contractions
- Tocolytic therapy
- Antepartum testing including biophysical profile, nonstress test, and amniotic fluid volumes
- Electronic fetal monitoring
- Fetal activity monitoring
- Maintaining a nutritional diet and adequate hydration
- Avoiding smoking and other substance use

PRACTICE/REVIEW QUESTIONS

After reviewing this module, answer the following questions.

1. *Preterm labor* is labor occurring less than _____ completed weeks' gestation.

2. The diagnosis of PTL is made when contractions less than 10 minutes apart are accompanied by:

    a. _____

    b. _____

    c. _____

3. The majority of perinatal morbidity and mortality in the United States are the result of:

    _____

4. Five *demographic* risk factors related to PTL are:

    a. _____

    b. _____

    c. _____

    d. _____

    e. _____

5. The single greatest risk factor for PTL is

    _____

6. List two of the four physiologic pathways related to the onset PTL.

    a. _____

    b. _____

7. Five *behavioral* risk factors related to PTL are:

    a. _____

    b. _____

    c. _____

    d. _____

    e. _____

8. List six warning signs of PTL.

    a. _____

    b. _____

    c. _____

    d. _____

    e. _____

    f. _____

9. A knowledgeable patient with an uncomplicated pregnancy who experiences symptoms of PTL with physical activity might be instructed to do the following:

    a. _____

    b. _____

    c. _____

    d. _____

    e. _____

10. _____ is the only biochemical marker with an excellent predictive value for preterm delivery.

11. Contraindications to collecting this biochemical marker (in question 10) are:

    a. _____

    b. _____

    c. _____

    d. _____

    e. _____

    f. _____

12. About half the time, preterm contractions will stop with _____ and _____.

13. List complications patients may develop when placed on bed rest.

    a. _____

    b. _____

    c. _____

    d. _____

    e. _____

    f. _____

    g. _____

14. List five clinical observations that should be noted when doing a cervical examination on a woman at risk for PTL.

    a. _____

    b. _____

    c. _____

    d. _____

    e. _____

15. List the initial nursing interventions when caring for the woman being admitted for PTL.

    a. _____

    b. _____

    c. _____

    d. _____

    e. _____

    f. _____

    g. _____

    h. _____

    i. _____

16. List candidates for neuroprotection therapy:

    a. _____

    b. _____

    c. _____

    d. _____

17. Drugs that have a depressant effect on the myometrium of the uterus are called _____.

18. The process of administering a drug for the purpose of inhibiting uterine contractions is called _____.

19. List seven contraindications to tocolytic therapy.

    a. _____

    b. _____

    c. _____

    d. _____

    e. _____

    f. _____

    g. _____

20. Two of the drugs that are commonly used for tocolysis are _____ and _____.

21. List five side effects of β-adrenergic drugs.

    a. _____

    b. _____

    c. _____

    d. _____

    e. _____

22. During tocolytic therapy with terbutaline, the physician should be notified if the maternal pulse exceeds _____ bpm.

23. The nurse should listen to the patient's breath sounds before tocolytic therapy begins and should monitor for signs of pulmonary edema, including _____, _____, _____, or _____.

24. MgSO$_4$, a central nervous system depressant, should never be administered in the absence of _____.

25. Seven potential side effects of MgSO$_4$ administration are:

    a. _____

    b. _____

    c. _____

    d. _____

    e. _____

    f. _____

    g. _____

26. Define premature rupture of membranes.

    _____

    _____

    _____

27. List eight nursing interventions when a woman is admitted with PROM.

    a. _____

    b. _____

    c. _____

    d. _____

    e. _____

    f. _____

    g. _____

    h. _____

28. List three possible complications resulting from PROM.

    a. _____

    b. _____

    c. _____

29. Name four signs of chorioamnionitis.

    a. _____

    b. _____

    c. _____

    d. _____

30. The management of PROM is determined by the gestational age of the fetus and the presence or absence of _____, _____, _____, and _____.

31. If the fetus is less than 34 weeks and the mother is not in active labor, her care should take place at _____.

32. Every fetus between 24 and 34 weeks' gestation at risk for preterm delivery should be considered a candidate for antenatal treatment with _____.

33. If chorioamnionitis develops or if there is evidence of fetal distress, _____ is indicated.

34. The benefits of antenatal administration of corticosteroids to the fetus at risk of preterm delivery include a reduction in the risks of _____, _____ and _____.

PRACTICE/REVIEW ANSWER KEY

1. 37
2. a. Progressive change in the cervix
   b. Cervical dilatation of 2 cm or more
   c. Cervical effacement of 80% or more
3. Preterm births
4. a. Age ≤20 or ≥35
   b. Race—African American especially
   c. Low socioeconomic status
   d. Unmarried
   e. Low level of education
5. Previous preterm birth
6. Any two of the following:
   a. Inflammation and infection
   b. Maternal or fetal stress
   c. Decidual hemorrhage or abruption
   d. Mechanical stretch of the uterus
7. Any five of the following:
   a. Smoking
   b. Alcohol and other substance abuse
   c. Poor nutritional status
   d. High altitude
   e. Domestic abuse
   f. Strenuous job activity
   g. High stress
   h. Lack of prenatal care
   i. Diethylstilbestrol (DES) exposure and other toxic exposures
8. a. Uterine contractions—five or more in hour
   b. Menstrual-like cramps
   c. Low, dull backache
   d. Pelvic pressure
   e. Abdominal cramping
   f. Increase or change in vaginal discharge
9. a. Empty her bladder
   b. Rest on her side
   c. Drink two to three glasses of water or juice
   d. Palpate for contractions
   e. Call back in 1 hour if symptoms persist or if symptoms recur with resumption of normal activities.
10. Fetal fibronectin (fFN)
11. a. Vaginal examination within past 24 hours
    b. Cervical dilation greater than 3 cm
    c. Ruptured membranes
    d. Cerclage in place
    e. Vaginal bleeding or placenta previa
    f. Sexual intercourse within the past 24 hours
12. Bed rest; hydration
13. a. Thromboembolic disease
    b. Muscle atrophy
    c. Bone loss
    d. Weight loss
    e. Cardiovascular deconditioning
    f. Endocrine changes
    g. Increased anxiety, depression, and somatic complaints
14. a. Position
    b. Consistency
    c. Effacement
    d. Dilation
    e. Station

15. a. Assessment of signs and symptoms of preterm labor
    b. Monitor uterine status
    c. Monitor fetal status
    d. Monitor maternal vital signs
    e. Instruct patient on initial bed rest and hydration
    f. Prepare for collection of urine/cervical cultures
    g. Baseline cervical examination
    h. Provide comfort measures and emotional support
    i. Prepare for the possibility of ultrasound, amniocentesis, tocolytic drug therapy, steroid therapy, baseline blood chemistry (complete blood count [CBC]). Educate patient and family about these procedures/therapies.
16. a. 23 0/7 to 31 6/7 weeks' gestation
    b. Preterm labor with high likelihood of birth within 12 hours
    c. PPROM
    d. Planned birth for maternal–fetal complications
17. Tocolytic drugs
18. Tocolytic therapy or tocolysis
19. a. Severe preeclampsia/eclampsia
    b. Placental abruption, acute hemorrhage, or active vaginal bleeding
    c. Intrauterine infection
    d. Lethal congenital or chromosomal abnormalities
    e. Evidence of fetal compromise or intrauterine demise
    f. Advanced cervical dilation
    g. Maternal hemodynamic instability or complications
20. Terbutaline; magnesium sulfate
21. Any five of the following:
    a. Tremors
    b. Maternal and fetal tachycardia
    c. Headache
    d. Palpitations
    e. Anxiety/nervousness
    f. Nausea and/or vomiting
    g. Hypotension
22. 120
23. Dyspnea; wheezing; coughing; rales
24. Patellar reflexes
25. a. Drowsiness
    b. Decreased sensorium
    c. Slurred speech
    d. Heavy eyelids
    e. Flushing
    f. Decreased gastrointestinal motility
    g. Respiratory depression
26. The spontaneous rupture of membranes before the onset of labor, regardless of gestational age
27. a. Confirm membrane status.
    b. Review dating criteria.
    c. Monitor fetal heart tones.
    d. Evaluate uterine activity.
    e. Observe for signs of infection.
    f. Determine the need for transport.
    g. Assess woman's understanding of the implications of PROM and provide support and education.
    h. Prepare for delivery of a high-risk infant.
28. a. Intrauterine infection (chorioamnionitis)
    b. Preterm labor
    c. Prolapsed umbilical cord

29. a. Maternal or fetal tachycardia
    b. Temperature higher than 100.4°F
    c. Uterine tenderness
    d. Foul-smelling, purulent amniotic fluid
30. Labor; chorioamnionitis; fetal distress; fetal lung maturity
31. A high-risk regional medical center
32. Corticosteroids (betamethasone)
33. Immediate delivery
34. Respiratory distress syndrome; intraventricular hemorrhage; mortality

REFERENCES

1. Martin, J., Hamilton, B., Osterman, J., et al. (2015). Birth: Final data for 2013. *National Vital Statistics Reports, 64*(1), 1–65.
2. March of Dimes. (2012). *Peristats. Infant mortality rates: United States,* 1997–2007. Retrieved from: http://www.mar-chofdimes.com/perstats/ViewSubtopic.aspx?reg+99&top+6&st op+91&lev+1&slev+1&obj+1&dv+ms
3. Behrman, R. E., & Butler, A. S. (Eds.), Institute of Medicine (US). (2007). *Committee on understanding premature birth and assuring healthy outcomes.* Washington, DC: National Academies Press (US).
4. Simhan, H., Iams, J., & Romero, R. (2012). Preterm labor. In Gabbe, S. G., Niebyl, J. R., Simpson, J. L., et al. (Eds.), *Obstetrics: Normal and problem pregnancies* (6th ed., pp. 627–658). Philadelphia, PA: Saunders Elsevier.
5. Cunningham, F., Leveno, K., Bloom, F., et al. (2013). Preterm labor. In *Williams obstetrics* (24th ed., pp. 829–861). New York, NY: McGraw Hill.
6. American College of Obstetricians and Gynecologists, Committee on Practice Bulletins—Obstetrics. (2012). ACOG practice bulletin no. 127: Management of preterm labor. *Obstetrics & Gynecology, 119*(6), 1308–1317.
7. Othman, M. (2013). Cervical anatomy in women at risk of preterm labor. *Obstetrics & Gynecology, 4*(4), WMC004206: doi: 10.9754/journal.wmc.2013.004206.
8. Maleki, Z., Bailis, A. J., Argani, C. H., et al. (2009). Periventricular leukomalacia and placental histopathologic abnormalities. *Obstetrics & Gynecology, 114*(5), 1115–1120.
9. Laxmi, U., Agrawal, S., Raghunandan, C., et al. (2012). Association of bacterial vaginosis with adverse fetomaternal outcome in women with spontaneous preterm labor: A prospective cohort study. *Journal of Maternal-Fetal and Neonatal Medicine, 25*(1), 64–67.
10. Greene, M. F., Creasy, R. K., Resnik, R., et al. (2008). *Creasy and Resnik's maternal-fetal medicine: Principles and practice.* Philadelphia, PA: Elsevier Health Sciences.
11. Torche, F. (2011). The effect of maternal stress on birth outcomes: Exploiting a natural experiment. *Demography, 48*(4), 1473–1491.
12. Shaw, J. G., Asch, S. M., Kimerling, R., et al. (2014). Posttraumatic stress disorder and risk of spontaneous preterm birth. *Obstetrics & Gynecology, 124*(6), 1111–1119.
13. Faramarzi, S., Kayisli, U. A., Kayisli, O., et al. (2013). Decidual cell expressed tissue factor promotes endometrial hemostasis while mediating abruption associated preterm birth. *Advances in Reproductive Sciences, 1*(3), 44–50.
14. Wiess, J. L., Malone, F. D., Vidaver, J., et al. (2004). Threatened abortion: A risk factor for poor pregnancy outcomes, a population-based screening study. *American Journal of Obstetrics & Gynecology, 190,* 745–750.
15. Goldenberg, R. L., Gravett, M. G., Iams, J., et al. (2012). The preterm birth syndrome: Issues to consider in creating a classification system. *American Journal of Obstetrics & Gynecology, 206*(2), 113–118.
16. Rose, C. H., McWeeney, D. T., Brost, B. C., et al. (2010). Cost-effective standardization of preterm labor evaluation. *American Journal of Obstetrics & Gynecology, 203*(3), 250.e1–e5.
17. March of Dimes. (2012). *Preterm labor assessment toolkit.* White Plains, NY: Author. Retrieved from https://www. prematurityprevention.org/portal/server.pt
18. Howard, E. (2013). Labor evaluation. In Angelini, D., & LaFontaine, D. (Eds.), *Obstetric triage and emergency care protocols* (pp. 159–167). New York, NY: Springer Publishing.
19. American Academy of Pediatrics, The American College of Obstetricians and Gynecologists. (2012). *Guidelines for perinatal care* (7th ed.).
20. Peaceman, A. M., Andrews, W. W., Thorp, J. M., et al. (1997). Fetal fibronectin as a predictor of preterm birth in patients with symptoms: A multicenter trial. *American Journal of Obstetrics & Gynecology, 177,* 13–18.
21. Stafford, I. P., Garite, T. J., Dildy, G. A., et al. (2008). A comparison of speculum and nonspeculum collection of cervicovaginal specimens for fetal fibronectin testing. *American Journal of Obstetrics & Gynecology, 199,* 131.e1–e4.
22. Owen, J., Szychowski, J. M., Hankins, G., et al. (2010). Does midtrimester cervical length >25 mm predict preterm birth in high-risk women? *American Journal of Obstetrics & Gynecology, 203*(4), 393.e1–e5.
23. Bolden, J. R. (2014). Acute and chronic tocolysis. *Clinical Obstetrics and Gynecology, 57*(3), 568–578.
24. U.S. Food and Drug Administration. (2011). *FDA Drug Safety Communication: New warnings against use of terbutaline to treat preterm labor.* Retrieved from: https://ww.fda.gove/Drugs/DrugSafety/ucm243539.htm
25. Reedy, N. (2014). Preterm labor and birth. In Simpson, K., & Creehan, P. (Eds.), *Perinatal nursing* (4th ed., pp. 166–202). Philadelphia, PA: Wolters Kluwer.
26. Institute for Safe Medicine Practices, High Alert Medications in Acute Care Settings. Retrieved from: https://www.ismp.org/tools/institutionalhighAlert.asp
27. Simpson, K. R., & Knox, G. E. (2004). Obstetrical accidents involving intravenous magnesium sulfate. Recommendations to promote patient safety. *Maternal Child Nursing, 29*(30), 161–169.
28. Chez, B. F., & Baird, S. M. (2011). Electronic fetal heart rate monitoring: Where are we now? *The Journal of Perinatal & Neonatal Nursing, 25*(2), 180–192.
29. Heitt, A. K., Devoe, L. D., Brown, H. L., et al. (1995). Effect of magnesium on fetal heart rate variability using computer analysis. *American Journal of Perinatology, 12*(4), 259–261.
30. Duffy, C., Odibo, A., Roehl, K., et al. (2012). Effect of magnesium sulfate on fetal heart rate patterns in the second stage of labor. *Obstetrics & Gynecology, 119*(6), 1129–1136.
31. Association of Womens' Health, Obstetric and Neonatal Nurses. (2010). *Guidelines for professional nurse staffing for perinatal units.* Available from: http://www.awhonn.org/awhonn/content.d o?name=04_ConsultingTraining/04_Staffing Guidelines.htm
32. Flenady, V., Wojcieszek, A. M., Papatsonis, D. N., et al. (2014). Calcium channel blockers for inhibiting preterm labor and birth. *The Cochrane Library, 6,* CDOO2255.

33. National Institutes of Health Consensus Development Panel. (2001). Antenatal corticosteroids revisited: Repeat courses—National Institutes of Health Consensus Statement, August 17–18, 2000. *Obstetrics & Gynecology, 98*(1), 144–150.

34. Verani, J. R., McGee, L., & Schrag, S. J., Division of Bacterial Diseases, National Center for Immunization and Respiratory Diseases, Centers for Disease Control and Prevention (CDC). (2010). Prevention of perinatal group B streptococcal disease. *Morbidity and Mortality Weekly Report, 59*(RR–10), 1–36.

35. American College of Obstetricians and Gynecologists. (2012). Magnesium sulfate before anticipated preterm birth for neuroprotection. Patient safety checklist no. 7. *Obstetrics & Gynecology, 120*, 432–433.

36. Constantine, M. M., & Weiner, S. J. (2009). Effects of antenatal exposure to magnesium sulfate on neuroprotection and mortality in preterm infants: A meta-analysis. *Obstetrics and Gynecology, 114*(2 pt 1), 354.

37. Reeves, S. A., Gibbs, R. S., & Clark, S. L. (2011). Magnesium for fetal neuroprotection. *American Journal of Obstetrics and Gynecology, 204*(3), 202.e1–e4.

38. Rouse, D., Hirtz, D., Thom, E., et al., Eunice Kennedy Shriver NICHD Maternal-Fetal Medicine Units Network. (2008). A randomized controlled trial of magnesium sulfate for the prevention of cerebral palsy. *New England Journal of Medicine, 359*(9), 895–905.

39. Mercer, B. M. (2012). Premature rupture of the membranes. In Gabbe, S. G., Niebyl, J. R., Simpson, J. L., et al. (Eds.), *Obstetrics: Normal and problem pregnancies* (6th ed., pp. 659–672). Philadelphia, PA: Saunders.

40. Mackeen, A. D., Seibel-Seamon, J., Muhammad, J., et al. (2014). Tocolytics for preterm premature rupture of membranes. *Cochrane Database of Systematic Reviews, 2*, CD007062.

41. Freeman, R. K., Garite, T. J., Nageotte, M. P., et al. (2012). *Fetal heart rate monitoring*. Philadelphia, PA: Lippincott.

Caring for the Laboring Woman with Hypertensive Disorders Complicating Pregnancy

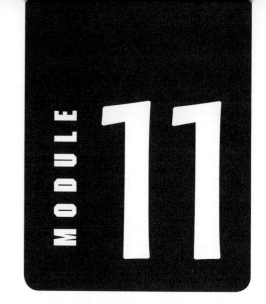

MODULE 11

PATRICIA M. WITCHER

Introduction

Hypertension is the most common medical condition in pregnant women and nonpregnant individuals,[1] affecting 10% of pregnancies world-wide.[2] Although hypertension was the second leading cause of pregnancy-related deaths in the United States from 1987 to 1997,[3–5] cardiovascular and other medical conditions have emerged as greater contributors to the causes of pregnancy-related death than the traditional pregnancy complications during the most recent surveillance period (2006–2009).[6] There remains an increasing trend for hospitalizations for hypertensive disorders of pregnancy in the United States[7] which suggests an opportunity for intervention to prevent the progression from morbidity to mortality for hypertensive women during pregnancy and postpartum.

Hypertension, along with other chronic conditions such as diabetes mellitus or chronic renal disease, increases the risk for preeclampsia, a pregnancy-specific hypertensive disorder that poses more significant risks to the woman and fetus[2] when it is superimposed upon pre-existing hypertension or presents alone. An understanding of the dynamic and progressive nature of the disease process, current diagnostic criteria, and management recommendations provide the foundation for reducing adverse outcomes. Astute and early assessments as well as patient education on premonitory signs and symptoms of preeclampsia are critical to appropriate diagnosis and early intervention. The etiology and pathophysiology of hypertension in pregnancy have been intensively researched over the years, and although a great deal is still unknown, there has been substantial improvement in the understanding of preeclampsia. This module presents what is currently reflected in the literature as well as guidelines from the American College of Obstetricians and Gynecologists (ACOG) Task Force on Hypertensive in Pregnancy.[2] The Task Force on Hypertensive in Pregnancy bases the guidelines for management of hypertensive disorders of pregnancy on evidence and consensus among obstetrical experts. This module reinforces prior understanding of pathophysiology and management guidelines and provides the changes in diagnostic criteria along with more precise recommendations that have evolved for management of hypertension.

Terminology and Classification

Different classification schemes and terminology in the literature have confused healthcare professionals and perpetuate imprecise diagnostic categories, which contributes to a lack of conformity in determining outcomes of hypertensive disorders complicating pregnancy in different research studies. The ACOG Task Force on Hypertension in Pregnancy currently uses the classification schema first introduced by ACOG in 1972[2] and modified reports of The National High Blood Pressure Education Program, Working Group Report on High Blood Pressure in Pregnancy (Working Group) published through the National Institutes of Health; and the National Heart, Lung, and Blood Institute; and outlines current accepted terminology for the hypertensive disorders of pregnancy[8–10] to classify hypertensive disorders in pregnancy.

A major goal of the classification system is to differentiate hypertensive disorders that precede pregnancy from those that develop during pregnancy or that are exacerbated by the pregnancy. Preeclampsia is peculiar to pregnancy and manifests with a wide range of clinical manifestations that arise from decreased end-organ perfusion secondary to arteriolar vasospasm, increased capillary permeability from endothelial injury, and hemostatic alterations.[11,12]

These pathophysiologic alterations typically progress in severity as pregnancy advances and do not resolve until after the infant's birth. Delivery at the optimal time requires a balanced consideration of the risks to the woman and fetus of continuing the pregnancy to a timeframe sufficient for fetal development and maturity. This timing is challenged by the dynamic and progressive nature of the disease and difficulty in differentiating worsening chronic hypertension versus superimposition of preeclampsia.[2]

Clarification of Terms

Preeclampsia versus Pregnancy-Induced Hypertension

The term, *pregnancy-induced hypertension* (PIH) has been used inconsistently to either broadly describe all new onset hypertension in pregnancy with or without accompanying proteinuria or it has been used interchangeably with the term, *preeclampsia*. Therefore, the term *pregnancy-induced hypertension* has been abandoned by classification systems used in the United States. This module incorporates this new classification system.[2]

Gestational Hypertension versus Transient Hypertension

The term, *transient hypertension* previously described a group of women with gestational hypertension that resolves during the postpartum period.[5] Gestational hypertension is defined as blood pressure elevation with onset after 20 weeks' gestation without proteinuria that often presents near term. Gestational hypertension may manifest for the first time postpartum, but resolves postpartum. Failure of blood pressure to normalize in the postpartum period (which is no longer specified to the specific postpartum day) constitutes chronic hypertension. The term, *transient hypertension* has been abandoned as well.[2]

Preeclampsia with or without Severe Features versus Mild and Severe Preeclampsia

Mild preeclampsia is no longer used to describe preeclampsia with the absence of severe manifestations because the Task Force on Hypertension in Pregnancy[2] believed it to misrepresent the dynamic and progressive nature of the disease. Even without severe manifestations, there remains a significant risk for morbidity and mortality. ACOG has further recommended that the term *severe preeclampsia* be replaced with *preeclampsia with severe features* for similar reasons.

Classification of Hypertensive Disorders Complicating Pregnancy

Each hypertensive disorder complicating pregnancy has distinguishing characteristics, diagnostic criteria, and risks of perinatal morbidity and mortality. The discussion in this module follows the Task Force on Hypertension in Pregnancy.[2]

1. Preeclampsia/eclampsia

NOTE: HELLP syndrome—preeclampsia subtype—is discussed within this category

2. Chronic hypertension
3. Chronic hypertension with superimposed preeclampsia
4. Gestational hypertension

Preeclampsia/Eclampsia

- Usually occurring after 20 weeks' gestation, preeclampsia is a pregnancy-specific syndrome with multiple organ system involvement from ischemia
- New onset hypertension plus new onset proteinuria
- Some women present with new onset hypertension without proteinuria. In the absence of proteinuria, preeclampsia may be diagnosed when new onset hypertension is accompanied by one of the following features that reflect the multisystem involvement:
  - Thrombocytopenia
  - Impaired liver function
  - New development of renal insufficiency

  - Pulmonary edema
  - New onset cerebral or visual disturbances
- **Eclampsia**—the onset of convulsions in the woman diagnosed with preeclampsia, which is a severe manifestation

Chronic Hypertension
- Hypertension known to be observed prior to pregnancy

OR
- Onset of elevated blood pressure before 20 weeks' gestation when prepregnancy blood pressure is unknown

Chronic Hypertension with Superimposed Preeclampsia
- Occurrence of preeclampsia in a woman with pre-existing hypertension

Gestational Hypertension
- New onset of hypertension after the 20th week of pregnancy in the absence of proteinuria

NOTE: Hypertension with an onset after 20 weeks' gestation that fails to normalize postpartum changes the diagnosis to chronic hypertension.

Observations that reflect current understanding of the hypertensive disorders in pregnancy include the following:
- Hypertension during pregnancy represents a continuum of disease processes. Hypertension may be the first sign, but the underlying pathophysiology can involve major organ systems.
- Hypertensive states are classified according to certain signs or symptoms based upon the timing in pregnancy in which they present. Women diagnosed with gestational hypertension established by onset of hypertension after 20 weeks without accompanying proteinuria, may actually have preeclampsia before either proteinuria or multisystem disturbances are manifested. These patients require surveillance for proteinuria and multisystem signs and symptoms, and should these develop, are no longer considered to have gestational hypertension, but preeclampsia.
- Chronic hypertension is associated with fetal morbidity, such as intrauterine fetal growth restriction and an increased risk for superimposed preeclampsia. Maternal and fetal morbidity increase substantially when preeclampsia is superimposed upon chronic hypertension.
- Chronic hypertension may not be accurately diagnosed until after childbirth in the setting of hypertension that initially manifests later in pregnancy because these women may have been presumed to have been normotensive prior to the pregnancy. These women may have had pre-existing hypertension, but experienced the normal physiologic decline in blood pressure during pregnancy; the return to a hypertensive state may reflect the physiologic return of blood pressure to prepregnancy levels. Postpartum follow-up is warranted in order to ascertain persistent elevations in blood pressure that may necessitate referral to a physician specializing in hypertension management.
- Preeclampsia may progress to severe disease rapidly, necessitating timely recognition of relevant signs and symptoms. Diagnosis of preeclampsia is not constrained to rigid criteria for diagnosis in order to optimize maternal and fetal management.
- HELLP syndrome is not included in the classification system because it is considered a preeclampsia subtype. HELLP syndrome is addressed later in this module.

NOTE: Although hypertensive disorders are discussed as separate diagnoses, recognition that preeclampsia may be superimposed upon gestational hypertension or chronic hypertension and progress to severe disease rapidly provides the foundation for ongoing assessment of these patients. Because the classification system is not precise and a missed diagnosis may lead to increased risk of adverse maternal and perinatal outcomes, a more prudent approach for clinical management is to overdiagnose preeclampsia.

Diagnosis of Preeclampsia and Eclampsia

- **How are hypertensive disorders specific to pregnancy diagnosed?[2]**

The Task Force on Hypertension in Pregnancy and others[9,10,13] identify reliable *diagnostic criteria* and guidelines for the evaluation of hypertensive disorders in pregnancy. Table 11.1 illustrates the diagnostic criteria for each.

TABLE 11.1	DIAGNOSTIC CRITERIA FOR HYPERTENSIVE DISORDERS OF PREGNANCY	
CLASSIFICATION	**DIAGNOSTIC CRITERIA**	**CHANGES IN CLASSIFICATION**
Gestational hypertension	New onset hypertension after the 20th week of gestation **Hypertension is defined as:** • SBP >140 mm Hg, **OR** • DBP >90 mm Hg	*Pregnancy induced hypertension* (PIH) and *transient hypertension* are abandoned terms
Preeclampsia	New onset hypertension after 20 wks' gestation **PLUS:** **Proteinuria defined as:** • >300 mg in 24-hour urine • Protein/creatinine ratio ≥0.3 • Urine dipstick ≥1+ (≥30 mg/dL) **OR IN THE ABSENCE OF PROTEINURIA:** Thrombocytopenia • Platelet count <100,000/mm³ Impaired liver function • ↑ ALT or AST New development of renal insufficiency • Serum creatinine >1.1 mg/dL, **OR** • Doubling of serum creatinine in the absence of other renal disease Pulmonary edema New onset cerebral or visual disturbances	*PIH* is an abandoned term and is not used interchangeably with preeclampsia *Mild preeclampsia* no longer used Proteinuria is not required for the diagnosis of preeclampsia HELLP syndrome (**H**emolysis, **E**levated **L**iver Enzymes, and **L**ow **P**latelets) is a subtype of preeclampsia and not included in the classification system
Eclampsia	New onset of grand mal seizure in woman with preeclampsia Eclampsia is the convulsive phase of preeclampsia	
Chronic hypertension	Pre-existing hypertension **OR** Onset of elevated blood pressure before 20 wks' gestation *Chronic hypertension is diagnosed when high blood pressure fails to normalize postpartum*	The postpartum period is not defined by a precise day or week following childbirth
Chronic hypertension with superimposed preeclampsia	Chronic hypertension **AND** Preeclampsia	
Preeclampsia with severe features	SBP ≥160 mm Hg DBP ≥110 mm Hg Thrombocytopenia • Platelet count <100,000 mm³ Impaired liver function • ↑ ALT or AST to twice the normal concentration • Severe, persistent RUQ or epigastric pain unresponsive to pain medication and not attributed to another medical diagnosis Progressive renal insufficiency • Serum creatinine >1.1 mg/dL • Doubling of serum creatinine in the absence of other renal disease Pulmonary edema Cerebral or visual disturbances	Severe preeclampsia is no longer used. Some clinical findings have been removed from the criteria for preeclampsia with severe features: • Proteinuria >5 g in 24 hours • Oliguria • Intrauterine fetal growth restriction

Diagnostic Criteria for Hypertensive Disorders of Pregnancy.

SBP, systolic blood pressure; DBP, diastolic blood pressure; ALT, alanine aminotransferase; AST, aspartate aminotransferase; RUQ, right upper quadrant.

Adapted from Task Force on Hypertension in Pregnancy. (2013). *Hypertension in Pregnancy* (pp. 1–89). Washington, DC: American College of Obstetricians and Gynecologists.

Preeclampsia

Preeclampsia is a syndrome with multiple organ system involvement that manifests in the second half of pregnancy with new onset hypertension and new onset proteinuria.

- Hypertension is defined by a persistent elevation in either the systolic blood pressure of 140 mm Hg or higher or the diastolic blood pressure of 90 mm Hg or higher on two occasions at least 4 hours apart.

- Proteinuria is defined as protein of greater than 300 mg in a 24-hour urine specimen. Alternatively, proteinuria may be defined as a protein/creatinine ratio of at least 0.3 (both measured in mg/dL) because this ratio has been demonstrated to be equivalent to or exceed a 24-hour urine protein collection of 300 mg. A urine dipstick reading of +1 may also be used to fulfill criteria for proteinuria in the absence of quantifiable tests.
- Proteinuria is not required for the diagnosis of preeclampsia. In the absence of proteinuria, new onset hypertension (as defined above) with any of the following constitutes preeclampsia:
  - Thrombocytopenia (less than 100,000/μL)
  - Impaired liver function (increase in blood levels of liver transaminases twice their normal value)
  - New development of renal insufficiency (serum creatinine greater than 1.1 mg/dL or doubling of serum creatinine
  - Pulmonary edema
  - New onset cerebral or visual disturbance

Hypertension is defined as either a systolic BP of 140 mm Hg or higher or diastolic BP of 90 mm Hg or higher on two occasions at least 4 hours apart.

NOTE: Preeclampsia is a syndrome that occurs only during pregnancy (the placenta plays a key role). Functional and structural changes in the developing placenta are believed to cause preeclampsia based upon the observation that the disease resolves after removal of the products of conception. Preeclampsia evolves from a complex interaction between placental-derived products and exaggerated adaptive mechanisms of normal pregnancy that lead to tissue ischemia.

Preeclampsia with Severe Features

Preeclampsia with severe features may be diagnosed with any of the following findings:
- Systolic blood pressure of 160 mm Hg or higher on two occasions at least 4 hours apart
- Diastolic blood pressure 110 mm Hg or higher on two occasions at least 4 hours apart
- Thrombocytopenia (less than 100,000/μL)
- Impaired liver function (increase in blood levels of liver transaminases twice their normal value or severe persistent right upper quadrant or epigastric pain unresponsive to medication and not accounted for by alternative diagnosis or both)
- New development of renal insufficiency (serum creatinine greater than 1.1 mg/dL or doubling of serum creatinine in the absence of other renal disease)
- Pulmonary edema
- New onset cerebral or visual disturbance

NOTE: Some clinical findings have been removed from the criteria for preeclampsia with severe features because they do not correlate with outcome or are not managed any differently than if the patient were not diagnosed with preeclampsia. The clinical findings that have been removed from consideration of severe disease include urine proteinuria greater than 5 g in 24 hours, intrauterine fetal growth restriction, and oliguria.

Preeclampsia is no longer categorized as mild or severe because of the progressive and dynamic nature of the disease. A woman who fulfills the basic criteria for hypertension (systolic blood pressure 140 to 159 mm Hg or diastolic blood pressure 90 to 109 mm Hg), but manifests with organ system derangements as outlined above are considered to have a severe form of the disease.

Early identification of worsening preeclampsia in a patient at a level I or II hospital is critical for timely transport to a high-risk regional center while the patient is stable and before a critical state is reached.

Eclampsia

- Eclampsia is defined as new onset grand mal seizure activity in the woman diagnosed with preeclampsia.
- Seizures can occur before, during, or after labor.

HELLP Syndrome

HELLP syndrome is a preeclampsia subtype; the acronym represents Hemolysis, Elevated Liver enzymes, and Low Platelets and is typically characterized by the following laboratory findings[11]:

- Hemolysis, defined as the presence of microangiopathic hemolytic anemia, which includes:
  - Abnormal peripheral blood smear (schistocytes, burr cells, echinocytes)
  - Elevated serum bilirubin (Serum bilirubin of 1.2 mg/dL or higher)
  - Low serum haptoglobin levels
  - Elevated lactate dehydrogenase (LDH) (usually greater than 600 U/L)
  - Significant decline in hemoglobin, unrelated to blood loss
- Elevated Liver Enzymes:
  - Aspartate transaminase (AST), twice the upper level of normal or greater
  - Alanine transaminase (ALT), twice the upper level of normal or greater
  - Elevated LDH
- Low platelets, less than 100,000/mm^3

Gestational Hypertension

- Gestational hypertension is new onset hypertension after 20 weeks' gestation without proteinuria.
- Multisystem features consistent with preeclampsia are also absent.
- Failure of hypertension to resolve postpartum fulfills the criteria for diagnosis of chronic hypertension.

NOTE: Some women will experience severe blood pressure elevations, yet not fulfill the criteria for diagnosis of preeclampsia but still experience similar outcomes to women with preeclampsia.

Women who present with hypertension initially during pregnancy, especially after 20 weeks' gestation, are presumed to have been normotensive prior to pregnancy and will usually be diagnosed with either gestational hypertension or preeclampsia based upon clinical presentation and fulfillment of diagnostic criteria, when in actuality, these patients may have pre-existing hypertension that was not diagnosed due the physiologic decline in blood pressure that normally occurs after the first trimester. This warrants further assessment of blood pressure postpartum in order to ensure that hypertension resolves. In the event that hypertension persists beyond the postpartum period, the patient more than likely has chronic hypertension that necessitates referral to a physician specializing in hypertension management. However, during the pregnancy, it is prudent to manage the patient in accordance with guidelines for preeclampsia in order to optimize the short-term outcomes for both mother and fetus.

Pathophysiology of Preeclampsia

Preeclampsia is believed to originate from abnormal implantation of the placenta. Normally, through a complex process early in placental development, placental trophoblast cells invade the uterine spiral arteries, converting them from small, high-resistance vessels to dilated, low-resistance vessels, to increase placental circulation. This process of vascular growth, termed angiogenesis, is essential to sustain the fetus throughout the pregnancy.[14] In pregnancies with preeclampsia, the partial invasion of trophoblasts into the superficial decidua fails to achieve this transformation, resulting in constricted and narrowed uterine arteries, compromising uteroplacental perfusion. Placental ischemia leads to the production of placental factors that enter the maternal circulation giving rise to widespread maternal endothelial dysfunction ensuing in a variety of manifestations of the disease from reduced end-organ perfusion.[2,11,14] Some of the placental factors released into the maternal circulation have received a great deal of attention; among them are inflammatory factors and antiangiogenic factors.[2] Antiangiogenic proteins (soluble fms-like tyrosine kinase-1 [sFlt-1] and soluble endoglin) antagonize proangiogenic proteins (vascular endothelial growth factor [VEGF] and placental like growth factor [PLGF]), thereby reducing free levels of these proangiogenic proteins that normally stimulate uteroplacental vascular growth and dilation and maintain endothelial integrity.[11] Increased circulating levels of sFLT-1 precede the development of preeclampsia by weeks to months and are accompanied by decreased circulating-free PLGF and VEGF levels.[2,14] Appearance of these biomarkers is being further studied to determine their value in predicting preeclampsia.[2]

The cause of preeclampsia remains unknown. Yet many mechanisms have been proposed to establish the pathophysiologic progression from abnormal placentation to development of the maternal syndrome. Predominant pathophysiologic mechanisms that have been implicated in the disease process include[2,11] oxidative stress, an exaggerated inflammatory response, and altered coagulation.

Oxidative Stress

Under normal conditions, maternal blood flow to the placenta increases oxygen tension along with an increase in antioxidant enzymes. In preeclampsia, there is a diminished antioxidant response to oxygen stimulation, leading to the generation of oxygen-free radicals that promote tissue damage with resultant neutrophil activation that extends the generation of cytotoxic superoxide ions and ultimately, activation of the vascular endothelium. Reduced antioxidant activity and increased oxidative stress in the placenta and in the maternal circulation[15] have instigated clinical trials that study the role of antioxidants, such as Vitamin C and Vitamin E, in preventing preeclampsia. Further study may conclude a risk reduction for preeclampsia; until definitive data demonstrate a clear benefit, Vitamin C and Vitamin E supplements are not currently recommended.[2] The lipid profile in preeclamptic women (increased concentrations of serum free fatty acids, triglycerides, and very-low density lipoprotein [VLDL]) may predispose to oxidative stress. The VLDL particles are smaller in preeclamptic women when compared to normotensive women, which may facilitate their oxidative degradation.[15]

Inflammatory Response

During normal pregnancy, the maternal immune system adaptations directed at establishing an immune tolerance to fetal antigens manifests as a systemic inflammatory response. Preeclampsia further enhances the immune response, as evidenced by elevated levels of proinflammatory mediators, interleukin-6, interleukin-8, tumor necrosis factor alpha (TNF-α), and monocyte chemoattractant protein 1 (MCR-1).[16] Neutrophil activation may contribute to vascular injury as a result of leukocyte adhesion to the endothelium, perpetuating the inflammatory response and promoting coagulation through uncontrolled activation of the complement system.[17]

Decreased placental perfusion and endothelial damage promote platelet aggregation and coagulation, resulting in an imbalance between vasoactive prostaglandins. Prostacyclin, a potent vasodilator and inhibitor of platelet aggregation, is normally produced by the vascular endothelium and renal cortex. In preeclampsia, a deficiency in prostacyclin is accompanied by an increase in thromboxane A_2 (TXA_2), a potent vasoconstrictor and platelet aggregator, which is produced by platelets and trophoblasts. The imbalance favoring TXA_2 suggests an exacerbation of the pathophysiologic derangements of preeclampsia,[11] leading to clinical trials examining the effects of low-dose aspirin in ameliorating the exaggerated inflammatory response by blocking the production of thromboxanes. Because of its protective effect, daily low-dose aspirin (60 to 80 mg) initiated in the late first trimester is recommended for women with significant risk for preeclampsia, primarily women with a medical history of early-onset preeclampsia and preterm birth at less than 34 0/7 weeks' gestation or women with a history of preeclampsia in more than one prior pregnancy.[2]

Daily low-dose aspirin is recommended for women with significant risk for preeclampsia, such as those women with a prior pregnancy complicated by preeclampsia and preterm birth prior to 34 completed weeks or women with more than one prior pregnancy complicated by preeclampsia.[2]

Altered Coagulation

The hypercoagulable state of normal pregnancy is potentiated in preeclampsia. Procoagulant proteins, such as tissue plasminogen activator (tPA), plasminogen activator inhibitor (PAI-1), and von Willebrand are elevated while proteins that inhibit the coagulation cascade, including anti-thrombin III, activated protein C, and protein S, are reduced. The compromise in placental perfusion may trigger fibrin deposition and formation of thrombi in the placental circulation, further worsening placental ischemia and resultant endothelial damage.[7]

• What are the major pathophysiologic events in preeclampsia that compromise end-organ perfusion?

Understanding the pathophysiology underlying the diagnostic signs and symptoms in pre-eclampsia facilitates a greater comprehension of the clinical manifestations and rationale for interventions. The primary pathophysiologic process underlying the multiorgan system involvement in preeclampsia is illustrated in Figure 11.1.

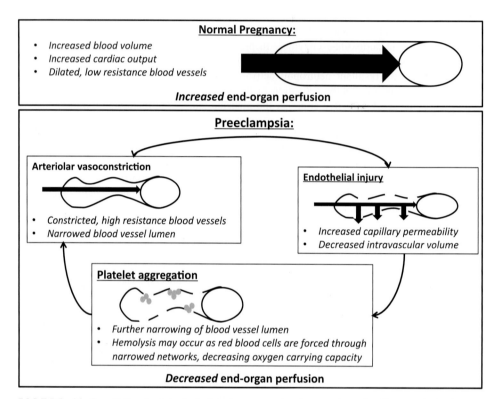

FIGURE 11.1   Pathophysiological alterations occurring in preeclampsia. (Source: Author)

Remember the pathologic process precedes the development of diagnostic signs by several weeks or months. Fetal circulation can be compromised by vasospasm within the placental vascular bed long before warning signs are evident.

The rationale for nursing interventions and medical management is directly related to the pathophysiologic and anatomic changes that occur in preeclampsia.

In response to the increased demands of normal pregnancy, significant physiologic adaptations occur in order to maintain maternal and fetal oxygenation. Among these physiologic changes are an increase in circulating blood volume, increase in cardiac output, and relaxation and dilation of systemic blood vessels; all directed at maximizing blood flow to maternal end-organs and the uteroplacental circulation.[18] There is decreased end-organ perfusion in preeclampsia arising from endothelial dysfunction which further propagates oxidative stress and systemic inflammation. The disease process is progressive, often resulting in:
   • Increased arterial pressure and vasospasm. Often a physiologic attempt at achieving hemostasis from vascular injury, it promulgates further endothelial injury.

- Fluid or fluid components escape out of the blood vessel into the interstitial compartment. These components include protein substances (e.g., albumin), fluid, or both. Loss of albumin from the intravascular space decreases colloid osmotic pressure (COP), or the pressure exerted to "pull" fluid within the blood vessels. A further compromise in circulating intravascular blood volume ensues.
- Platelets aggregate at the sites of endothelial injury, narrowing the blood vessel lumen further. The decline in platelet count reflects the consumption of platelets.
- Arterial blood flow to end-organs is compromised. The flow of blood under high pressure through narrowed blood vessels may result in hemolysis, compounding the state of decreased oxygen delivery from reduced oxygen carrying capacity.

- **What clinical findings are associated with the pathophysiologic changes?**

The spectrum of multisystem manifestations of preeclampsia include the following[11]:
- *Cardiovascular:* hypertension, hypovolemia, dependent edema
- *Hematologic:* thrombocytopenia, abnormal peripheral blood smear (schistocytes, burr cells, echinocytes), elevated lactate dehydrogenase (LDH), or significant decline in hemoglobin, unrelated to blood loss
- *Renal system:* proteinuria, increased serum creatinine, increased serum uric acid, oliguria
- *Hepatic system:* elevated serum bilirubin (serum bilirubin of 1.2 mg/dL or higher)—rarely increased, low-serum haptoglobin levels, elevated liver enzymes (AST and ALT) twice the upper level of normal or greater, right upper quadrant or epigastric pain (which may be indicative of subcapsular liver hematoma)[19]
- *Neurologic system:* visual disturbances, cerebral disturbances, eclampsia
- *Uteroplacental unit:* intrauterine fetal growth restriction, fetal surveillance findings that may indicate fetal hypoxemia (abnormal FHR, low biophysical profile score, abnormal Doppler velocimetry)
- *Pulmonary system:* pulmonary edema from increased capillary permeability and resultant interstitial edema

Etiology of Preeclampsia

Most cases of preeclampsia occur in healthy nulliparous women and the ability to assess the risk for preeclampsia by socioeconomic and cultural factors has been difficult.[2] Multiple factors that predispose the woman to the disease may further an understanding of what causes the disease. The etiology, however, remains unknown.

- **Paternal factors** may play a significant role in the pathogenesis of preeclampsia. Long-term exposure to sperm from the same partner may offer protective effects against the physiologic events that lead to preeclampsia. This protective effect is lost when exposure to sperm from the same partner is of short duration, which might explain the increased incidence of preeclampsia in younger, nulliparous women less than 20 years of age, use of condoms, or conception with donor sperm. Conversely, a prior normal pregnancy with the same partner reduces the risk of preeclampsia. In addition, there are observations that demonstrate that the risks for preeclampsia are not entirely unique to women. A man who fathered a preeclamptic pregnancy is almost twice as likely to father another pregnancy in a new partner who develops preeclampsia, even if the woman herself has had a prior normal pregnancy with another partner.[11]
- **Genetic predisposition** is thought to play a role based upon the observation that women whose mothers and sisters have had preeclampsia are more likely to have the disease compared to women without this family history.[20]
- **Women with pre-existing vascular disease or metabolic abnormalities** are at increased risk for preeclampsia. The exact mechanism is not precisely understood. Some of the risk factors for preeclampsia are also associated with cardiovascular disease risk factors, such as maternal age older than 40 years, pregestational diabetes, pre-existing hypertension, and obesity.[2,7] The "acute atherosis" of placental vessels encountered in preeclampsia closely resemble atherosclerotic plaques. In addition, levels of an adipocyte-derived hormone, leptin, are also observed in preeclampsia and coronary vascular disease. Obesity is also characterized by lipid abnormalities, which may explain why obese women are at higher risk for preeclampsia.[7]

• Are certain pregnant women at risk for developing preeclampsia?

The prevailing risk factors for preeclampsia include the following[2]:
- Primiparity
- Prior pregnancy complicated by preeclampsia
- Chronic hypertension
- Chronic renal disease
- History of thrombophilia
- Multifetal pregnancy
- Family history of preeclampsia
- Type I or type II diabetes mellitus
- Obesity
- Collagen vascular disease, such as systemic lupus erythematosus (SLE)
- Maternal age greater than 40, or maternal age greater than 35 with co-morbid conditions

Complications of Preeclampsia

Decreased end-organ perfusion contributes to organ system derangements in preeclampsia, which are observed on a continuum that extends from a presentation without severe features to catastrophic organ system failure. Signs and symptoms that may possibly indicate progression in severity of the disease and that potentially end with adverse outcomes necessitate vigilant assessment.

WATCH FOR SIGNS OF THE FOLLOWING[21]:
- Eclampsia
- Abruptio placentae
- Hemorrhage or disseminated intravascular coagulation (DIC)
- Acute renal failure
  - Subcapsular liver hematoma or hepatic rupture
  - Cerebrovascular accident
  - Pulmonary edema
  - Hypertensive cardiomyopathy

Eclampsia

- Eclampsia is defined as the new onset of grand mal seizure activity in the woman diagnosed with preeclampsia, with no history of pre-existing neurologic pathology.[2]
- In 2010 to 2011, the Division of Reproductive Health at the Centers for Disease Control and Prevention on severe maternal morbidity and mortality reported an incidence in eclampsia of 7 per 100,000 births in the United States.[6] About 2% to 3% of women with preeclampsia develop eclampsia.[22]
- Eclamptic seizures are usually accompanied by fetal bradycardia as a result of decreased uteroplacental perfusion from interrupted maternal oxygenation. The bradycardia usually resolves with abatement of the seizure, but intrauterine fetal resuscitation measures directed at increasing uteroplacental perfusion are warranted.[21]
- Perinatal morbidity and mortality is associated with abruption placentae, DIC, acute renal failure, pulmonary edema, aspiration pneumonia, cardiopulmonary arrest, or intracerebral hemorrhage (rare).[11]
- While the majority of eclamptic seizures occur prior to delivery, the onset has been reported weeks after childbirth.[21] However, further evaluation for causes other than preeclampsia is warranted when new-onset seizure occurs after the first 48 hours postpartum.[11]

NOTE: Eclamptic convulsions can occur in women without any preceding signs or symptoms and are unpredictable.[21]

Immediate care during a seizure is supportive and directed at promoting maternal and fetal oxygenation. Establishing a patent airway along with administration of supplemental oxygen is a priority. Supportive therapy is continued and focuses on minimizing the risk of aspiration, preventing recurrent seizure activity, and controlling blood pressure. Once the patient has been stabilized, management is directed toward delivery of the infant.

• What are the typical features of eclampsia?

Eclampsia has a variable clinical presentation, ranging from no signs and symptoms of pre-eclampsia without any cerebral or visual disturbances to preeclampsia with severe features. Although not predictive of impending seizure, some signs and symptoms are helpful in indicating the potential for eclampsia and include the following[2]:

- Persistent occipital or frontal headache
- Blurred vision
- Photophobia
- Epigastric or right upper quadrant pain, or both
- Altered mental status

Eclamptic seizures usually resolve within a few minutes. Continued loss of consciousness, coma, or progression to respiratory or cardiopulmonary arrest is unusual and should elicit further evaluation for magnesium toxicity secondary to magnesium sulfate infusion.[11] Immediately following the seizure, assessment focuses on the return of spontaneous respirations, assessment of hemoglobin arterial oxygen saturation (SaO_2), and level of consciousness. Electronic fetal heart rate (FHR) monitoring is resumed or initiated as soon as efforts directed at restoring maternal oxygenation have been initiated in order to evaluate return of the FHR to baseline and subsequent patterns that might indicate potential fetal acidemia. Despite appropriate magnesium sulfate therapy, eclamptic seizure may recur, even in the setting of a therapeutic magnesium level.[21] Therefore, maternal and fetal assessment is ongoing and the woman optimally remains in the labor and delivery area for observation for at least 24 hours after childbirth.

Aspiration is a significant contributor to maternal morbidity after an eclamptic seizure. The woman should be in a lateral decubitus position to minimize the risk of aspiration if vomiting occurs. Emergency airway equipment, including endotracheal tube and suctioning, should be readily available.

NOTE: Preeclampsia without severe features can progress to eclampsia. Or, eclampsia can be the initial manifestation of preeclampsia without premonitory signs and symptoms.

Chronic Hypertension with Superimposed Preeclampsia

- Preeclampsia that complicates hypertension that was known to exist prior to pregnancy, or hypertension before 20 weeks' gestation when prepregnancy blood pressures are unknown is diagnosed as chronic hypertension with superimposed preeclampsia.
- Superimposed preeclampsia develops in up to 40% of women with chronic hypertension.[2]
- *The prognosis for both the woman and fetus is much worse than with chronic hypertension alone.*
- There is a strong association between hypertension (chronic) and cardiovascular disease risk; the higher the blood pressure, the greater the risk for kidney disease, along with other cardiovascular disease events.[23] Pre-existing hypertension with proteinuria may actually reflect the progression of the end-organ damage associated with elevated blood pressure, making the diagnosis of superimposed preeclampsia uncertain. The diagnosis of superimposed preeclampsia is highly likely with the new onset of proteinuria after 20 weeks' gestation or in women who had proteinuria prior to 20 weeks' who develop one of the following findings[2]:
  - Sudden exacerbation of hypertension or need to escalate antihypertensive medication dose, especially when previously controlled on these medications
  - Substantial increase in proteinuria that is sustained
  - Renal insufficiency (either serum creatinine greater than 1.1 mg/dL or doubling in the serum level)
  - *Thrombocytopenia* (platelet count less than 100,000 cells/mm[3])
  - Sudden presentation of other signs and symptoms of preeclampsia, such as right upper quadrant or epigastric pain, increase in liver enzymes to abnormal levels, or severe headache
  - Pulmonary edema or congestion
- The fetus is at even greater risk of growth restriction than with preeclampsia or chronic hypertension alone.

Chronic Hypertension

- Chronic hypertension is defined as hypertension that is present and observable before pregnancy or that is diagnosed before the 20th week of gestation.[2]
- When hypertension is observed during pregnancy without a prior history, distinguishing chronic hypertension from gestational hypertension, can be challenging.[2]
- Pregnancy imposes a physiologic stress that generates physiologic adaptations directed at fulfilling the increased metabolic demands of pregnancy.[18] The physiologic response to these changes may bare a pre-existing condition that was not appreciated before the pregnancy. Furthermore, transient blood pressure elevations are common postpartum because of volume redistribution, administration of intravenous crystalloids, alterations in vascular tone, and use of nonsteroidal anti-inflammatory agents for pain management.[24] Hypertension that persists beyond the postpartum period warrants categorization and treatment in accordance with adult guidelines on hypertension.[2,24]
- Hypertension may co-exist with other medical conditions, such as diabetes mellitus or may produce consequences to target organs directly, such as chronic kidney disease (Chobanian, 2003). Proteinuria that accompanies chronic hypertension may reflect the renal system involvement of a chronic nature rather than superimposed preeclampsia.

Approximately 30% of individuals are unaware of their hypertension and more than 40% of individuals with hypertension are not being treated.[24] Therefore, women may be diagnosed with gestational hypertension or preeclampsia and presumed to have been normotensive,[2] when in actuality, are provided with an opportunity for diagnosis of a pre-existing hypertension during routine obstetrical care.

NOTE: Hypertension diagnosed for the first time during pregnancy that does not resolve postpartum, is diagnosed as chronic hypertension. The Task Force on Hypertension in Pregnancy[2] does not specify the timing for the postpartum period, but indicates a timeframe of up to 6 months postpartum to the first year after childbirth for blood pressure to normalize.

- Causal factors for hypertension, such as obesity, are becoming increasingly more prevalent[23] in the general population, affecting women at a disproportionately higher rate than men.[24] Birth rates in women 30 years and older have consistently increased in the United States.[25] Given the trend of childbearing at an older age, an increase in the incidence of chronic hypertension in pregnancy is anticipated.
- Of all chronic hypertensive pregnant women, 90% have primary (or essential) hypertension The remaining percentage of hypertension (secondary hypertension) may be attributed to underlying medical conditions, such as renal or endocrine disorders.[2]
- Chronic hypertension is associated with increased rates of adverse outcomes such as intrauterine fetal death, intrauterine fetal growth restriction, small-for-gestational-age infants, premature birth, and placental abruption. Superimposed preeclampsia further increases the risk for these adverse outcomes.[26]
- Target organ damage (heart, brain, and kidneys) is uncommon with hypertension without superimposed preeclampsia. The risk of stillbirth is 2.3-fold higher for women with chronic hypertension when accompanied by other co-morbid conditions, such as diabetes mellitus or renal disease.[2]
- Chronic hypertension is a risk factor for preeclampsia. Women with chronic hypertension require enhanced surveillance for signs and symptoms of preeclampsia and evaluation of fetal well-being.[2]

NOTE: Sodium restriction, bedrest, antioxidant supplementation with Vitamin C and Vitamin E, and calcium supplementation in women who do not have a nutritional deficiency of calcium have not shown any benefit in reducing the risk of preeclampsia and are not recommended.[2]

Evidence-Based Findings on Clinical Management of Chronic Hypertension

- Initial evaluation of the woman with chronic hypertension includes a review of laboratory and diagnostic studies performed prior to pregnancy in order to establish her baseline status,[2] such as 12-lead ECG, urinalysis, blood glucose and hematocrit, serum potassium and creatinine, and lipoprotein profile.[23] This baseline evaluation may provide value in differentiating superimposed preeclampsia from exacerbation of target organ damage from pre-existing hypertension. Performance of these studies may be indicated if baseline data are not available during prenatal care.

- Chronic hypertension is associated with an increased risk for acute renal failure, pulmonary edema,[27] gestational diabetes mellitus, and placental abruption[2] during pregnancy, which necessitates review of baseline health status before the pregnancy and evaluation for progression of the disease or development of complications throughout the pregnancy.

- Sudden onset of hypertension, sudden increase in blood pressure despite antihypertensive medications, or poorly controlled blood pressures suggests secondary hypertension, which necessitate further workup. Secondary hypertension arises from other disease processes, such as pheochromocytoma, coarctation of the aorta, Cushing syndrome, primary aldosteronism, or renal parenchymal disease.[23] Consultation with a physician who specializes in hypertension management may be warranted.

- Women with chronic hypertension are at higher risk for heart failure if the heart is incapable of augmenting blood flow sufficient for the increased metabolic demands of pregnancy and the larger body mass. Echocardiography may be indicated to assess left ventricular function, especially if there has been severe hypertension (systolic BP ≥160 or diastolic BP ≥100)[23] of a long duration (more than 4 years).[2]

- Although antihypertensive agents are associated with preterm birth, low birth weight infant, low apgar, intrauterine fetal growth restriction, and preeclampsia, these risks are lower when compared to hypertensive women who are not treated with antihypertensives.[28]

- The goal of antihypertensive therapy for women with chronic hypertension during pregnancy is systolic blood pressure of 130 to 155 mm Hg and diastolic blood pressure of 80 to 105 mm Hg.[24]

- Angiotensin converting enzyme (ACE) inhibitors are contraindicated because of their association with congenital malformations, affecting both the cardiovascular and central nervous systems during exposure in the first trimester and with oligohydramnios and neonatal renal failure with administration during the second trimester.[29] Although data are not available on the use of angiotensin II receptor antagonists during pregnancy, adverse effects are likely to be similar to ACE inhibitors. These agents should be avoided. See Table 11.2 for the antihypertensive agents used for chronic hypertension complicating pregnancy.[9,29]

TABLE 11.2	ANTIHYPERTENSIVE AGENTS FOR CONTINUOUS MANAGEMENT OF CHRONIC HYPERTENSION		
MEDICATION	**MECHANISM OF ACTION**	**DOSAGE**	**PRECAUTIONS**
Labetalol	Nonselective beta blocker with alpha receptor blockade.	200–2,400 mg orally in 2–3 divided doses per day	Potential bronchoconstriction; avoid in patients with asthma Avoid in patients with heart disease or congestive heart failure Maternal side effects include lethargy, fatigue, sleep disturbances May be associated with small for gestational age infant
Methyldopa	Central activity alpha-2 adrenergic agonist	500–3,000 mg in 2–3 divided doses per day	No reports of adverse effects on uteroplacental perfusion or neonatal adverse outcome Maternal side effects include hepatic dysfunction and necrosis and hemolytic anemia
Nifedipine		30–120 mg in 2–3 divided doses of slow release form per day	Avoid immediate release or sublingual form due to increased risk for profound maternal hypotension
Thiazide diuretics	Depends upon agent	Depends upon agent	Typically not initiated during the pregnancy, but rather administration may be continued if the woman was taking diuretics before the pregnancy Theoretical concern for decreased circulating blood volume with resultant decreased uteroplacental perfusion and decreased fetal growth, but this has not been established Monitor and report hypokalemia

Adapted from Task Force on Hypertension in Pregnancy. (2013). *Hypertension in Pregnancy* (pp. 1–89). Washington, DC: American College of Obstetricians and Gynecologists.

Expert Clinical Assessment

Measuring Blood Pressure

Although the auscultatory method using mercury sphygmomanometer remains the preferred method for assessing blood pressure, it has been replaced by other devices, such as aneroid sphygmomanometers and automated equipment, in most clinical settings due to the elimination of mercury-containing waste in health care.[30–32] Aneroid sphygmomanometers record blood pressure in a similar manner as mercury devices in that the examiner auscultates with a stethoscope over the artery just below the cuff, typically the brachial artery, for Korotkoff sounds, which return as pulsatile blood flow in the artery is re-established and then become progressively absent as the cuff pressure is gradually deflated. Korotkoff sounds have been classified into five phases: phase I (first appearance of sound) corresponds to systolic blood pressure; phases II and III, are clinically insignificant; and disappearance of sounds, phase IV (muffling of sound) and phase V (last audible sound) correspond to diastolic blood pressure. Currently, there is general consensus that Korotkoff V should be used to determine diastolic blood pressure,[32] except in situations when audible sounds can be heard even after complete deflation of the cuff. In this situation, it is recommended to use Korotkoff IV.[31] Automated devices evaluate oscillations created by arterial pulsatile pressures that correspond to changes in arterial blood flow arising from inflation and deflation of the cuff and estimate systolic and diastolic blood pressure using computerized algorithms.[33] Automated oscillometric devices are useful when frequent blood pressures are required, but may underestimate mean arterial pressure in individuals with widened pulse pressure.[32]

The diagnosis, evaluation, and treatment of hypertension depend upon correct measurement of blood pressure. Appropriate use of electronic devices requires periodic calibration and validation in accordance with manufacturer's guidelines to ensure accuracy of measurements. In addition, there are a number of recommendations provided by the American Heart Association (AHA) that promote the accuracy of blood pressure measurement[32]:

- Measure blood pressure over the brachial artery whenever possible in order to allow for trending of values across the continuum of care. Systolic blood pressure typically increases in more distal arteries whereas diastolic blood pressure decreases.
- Ensure appropriate cuff size as this is critical to accurate blood pressure measurements. Ideal cuff has a bladder length that is 80% and a width that is 40% of the arm circumference (length-to-width ratio of 2:1).
- Ensure that devices are validated and calibrated in accordance with manufacturer guidelines.
- When possible, record blood pressure with the patient in a sitting position, with her back supported. Feet should be planted on a flat surface. Diastolic blood pressure is higher in the sitting position than in the supine position and increases when the back is not supported. In addition, ensure that the patient's legs are uncrossed as crossing the legs may raise the systolic blood pressure.
- Support the weight of the patient's arm and place the arm at heart level. Blood pressure will be higher when the patient holds up her arm. Blood pressure decreases when the arm is above the heart and increases when the arm is below the level of the heart. When blood pressure is measured with the patient in a lateral recumbent position, support the arm at heart level.

Keep in mind that the clinical onset of preeclampsia can be insidious and might not be accompanied by overt symptoms.

An increase of 30 mm Hg systolic blood pressure or 15 mm Hg diastolic blood pressure over baseline readings ("30/15 rule") has limited value in diagnosing new onset hypertension. Increases in blood pressure may reflect normal physiologic return to prepregnancy blood pressure values after the initial decrease in blood pressure from progesterone-mediated smooth muscle relaxation in early pregnancy[18] or signs of developing pathology. Furthermore, gestational age and position of the patient affect increases in blood pressure. Diagnosis of hypertension is based upon sustained elevation of 140 mm Hg or more systolic or 90 or higher diastolic. Although not diagnostic, the "30/15 rule" does warrant further evaluation for signs and symptoms heralding the development of preeclampsia.[2]

NOTE: Relative, gradual increases in BP throughout a pregnancy signify a need to remain alert to risk factors, to the possibility of an increase in the presence of existing hypertension, and to the development of additional signs and symptoms.

Evaluating Proteinuria

Until recently, the diagnosis of preeclampsia required the presence of proteinuria. Proteinuria is no longer required for the diagnosis of preeclampsia when other signs of organ system involvement accompany new onset hypertension.

When renal function is normal in pregnancy, up to 300 mg of protein may be excreted in the urine each day due the increase in glomerular filtration. Greater than 300 mg in 24 hours exceeds the threshold for what would be considered normal urinary protein excretion, and may signify increased glomerular permeability from endothelial damage.[34]

Clinical Significance of Proteinuria[2]

- Although more substantial proteinuria has historically been considered to worsen the prognosis, the degree of proteinuria (above 5 g in 24 hours) has not demonstrated an effect upon the clinical course of the patients. Consequently, proteinuria has been eliminated from the criteria for consideration of preeclampsia as severe.
- Proteinuria is not required for the diagnosis of preeclampsia.
- Once preeclampsia is diagnosed, and after the initial finding of proteinuria, further evaluation of protein excretion in the urine is not necessary.

Measurement of Proteinuria

There are currently three methods for determining protein excretion: 24-hour urine collection, protein/creatinine ratio on a single-voided urine specimen, and urine dipstick. The 24-hour urine collection is considered the "gold standard."[34] Alternatively, a protein/creatinine (each measured as mg/dL) ratio of at least 0.3 is considered a threshold for the establishment of proteinuria in pregnancy.[2] Urine dipstick analysis is only moderately reliable. Readings can be falsely positive or falsely negative based on how it is performed and interpreted. In addition, a dipstick analysis of proteinuria on a urine specimen may not accurately represent protein excretion over a 24-hour period.[35]

- Interpretation when using a multiple reagent strip (dipstick) is as follows[36]:

Qualitative Interpretation	mg/dL
Negative	<10
Trace	10–20
1+	30
2+	100
3+	300
4+	1,000

Avoid "rounding up" of color assignments when reading the dipstick. This can lead to inaccurate readings.[35]

- Urine dipstick reading of 1+ of higher indicates proteinuria.
- Obtain clean urine samples. Aspirate fresh urine from the tubing of the retention catheter rather than from the collection bag. Or, preferably, obtain a sample of fresh urine from the urometer of a Foley catheter.
- When using a multiple reagent strip, test for specific gravity (SG) and pH.

NOTE: Urine SG less than 1.010 indices diluted urine, which may yield a false-negative value. Urine SG of 1.030 or more indicates concentrated urine, which may produce a false-positive value. Sulfosalicylic acid (very alkaline) or urine pH 8.0 or higher, may provide a false-negative test result.

• Increased urinary excretion of protein may be observed in the absence of renal pathology or preeclampsia with increased physical activity, upright position, increased catecholamine levels observed with emotional stress, corticosteroids, hematuria, or bacteriuria.[34]

Enhanced Surveillance of Women with Gestational Hypertension or Women with Preeclampsia without Severe Features

Women diagnosed with gestational hypertension may either have preeclampsia that has not been diagnosed due to the absence of fulfillment of the criteria for diagnosis of preeclampsia or may progress to preeclampsia. In addition, women with preeclampsia without severe features at less than 34 completed weeks' gestation may be managed as outpatient. These patients require enhanced surveillance for either onset of preeclampsia, in the setting of gestational hypertension, or progression to severe disease, in the setting of preeclampsia. The surveillance of these patients typically includes weekly determinations of platelet count and blood transaminases, CBC, and serum creatinine; twice weekly assessment of blood pressure (one of these blood pressures may be measured at home in gestational hypertensive patient); daily self-monitoring by the woman for symptoms of preeclampsia and fetal movement; measurement of urinary protein excretion at each obstetrical visit; and fetal surveillance (amniotic fluid volume, nonstress test, or biophysical profile) once to twice weekly.[2]

• **What are the symptoms of preeclampsia that the woman should be educated to report?[2]**

- Severe headache
- Visual disturbances
- Epigastric pain or right upper quadrant pain
- Shortness of breath
- Symptoms that indicate onset of labor or possible indication for induction of labor:
  - Persistent abdominal pain or uterine contractions
  - Vaginal spotting
  - Rupture of membranes
  - Decreased fetal movement

Assessment of Signs or Symptoms Reflecting Pathologic Alterations

- Systolic BP ≥140 mm Hg or diastolic BP ≥90 mm Hg. An elevation to this extent in a woman beyond 20 weeks' gestation on two occasions 4 hours or more apart may indicate preeclampsia or gestational hypertension. Failure of blood pressure to normalize postpartum indicates chronic hypertension.

Look for the following:
- Systolic BP ≥140 mm Hg or diastolic BP ≥90 mm Hg.
- Further elevation in systolic BP ≥160 mm Hg OR diastolic BP ≥110 mm Hg. Repeat blood pressure measurement in 15 minutes. Blood pressure sustained at either systolic BP ≥160 mm Hg or diastolic BP ≥110 mm Hg in a preeclamptic patient constitutes a hypertensive emergency that necessitates urgent administration of antihypertensive agents.
- Scrutinize BP and laboratory values with development of other signs and symptoms.

- Endothelial injury and increased capillary permeability promote the shift of fluids from the intravascular compartment to the interstitium, decreasing intravascular volume. Despite the observation of peripheral edema, women with preeclampsia, especially with severe features, often have intravascular volume depletion.
- Preeclamptic women are more likely to sustain epidural-mediated hypotension with resultant abnormal FHR following initiation of epidural analgesia or anesthesia. Sympathetic blockade from the anesthetic dilates the systemic vasculature, which decreases venous return of blood to the heart and decreases cardiac output, manifested as hypotension. These patients may require more than the typical 500-mL intravenous fluid bolus prior to initiating the epidural.[37]

Look for the following:
- New onset minimal FHR variability or FHR decelerations
- Hypotension after initiation of epidural analgesia or anesthesia

- Blood loss at birth or from placental abruption further exacerbates the state of decreased circulating blood volume, predisposing the women with preeclampsia to acute renal failure.

Look for the following:
- Fetal bradycardia
- New onset minimal FHR variability or FHR decelerations
- Vaginal bleeding
- Decreased urine output or oliguria
- Signs of maternal hypovolemic shock (tachycardia which often precedes hypotension, decreased peripheral perfusion)

- The shift of intravascular fluid volume into the interstitium, predisposes women with preeclampsia to the development of pulmonary edema, which presents postpartum more often than before birth.[21] Optimal intravascular volume management is often difficult to achieve because of the intravascular volume depletion from the disease process and indications for fluid volume expansion in labor. Intravascular volume expansion with intravenous fluids beyond what is necessary to correct oliguria, abnormal FHR patterns, or hemodynamic instability should be avoided, when possible, because of the potential for development of pulmonary edema postpartum.

Look for the following:
- Decreased hemoglobin arterial oxygen saturation (SaO_2)
- Shortness of breath, dyspnea, orthopnea, or adventitious lung sounds

NOTE: Pulmonary edema in preeclampsia is attributed more often to endothelial capillary injury (noncardiogenic) rather than fluid overload or left ventricular failure (cardiogenic). Even with optimal intravascular fluid volume management, women with preeclampsia are at risk for developing pulmonary edema, most often postpartally.[21]

- Hemoconcentration may reflect decreased intravascular blood volume. A decline in hematocrit values may reflect normalization of circulating blood volume, but may likely indicate either excessive blood loss or hemolysis.[11]

Look for the following:
- Elevated hematocrit values
OR
- Falling hematocrit values if there is excessive blood loss or hemolysis. Evaluate hematocrit and hemoglobin values in light of heart rate, blood pressure, or other signs of decreased peripheral perfusion

- Thrombocytopenia suggests platelet aggregation and consumption.

Look for the following:
- Decreasing platelets; thrombocytopenia is defined by a platelet count of less than 100,000/mm[3,11]

- **In normal pregnancies,** renal blood flow increases by 50% during early pregnancy and remains at this level until late into the third trimester. The resultant increase in the glomerular filtration rate leads to an *increase* in *urinary* excretion of creatinine with a concomitant *decrease* in *serum* creatinine, blood urea nitrogen (BUN), and uric acid levels.
- In **preeclampsia,** renal perfusion and glomerular filtration are reduced. *Urinary excretion of creatinine decrease and serum creatinine and BUN levels increase.* Plasma uric acid concentration tends to be high in some women with preeclampsia.

Look for the following:
- Proteinuria greater than 300 mg/L per 24 hours or protein/creatinine ratio of 0.3
- Elevated BUN
- Elevated uric acid
- Elevated serum creatinine (serum values may increase several times over nonpregnant values in the setting of significant renal insufficiency)

NOTE: As urine urea nitrogen and creatinine levels fall, blood levels rise.

- Headache and visual disturbances (blurred vision, diplopia, scotomata, visualizing flashes of light) associated with preeclampsia herald seizures in some women with preeclampsia. The pathophysiologic mechanism inciting eclampsia has not been determined with precision.[22]

Look for the following:
- A complaint of dizziness or visual disturbances, such as blurred vision, scotomata, visualizing flashes of light, or diplopia
- Persistent, sometimes severe headache

- Systemic arteriolar vasospasm may produce hepatic infarction with subsequent hemorrhage in the liver capsule, or subcapsular hematoma, which may rupture into the peritoneal space (hepatic rupture) ensuing with shock and potentially, death.[21]

Look for the following:
- Elevated serum transaminase levels, such as increase in AST or ALT more than two times the upper limit of normal
- A complaint of *epigastric or right upper quadrant pain*
- Signs of hypovolemic shock, including tachycardia, which often precedes, oliguria, decreased peripheral perfusion (sluggish capillary refill, cool extremities, inability to register SaO_2, cool, clammy skin), hypotension, or reduced level of consciousness

NOTE: The physiologic compensatory response to hypovolemic shock (vasoconstriction) preferentially perfuses the heart and brain at the expense of nonessential organs (kidneys, peripheral tissues, uteroplacental unit). Tachycardia often precedes other signs of hemodynamic compromise (hypotension and end-organ disturbances). In addition, the patient may remain alert, talk appropriately, and appear "stable" despite hemodynamic compromise. Efforts to stabilize the woman should occur with appearance of unstable vital signs and clinical signs of decreased end-organ perfusion. The ability of the woman to be conversant should not reassure care providers that she is stable.

- Decreased uteroplacental blood flow may produce abnormal FHR patterns or other clinical findings associated with hypoxemia.

Look for the following:
- New onset absent or minimal fetal heart rate variability, recurrent decelerations of the fetal heart rate, fetal tachycardia
- Reduced amniotic fluid index by ultrasound
- Reported findings of intrauterine fetal growth restriction, low biophysical profile score, abnormal Doppler velocimetry findings

NOTE: Nonstress testing (NST), ultrasound assessment of fetal activity (BPP), and amniotic fluid index are recommended antenatal fetal surveillance methods for the evaluation of gestational hypertension or increasing severity of manifestations of preeclampsia (Task Force, 2013).

Detecting Symptoms of Preeclampsia While Admitting the Laboring Woman

- Conduct a comprehensive review of the laboring woman's prenatal record, as well as evaluating her current clinical presentation.

- Review her past medical and obstetric history to identify predisposing factors.
- Evaluate blood pressure.
- Note sudden, considerable weight gain or excessive overall weight gain.

Although not diagnostic of preeclampsia, SUDDEN, EXCESSIVE WEIGHT GAIN may indicate IMPENDING PREECLAMPSIA. Further assessment of blood pressure, proteinuria, and other signs and symptoms of preeclampsia will determine the diagnosis of preeclampsia.

- A history of or current complaints of headache or blurred vision.
- Assess deep tendon reflexes (patellar reflex). This serves as a baseline for comparison to determine if deep tendon reflexes have decreased as an early sign of magnesium sulfate toxicity.
- Obtain a clean-catch or catheterized urine specimen for proteinuria.
- Inquire about vague symptoms that may have an association with preeclampsia, such as nausea and vomiting, malaise, or "just not feeling right."

Detecting Severe Features of Preeclampsia[2]

Severe features of preeclampsia include the following:
- Either systolic BP of 160 mm Hg or higher OR diastolic BP of 110 mm Hg or higher on two occasions, 4 hours apart

After any initial systolic BP of 160 mm Hg or higher OR any initial diastolic BP of 110 mm Hg or higher, REPEAT BP MEASUREMENT IN 15 MINUTES. If blood pressure remains elevated at this level, NOTIFY THE PHYSICIAN IMMEDIATELY to facilitate immediate administration of antihypertensive therapy.

- Visual disturbances
- Cerebral disturbances, such as altered level of consciousness, irritability, restlessness, or apprehension
- Severe, persistent epigastric pain or right upper quadrant pain or pain unresponsive to pain medication
- Renal insufficiency, defined by either serum creatinine greater than 1.1 mg/dL or doubling of serum creatinine

Look for oliguria:
- Urine output less than 30 mL per hour for 2 consecutive hours
- Urine output less than 100 mL over 4 hours
- Urine output less than 400 mL in 24 hours

- Thrombocytopenia
- Elevated blood transaminases (ALT or AST) to twice the upper limit of normal
- Pulmonary edema

Early identification of worsening preeclampsia in a patient at a level I or II hospital is critical in order to ensure timely transport of the woman to a tertiary hospital.

Preeclampsia with severe features can result in acute and long-term complications in both the woman and fetus or newborn. For women with preeclampsia with severe features at or above 34 weeks' gestation, delivery after maternal stabilization is recommended. Delivery after initial maternal stabilization is warranted at any gestational age when either the mother or fetus is unstable.

- **What are the complications that compel urgent delivery irrespective of gestational age?[2]**

- Abruptio placentae
- Eclampsia or other persistent cerebral symptoms

- DIC
- Severe thrombocytopenia
- Acute renal failure
- Pulmonary edema
- Abnormal FHR or abnormal fetal surveillance
- Intrauterine fetal demise

Detecting HELLP Syndrome

HELLP syndrome is not a separate disease entity, but a subtype of preeclampsia. It is characterized by laboratory features that include hemolysis, elevated liver enzymes, and low platelets. The underlying pathophysiology as described earlier includes the following:
- Endothelial injury and arteriolar vasospasm.
- Platelet aggregation at sites of endothelial injury. The clotting cascade may be activated with fibrin deposition.
- Red blood cells are forced through narrowed network under high pressure, resulting in hemolysis, which damages erythrocytes (schistocytes, Burr cells).

H—hemolysis as detected with the following:
- Abnormal red blood cells on a peripheral smear
- Elevated LDH
- Falling hematocrit in the absence of blood loss
- Bilirubin greater than 1.2 mg/dL

- Maternal liver dysfunction results from microemboli in the hepatic vasculature, which causes ischemia and tissue damage within the liver.

EL—elevated liver enzymes
- AST greater than twice the upper limit of normal
- ALT greater than twice the upper limit of normal
- LDH greater than 600 IU/L

In addition to review of laboratory results, assess for symptoms:
- Feelings of malaise
- Viral-like syndrome
- Right upper quadrant pain or epigastric pain

- Thrombocytopenia occurs because of increased platelet consumption.

LP—low platelets
- Low, less than 100,000/mm^3
- Severe, less than 50,000/mm^3

In the setting of intrauterine fetal demise or placental abruption, also evaluate the following:
- Coagulation studies
- Hematuria
- Mucosal bleeding, bleeding around IV sites or incision
- Petechiae
- Easy bruising

NOTE: Coagulation studies, such as prothrombin time, partial thromboplastin time, fibrinogen, and bleeding times are typically normal in the absence of placental abruption or intrauterine fetal demise.[21]

Priorities for Treatment and Nursing Management

Management of Preeclampsia

The primary goals in the management of the preeclamptic woman are as follows:
1. Control of hypertension
2. Optimizing end-organ perfusion

3. Prevention of seizures in women with severe features of preeclampsia
4. Stabilization of the woman and fetus so that a vaginal or cesarean birth can be accomplished

The *definitive treatment* for preeclampsia is delivery. Clinical management of preeclampsia without severe features usually involves a conservative approach, with weekly or twice weekly office visits (refer to assessments included in Enhanced Surveillance of Women with Gestational Hypertension or Women with Preeclampsia without Severe Features in the section, "Expert Clinical Assessment"), in order to perform frequent laboratory and physical assessments. Fetal surveillance includes tests, such as fetal movement counting, nonstress testing, and biophysical profile. Hospitalization is required for the following findings[2]:

- Systolic blood pressure of 160 mm Hg or higher or diastolic blood pressure of 110 mm Hg or higher
- Nonreassuring fetal surveillance
- Intrauterine growth restriction
- Elevated liver function tests
- Decreased platelets
- Labor onset or rupture of membranes

Once the woman achieves 37 0/7 weeks' gestation and remains stable without severe features of preeclampsia, onset of labor, or premature rupture of membranes, it is recommended that the patient be delivered, even if cervical ripening agents are necessary.[2]

Management of Preeclampsia with Severe Features

Management focuses on monitoring for progression of severity of preeclampsia or any maternal–fetal instability. Expectant management (continued observation without movement toward delivery unless there is a change in maternal or fetal condition) versus proceeding with delivery is based upon gestational age and whether there is any maternal or fetal instability. Delivery is recommended for any woman with preeclampsia with severe features with any of the following[2]:

- Gestational age of 34 0/7 weeks or greater
- Following maternal stabilization, regardless of gestational age when one of the following complications presents:
  - Eclampsia
  - Pulmonary edema
  - DIC
  - Uncontrolled, severe hypertension
  - Nonviable fetus
  - Abnormal fetal surveillance
  - Placental abruption
  - Intrauterine fetal demise

The American College of Obstetricians and Gynecologists[2] recommends hospitalization in a tertiary care center with delivery after 48 hours of antenatal corticosteroids for stable women less than 34 0/7 weeks' gestation with any of the following:

- Persistent symptoms of severe disease
- HELLP syndrome
- Intrauterine fetal growth restriction with estimated fetal weight less than the fifth percentile
- Severe oligohydramnios
- Reversed umbilical artery end-diastolic flow (Doppler velocimetry studies)
- Labor
- Premature rupture of membranes
- Significant renal dysfunction

During antepartum observation in the hospital, assessment should include the following:

- Vital signs and intake and output at least every 8 hours
- Monitoring for symptoms that indicate progressing severity every 8 hours: headaches, visual changes, epigastric or right upper quadrant pain or pressure, shortness of breath, nausea and vomiting
- Monitoring at least 8 hours for onset of labor or rupture of membranes
- Daily laboratory evaluation of CBC (includes platelet count), blood transaminases, and serum creatinine (these may be evaluated every other day if they remain stable and the patient remains asymptomatic)

- Nonstress test with uterine contraction monitoring along with evaluation of fetal movement daily
- Biophysical profile twice weekly
- Ultrasound every 2 weeks for assessment of fetal growth. Umbilical artery Doppler velocimetry is typically added to the assessment if growth restriction is suspected

Hospitalization facilitates timely administration of antihypertensives for severe, elevated blood pressures and timely delivery of the infant should the woman or fetus become unstable or if the symptoms of severe disease become more progressive and persistent.

- Obtain standardized BP readings by practicing the following steps:
  - Keep the arm supported in a horizontal position at the level of the heart.
  - Ensure that BP readings are taken with the woman in the same posture each time, when possible.
  - Use the sitting position when possible. If the blood pressure is taken in the lateral position, the blood pressure cuff is placed on the arm at the level of the heart.

BP readings are as follows:
- Highest when supine or standing
- Higher when the blood pressure is taken in the arm below heart level
- Intermediate when sitting (recommended when possible)
- Lower in the lateral recumbent position
- Lower when the blood pressure is taken in the arm above heart level

- When auscultating the blood pressure, use the fifth phase disappearance of the sound (the K5 sound). Use the muffled sound (K4) if Korotkoff sound persists after full blood pressure cuff deflation.
- Bedrest during the antepartum period is not recommended unless there is another clinical condition that warrants bedrest. During labor, place the woman in a lateral recumbent or semirecumbent position. This alleviates compression of the maternal vena cava and aorta; and enhances uteroplacental perfusion, thus benefiting the fetus. Continuous electronic fetal monitoring is recommended during labor.
- During labor, record hourly intake and output using a Foley catheter with a urometer.

Oliguria (less than 30 mL/hr for 2 hours) can result from intravascular volume depletion, renal vasospasm, or cardiac failure. Oliguria is an indication of renal insufficiency that necessitates physician notification.

- Administer intravenous fluid judiciously, reserving intravenous fluid boluses for initiation of epidural analgesia, maternal tachycardia or hypotension, oliguria, or intrauterine fetal resuscitation. Limit maintenance rate of fluid administration to no more than 150 mL/hr.

The woman is at risk for pulmonary edema postpartum because of endothelial injury and increased capillary permeability. Even with judicious administration of intravenous fluids, she may develop pulmonary edema. Intravenous fluid boluses should not be withheld when there is an indication for intravascular volume expansion, but should be reserved for signs suggestive of decreased circulating blood volume.

- Use side rails when the patient is in bed.
- Obtain appropriate laboratory workup, which includes the following:
  - Complete blood count (CBC) with platelets and type and screen
  - Liver function tests
  - DIC profile, when indicated by bleeding, such as from placental abruption
- When testing urine for protein excretion, *use a fresh specimen* from the Foley catheter tubing or urometer.
- Assess deep tendon reflexes hourly to determine an early sign of magnesium sulfate toxicity.
- Certain premonitory signs and symptoms may indicate an elevated risk for eclampsia and the physician may consider magnesium sulfate infusion. Monitor the patient for headache, altered mental status, blurred vision, scotomata, clonus, and RUQ pain. Report these symptoms to the physician.

- HAVE EMERGENCY EQUIPMENT READY—SEIZURE PRECAUTIONS.
  - Oxygen and suctioning equipment. Check that the equipment is in operating order.
  - Be able to immediately locate an emergency cart with airway and other resuscitation supplies.
- Administer magnesium sulfate according to the physician's orders. Intrapartum parenteral magnesium sulfate is recommended for preeclampsia with severe features. Although routinely administered as an intravenous infusion, it may be given intramuscularly.

Intravenous administration of magnesium sulfate is recommended because it permits more precise control of serum magnesium blood levels in the woman. Also, the pain of an intramuscular injection is avoided.

- Evaluate the patient for signs of pulmonary edema (shortness of breath, orthopnea, decreased SaO_2) and report them to the physician immediately in order to expedite an order for a chest x-ray.[38]

The woman with preeclampsia requires ongoing assessment for progression in severity of the disease.

Intrapartum Pain Management[2,8,9]

- Vaginal birth is preferable to cesarean delivery. Cesarean delivery is typically reserved for obstetric indications (such as breech presentation, arrest of dilatation or fetal descent disorders, category III FHR tracings or some category II FHR tracings).
- Continuous epidural analgesia for pain relief during labor in women with severe hypertensive disease does not appear to increase cesarean birth rates, maternal pulmonary edema, or acute renal failure.
- Coagulopathy or thrombocytopenia predisposes the patient to epidural or spinal hematoma with regional anesthesia.

Either a systolic BP of 160 mm Hg or higher or a diastolic BP of 110 mm Hg or higher predisposes the woman with preeclampsia to hemorrhagic stroke.[39] Blood pressure elevation that is sustained at this level for 15 minutes necessitates immediate administration of an intravenous antihypertensive agent,[38] even if the elevated blood pressure is attributed to pain.

Anticonvulsant Therapy

- **What is the current recommended treatment schedule for administering magnesium sulfate to the woman with preeclampsia with severe features?**

Magnesium sulfate is given for seizure prophylaxis. Although the smooth muscle relaxation may initially decrease blood pressure, **it is not given to treat hypertension**.

Magnesium sulfate is the drug of choice for seizure prophylaxis in preeclamptic women.[2] It is recognized as a high-risk medication and medication errors with the potential to cause adverse outcome are common.[40,41] The following recommendations represent currently accepted practices in the treatment of the preeclamptic woman with magnesium sulfate.[2,40,41]

- Indications for magnesium sulfate include the following[2]:
  - Preeclampsia with severe features
  - Eclampsia
- When given for seizure prophylaxis, an intravenous loading dose of 4 to 6 g is given over 20 to 30 minutes followed by a maintenance infusion of 1 to 2 g/h for at least 24 hours.
  - Women may sustain an eclamptic seizure despite magnesium sulfate therapy, usually as a result of subtherapeutic levels which necessitates ongoing assessment for seizures in addition to magnesium toxicity.

* Some women may require a higher infusion rate in order to achieve therapeutic magnesium levels.
* When given for eclampsia, a loading dose followed by maintenance infusion as described above for seizure prophylaxis is typically recommended if the patient has an eclamptic seizure prior to initiating magnesium sulfate. An eclamptic seizure during magnesium sulfate infusion may be treated with an additional 2 g intravenous bolus infusion of magnesium sulfate.[21]
    * Seizures refractory to magnesium sulfate infusion may be treated with 100 mg thiopental sodium (Pentothal), 1 to 10 mg diazepam (Valium), or sodium amobarbital up to 250 mg IV.[21]
    * Anticipate respiratory depression with higher doses of magnesium sulfate or when other anticonvulsant agents are administered. Ensure immediate access to airway supplies and be prepared to assist with endotracheal intubation and mechanical ventilation.

Recurrent seizure activity despite adequate magnesium sulfate therapy may indicate other neurologic pathology, such as cerebral edema or cerebral venous thrombosis. Therefore, anticipate CT evaluation of the brain once the patient has been stabilized.[21]

Magnesium sulfate should be continued during the intrapartum or intraoperative period. Despite the prolongation of the duration of nondepolarizing muscle relaxants used for anesthesia, ACOG recommends against discontinuing magnesium sulfate during delivery for the following reasons[2]:
* The half-life of magnesium sulfate is 5 hours. Discontinuing magnesium sulfate during delivery will have minimal benefit on the desired intent to avoid anesthetic interactions.
* Discontinuing magnesium sulfate may lead to eclampsia from subtherapeutic magnesium serum level.
* The physiologic stress of anesthesia induction and delivery escalates the risk for eclampsia.

Universal prophylaxis to women with preeclampsia is not recommended unless systolic BP is 160 mm Hg or higher, diastolic BP is 110 mm Hg or higher, there are severe features, or there are premonitory maternal symptoms for eclampsia.[2]

---

* **What are the recommended practices for administration of magnesium sulfate as a high-risk medication to promote patient safety?[40,41]**

---

* Use standardized concentration of magnesium sulfate, prepared by a central pharmacy.
* Use a controlled infusion device with free-flow protection for all infusions of magnesium sulfate.
* Clearly label IV bags with easy-to-read large print and colored labels.
* Use a separate IV bag for the bolus dose rather than bolusing from the IV bag used for maintenance infusion. The loading dose should be delivered via a 100- to 150-mL IV solution. The maintenance infusion should employ a separate, 500-mL IV solution.
* Ensure that institutional practice incorporates double-checks of the magnesium sulfate solution and programmed rate during initiation, any time the dose is adjusted, and during hand-offs to other care providers.
* Monitor hourly for signs of magnesium toxicity.
* Ensure rapid access to calcium gluconate.
* Refrain from abbreviating magnesium sulfate as $MgSO_4$ anywhere in the medical record.

---

* **What special monitoring of the patient is required during administration of magnesium sulfate?**

The precise mechanism of action for magnesium sulfate as an anticonvulsant agent is unknown. In therapeutic ranges, magnesium sulfate slows neuromuscular conduction and may depress central nervous system irritability.[40] The purpose of the drug is to prevent the recurrence of eclamptic seizures. During the loading dose, ensure continuous nursing presence at the bedside to assess maternal and fetal status.

- Review or obtain baseline assessment data prior to initiating the loading dose, to include:
  - Maternal vital signs
  - SpO_2
  - Level of consciousness
  - FHR parameters, to include baseline FHR, baseline FHR variability, accelerations, and/or the presence of decelerations
  - Uterine activity
- Observe and document the following assessments every 15 minutes for the first hour, every 30 minutes during the second hour, and at least hourly during the maintenance infusion:
  - Respiratory rate
  - SpO_2
  - Deep tendon reflexes (may be monitored every 2 hours after the initial few hours)
  - Level of consciousness
  - Urine output
  - Toleration of the medication and any side effects

The therapeutic range for magnesium sulfate is a serum magnesium level of 3 to 7 mEq/L (4 to 8 mg/dL). Concentrations greater than 7 mEq/L (8 mg/dL) suggest magnesium toxicity. Signs of magnesium toxicity include:

- Loss of deep tendon reflexes
- Respiratory depression
- Loss of consciousness

Respiratory and cardiac arrest may ensue if toxicity is not remedied with calcium gluconate.

- Protocols for nursing supervision of patients on magnesium sulfate typically incorporate a 1:1 nurse-to-patient ratio.
- Magnesium sulfate is excreted by the kidneys. Oliguria increases the risk for magnesium toxicity.

TO AVOID THE RISK OF TOXICITY:
Vigilantly monitor DTRs and respiratory rate. Ensure that respiratory rate is at least 12 breaths per minute and that patellar reflexes are present. Obtain serum magnesium level if signs of toxicity are present. Discontinue magnesium sulfate for respiratory depression or decreased level of consciousness while awaiting serum magnesium level results. Monitor urine output.

The most common causes of toxicity are
1. Iatrogenic overdosage
2. Decreased urinary excretion of magnesium, which may occur in the setting of renal insufficiency.

- **How is a magnesium sulfate overdose managed?**

Calcium gluconate is the antidote to magnesium toxicity.

- Administer 1 g of calcium gluconate intravenously slowly over 3 minutes (each milliliter of 10 mL vial of 10% calcium gluconate solution contains 0.1 g of calcium gluconate).[40]
- Establish airway and provide ventilatory support for respiratory arrest.

Antihypertensive Therapy: Current Recommendations

There is consensus to treat severe hypertension (systolic BP ≥160 mm Hg or diastolic BP ≥110 mm Hg) in order to reduce the risk of end-organ complications, such as placental abruption, stroke, and pulmonary edema.[1,2,42] The higher threshold for treating acute onset of hypertension during pregnancy is based upon the lack of evidence that "mild" hypertension of short duration (usually about 4 to 5 months) adversely affects maternal outcomes. In addition, antihypertensive therapy may compromise uteroplacental perfusion.[1] Rather than normalizing blood pressure, the goal of treatment is to achieve both a systolic blood pressure in the range of 140 to less than 159 mm Hg and a diastolic blood pressure in the range of 90 to 100 in order to avoid prolonged, repeated exposure to severe systolic hypertension with subsequent loss of cerebral vascular autoregulation.[42]

First-Line Antihypertensive Therapy for Acute Management of Hypertension

Either a systolic BP of 160 mm Hg or higher OR a diastolic BP of 110 mm Hg or higher constitutes an obstetric emergency and warrants immediate administration of intravenous antihypertensive medication.[38,42] Either parenteral labetalol or hydralazine or oral nifedipine are considered first-line therapy for the control of severe hypertension in the pregnant or postpartum patient with preeclampsia. The current guidelines for emergent therapy for acute onset, severe hypertension with preeclampsia or eclampsia are as follows[42]:

- After initial reading of either a systolic BP ≥160 mm Hg or diastolic BP ≥110 mm Hg, repeat BP measurement in 15 minutes. Notify physician immediately if BP values remain in this range and anticipate an order for an intravenous antihypertensive.
- Administer the intravenous antihypertensive in accordance with the physician's order with anticipation that the order will reflect the following guidelines:

*NOTE: Target BP threshold includes **both**:*
- *Systolic BP 140 to 159 mm Hg*
- *Diastolic BP 90 to 100 mm Hg*

Labetalol	**Hydralazine**
Initial dose: 20 mg IV push over 2 minutes	Initial dose: 5–10 mg IV push over 2 minutes
Take BP 10 minutes after dose. If BP is still elevated, proceed to next dose	*Take BP 20 minutes after dose. If BP is still elevated, proceed to next dose.*
Second dose: 40 mg IV push over 2 minutes	Second dose: 10 mg IV push over 2 minutes
Take BP 10 minutes after dose. If BP is still elevated, proceed to next dose	*Take BP 20 minutes after dose. If BP is still elevated, proceed to labetalol.*
Third dose: 80 mg IV push over 2 minutes	**Change medication to labetalol.** Give 20 mg IV push over 2 minutes
Take BP 10 minutes after dose. If BP is still elevated, proceed to hydralazine.	*Take BP 10 minutes after dose. If BP is still elevated, proceed to next dose*
Change medication to hydralazine. Give 10 mg IV push over 2 minutes	Second dose of labetalol: give 40 mg IV push over 2 minutes
Take BP 20 minutes after hydralazine. Notify provider if BP is still elevated.	*Take BP 10 minutes after dose. Notify provider if BP is still elevated.*

OR

Nifedipine

Initial dose: 10 mg orally
> *Take BP 20 minutes after dose. If BP is still elevated proceed to next dose*

Second dose: 20 mg orally
> *Take BP 20 minutes after dose. If BP is still elevated proceed to next dose*

Third dose: 20 mg orally
> *Take BP 20 minutes after dose. If BP is still elevated proceed to next dose*

Change medication to labetalol. Give 40 mg IV push over 2 minutes.
> *Take BP 10 minutes after dose. If BP still elevated, notify provider*

- Once target BP is achieved, ACOG recommends the following frequency for assessment of blood pressure:
  - Every 10 minutes for 1 hour
  - Every 15 minutes for 1 hour
  - Every 30 minutes for 1 hour
  - Every 4 hours thereafter
- Initiate electronic FHR monitoring if appropriate for gestational age of fetus (i.e., fetal viability).
- In the event that intravenous access has not yet been obtained and acute therapy is warranted, anticipate order for 200 mg of labetalol orally to be repeated in 30 minutes if target

blood pressure is not achieved. The guideline for administration of labetalol is illustrated in Figure 11.2 and the guideline for administration of hydralazine is illustrated in Figure 11.3.

Oral nifedipine has been compared to intravenous labetalol for the treatment of acute, severe hypertension[43,44] and has lowered blood pressure effectively in these studies. Short-acting, or immediate-release, nifedipine significantly increases the risk of a precipitous fall in maternal blood pressure and is therefore not recommended for the acute treatment of hypertension in pregnancy.[1,2]

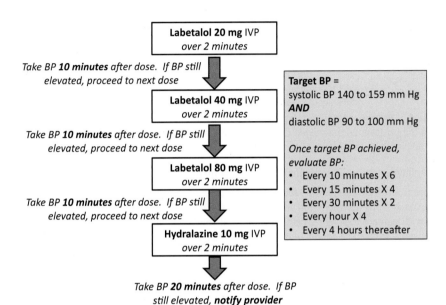

FIGURE 11.2 Guideline for administering intravenous labetalol for acute, severe hypertension in preeclampsia. (Source: Author. Adapted from Task Force on Hypertension in Pregnancy. (2013). *Hypertension in Pregnancy* (pp. 1–89). Washington, DC: American College of Obstetricians and Gynecologists.)

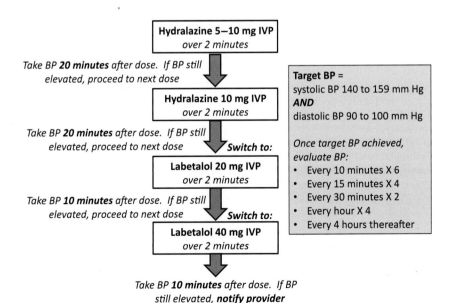

FIGURE 11.3 Guidelines for administering intravenous hydralazine for acute, severe hypertension in preeclampsia. (Source: Author. Adapted from Task Force on Hypertension in Pregnancy. (2013). *Hypertension in Pregnancy* (pp. 1–89). Washington, DC: American College of Obstetricians and Gynecologists.)

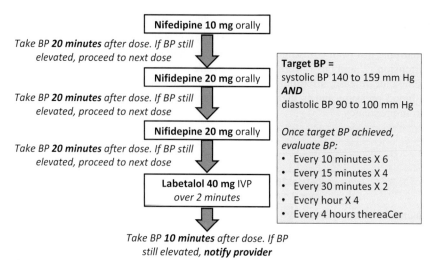

*Take BP **20 minutes** after dose. If BP still elevated, proceed to next dose*

Nifedipine 10 mg orally

Nifidepine 20 mg orally

*Take BP **20 minutes** after dose. If BP still elevated, proceed to next dose*

Nifidepine 20 mg orally

*Take BP **20 minutes** after dose. If BP still elevated, proceed to next dose*

Labetalol 40 mg IVP
over 2 minutes

Target BP =
systolic BP 140 to 159 mm Hg
AND
diastolic BP 90 to 100 mm Hg

Once target BP achieved, evaluate BP:
• Every 10 minutes X 6
• Every 15 minutes X 4
• Every 30 minutes X 2
• Every hour X 4
• Every 4 hours thereaCer

*Take BP **10 minutes** after dose. If BP still elevated, **notify provider***

FIGURE 11.4 Source: ACOG. Emergent therapy for acute-onset, severe hypertension during pregnancy and the postpartum period. ACOG Committee Opinion, 2015; No 514.

Second-Line Antihypertensive Therapy for Acute Management of Hypertension

Failure of parenteral hydralazine or labetalol to achieve adequate control of blood pressure is rare. However, if both regimens fail to achieve target threshold blood pressure, emergency consultation with a maternal–fetal specialist, internal medicine or critical care specialist, or anesthesiologist is advised. Second-line agents include continuous intravenous infusion of labetalol or continuous intravenous infusion of nicardipine. Sodium nitroprusside is reserved for extreme emergencies where duration of therapy is short in order to avert fetal cyanide and thiocyanate toxicity.[42]

Antihypertensive Agents Used for Continuous Management of Hypertension during Pregnancy

Women with chronic hypertension or preeclamptic women before 34 weeks' gestation who are closely observed and managed expectantly may receive antihypertensive medications during pregnancy. A women with chronic hypertension who has been taking antihypertensive medications may require medication adjustments in order to ensure that she is receiving the safest medication possible to produce the desired effect of controlling hypertension. The two most common categories for antihypertensive medications used to manage chronic hypertension before pregnancy, are angiotensin-converting enzyme (ACE) inhibitors and diuretics. ACE inhibitors are contraindicated during pregnancy.[29] They are associated with congenital malformations in the first trimester, effecting primarily the fetal cardiovascular and central nervous systems[2,29] and later in pregnancy they are associated with fetal anuria, fetal renal failure, oligohydramnios,[29] fetal pulmonary hypoplasia, and intrauterine fetal growth restriction.[2] These patients will require conversion to an alternate medication. Women who were taking diuretics prior to pregnancy may be continued on diuretic therapy during the pregnancy, despite the increased risk for decreasing maternal circulating blood volume, which may potentially compromise uteroplacental perfusion.[29] Antihypertensive agents that are most commonly used during pregnancy include labetalol, slow-release nifedipine, and methyldopa.[2] An overview of the medications that may be encountered during care of the woman requiring continuous management of hypertension follows. Common antihypertensives used for ongoing management of hypertension in pregnancy are summarized in Table 11.2.

Alpha-Adrenergic Agonists

Methyldopa (Aldomet) is the most widely used antihypertensive pharmacologic agent for the management of chronic hypertension in pregnancy.[2,29,45] This medication is metabolized to alpha methylnorepinephrine, which replaces norepinephrine at its site of action, thereby blocking alpha-2 receptors.[45] As a result of alpha-2 receptor blockade, sympathetic tone is reduced, promoting vasodilation and gradually lowering blood pressure.[29] Side effects, such as decreased mental alertness, fatigue, and impaired sleep are attributed to the central alpha-2 blockade.[45]

Nonselective Beta-Adrenergic Blockers

Labetalol has become a more favored antihypertensive agent in pregnancy[29] and lowers blood pressure by antagonizing both beta and peripheral alpha-1 receptors.[2,29] Its nonselective beta-receptor antagonist activity makes it more favorable to pure beta-1 antagonists, such as atenolol. Pure beta-1 blockers lower cardiac output by blocking beta-1 receptors in the heart with potential negative effect upon uteroplacental perfusion and fetal growth.[29] Labetalol's effects upon beta-1 receptors are moderated by its alpha-1 blocking activity, which promotes peripheral vasodilation. Beta-1 antagonist mediated effects of decreased cardiac output, decreased heart rate, and bronchoconstriction explain why it should be avoided in patients with asthma or cardiac disease.

Calcium Channel Blockers

Nifedipine promotes vasodilation primarily by blocking calcium entry into the arterial muscle cells. Nifedipine does not appear to negatively impact uteroplacental perfusion and is considered an acceptable medication for the treatment of hypertension in pregnancy.[2] The sublingual form is discouraged for the treatment of hypertension.

Diuretics

A possible side effect of diuretics is the reduction of circulating blood volume, which may negatively impact uteroplacental perfusion.[29] They are generally discouraged during pregnancy[46] unless the woman was already managed with diuretic therapy prior to pregnancy.

Special Delivery Preparation

Administration of corticosteroids for 48 hours prior to birth in order to promote fetal lung maturity is recommended for women with preeclampsia accompanied by severe features less than 34 weeks' gestation unless they require immediate delivery for either maternal or fetal instability. These patients should be cared for in a facility with adequate maternal and neonatal intensive care resources (typically tertiary facility). It is further recommended that any patient with severe features of preeclampsia who are candidates for continued observation during pregnancy be cared for at a tertiary hospital as well.[2]

The dynamic and progressive nature of preeclampsia may lead to rapid clinical deterioration of the woman and/or fetus. These women remain at risk for eclampsia, cerebrovascular accidents in the setting of severe, acute elevations in blood pressure, placental abruption, and renal insufficiency. Frequent monitoring for maternal, cerebral, and neurologic symptoms, FHR changes, urine output, vital signs, and new onset of symptoms such as epigastric or right upper quadrant pain throughout the intrapartum period is warranted.

Recognize that any significant fall in BP soon after delivery in these women often reflects excessive blood loss and not a return to a more normotensive state.

Oliguria soon after delivery may signify blood loss. Hemoglobin and hematocrit should be evaluated if there is oliguria that does not respond to an intravenous fluid bolus or that is accompanied by maternal tachycardia, drop in blood pressure, or other signs of decreased end-organ perfusion. Ascertainment of hemoglobin and hematocrit status will enable the identification of anemia from blood loss, which will facilitate optimizing end-organ perfusion with blood transfusion.

- Epidural analgesia/anesthesia is considered safe and is the anesthetic of choice in preeclampsia, if preceded by volume preloading, to prevent maternal hypotension. An intravenous fluid bolus of 500 mL may not be insufficient to prevent the onset of hypotension. Maintenance of intravenous fluid management consists of normal saline or lactated Ringer's solution at a rate of 100 to 125 mL/hr, but no more than 150 mL/hr.
- Intravenous fluid boluses should only be administered when the need for intravascular volume expansion is evident (i.e., FHR abnormality associated with intravascular volume depletion, oliguria, maternal hypotension, or tachycardia). Intravenous fluids decrease COP

through hemodilution of circulating plasma proteins. This, combined with increased capillary permeability from endothelial injury, may lead to pulmonary edema. Pulmonary edema most often presents postpartum, after the intravenous fluids were administered, necessitating vigilant monitoring for signs and symptoms consistent with pulmonary edema.

Postpartum Care and Education, Including Long-Term Outcomes

Women with preeclampsia continue to be at risk for adverse events postpartum, such as eclampsia, hypertensive encephalopathy, pulmonary edema, and stroke.[2] Women with preeclampsia, particularly those women with severe features accompanying preeclampsia, recurrent preeclampsia (preeclampsia in two or more pregnancies), or preeclampsia prior to 34 weeks' gestation[7,47,48] have an increased risk also for cardiovascular disease, including ischemic heart disease and stroke[49,50] later in life that necessitates further evaluation following childbirth and life-style modifications. Effective patient education on the complications of preeclampsia and when to seek medical care is imperative to empower the woman in identifying signs and symptoms that necessitate timely access to medical care should complications ensue.

- Postpartum preeclampsia is associated with a high risk for stroke, which may be the underlying cause of severe headache.[24] Instruct the patient to contact her medical provider or seek emergency medical care for severe headache.
- Women with preeclampsia are optimally encouraged to discuss the long-term risk of cardiovascular disease with their medical provider following childbirth in order to engage in health behaviors that modify the risk, including achieving and maintaining an ideal body weight, aerobic exercise, smoking cessation, and dietary intake of high-fiber, lower-fat foods with vegetables and fruits.[2]

PRACTICE/REVIEW QUESTIONS
After reviewing this module, answer the following questions.

1. Hypertension complicates _____% of all pregnancies world-wide.

2. A term that describes new onset of hypertension without proteinuria after 20 weeks' gestation is _____.

   _____

3. The occurrence of preeclampsia in a woman with pre-existing hypertension is termed_____.

4. A hypertensive state in pregnancy occurring after the 20th week that may include a convulsive phase of the disorder is _____.

5. New onset hypertension with new onset proteinuria is called _____.

6. Match the terms in Column B with the descriptions given in Column A.

Column A

_____ 1. Hypertension with the onset during the last 20 weeks of pregnancy or postpartum without proteinuria or other signs of preeclampsia

_____ 2. Elevated blood pressure that fails to normalize postpartum

_____ 3. A subset of preeclampsia characterized by certain laboratory findings

_____ 4. May be initially observed in previously normotensive woman following childbirth but resolves postpartum

_____ 5. The development of a BP of 140/90 mm Hg or higher after the 20th gestational week and accompanied by new onset proteinuria

Column B

a. Preeclampsia
b. Eclampsia
c. Chronic hypertension
d. HELLP syndrome
e. Chronic hypertension with superimposed preeclampsia
f. Gestational hypertension

_____ 6. The disease process, occurs before the observation of clinical manifestations, typically presenting after the 20th week

_____ 7. A disorder that involves abnormal placental implantation weeks or months before overt signs or symptoms

_____ 8. BP of 160/110 mm Hg or higher is considered a severe manifestation of this disease

_____ 9. Can develop in women who enter pregnancy with pre-existing hypertension

_____ 10. Has as its underlying pathophysiology arterial vasospasm leading to microangiopathic hemolytic anemia

_____ 11. Is characterized by grand mal seizure not attributed to other neurologic disease

_____ 12. Is diagnosed by persistent BP elevation of at least 140/90 mm Hg before the 20th gestational week

_____ 13. Convulsion may be the initial clinical manifestation of this disease

_____ 14. This hypertensive disorder may co-exist with diabetes, renal disease, or a cardiac condition

7. The following statements elicit your understanding of the current thinking about hypertensive states in pregnancy.

a. Perinatal morbidity increases with increasing proteinuria.
   1. True
   2. False

b. Chronic hypertension and preeclampsia have the same etiology.
   1. True
   2. False

c. Urinary protein excretion greater than 5 g in 24 hours is considered to be a severe feature of preeclampsia.
   1. True
   2. False

d. Eclampsia can be predicted by an aura or other cerebral or visual disturbances
   1. True
   2. False

e. A diagnostic criterion for hypertension is a BP of 140/90 mm Hg.
   1. True
   2. False

f. Severe hypertension is diagnosed when the BP reaches 150/100 mm Hg.
   1. True
   2. False

g. A woman with new onset hypertension after 20 weeks' gestation without proteinuria whose blood pressure normalizes postpartum is described under the current classification to have transient hypertension.
   1. True
   2. False

h. A BP of 146/100 mm Hg in a laboring woman with no previous hypertension history and with no proteinuria can indicate gestational hypertension.
   1. True
   2. False

i. If the laboring woman mentioned above in "h" manifested with BP elevation without proteinuria for the first time postpartum, the same diagnosis would be anticipated.
   1. True
   2. False

8. Name the two principal signs present in preeclampsia:
   a. _____
   b. _____

9. Select the hypertensive state that fits the descriptions given in a through j.
   G = Gestational hypertension
   P = Preeclampsia
   H = Chronic Hypertension
   E = Eclampsia

   a. _____ Is typically not accompanied by adverse fetal outcomes
   b. _____ Progresses in severity as pregnancy advances

c. _____ Is characterized by endothelial injury and increased capillary permeability

d. _____ Hypertension onset after 20 weeks' gestation without proteinuria or other organ system disturbances

e. _____ Elevated blood pressure that does not normalize in the postpartum period

f. _____ May not be accurately diagnosed until after the postpartum period

g. _____ The only definitive cure is delivery of the infant

h. _____ May involve microvascular damage to the endothelial lining of blood vessels and platelet activation diagnosed in laboratory studies

i. _____ Typically unpredictable and often accompanied by fetal bradycardia

j. _____ Associated with poor maternal and perinatal outcomes

10. List at least five predisposing risk factors for developing preeclampsia:

   a. _____

   b. _____

   c. _____

   d. _____

   e. _____

11. Proteinuria is defined as:

   a. Protein/creatinine ratio of 0.3

   b. 10 mg/dL in any single voided specimen

   c. Trace or higher on dipstick tested twice 4 hours apart

   d. Elevated serum creatinine to 1.1 mg/dL

12. Which of the following is required for the diagnosis of preeclampsia?

   a. New onset hypertension after 20 weeks' gestation

   b. Proteinuria

   c. 30 mm Hg increase in systolic blood pressure

   d. All of the above

13. Place an "X" next to any statement below that accurately characterizes chronic hypertension.

   a. _____ Most pregnant women with chronic hypertension have primary or essential hypertension.

   b. _____ Increased occurrence of chronic hypertension is associated with the increased incidence of obesity in women of childbearing age.

   c. _____ It rarely leads to intrauterine fetal growth restriction or small for gestational age newborn.

   d. _____ Is associated with worse maternal and fetal morbidity when compared to preeclampsia.

e. _____ Pregnancy requires discontinuation of diuretics that were being administered prior to pregnancy.

f. _____ Sodium restriction is advocated to reduce the potential for edema.

14. Hypertensive disorders of pregnancy that resolve postpartum:

   _____ and _____.

15. New onset hypertension after 20 weeks may be diagnosed as preeclampsia in the absence of proteinuria when one of the following is manifested:

   a. Anemia

   b. Intrauterine growth restriction

   c. Oliguria

   d. Thrombocytopenia

16. Which of the following most likely indicates superimposed preeclampsia in a woman with chronic hypertension?

   a. Elevated LDH

   b. Fetal intrauterine growth restriction

   c. Oliguria

   d. Pulmonary edema

17. The underlying disease process in preeclampsia is

   a. Unknown

   b. Neurologic irritability

   c. Endothelial dysfunction

   d. DIC

18. In preeclampsia, hypertension is the:

   a. Primary clinical feature

   b. Cause of the disease

   c. Earliest symptom

   d. Latest symptom

19. Which of the following reflect the current understanding of preeclampsia? Circle all that apply.

   a. Is a dynamic and progressive disease

   b. May involve a genetic predisposition

   c. Predominantly affects women of lower socioeconomic status

   d. Rarely occurs in primigravas

20. Pathophysiologic processes of preeclampsia include all of the following except:

   a. A balance in two potent vasoactive substances

   b. Endothelial dysfunction

   c. Incomplete invasion of the uterine spiral arteries

   d. Placental ischemia

21. Match the descriptions given in Column A to the terms in column B.

    Column A

    _____ 1. Vasodilator

    _____ 2. VEGF

    _____ 3. Generation of oxygen-free radicals

    _____ 4. Enhanced immune response

    _____ 5. Antiangiogenic proteins

    _____ 6. Diminished anti-oxidant response

    _____ 7. Inhibits platelet aggregation

    Column B

    a. Biomarker associated with preeclampsia
    b. Prostacyclin
    c. Oxidative stress
    d. Inflammatory response

22. Fill in the blanks from the following list of terms:

    Antioxidant

    Coagulation

    Endothelium

    Inflammatory

    Oxygen stimulation

    Platelet consumption

    Vasodilation

    In preeclampsia there is diminished _____ response to oxygen stimulation, leading to generation of oxygen-free radicals that produce tissue damage with eventual activation of the vascular _____. Neutrophils from vascular activation perpetuate the _____ response, promoting _____ through initiation of the complement system.

23. What are mechanisms for pulmonary edema in preeclampsia?

    _____ and _____

24. List clinical or laboratory manifestations that correspond to the underlying pathophysiologic features of preeclampsia.

    a. Arteriolar vasospasm: _____

    b. Increased capillary permeability: _____

    c. Platelet aggregation: _____

25. Fill in the blanks from the following list of terms:

    Angiogenic

    Coagulation

    Endothelial

    End-organ

    Neutrophil

    Inflammatory

    Ischemia

    In preeclampsia, placental _____ leads to the production of placental factors, such as antiangiogenic proteins and _____ mediators that enter the maternal circulation and perpetuate widespread _____ dysfunction, leading to reduced _____ perfusion.

26. Preeclampsia potentiates the normal, hypercoagulable state of pregnancy with a(n) _____ in procoagulant proteins and a(n) _____ proteins that inhibit the coagulation cascade.

27. In order to promote hemostasis, platelets aggregate at sites of endothelial injury, resulting in the consumption of platelets, which may manifest as _____.

28. List the features of the HELLP syndrome that comprise the acronym.

    a. _____

    b. _____

    c. _____

29. It is recommended that women who are at significant risk for preeclampsia receive which of the following prescriptions after the first trimester? Check all that apply.

    a. Low-dose aspirin

    b. Vitamin C

    c. Vitamin E

    d. Bedrest

30. An increase in the systolic blood pressure by 30 mm Hg or more or increase in the diastolic blood pressure by 15 mm Hg or more indicates which of the following?

    a. Diagnosis of hypertension

    b. Immediate hospitalization and further observation

    c. Risk for hypertension warranting enhanced surveillance

    d. Normal finding in pregnancy that does not warrant further evaluation

31. Which of the following laboratory values might reflect hemoconcentration from intravascular volume depletion in a woman with preeclampsia?

    a. Decreased hematocrit

    b. Elevated hematocrit

    c. Elevated blood urea nitrogen

    d. Proteinuria

32. List two laboratory findings that indicate decreased renal perfusion in preeclampsia.

_____

_____

33. Thrombocytopenia is defined as a platelet count less than _____/mm^3

34. Proteinuria (check all that apply):

   a. Is required for the diagnosis of preeclampsia

   b. Indicates severe disease when it exceeds 5 g in 24 hours

   c. Generally reflects injury to the glomerular basement membrane

   d. Offers prognosis based upon the amount excreted

35. List four visual disturbances that may be observed with preeclampsia

   a. _____

   b. _____

   c. _____

   d. _____

36. Ischemia and tissue damage within the liver capsule predispose the patient to the development of _____.
   Complains of _____ therefore warrant further evaluation.

37. Persistent, severe headache in a patient with preeclampsia indicates _____ involvement

38. Hypertension in pregnancy can compromise blood supply to the placenta and lead to fetal _____.

39. Increases in systolic and diastolic pressures indicate pathology with only an occasional exception.

   a. True

   b. False

40. Relative gradual increases in BP can be interpreted as "normal" and further screening is not necessary.

   a. True

   b. False

41. The diagnosis of preeclampsia requires the presence of proteinuria and edema.

   a. True

   b. False

42. Edema is not diagnostic of preeclampsia.

   a. True

   b. False

43. Most pregnant women exhibit some edema.

   a. True

   b. False

44. Massive proteinuria (greater than 5 g in 24 hours) is one of the criteria for diagnosis of preeclampsia with severe features.

   a. True

   b. False

45. Women with preeclampsia are more likely to exhibit epidural-mediated hypotension with epidural analgesia/anesthesia because of intravascular volume depletion.

   a. True

   b. False

46. A woman whose blood pressures ranged in the 150s to 160s systolic with diastolic blood pressures of 100s to 110s during labor now has a blood pressure of 110/68 about 6 hours after vaginal birth. This should be recognized as a return of the patient's blood pressure to normal following delivery.

   a. True

   b. False

47. A 19-year-old nulliparous woman at 37 weeks' gestation presents with a BP of 150/100 mm Hg and a 24-hour urine specimen reported to have 5.3 g of protein. By definition, the diagnosis is _____

48. Fill in the blank.

   Women less than _____ weeks' gestation should be cared for in a tertiary care center when there are persistent severe features of preeclampsia, they are in labor, or demonstrate features consistent with significant uteroplacental insufficiency.

49. Fill in the blank.

   It is recommended that any woman with preeclampsia (without severe features) be delivered at _____ weeks' gestation, even if cervical ripening agents are necessary for induction of labor.

50. Fill in the blank.

   Women with severe features of preeclampsia should be delivered at _____ weeks' gestation, unless maternal or fetal instability require earlier delivery.

51. Fill in the blanks.

   A systolic blood pressure of _____ mm Hg or higher or diastolic blood pressure of _____ mm Hg or higher should be measured again in _____. If still elevated in this range, the physician should be notified _____.

52. List four signs and symptoms of preeclampsia that the patient should be educated to report to her medical provider.

    a. _____

    b. _____

    c. _____

    d. _____

53. Match the position of the patient in Column A with the effect on blood pressure in Column B.

    Column A

    _____ 1. Arm above heart level

    _____ 2. Arm below heart level

    _____ 3. Arm supported at heart level

    Column B

    a. Higher

    b. Lower

    c. Most accurate

54. Following cesarean birth for breech presentation, a woman with preeclampsia presents with urine output of 20 to 30 mL/hr over the last 2 hours. In the next hour following a 500-mL fluid bolus, her urine output is 20 mL/hr. Which of the following interventions is most appropriate?

    a. Administer 10 mg of Lasix IV

    b. Obtain a hemoglobin and hematocrit level

    c. Observe urine output for one additional hour

    d. Transfuse 1 to 2 units of packed red blood cells

55. List at least five complications of preeclampsia that warrant delivery regardless of gestational age.

    a. _____

    b. _____

    c. _____

    d. _____

    e. _____

56. List both indications that serve as rationale for assessing deep tendon reflexes in the patient with preeclampsia.

    a. _____

    b. _____

57. Fill in the blanks with the any of the following terms:

    Cardiogenic

    Endothelial injury

    Fluid overload

    Intrapartum

    Noncardiogenic

    Postpartum

Women are more often predisposed to _____ pulmonary edema rather than _____ pulmonary edema due to _____. Pulmonary edema is more likely to present in the _____ period.

58. Fill in the blank.

    When evaluating blood pressure with the auscultatory method, the examiner should use the _____ Korotkoff sound to determine diastolic blood pressure.

59. Which of the following signs provides the earliest indicator of hemodynamic compromise?

    a. Cool, clammy skin

    b. Decreased level of consciousness

    c. Pallor

    d. Tachycardia

60. Using current recommendations, magnesium sulfate is indicated in which of the following patients? Circle all that apply.

    a. Eclamptic seizure

    b. Mild preeclampsia

    c. Myasthenia gravis

    d. Preeclampsia with severe features

61. The antidote for magnesium toxicity is _____

62. A woman with preeclampsia has received a loading dose of magnesium sulfate and is now receiving the maintenance infusion. Which of the following is an indication for an additional 2 g bolus infusion? Check all that apply.

    a. Diuresis

    b. Grand mal seizure

    c. Diastolic blood pressure 168 mm Hg

    d. None of the above

63. Some women may require a higher infusion rate of magnesium sulfate than what is typically encountered to achieve a therapeutic magnesium level.

    a. True

    b. False

64. Recurrent seizure activity despite adequate magnesium sulfate may indicate other neurologic pathology.

    a. True

    b. False

65. Universal seizure prophylaxis is recommended for all patients with the diagnosis of preeclampsia.

    a. True

    b. False

66. List at least two reasons why magnesium sulfate should not be discontinued during the delivery?

    a. _____

    b. _____

67. A woman has been given a loading dose of magnesium sulfate from a 20 g/500 mL bag of magnesium sulfate during an eclamptic seizure. Immediately following the seizure, she is breathless and pulseless, which would lead the care providers to suspect which of the following as the most likely contributor?

    a. Amniotic fluid embolism

    b. Heart failure

    c. Magnesium overdose

    d. Myocardial infarction

68. Which of the following increase the risk for magnesium toxicity? Circle all that apply.

    a. Calculation error

    b. Hypotension

    c. Oliguria

    d. Pulmonary edema

69. What are the blood pressure indices that warrant urgent administration of first-line antihypertensive therapy if sustained for 15 minutes?

    _____

    _____

70. A woman who is being induced at 37 weeks for pre-eclampsia is now in active labor and verbalizes a pain score of 5/10. Her blood pressures over the past hour are 168/99, 162/100, 167/90, and 160/100. Upon notifying the physician, the nurse would anticipate which of the following orders based upon current guidelines?

    a. IV fluid bolus of 500 mL

    b. Labetalol 20 mg IV push

    c. Nifedipine 10 mg sublingual

    d. Morphine sulfate 5 mg IV push

71. The physician has ordered IV hydralazine 5 mg to a patient with chronic hypertension with superimposed preeclampsia whose blood pressure is 178/112. When should the nurse measure the patient's blood pressure?

    _____

72. What is the target threshold blood pressure for acute, emergent IV antihypertensive medications?

    Systolic BP: _____

    Diastolic BP: _____

73. The initial 5 mg dose of hydralazine did not achieve the target threshold. What should the nurse anticipate the next order for medication and dose to be?

    _____

74. The patient's blood pressure did not reach the target threshold after receiving the medication listed in question 73 above. What should the nurse anticipate the next order for medication and dose to be?

    _____

75. Match the mechanism of action provided in Column B for the medication listed in Column A.

    Column A   **Column B**

    _____ 1. Methyldopa   a. Blocks intracellular entry of calcium

    _____ 2. Labetalol   b. Blocks alpha-2 receptors

    _____ 3. Nifedipine   c. Blocks alpha-1 and beta receptors

76. Which of the following medications should not be administered for the long-term management of hypertension during pregnancy? Check all that apply.

    a. ACE-inhibitors

    b. Calcium channel blockers

    c. Central alpha-adrenergics

    d. Diuretics

77. Which of the following antihypertensive agents should not be administered to the woman with asthma?

    a. Hydralazine

    b. Labetalol

    c. Methyldopa

    d. Nifedipine

PRACTICE/REVIEW ANSWER KEY
1. 10%
2. Gestational hypertension
3. Chronic hypertension with superimposed preeclampsia
4. Eclampsia
5. Preeclampsia
6. 1. f
   2. c
   3. d
   4. f
   5. a
   6. a
   7. a
   8. a
   9. e
   10. a or d
   11. b
   12. c
   13. a or b
   14. c
7. a. 2, False
   b. 2, False
   c. 2, False
   d. 2, False
   e. 1, True

f. 2, False
g. 2, False
h. 1, True
i. 1, True

8. a. Elevated BP: 140/90 mm Hg or higher
   b. Proteinuria

9. a. G
   b. P
   c. P
   d. G
   e. H
   f. H
   g. P
   h. P
   i. E
   j. P

10. Any five of the following:
    a. Primiparity
    b. Prior pregnancy complicated by preeclampsia
    c. History of chronic hypertension
    d. Multifetal pregnancy
    e. Chronic renal disease
    f. History of thrombophilia
    g. Family history of preeclampsia
    h. Diabetes mellitus
    i. Obesity
    j. Systemic lupus erythematosus
    k. Maternal age greater than 40 years
    l. Maternal age greater than 35 years in a woman with co-morbid conditions

11. a
12. a
13. both a and b are correct
14. Gestational hypertension and preeclampsia
15. d
16. d
17. c
18. a
19. a and b
20. a
21. 1. b
    2. a
    3. c
    4. d
    5. a
    6. c
    7. b
22. Antioxidant, endothelium, inflammatory, coagulation
23. Increased capillary permeability (from endothelial injury) and iatrogenic fluid overload
24. a. Hypertension
    b. Interstitial edema
    c. Thrombocytopenia
25. Ischemia, inflammatory, endothelial, end-organ
26. Increase, decrease
27. Thrombocytopenia
28. Hemolysis, elevated liver enzymes, low platelets
29. a

30. c
31. b
32. Serum creatinine >1.1 mg/dL, doubling of serum creatinine
33. 100,000 mm^3
34. c
35. a. Blurred vision
    b. Diplopia
    c. Scotomata
    d. Flashes of light
36. Subcapsular hematoma, epigastric or right upper quadrant pain
37. Central nervous system
38. Intrauterine growth restriction
39. b, False
40. b, False
41. b, False
42. a, True
43. a, True
44. b, False
45. a, True
46. b, False
47. Preeclampsia
48. 34
49. 37
50. 34
51. 160, 110, 15, immediately
52. Any four of the following: severe headache, visual disturbances, epigastric or right upper quadrant pain, shortness of breath, persistent abdominal pain, vaginal spotting, rupture of membranes, decreased fetal movement
53. 1. b
    2. a
    3. c
54. b
55. Any five of the following: eclampsia, pulmonary edema, DIC, severe hypertension that is uncontrolled, nonviable fetus, abnormal fetal surveillance, abruptio placentae, intrauterine fetal demise.
56. To establish a baseline, to monitor for magnesium toxicity
57. Noncardiogenic, cardiogenic, endothelial injury, postpartum
58. Fifth
59. d
60. both a and d
61. calcium gluconate
62. b
63. a, true
64. a, true
65. b, false
66. At least two of the following: Discontinuing magnesium sulfate will not avoid anesthetic interactions because of long half-life (5 hours), will produce subtherapeutic levels of magnesium, or the physical stress of labor or delivery increases the risk for eclampsia
67. c
68. Both a and c
69. Systolic BP ≥160 mm Hg, diastolic BP ≥110 mm Hg

70. b
71. 20 minutes
72. Systolic BP 140 to 159 mm Hg and diastolic BP 90 to 100 mm Hg
73. Hydralazine 10 mg
74. Labetalol 20 mg
75. 1. b
    2. c
    3. a
76. a
77. b

REFERENCES

1. Scantlebury, D. C., Schwartz, G. L., Acquah, L. A., et al. (2013). The treatment of hypertension during pregnancy: When should blood pressure medication be started? *Current Cardiology Reports, 15*(412), 4–10.

2. Task Force on Hypertension in Pregnancy. (2013). *Hypertension in pregnancy* (pp. 1–89). Washington, DC: American College of Obstetricians and Gynecologists.

3. Berg, C. J., Atrash, H. K., Koonin, L. M., et al. (1996). Pregnancy-related mortality in the United States, 1987–1990. *Obstetrics and Gynecology, 88*(2), 161–167.

4. Berg, C. J., Chang, J., Callaghan, W. M., et al. (2003). Pregnancy-related mortality in the United States, 1991–1997. *Obstetrics and Gynecology, 101*(2), 289–296.

5. Berg, C. J., Callaghan, W. M., Syverson, C., et al. (2010). Pregnancy-related mortality in the United States, 1998–2005. *Obstetrics and Gynecology, 116*(6), 1302–1309.

6. Creanga, A. A., Berg, C. J., Ko, J. Y., et al. (2014). Maternal mortality and morbidity in the United States: Where are we now? *Journal of Women's Health, 23*(1), 3–9.

7. Garovic, V. D., & August, P. (2013). Preeclampsia and the future risk of hypertension: The pregnant evidence. *Current Hypertension Reports, 15*(2), 114–121.

8. National High Blood Pressure Education Program Working Group on High Blood Pressure in Pregnancy. (2000). Report of the National High Blood Pressure Education Program Working Group on high blood pressure in pregnancy. *American Journal of Obstetrics and Gynecology, 183*(1), S1–S22.

9. National High Blood Pressure Education Program. (2000). *Working group report on high blood pressure in pregnancy.* Bethesda, MD: Heart Lung and Blood Institute.

10. Gifford, R., August, P., Cunningham, G., et al. (2000). *National high blood pressure education program working group national high blood pressure in pregnancy* [NIH Publication No. 00–3029]. Bethesda, MD: National Institutes of Health, National Heart, Lung, Blood Institute.

11. Sibai, B. M. (2012). Hypertension. In Gabbe, S. G., Niebyl, J. R., Simpson, Jl. L., et al. (Eds.), *Obstetrics: Normal and problem pregnancies* (6th ed., pp. 779–824). Philadelphia, PA: Saunders.

12. Cunningham, F. G., Levelo, K. J., Bloom, S. L., et al. (2010). Pregnancy hypertension. In *Williams obstetrics* (23rd ed., pp. 706–756). New York: McGraw-Hill.

13. Magee, L. A., Pels, A., Helewa, M., et al., Hypertensive Guideline Committee. (2014). Diagnosis, evaluation, and management of the hypertensive disorders of pregnancy: Executive summary. *Journal of Obstetrics and Gynaecology Canada, 36*(5), 416–438.

14. Maynard, S. E., & Karumanchi, S. A. (2011). Angiogenic factors and preeclampsia. *Seminars in Nephrology, 31*(1), 33–46.

15. Raijmakers, M. T., Dechend, R., & Poston, L. (2004). Oxidative stress and preeclampsia. Rationale for antioxidant clinical trials. *Hypertension, 44*(4), 374–380.

16. Schramm, A. M., & Clowse, M. E. B. (2014). Aspirin for prevention of preeclampsia in lupus pregnancy. *Autoimmune Disease, 2014*:920467.

17. Ramma, W., & Ahmed, A. (2011). Is inflammation the cause of pre-eclampsia? *Biochemical Society Transactions, 39*(6), 1619–1627.

18. Norwitz, E. R., & Robinson, J. N. (2010). Pregnancy-induced physiologic alterations. In Belfort, M. A., Saade, G., Foley, M. R., et al. (Eds.), *Critical care obstetrics* (5th ed., pp. 30–52). Hoboken, NJ: Wiley-Blackwell.

19. Karateke, A., Silfeler, D., Karateke, F., et al. (2014). HELLP syndrome complicated by subcapsular hematoma of the liver: A case report and review of the literature. *Case Reports in Obstetrics and Gynecology, 2014*, 585672.

20. Harvey, C. J., & Sibai, B. M. (2013). Hypertension in pregnancy. In Troiano, N. H., Harvey, C. J., & Chez, B. F. (Eds.), *High risk & critical care obstetrics* (3rd ed., pp. 109–124). Philadelphia, PA: Lippincott Williams & Wilkins.

21. Dildy, G. A., & Belfort, M. A. (2010). Complications of preeclampsia. In Belfort, M. A., Saade, G., Foley, M. R., et al. (Eds.), *Critical care obstetrics* (5th ed., pp. 438–465). Hoboken, NJ: Wiley-Blackwell.

22. Kane, S. C., Dennis, A., Da Silva Costa, F., et al. (2013). Contemporary clinical management of the cerebral complications of preeclampsia. *Obstetrics and Gynecology International, 2013*, 985606.

23. Chobanian, A. V., Bakris, G. L., Black, H. R., et al., the National High Blood Pressure Education Program Coordinating Committee. (2003). Seventh Report of the Joint National Committee on Prevention, Detection, Evaluation, and Treatment of High Blood Pressure. *Hypertension, 42*(6), 1206–1252.

24. Bushnell, C., McCullough, L. D., Awad, I. A., et al. (2014). Guidelines for the prevention of stroke in women. A statement for healthcare professionals from the American Heart Association/American Stroke Association. *Stroke, 45*, 1545–1588.

25. Ventura, S. J., Mosher, W. D., Curtin, S. C., et al. (2000). Trends in pregnancies and pregnancy rates by outcome. Estimates for the United States, 1976–96. *National Center for Health Statistics. Vital Health Stat, 21*(56).

26. Yanit, K. E., Snowden, J. M., Cheng, Y. W., et al. (2012). Prevalence, trends, and outcomes of chronic hypertension: A nationwide sample of delivery admissions. *American Journal of Obstetrics and Gynecology, 206*(2), 333.e1–e6.

27. Bateman, B. T., Bansil, P., Hernandez-Diaz, S., et al. (2012). Prevalence, trends, and outcomes of chronic hypertension: A nationwide sample of delivery admissions. *American Journal of Obstetrics and Gynecology, 206*(2), 134–141.

28. Orbach, H., Motok, I., Gorodischer, R., et al. (2013). Hypertension and antihypertensive drugs in pregnancy and perinatal outcomes. *Obstetrics and Gynecology, 208*(4), 301.e1–e6.

29. Kattah, A. G., & Garovic, V. D. (2013). The management of hypertension in pregnancy. *Advances in Chronic Kidney Disease, 20*(3), 229–239.

30. Ma, Y., Temprosa, M., Fowler, S., et al., The Diabetes Prevention Program Research Group. (2009). Evaluating the accuracy of an aneroid sphygmomanometer in a clinical trial setting. *American Journal of Hypertension, 22*(3), 263–266.

31. Ogedegbe, G., & Pickering, T. (2010). Principles and techniques of blood pressure measurement. *Cardiology Clinics, 28*(4), 571–586.

32. Pickering, T. G., Hall, J. E., Appel, L. J., et al. (2005). Recommendations for blood pressure measurement in humans

and experimental animals: Part I: Blood pressure measurement in humans: A statement for professionals from the Subcommittee of Professional and Public Education of the American Heart Association Council on High Blood Pressure Research. *Hypertension, 45*(1), 142–161.

33. Babbs, C. F. (2012). Oscillometric measurement of systolic and diastolic blood pressures validated in a physiologic mathematical model. *Biomedical Engineering Online, 11*, 56.

34. Lindheimer, M. D., & Kanter, D. (2010). Interpreting abnormal proteinuria in pregnancy. The need for a more pathophysiological approach. *Obstetrics and Gynecology, 115* (2 pt 1): 365–375.

35. Bell, S. C., Halligan, A. W., Martin, A., et al. (1999). The role of observer error in antenatal dipstick proteinuria analysis. *British Journal of Obstetrics and Gynecology, 106*(11), 1177–1180.

36. Carroll, M. F., & Temte, J. L. (2000). Proteinuria in adults. A diagnostic approach. *American Family Physician, 62*(6), 1333–1340.

37. Vricella, L. K., Louis, J. M., Mercer, B. M., et al. (2012). Epidural-associated hypotension is more common among severely preeclamptic patients in labor. *American Journal of Obstetrics and Gynecology, 207*(4), 335–341.

38. Clark, S. L., & Hankins, G. D. (2012). Preventing maternal death. 10 clinical diamonds. *American Journal of Obstetrics and Gynecology, 119*(2 pt 1), 360–364.

39. Martin, J. M., Thigpen, B., Moore, R., et al. (2005). Stroke and severe preeclampsia and eclampsia: A paradigm shift focusing on systolic blood pressure. *Obstetrics and Gynecology, 105*(2), 246–254.

40. Simpson, K. R., & Knox, G. E. (2004). Obstetrical accidents involving intravenous magnesium sulfate. Recommendations to promote patient safety. *Maternal Child Nursing, 29*(30), 161–169.

41. Joint Commission on Accreditation of Healthcare Organizations. (2003). *National patient safety goals.* Oakbrook, IL: Author.

42. American College of Obstetricians and Gynecologists (2015). *Emergent therapy for acute-onset, severe hypertension during pregnancy and the postpartum period. ACOG Committee Opinion, 514.* Washington, DC: Author.

43. Giannubilo, S. R., Bezzeccheri, V., Cecchi, S., et al. (2012). Nifedipine versus labetalol in the treatment of hypertensive disorders in pregnancy. *Archives of Gynecology and Obstetrics, 286*(3), 637–642.

44. Shekhar, S., Sharma, C., Thakur, S., et al. (2013). Oral nifedipine or intravenous labetalol for hypertensive emergency in pregnancy. A randomized controlled trial. *Obstetrics and Gynecology, 122*(5), 1057–1063.

45. Mustafa, R., Ahmed, S., Gupta, A., et al. (2012). A comprehensive review of hypertension in pregnancy. *Journal of Pregnancy, 2012*, 105918.

46. Al Khaja, K. A., Sequeira, R. P., Alkhaja, A. K., et al. (2014). Drug treatment of hypertension in pregnancy: A critical review of adult guideline recommendations. *Journal of Hypertension, 32*(3), 454–463.

47. Mannisto, T., Mendola, P., Vaarasmaki, M., et al. (2013). Elevated blood pressure in pregnancy and subsequent chronic disease risk. *Circulation, 127*, 681–690.

48. Melchiorre, K., Sutherland, G. R., Liberati, M., et al. (2011). Preeclampsia is associated with persistent postpartum cardiovascular impairment. *Hypertension, 58*, 709–715.

49. Berks, D., Hoedjes, M., Raat, H., et al. (2013). Risk of cardiovascular disease after preeclampsia and the effect of lifestyle interventions: A literature-based study. *British Journal of Obstetrics and Gynecology, 120*(8),924–931.

50. Drost, J. T., van der Schouw, Y. T., Mass, A. H., et al. (2013). Longitudinal analysis of cardiovascular risk parameters in women with a history of hypertensive pregnancy disorders: The Doetinchem Cohort Study. *British Journal of Obstetrics and Gynecology, 20*(11), 1333–1339.

Intrapartum Infections

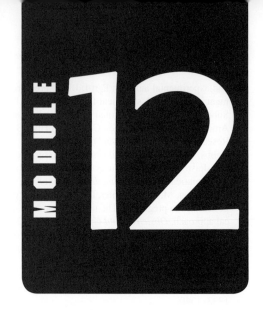

MODULE 12

As you complete this module, you will learn:

1. Risk factors for chorioamnionitis
2. Effects of chorioamnionitis on uterine contractions and labor progress
3. Management of chorioamnionitis
4. Potential perinatal consequences of chorioamnionitis
5. Group B Streptococcus (GBS) perinatal transmission and potential neonatal consequences of GBS
6. Screening, diagnosis, and antibiotic management for GBS
7. Procedure for obtaining GBS cultures
8. The definition and phases of HIV infection
9. Common opportunistic infections in those infected with HIV
10. The state of the HIV/AIDS epidemic
11. Risk factors for HIV infection
12. Methods of HIV transmission
13. Screening and diagnosis of HIV infection
14. Effects of pregnancy on HIV and HIV on pregnancy, and methods to minimize risk of perinatal transmission
15. Pharmacotherapeutic treatment recommendations during pregnancy and potential side effects of antiretroviral (ARV) medications
16. Intrapartum and immediate postpartum management of the HIV-infected mother and newborn
17. Psychosocial and ethical issues in the care of the HIV-infected mother
18. Education of the HIV-infected mother
19. Epidemiology, clinical features, perinatal consequences, and treatments for sexually transmitted infections.

When you have completed this module, you should be able to recall the meaning of the following terms. You should also be able to use the terms when consulting with other health professionals.
The terms are defined in this module or in the glossary at the end of this book.

amnion
acquired immunodeficiency
  syndrome (AIDS)
antibody
antigen
ARV therapy
CD4 cell
chorioamnionitis
chorion
fetal inflammatory response
  syndrome (FIRS)
funisitis
group B Streptococcus (GBS)
human immunodeficiency virus
  (HIV)

horizontal transmission
immunoassay
lactobacilli
leukocytosis
opportunistic infection
opt-out HIV screening
perinatal transmission
protease inhibitor
seroconversion
transplacental transmission
vertical transmission
viral load
viral suppression
zidovudine

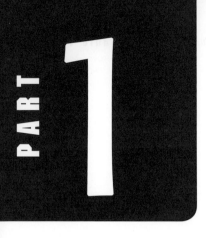

Chorioamnionitis

SUZANNE McMURTRY BAIRD

Introduction

• What is chorioamnionitis?

Chorioamnionitis (intra-amniotic infection, amnionitis) occurs in approximately 1% to 10% of all term pregnancies, but approaches 40% to 70% in women with preterm labor (PTL) and birth.[1,2] Risk factors include the following[1,3]:

- Psychosocial factors
  - Young age (<21 years old)
  - Low socioeconomic status
  - Alcohol use
  - Smoking
- Neuraxial anesthesia[4]
- Prolonged labor
  - Active labor >12 hours[5]
  - Second stage of labor >2 hours[4]
- Prolonged rupture of membranes (>18 hours)[4]
- Multiple cervical exams during labor in women with ruptured membranes
- Pre-existing infections of the lower genital tract
- GBS bacteriuria
- Internal fetal and/or uterine monitoring

NOTE: Combination of risk factors increases the likelihood of infection.

Chorioamnionitis is a broad term that includes any acute, bacterial infection of the chorion (outer fetal membrane), amnion (encloses the fetus), placenta, or the amniotic fluid.[3] The most common causative organisms are *Escherichia coli,* anaerobic gram-positive cocci, GBS, and genital mycoplasmas.[1,3] These organisms can enter the amniotic membranes/fluid from maternal dissemination, invasive procedures (amniocentesis), but more likely ascend from the vaginal flora when the fetal membranes are ruptured. With less frequency, the inflammatory process of chorioamnionitis can occur with intact membranes and is usually due to genital mycoplasmas such as Ureaplasma species and Mycoplasma hominis, found in the lower genital tract of over 70% of women.[6]

• How is chorioamnionitis diagnosed?

The diagnosis of chorioamnionitis is based on the clinical signs and symptoms—*clinical chorioamnionitis.* Initial signs and symptoms are maternal fever (temperature >100.4°F) and tachycardia in both the mother (>100/min) and fetus (>60/min for 10 minutes or more). As the infection progresses, other abnormal assessment parameters may include uterine tenderness and purulent, foul-smelling amniotic fluid.[1,3] Diagnosis is made based on clinical findings, in the absence of other infections of the urinary tract, respiratory system, appendix, or a viral syndrome.[1] Other diagnostic screening may be helpful in the preterm woman in order to determine the need for tocolysis and corticosteroids. The provider may determine the need to perform a transabdominal amniocentesis and directly test the amniotic fluid for infection. Laboratory assessments are listed in Table 12.1.

TABLE 12.1	LABORATORY TESTS FOR CHORIOAMNIONITIS		
TEST	**SOURCE**	**ABNORMAL FINDING**	**NOTE**
WBC count	Maternal serum	≥15,000 cells/mm³	Labor and/or corticosteroids may also increase WBC count.
WBC differential	Maternal serum	Leukocytosis (occurs in 70–90% of clinical chorioamnionitis cases) Left shift Bandemia	Isolated leukocytosis may occur in labor and with steroid administration
Glucose	Amniotic fluid	≤10–15%	Excellent correlation with clinical infection and positive amniotic fluid culture
Interleukin-6	Amniotic fluid	≥7.9 ng/mL	Excellent correlation with clinical infection and positive amniotic fluid culture
Leukocyte esterase	Amniotic fluid	>1 + reaction	Good correlation with clinical infection and positive amniotic fluid culture
Gram stain	Amniotic fluid	Any organism	Can identify GBS, but not mycoplasmas
Culture	Amniotic fluid	Growth of aerobic or anaerobic microorganism	Requires incubation time; final results in 3 d.
Blood cultures	Maternal serum; two peripheral sites required	Growth of aerobic or anaerobic microorganism	Positive in 5–10% of patients; requires incubation time; treatment based on clinical diagnosis and should not wait on cultures.

From Duff, P. (2012). Maternal and perinatal infection–bacterial. In Gabbe, S. G., Niebyl, J. R., Simpson, J. L., et al. (Eds.), *Obstetrics: Normal and problem pregnancies* (6th ed., pp. 1140–115). Philadelphia, PA: Saunders; Tita, A. T., Andrews, W. W. (2010). Diagnosis and management of clinical chorioamnionitis. *Clinical Perinatology, 37*(2), 339–354.

Maternal fever may occur in a woman with neuraxial anesthesia—"epidural fever"—making it difficult to determine a diagnosis of clinical chorioamnionitis. In addition, neuraxial anesthesia rates are higher in nulliparous women, prolonged labor, and decrease the nurse's ability to assess uterine tenderness. Medications (ephedrine, neo-synephrine) given for hypotension associated with neuraxial anesthesia also increase the maternal and fetal heart rates. The exact physiologic mechanism of "epidural fever" is unknown. It is theorized that medications used for neuraxial anesthesia block the thermoregulatory processes. However, there is some evidence that suggests higher incidence in the presence of placental inflammation.[7]

NOTE: It is not the nurse's responsibility to diagnose chorioamnionitis. If the woman becomes febrile or maternal or fetal tachycardia is assessed, notify the provider.

If chorioamnionitis is suspected or diagnosed in the intrapartum period, the placenta and umbilical cord should be sent for pathological examination. In addition, if there is unexpected newborn compromise, histologic examination of the placenta may reveal a diagnosis of inflammation, even in the absence of maternal or fetal symptoms.

• **What are the potential complications of chorioamnionitis?**

Maternal, fetal, and neonatal complications of chorioamnionitis can result in morbidity and morality. If inadequately or untreated, progression of the disease process can occur and lead to fetal inflammatory response syndrome (FIRS).[3,8] (See Fig. 12.1.) FIRS is the immune response in the fetus in response to infection- or injury-mediated release of inflammatory mediators such as interleukins, TNF-alpha, C-reactive protein, etc.[1,8,9] FIRS increases fetal and neonatal morbidity and mortality, including the following[1,3,8,9]:
  • Preterm labor and birth
  • Hematologic abnormalities
  • Endocrine activation
  • Cardiac dysfunction
  • Pulmonary injury
  • Renal dysfunction
  • Brain injury (cerebral white matter)
  • Perinatal death

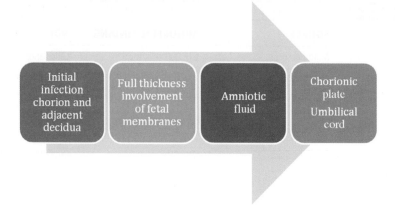

FIGURE 12.1 Chorioamnionitis progression. From Duff, P. (2012). Maternal and perinatal infection–bacterial. In Gabbe, S. G., Niebyl, J. R., Simpson, J. L., et al. (Eds.), *Obstetrics: Normal and problem pregnancies* (6th ed., pp.1140–115). Philadelphia, PA: Saunders; Tita, A. T., & Andrews, W. W. (2010). Diagnosis and management of clinical chorioamnionitis. *Clinical Perinatology, 37*(2), 339–354.

Funisitis, inflammation of the umbilical cord, occurs with leukocyte infiltration into the umbilical cord or Wharton's jelly and may include chorionic vasculitis. Up to 60% of chorioamnionitis cases involve funisitis, but the diagnosis of chorioamnionitis is made in all cases of funisitis (Fig. 12.1).[9]

Maternal complications[1,3]:
- Postpartum infections
- Sepsis
- Maternal death

Neonatal complications[1,3,8,9]:
- Stillbirth
- Preterm birth
- Pneumonia
- Bacteremia
- Meningitis
- Neonatal sepsis
- Chronic lung disease
- Brain injury leading to neurodevelopmental disabilities

Management of Chorioamnionitis

- **How is chorioamnionitis managed?**

Early Recognition of Signs and Symptoms

The nurse should provide timely assessments of maternal vital signs and fetal status. Early recognition and communication to the provider regarding abnormal assessment parameters (tachycardia, fever), uterine tenderness, or fetal tachycardia expedites diagnosis and intrapartum treatment.

Antibiotic Administration

Intravenous antibiotics that target the most common causative organisms (*E. coli* and GBS) improve outcomes for the mother and newborn. Evidence demonstrates decreased duration of maternal fever and hospitalization, neonatal bacteremia, and pneumonia with prompt and adequate intrapartum antibiotic treatment versus treatment after birth. The following are the most tested and recommended antibiotic dosing regimes[1]:
- Ampicillin 2 g IV every 6 hours **OR** penicillin 5 million units every 6 hours plus gentamicin 1.5 mg/kg every 8 hours.

- If the woman is allergic to penicillin or betalactam antibiotics, clindamycin 900 mg every 8 hours should be given.

Antibiotics are usually discontinued after birth or when the mother has been without fever for 24 hours. The provider will individualize the treatment regime for each woman.

NOTE: Even though many cases of chorioamnionitis are caused by ureaplasma species, there are no data to support the use of additional antimicrobial coverage (macrolide antibiotics) to improve outcomes.[3]

Labor and Birth

Chorioamnionitis increases the risk of dysfunctional labor requiring oxytocin augmentation in 75% of infected women.[1] Every effort should be made to optimize uterine activity while monitoring the fetal response in labor. Fetal tachycardia occurs in greater than three fourths of all cases, and may decrease baseline variability depending on the rate. Therefore, intermittent fetal scalp stimulation may be done to assess fetal acid–base status.[1] Cesarean birth places the woman at increased risk of postpartum complications for wound infection (up to 8%), pelvic abscess (1%), thromboembolism, increased blood loss, and maternal death. In addition, there is no evidence to show improvements in neonatal outcomes.[3]

NOTE: In isolation, chorioamnionitis is not an indication for cesarean birth.[3]

If the woman requires a cesarean birth for obstetric reasons, additional antimicrobial coverage for anaerobic organisms is recommended such as clindamycin (900 mg) or metronidazole (500 mg).[1] Antipyretics (acetaminophen) may be given to reduce maternal symptoms such as fever and tachycardia thereby improving the ability for the nurse to assess fetal status. However, the absence of symptoms due to medication does not mean the newborn will not need the presence of the neonatal team at birth or the possibility of assessment and treatment in the nursery.

Newborn Care

With the potential for newborn compromise, the neonatal team should be present at birth for resuscitation needs. Information regarding the mother's temperature, fetal heart rate monitoring patterns during labor, and antibiotics given during labor should be provided to the team in order for newborn care planning. All well-appearing newborns born to women diagnosed with chorioamnionitis should undergo limited diagnostic evaluation (without a lumbar puncture) and prophylactic antibiotic therapy.[10]

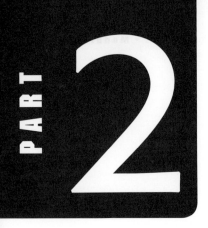

PART 2

Group B Streptococcus Infections in Pregnancy

BETSY BABB KENNEDY

Introduction

- **What is group B streptococcus?**

GBS is a naturally occurring gram-positive bacteria with several different serotypes, and one of the leading infectious causes of morbidity and mortality among newborns.[1]

When clinical signs and symptoms appear within the first 24 hours through week of life, it is referred to as *early-onset disease*, and when signs and symptoms present after 1 week, usually evident in the first 3 months of life, it is referred to as *late-onset disease*. Although screening and intrapartum antibiotic prophylaxis treatment recommendations have significantly reduced the incidence of *early-onset* disease, the rate of maternal colonization remains steady.[1]

Terminology

- **Colonization**—The presence of microorganisms in an organ or tissue of the body with or without any pathology. The presence of the organism is determined by culture. A positive culture does not indicate infection, but rather that the individual harbors or carries the organism without adverse consequences. For example, if the organism is obtained from surfaces such as skin, ears, or umbilical cord or from gastric contents in a healthy individual, exposure to the organism and colonization are documented. However, infection is not necessarily present. Women who are colonized with GBS may be asymptomatic.
- **Infection**—The invasion by microorganisms of a body site that is normally considered sterile (e.g., bladder, amniotic fluid, blood, lungs, cerebrospinal fluid), causing disease by local cellular injury, secretion of toxins, and other pathologic mechanisms.
- **Invasive disease**—High bacterial load affecting major body systems and inducing serious pathologic events, such as meningitis and respiratory distress.

NOTE: GBS resides in the gastrointestinal tract of many individuals (men and women) without causing any complications. However, close approximation of the anus to the introitus and urethra facilitates colonization of the vagina and urinary tract with GBS. Antibiotic treatment sufficient to eliminate GBS in the gastrointestinal tract of a colonized individual is not possible. Treatment eradicates the organism or, in instances of heavy colonization, lowers the colony count, for locally colonized or infected sites such as the cervix, vagina, or bladder. Colonization can be (1) transient, (2) intermittent, or (3) persistent. GBS colonization of the maternal genital tract involves the most risk to the newborn because of exposure during the birth process. The management goal for the woman with GBS is to reduce infection risks for both mother and neonate.

Epidemiology[1-5]

- It is estimated that 10% to 30% of all pregnant women are GBS carriers.[1,2]
- GBS is a common cause of sepsis, pneumonia, and meningitis in neonates and young infants.
- Most neonatal infections occur in the first few days of life (**early onset**).
- Reinfection can occur in a small percentage of neonates, and often this is at a new site.
- The lower female genital tract, that is, the lower third of the vagina, the vaginal introitus, and the rectum are the most common sites of colonization. The upper third of the vagina and

cervix are less commonly colonized. The urethra can be colonized, leading to urinary tract involvement.

- Colonization of the lower maternal genital tract may lead to chorioamnionitis, postpartum endometritis, and neonatal infection.
- GBS is a common cause of bacteremia from a urinary tract infection in pregnant women. This can be asymptomatic in a small percentage of women and can lead to pyelonephritis if untreated.
- GBS is among the most common causes of intrapartal acute chorioamnionitis.

• How is GBS transmitted?[1]

- Early-onset GBS infection is caused by vertical transmission whereby the organism invades the amniotic membranes and infects the fetus in utero. Many newborns are infected before birth.
- Although perhaps half of newborns are exposed to GBS when membranes rupture or during the birth process, only a small percentage (1% to 2%) develops the *disease.*

• What are the risk factors for GBS?

- Maternal risk factors associated with *early-onset newborn disease* include a positive vaginal/rectal culture, prolonged rupture of membranes, gestational age before 37 weeks' gestation, intra-amniotic infection, young maternal age, black race.[2]
- Heavy maternal colonization and having an previously given birth to a GBS infected infant increase the risk of neonatal infection.[2]
- Maternal risk factors associated with *late-onset neonatal infection* are thought to be vertical transmission and hospital-acquired infection.[4]

NOTE: When a GBS-positive infant has been identified, isolation of the infant is not recommended. Outbreaks in nurseries do not occur.[6]

• What are the perinatal consequences of GBS for the mother and baby?[1]

- Colonization in women can lead to spontaneous abortion, sepsis, stillbirth, preterm premature rupture of membranes (PPROM), preterm birth, and postpartum endometritis.
- Most newborns who develop *early-onset invasive GBS disease* are term infants.
- Preterm infants are more susceptible to *early-onset infection.*
- Signs and symptoms of *early-onset* infection are generally seen within the first 24 to 48 hours of life (even within the first hour) and include septicemia, pneumonia, and meningitis. Respiratory distress is the most common sign. Infants may be lethargic, have labile temperatures, exhibit poor feeding, and have glucose intolerance.
- *Signs of severe infection include fetal asphyxia (indicating in utero infection), newborn hypotension, accelerating signs of respiratory distress, and persistent pulmonary hypertension. This requires immediate attention.*
- The case fatality rate of *early-onset* disease has dropped dramatically due to implementation of universal screening and subsequent treatment to 4% to 6%. Preterm infants have a higher case fatality rate of 20% of 30%.[1]
- The mortality rate for *late-onset* disease is 4% to 6%.[1]

Screening[1-4]

In 2002, the American College of Obstetricians and Gynecologists (ACOG), American Academy of Pediatrics (AAP), the Association of Certified Nurse Midwives (ACNM), and the Centers for Disease Control (CDC) adopted national prevention guidelines, recommending a single strategy for *universal antenatal culture based screening at 35 to 37 weeks' gestation.* Updated guidelines from the CDC, AAP, and ACOG continue to support universal screening but have the following key differences[1]:
- Expanded recommendations on laboratory methods for the identification of GBS
- Clarification of the colony-count threshold required for reporting GBS detected in the urine of pregnant women
- Updated algorithms for GBS screening and intrapartum chemoprophylaxis for women with PTL or PPROM

- A change in the recommended dose of penicillin-G for chemoprophylaxis
- Updated prophylaxis regimens for women with penicillin allergy
- Revised algorithm for management of newborns with respect to risk for early-onset GBS disease

Updated recommendations include the following:
- Continued culture-based screening
  - Vaginal and rectal cultures should be performed at 35 to 37 weeks' gestation on all pregnant women.
  - Cultures done earlier in pregnancy do not predict that colonization will be present at birth. All culture-positive women are treated in the intrapartum period. It is NOT recommended to treat antepartum.[1]
  - Cervical, perianal, perirectal, or perineal cultures are not recommended, and specula should not be used for specimen collection.

NOTE: A GBS-positive urine culture (in any concentration) in the prenatal period indicates heavy colonization and an increased risk for infection or invasive disease. This requires immediate antibiotic treatment.[1]

- **What if the mother's GBS status is unknown at admission?**

Risk based approach—*When culture results are unknown in the intrapartum period, treat all women with a known risk factor.*
Any woman with one or more of the following risk factors in the intrapartum period should be considered for antibiotic treatment:
- A history of a previous newborn with invasive GBS infection
- A history of GBS bacteriuria during the current pregnancy
- Delivery predicted to occur before 37 weeks' gestation
- Rupture of membranes for 18 hours or more
- Presence of maternal fever of 38°C (100.4°F) or higher

Maternal Treatment[1-4]

- **How is the mother treated in labor?**

- Intrapartal treatment is targeted for women documented as being GBS positive (by history or antenatal culture) or for women with intrapartal risk factors.
- *The CDC recommends treatment must be completed at least 4 hours before the birth so that adequate antibiotic levels are reached in serum and amniotic fluid, thus reducing the risk of newborn colonization.*

- **What if the mother will deliver before 4 hours of treatment are completed?**

- *Antibiotics used in GBS treatment (bactericidal) are known to rapidly reach effective levels in amniotic fluid. Therefore, treatment given less than 4 hours before birth is likely beneficial, with reports that as little as 1 to 2 hours of prophylaxis may offer protection for vertical transmission.*[1,3]

- **What if the mother is allergic to penicillin?**[1-4]

- Intrapartum chemoprophylaxis includes penicillin-G or ampicillin, with clindamycin, vancomycin, or cefazolin as alternatives for women with penicillin allergy.

Recommended regimen	→ Penicillin-G	First dose 5 million units IV, subsequent doses 2.5–3 million units q4h until birth
Alternative (Penicillin not available)	→ Ampicillin	First dose 2 g IV, subsequent doses 1 g q4h until birth

Penicillin-allergic (high risk for anaphylaxis)	→ Clindamycin	900 mg IV q8h until birth
Penicillin-allergic (high risk for anaphylaxis, susceptibility unknown)	→ Vancomycin	1 g IV q12h until birth
Penicillin-allergic (low risk for anaphylaxis)	→ Cefazolin	First dose 2 g IV, subsequent doses 1 g q8h until birth

---

- **What if the mother is having a cesarean birth?[4]**

- Antibiotic prophylaxis is not indicated in women undergoing a planned cesarean birth in the absence of labor or ruptured membranes due to the low incidence of acquiring disease, but the woman should still have cultures completed at 35 to 37 weeks' gestation due to the possibility of PPROM and labor beginning prior to the schedule cesarean.

- **What if the woman does not have or want an IV?**

- *There is currently no alternative oral or intramuscular regimen that is recommended for prophylaxis.*[1,2]

- **Should cervical examinations be limited on women who are GBS positive?**

- *Obstetric procedures such as cervical exams and internal electronic fetal and uterine monitoring should not be avoided solely on the basis of positive GBS status.*[1,2,5]

Onset of Labor or ROM before 37 Weeks' Gestation[4]

- **What if the woman is in PTL or has PPROM?**

- The preterm infant is at significantly higher risk for GBS sepsis.
- If maternal GBS status is negative (in the previous 5 weeks), no antibiotic prophylaxis is needed.
- If maternal GBS status is known and positive, antibiotic prophylaxis should be started and continued for at least 48 hours during tocolysis and during labor.
- If maternal GBS status is unknown or there has been no culture in the previous 5 weeks, a rectovaginal culture should be obtained. Antibiotic prophylaxis should be started, but may be discontinued when negative results are confirmed or if it is determined the woman is **NOT** in labor.
- If the woman has a GBS culture that is negative at the time of threatened preterm delivery, but does not deliver, repeat cultures should be done again at 35 to 37 weeks' gestation or upon repeated admission if the prior cultures were completed more than 5 weeks prior.
- In the case of PPROM, if antibiotics are being given for latency, that include ampicillin 2 g intravenously (IV) once, followed by 1 g IV every 6 hours for at least 48 hours are adequate for GBS prophylaxis. If other regimens are used, GBS prophylaxis should be initiated in addition.
- GBS prophylaxis should be discontinued at 48 hours for women with PPROM who are not in labor. If results from an admission GBS culture become available during the 48-hour period and are negative, GBS prophylaxis should be discontinued at that time.
- If the woman with PPROM begins labor and previous culture were done more than 5 weeks previous, she should be rescreened and managed accordingly.

Neonatal Treatment[3,4]

- **How is the baby treated?**

- The CDC algorithm for management of the newborn was revised to apply to all newborns, providing recommendations that depend upon clinical appearance of the neonate and other risk factors (such as maternal chorioamnionitis, adequacy of intrapartum antibiotic prophylaxis if indicated for the mother, gestational age, and duration of membrane rupture). The algorithm was revised to address unnecessary evaluations in well-appearing newborns at relatively low risk for early-onset GBS disease (see Fig. 12.2 and Table 12.2).[3]

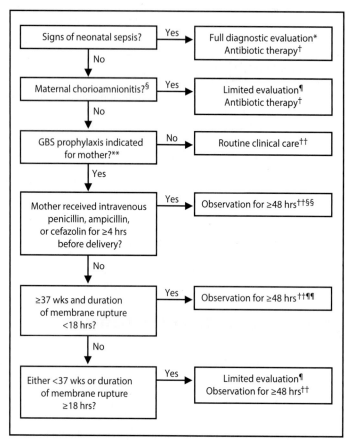

* Full diagnostic evaluation includes a blood culture, a complete blood count (CBC) including white blood cell differential and platelet counts, chest radiograph (if respiratory abnormalities are present), and lumbar puncture (if patient is stable enough to tolerate procedure and sepsis is suspected).

† Antibiotic therapy should be directed toward the most common causes of neonatal sepsis, including intravenous ampicillin for GBS and coverage for other organisms (including *Escherichia coli* and other gram-negative pathogens) and should take into account local antibiotic resistance patterns.

§ Consultation with obstetric providers is important to determine the level of clinical suspicion for chorioamnionitis. Chorioamnionitis is diagnosed clinically and some of the signs are nonspecific.

¶ Limited evaluation includes blood culture (at birth) and CBC with differential and platelets (at birth and/or at 6–12 hrs of life).

** See Table 12.3 for indications for intrapartum GBS prophylaxis.

†† If signs of sepsis develop, a full diagnostic evaluation should be conducted and antibiotic therapy initiated.

§§ If ≥37 wks' gestation, observation may occur at home after 24 hours if other discharge criteria have been met, access to medical care is readily available, and a person who is able to comply fully with instructions for home observation will be present. If any of these conditions is not met, the infant should be observed in the hospital for at least 48 hours and until discharge criteria are achieved.

¶¶ Some experts recommend a CBC with differential and platelets at age 6–12 hrs.

November 2010

FIGURE 12.2 Algorithm for secondary prevention of early-onset group B streptococcal (GBS) disease among newborns. (With permission from the CDC—http://www.cdc.gov/mmwr/preview/mmwrhtml/rr5910a1. htm?s_cid = rr5910a1_w)

TABLE 12.2 GBS INTRAPARTUM ANTIBIOTIC PROPHYLAXIS

Indications and nonindications for intrapartum antibiotic prophylaxis to prevent early-onset group B streptococcal (GBS) disease

INTRAPARTUM GBS PROPHYLAXIS INDICATED	INTRAPARTUM GBS PROPHYLAXIS NOT INDICATED
Previous infant with invasive GBS disease	Colonization with GBS during a previous pregnancy (unless an indication for GBS prophylaxis is present for current pregnancy)
GBS bacteriuria during any trimester of the current pregnancy	GBS bacteriuria during previous pregnancy (unless an indication for GBS prophylaxis is present for current pregnancy)
Positive GBS vaginal-rectal screening culture in late gestation during current pregnancy	Negative vaginal and rectal GBS screening culture in late gestation during the current pregnancy, regardless of intrapartum risk factors
Unknown GBS status at the onset of labor (culture not done, incomplete, or results unknown) and any of the following: • Delivery at <37 wks' gestation • Amniotic membrane rupture ≥18 hrs • Intrapartum temperature ≥100.4°F (≥38.0°C) • Intrapartum nucleic acid amplification test (NAAT) positive for GBS	Cesarean birth performed before onset of labor on a woman with intact amniotic membranes, regardless of GBS colonization status or gestational age

Intrapartum antibiotic prophylaxis is not indicated in this circumstance if a cesarean birth is performed before onset of labor on a woman with intact amniotic membranes

Optimal timing for prenatal GBS screening is at 35–37 wks' gestation

If amnionitis is suspected, broad-spectrum antibiotic therapy that includes an agent known to be active against GBS should replace GBS prophylaxis

SKILL UNIT OBTAINING A GBS CULTURE

Step 1	Informed the woman about the testing procedure and rationale for testing	
Step 2	Swab the lower vagina (vaginal introitus)	A speculum should not be used for culture collection
Step 3	Swab the rectum by inserting through the anal sphincter	The same swab or a different swab may be used; cervical, perianal, perirectal, or perineal specimens are not acceptable
Step 4	Place the swab(s) into a nonnutritive transport medium	Appropriate transport systems (e.g., Stuart's or Amies with or without charcoal) are commercially available. GBS isolates can remain viable in transport media for several days at room temperature; however, the recovery of isolates declines over 1–4 d, especially at elevated temperatures, which can lead to false-negative results. When feasible, specimens should be refrigerated before processing
Step 4	Label the specimen	Specimen requisitions should indicate clearly that specimens are for GBS testing

From Centers for Disease Control and Prevention. (2010). Prevention of perinatal group B streptococcal disease. *Morbidity and Mortality Weekly Report, 59*(RR-10). Retrieved from: http://www.cdc.gov/mmwr/preview/mmwrhtml/rr5910a1.htm?s_cid= rr5910a1_w.

NOTE: *A woman may obtain her own culture if appropriately instructed on the procedure.*

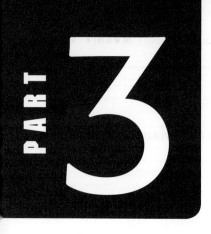

Human Immunodeficiency Virus (HIV) Infection or Acquired Immunodeficiency Syndrome (AIDS)

CYNTHIA F. KRENING

Introduction

- **What is the human immunodeficiency virus (HIV)?**

HIV is the virus that can lead to acquired immunodeficiency syndrome, or AIDS. Unlike some other viruses, the human body cannot get rid of HIV once infected. The HIV virus destroys the body's natural immune system over a number of years. It is transmitted primarily through blood and genital fluids, and to newborn infants from infected mothers. A healthy immune system destroys bacteria, parasites, viruses, and molds that it's exposed to, preventing damaging effects to the human body. The CD4 cell, also known as the T4 cell or T-helper cell, plays an essential role in orchestrating the body's immune responses. When the HIV virus invades the body, it uses the CD4 cell for replication. With CD4 lymphocytes, HIV replication can cause cell death; while in other cells, such as macrophages, persistent infection can occur, creating hosts for the virus in many cells and tissues. HIV produces cellular immune deficiency characterized by the depletion of helper T lymphocytes (CD4 cells).

Initially, antibodies are produced in reaction to the penetration of HIV in the cells, and there is a balance between the destruction of CD4 cells during HIV replication and the production of new CD4 cells. Over time though, the individual's immune system is no longer capable of producing enough new CD4 cells to compensate for the loss of those cells to the virus. Declining numbers of CD4 cells result in the progressive decline of the individual's immune response and the development of opportunistic infections and neoplastic processes. The HIV virus causes AIDS by interacting with a large number of different cells in the body and escaping the host immune response against it. The host reaction against HIV, through neutralizing antibodies and particularly through strong cellular immune responses, can keep the virus suppressed for many years. Long-term survival appears to involve infection with a relatively low-virulence strain that remains sensitive to the immune response.

Phases of HIV Infection

- **What are the phases of HIV infection?**

There are three distinct phases of HIV infection: acute infection and seroconversion, asymptomatic infection and AIDS[1].

Acute Infection and Seroconversion

In humans, 4 to 11 days after mucosal entrance of the virus, there is a rapid onset of plasma viremia with widespread dissemination of the virus.[1] *Viral load*—the amount of HIV in the blood—expressed by the number of virus copies per milliliter of blood is typically very high at this point. The greater the viral load, the more chance that the CD4 cell count will fall as the virus uses CD4 cells to make copies of itself and destroys those cells in the process. With a high viral load, the risk of transmission of the virus to others is the highest. Symptoms of seroconversion can include fever, flu symptoms, lymphadenopathy, and rash. These symptoms occur in approximately half of all people infected with HIV. Seroconversion can take a few weeks to several months.[1] Eventually, the immune response will begin to bring the amount of virus back down to a stable level. At this point, CD4 counts will begin to increase, but may not return to pre infection levels.

Asymptomatic Infection

During this phase, HIV is still active, but reproduces at very low levels. Those infected will have few or no symptoms at all for a number of years. This is because the immune response against the virus is effective and vigorous. Those on ARV therapy may live with clinical latency for several decades. If not taking ARVs, this period can last up to a decade, but some may progress through this phase faster. During this phase of clinical latency, those with HIV can still transmit it, even if on ARV therapy, although the medications greatly reduce the risk. Near the end of this phase, the viral load again begins to rise, and the CD4 count begins to drop. Symptoms of HIV infection reappear, as the weakened immune system is unable to provide protection.

AIDS

AIDS occurs when the immune system is damaged enough that it's vulnerable to opportunistic infections and infection-related cancers. In the United States, a CD4 cell count less than $200/\mu L$ is also used as a test to indicate AIDS, although some opportunistic infections develop when CD4 cell counts are higher than $200/\mu L$, and some with CD4 counts under $200/\mu L$ may remain relatively healthy. A diagnosis of AIDS is also made when one or more opportunistic illnesses are present, regardless of the CD4 count. Many opportunistic infections and conditions are used to mark when HIV infection has progressed to AIDS. All of these infections and conditions are uncommon or mild in immunocompetent persons. When one of these is unusually severe or frequent in a person infected with HIV, and no other causes for immune suppression can be found, AIDS is diagnosed.[2] Without treatment, those who are diagnosed with AIDS usually survive about 3 years. In the presence of a dangerous opportunistic illness, life expectancy without treatment falls to an average of 1 year.

• **What are opportunistic infections?**

Opportunistic infections are caused by organisms that a healthy immune system, under normal situations, could easily destroy on its own or manage to overcome with the assistance of medication. However, with HIV infection, the immune system is compromised, and an opportunistic infection can be life threatening. Opportunistic infections are more frequent or more severe because of immunosuppression in those living with HIV infection. Prior to the widespread use of potent combination ARV therapy, opportunistic infections were the primary cause of morbidity and mortality in this population. Since the early 1990s, better strategies for managing acute infections, chemoprophylaxis, and immunizations have improved quality of life and survival rates.[3] Table 12.3 outlines the most common opportunistic infections that occur if the woman has HIV infection.

TABLE 12.3 OPPORTUNISTIC INFECTIONS IN HIV

Early in HIV Infection

• Thrush	• Pneumococcal pneumonia
• Shingles	• Oral hairy leukoplakia
• Herpes simplex	• Thrombocytopenic purpura

Late in the Course of HIV Infection

• *Pneumocystis carinii* pneumonia (PCP)	• Toxoplasmosis
• Kaposi sarcoma	• Cryptococcosis
• Tuberculosis	• Cryptosporidiosis

From COHIS. (2000). *AIDS/HIV opportunistic infections* [Online]. Retrieved from: www.medvalet.com/index.html.

• What is the state of the HIV/AIDS epidemic?

HIV and AIDS were the first identified in the early 1980s. In the past 30 years, this disease has become the worst international pandemic of the 20th century. At the end of 2012, 35 million people were living with HIV, although the prevalence of this epidemic continues to vary widely around the world.[5,6] Currently, more than 1.1 million people in the United States are living with HIV infection.[7] Over the past decade, the annual number of new HIV infections in the United States has remained relatively stable, although the number of people living with HIV has increased due to prolonged survival.[7] An estimated 15,529 people with an AIDS diagnosis died in the United States in 2010.[7] The distribution of people living with HIV and AIDS is concentrated in the southern states, urban communities, and is most prevalent in Black/African-American and Hispanic/Latinos.[8] In 2011, 25% of HIV-infected people in the United States were women, and 20% of new infections were in women.[9] Almost 85% of new HIV infections in women are attributed to heterosexual contact. Only about one half of women with an HIV diagnosis were receiving treatment for their condition in 2010, and even less had the virus under control.[9] The number of women with HIV giving birth in the United States increased approximately 30%, from 2000 to 2006. Despite the increase in the number of women infected with HIV giving birth, the estimated number of perinatal HIV infections per year continues to decline. In 2010, 75% of children infected with HIV acquired it perinatally.[10] This reflects a decline in perinatal transmission from the beginning of the epidemic.[10] The number of children newly infected with HIV in 2012 had declined 35% in 3 years.[10]

Risk Factors and Transmission

• What are some risk factors for acquiring HIV infection?

Some of the factors that place women at increased risk for HIV infection include the following:
- Lack of knowledge about male partner's risk factors for HIV
- Vaginal or anal sex without a condom
- Fear of talking with male partner about need for condom use
- Sexually transmitted diseases (STDs) such as gonorrhea and syphilis
- History of sexual abuse
- Injection drug and other substance use
- Sex with Black/African-American or Hispanic/Latino, due to the high prevalence of people living with HIV in African-American and Hispanic/Latino communities[9]

• What are the methods of HIV transmission?

The risk of acquiring HIV varies with the type of exposure, with some carrying a much higher risk of transmission than others.[11] See Table 12.4.

Currently, the most common methods of HIV transmission are the following:
- Sexual transmission; homosexual and heterosexual
- Perinatal transmission
- Parenteral transmission; injection drug users[12]

HIV is transmitted through the following[13]:
- Blood
- Semen
- Pre seminal fluid
- Rectal fluid
- Vaginal secretions
- Breast milk

Fluids must come in contact with a mucous membrane or damaged tissue or be directly injected into the bloodstream (from a needle or syringe) for transmission to occur. HIV transmission occurs vertically or horizontally.

| **TABLE 12.4** | HIV TRANSMISSION RISK |

June 2014

The risk of getting HIV varies widely depending on the type of exposure. Some exposures, such as exposure to HIV during a blood transfusion, carry a much higher risk of transmission than other exposures, such as oral sex. For some exposures, risk of transmission, while biologically plausible, is so low that it is not possible to provide a precise number.

Different factors can increase or decrease transmission risk. For example, taking antiretroviral therapy (i.e., medicines for HIV infection) can reduce the risk of an HIV-infected person transmitting the infection to another by as much as 96%[1], and consistent use of condoms reduces the risk of getting or transmitting HIV by about 80%[2]. Using both condoms and antiretroviral therapy reduces the risk of HIV acquisition from sexual exposure by 99.2%[3]. Conversely, having a sexually transmitted infection or a high level of HIV virus in the blood (which happens in early and late-stage infection) may increase transmission risk.

The table below lists the risk of transmission per 10,000 exposures for various types of exposures.

Estimated Per-Act Probability of Acquiring HIV from an Infected Source, by Exposure Act*

TYPE OF EXPOSURE	RISK PER 10,000 EXPOSURES
Parenteral[3]	
Blood Transfusion	9,250
Needle-sharing during injection drug use	63
Percutaneous (needle-stick)	23
Sexual[3]	
Receptive anal intercourse	138
Insertive anal intercourse	11
Receptive penile-vaginal intercourse	8
Insertive penile-vaginal intercourse	4
Receptive oral intercourse	low
Insertive oral intercourse	low
Other ^	
Biting	negligible[4]
Spitting	negligible
Throwing body fluids (including semen or saliva)	negligible
Sharing sex toys	negligible

Reprinted with permission from the CDC.

* Factors that may increase the risk of HIV transmission include sexually transmitted diseases, acute and late-stage HIV infection, and high viral load. Factors that may decrease the risk include condom use, male circumcision, antiretroviral treatment, and pre-exposure prophylaxis. None of these factors are accounted for in the estimates presented in the table.

^ HIV transmission through these exposure routes is technically possible but unlikely and not well documented.

[1] Cohen MS, Chen YQ, McCauley M, et al; HPTN 052 Study Team. Prevention of HIV-1 Infection with early antiretroviral therapy. N Engl J Med 2011;365(6):493–505.

[2] Weller SC, Davis-Beaty K. Condom effectiveness in reducing heterosexual HIV transmission (Review). The Cochrane Collaboration. Wiley and Sons, 2011.

[3] Patel P, Borkowf CB, Brooks JT. Et al. Estimating per-act HIV transmission risk: a systematic review. AIDS. 2014. doi: 10.1097/QAD.0000000000000298.

[4] Pretty LA, Anderson GS, Sweet DJ. Human bites and the risk of human immunodeficiency virus transmission. Am J Forensic Med Pathol 1999;20(3):232–239.

Horizontal Transmission of HIV

In horizontal transmission, the virus is transmitted from an HIV-infected person to another by direct contact. Examples of such contact include the following:

- **Intimate sexual contact (oral, anal, or vaginal) with someone infected with the HIV.**
- **Sharing of drug needles and syringes with an infected individual.**
- **Receipt of a blood transfusion that contains HIV**—Risk from blood transfusions has been virtually eliminated through careful screening procedures now done on all donated blood and plasma.
- Inadvertent contamination of mucous membranes or breaks in the skin (e.g., of a nurse or other healthcare provider) by the blood or body fluid of the infected person.

Vertical Transmission of HIV

Vertical transmission of HIV occurs when the virus is passed from the mother to her infant during the perinatal period. Transmission can occur during the antepartum, intrapartum, or postpartum period. HIV has been isolated from many sources (early gestational embryo, blood, breast milk, amniotic fluid, cord blood, and the placenta), which indicates multiple potential routes of fetal or neonatal transmission. The virus has been isolated in 13- to 20-week-old fetuses, but **transmission is generally believed to occur most often in late pregnancy.**[14,15] In the United States, the extensive implementation of the Public Health Service guidelines for universal counseling and testing, and the use of a combination of ARV agents have sharply reduced transmission risk and the number of mother-to-infant transmissions. **Risk factors for vertical transmission include the following:**

- Immunologically or clinically advanced HIV disease
- Increased plasma viral load
- Injected drug use during pregnancy
- Low CD4 cell count
- Breastfeeding
- Lack of ARV therapy in pregnancy
- Invasive procedures; for example, amniocentesis, fetal scalp electrode, fetal scalp sampling

NOTE: The Public Health Service provides specific management guidelines for postexposure ARV intervention. Every institution should use these guidelines.

Diagnosis of HIV

• How is the diagnosis of HIV infection made?

The antibody screening test (immunoassay) is the most common test for the presence of HIV. It tests for antibodies that the body makes against HIV. The immunoassay may be conducted in a lab or as a rapid test. Most blood-based lab tests find infection sooner after exposure than rapid HIV tests. Other tests can detect both antibodies and antigen (part of the virus itself). These tests identify recent infection earlier than tests that detect only antibodies. As soon as 3 weeks after exposure to the virus, the antigen/antibody combination tests can find HIV in the bloodstream. The rapid test is an immunoassay used for screening, producing quick results, usually within an hour or less. Rapid tests detect HIV antibodies in the blood. If an immunoassay (lab test or rapid test) is conducted during the window period (the period after exposure but before the test can detect antibodies), a false-negative result may be reported.

All immunoassays that are positive require follow-up diagnostic testing to confirm the result. Follow-up tests include the following:

- antibody differentiation test, which distinguishes HIV-1 from HIV-2;
- HIV-1 nucleic acid test, which looks for virus directly; or the
- Western blot or indirect immunofluorescence assay, which detect antibodies.

Although immunoassays are generally very accurate, follow-up testing is routine.[16] The CDC has published updated recommendations for HIV testing by US laboratories. The revised algorithm is a sequence of tests used in combination to improve the accuracy of the laboratory diagnosis of HIV. These updated guidelines include tests for HIV antigens and nucleic acid. Studies have shown that antibody testing alone may miss a considerable percentage of HIV infections detectable by virologic tests.[17]

• What are the recommendations for HIV testing in pregnancy?

All pregnant women should be offered routine, universal HIV testing early in pregnancy. ACOG, the Institute of Medicine, CDC, other leading professional organizations, and most states support *opt-out HIV screening.* With this approach to testing, the patient is notified that HIV testing will be performed as a routine part of obstetric care and written consent is not required. As with any testing, the woman has the option to opt out and decline testing. This approach helps to reduce barriers to testing that may result from extensive counseling or from perceptions of stigmatization associated with HIV status. If a woman initially declines testing, education should be provided, and she should continue to be encouraged to be tested. Women with an acute infection who have symptoms of acute retroviral syndrome or who suspect recent HIV exposure should be offered repeat testing. Repeat testing should also be offered during the third trimester of pregnancy to women who had an earlier negative HIV test but who have continued high-risk behaviors. If a woman presents with symptoms of labor and an unknown HIV status, rapid HIV testing should be done (using an opt-out consent strategy when allowed by jurisdiction).[18]

Newborns of women who decline HIV testing or whose infection status remains unknown at birth should have rapid antibody testing as soon as possible after birth. The mother should be informed that a positive newborn test indicates maternal HIV infection but not necessarily an infant infection.[18] Screening all pregnant women for HIV, and giving them appropriate medical care, helped to decrease the number of babies born with HIV from a high of 1,650 in 1991 to 127 in 2011.[16]

• What is the effect of pregnancy on HIV infection?

Even though pregnancy is accompanied by a mildly immunosuppressive state, **no conclusive evidence exists that pregnancy aggravates the health of the expectant woman who has HIV infection.**[19] Evidence has shown no overall significant differences in HIV disease progression, progression to AIDS, fall in CD4 count to below 200 or death comparing pregnant women and nonpregnant women with HIV infection.[20] In addition, there is no difference in viral load, CD4, or progression of clinical disease in women who had one pregnancy when compared with women with more than one pregnancy.[21]

During pregnancy, a decline in absolute CD4 cell counts is seen in both HIV-positive and HIV-negative women. It is thought to be secondary to hemodilution of pregnancy. Therefore, the use of a percentage of CD4 cells, rather than an absolute number of CD4 cells, is the most accurate method to measure immune function. Pregnancy does not accelerate a decline in CD4 cells, and HIV RNA (viral load) levels remain relatively stable during pregnancy.[22]

There is some evidence that during the postpartum period viral load levels increase despite ARV therapy, possibly due to immune activation associated with hormonal changes, or the end of pregnancy-related viral load suppression. Transmission risk and treatment recommendations have not been clarified for this increase in viral load.[23–25] This postpartum increase in viral load does not appear to be long-lasting.[21,25]

• What is the effect of HIV infection on pregnancy?

Some studies suggest that HIV-infected women may have multiple coexisting risk factors for adverse pregnancy outcome including sexually transmitted infections (STIs), malnutrition, poverty, substance abuse, domestic violence, and inadequate or no prenatal care. If these problems are controlled for, there is no independent effect of HIV on adverse outcomes.[26] Risk factors for adverse pregnancy outcomes in women receiving ARV therapy are similar to those reported in uninfected women.[26] There may be a slightly increased risk for preterm delivery prior to 37 weeks' gestation in women taking protease inhibitors (PIs), but data are conflicting.[27] The clear benefits of ARV agents in reducing perinatal transmission of HIV outweigh the conflicting data regarding preterm birth.

Reducing Perinatal Transmission

• How is the risk of perinatal HIV transmission reduced?

NOTE: NO Therapies Guarantee A 0% Risk Of Vertical Transmission. The Highest Risk for Vertical Transmission is Among Women With Relatively High Plasma Viral Loads.

Every infant that is born HIV infected is a sentinel health event as a result of either a missed prevention opportunity or, rarely, prophylaxis failure.[5]

Strategies to Prevent Transmission

- Early prenatal care
- Universal HIV testing
- In the HIV-positive woman:
  - Reducing viral load
  - ARV regimen
  - Minimizing exposure of fetus to HIV during the intrapartum period
  - Preventing exposure to HIV infection during the postpartum period

Transmission rate can be reduced to less than 2% with universal screening of women in combination with ARV prophylaxis, scheduled cesarean birth when indicated, and avoidance of breastfeeding.[28]

• How is the viral load reduced?

The viral load (also called the HIV RNA test) is a measurement of the magnitude of active HIV replication. The viral load assesses the relative risk for disease progression and the efficacy of ARV therapies. The CD4 cell count is an indicator of the extent of immune system damage. The CD4 cell count assesses the risk for developing specific opportunistic infections and other sequelae of HIV infection. When the viral load and the CD4 cell count are used together, the risk for disease progression can be predicted.

NOTE: The viral load correlates with the risk of perinatal transmission.

Mother-to-child transmission of HIV is the most common way that children become infected with the virus. Although perinatal HIV transmission can occur during pregnancy, labor, and birth, or during breastfeeding, currently the risk of perinatal transmission is less than 2% in the United States and Europe. HIV-infected pregnant women should be educated that ARV drug regimens during pregnancy are highly recommended because viral suppression significantly decreases the risk of transmission to the fetus. Full viral suppression decreases the risk of perinatal HIV transmission to around 1%,[29] while those with a viral load greater than 30,000 copies/mL have a transmission rate of up to 23%.[30] Unfortunately, data indicate that even some women with an undetectable viral load are still able to transmit the virus to their newborn. Because the low residual risk may be due to the presence of HIV in the genital secretions, ARV prophylaxis is recommended for all pregnant women regardless of their viral load.

The current standard of care is the simultaneous use of three ARV drugs for full viral suppression. In making decisions regarding treatment in a pregnant woman, the following must be considered:

- The treatment of HIV infection
- Reduction of the risk of perinatal transmission
- The known and unknown benefits and risks of therapy as well as nontherapy

Careful medication selection is important to avoid toxicity in the woman and developing fetus. Combination ARV regimens are more effective in reducing transmission than a single-drug regimen. Prophylaxis antepartal, and during the intrapartum and postpartum period, combined with newborn prophylaxis is more effective than only intrapartum and postpartum treatments. The earlier in pregnancy prophylaxis is initiated, the more effective the regimen is in reducing perinatal transmission.

Pregnancy is not a reason to delay standard HIV treatment for maternal health. In 2012, 62% of pregnant women living with HIV were receiving ARV treatment.[5] Recommended treatments for viral suppression during pregnancy are outlined in Table 12.5.

TABLE 12.5 RECOMMENDED STRATEGIES FOR VIRAL LOAD SUPPRESSION	
	PREGNANCY RECOMMENDATIONS
On antiretroviral therapy with viral suppression	Continue antiretroviral medications if tolerating regime Certain agents may require dosing changes
On antiretroviral therapy without viral suppression	Evaluate reason viral suppression has not been achieved (nonadherence, drug resistance) Consider drug resistance testing and new antiretroviral medication regime tailored to the resistance profile and medication tolerance of the woman

---

NOTE: The standard of care is the simultaneous use of multiple ARV drugs to suppress the viral load below detectable limits regardless of CD4 cell count or plasma HIV RNA copy number, in order to prevent perinatal transmission of HIV.

Treatment Naïve (Treatment in Someone Who Has Never Taken HIV Drugs Before as Opposed to Someone Who Is "Treatment-Experienced")

Perinatal transmission of HIV is decreased with initiation of an ARV regimen early in pregnancy, so that viral suppression is attained by the time of birth.[31,32] However, the benefits of any medication regimen must be weighed against any known fetal teratogenic effects of drug exposure in the first trimester. In the first trimester of pregnancy, women who have not begun ARV therapy may wish to delay initiation of therapy until after completion of organogenesis at 10 to 12 weeks' gestation. Delaying initiation of medications until the second trimester is an option if CD4 cell count is greater than 350 cells/µL. ARV prophylaxis should be initiated regardless of gestational age if the CD4 cell count is less than 350 cells/mm,[3] symptoms of HIV disease, or a co-infection, a high viral load or AIDS are present.[27]

• What are the pharmacotherapeutic treatments for HIV infection in pregnancy?

The drug regimen for HIV treatment and prevention of perinatal transmission is based on efficacy and safety for both the woman and fetus. Few comparative data are available on the most efficacious agents to use during pregnancy. The discussion about antiviral regimens should include the following:
- Potential impact of therapy on the fetus and newborn
- Ability to adhere to the prescribed regimen
- Long-term treatment plans for the woman

Most available studies have focused on prevention of infant transmission instead of efficacy of the medication in treatment of HIV during pregnancy. The mean half-life of plasma virions (a complete virus particle) is estimated at only 6 hours, so the focus of intervention is to initiate aggressive combination ARV regimens quickly to maximally suppress viral replication, preserve immune function, and reduce the development of drug resistance.[22,33] In the pregnant HIV-infected woman, administration of a three-drug ARV regimen continues HIV treatment while preventing mother-to-child transmission of the disease. In most patients, viral suppression is generally achieved in 12 to 24 weeks.

For the majority of women, the HIV regimen used in pregnancy includes two nucleoside reverse-transcriptase inhibitors (NRTIs) which easily cross the placenta, plus a nonnucleoside reverse-transcriptase inhibitor (NNTRI), or one or more PIs.[34] Nucleoside analog reverse-transcriptase inhibitors inhibit viral replication in the cells by targeting the HIV reverse-transcriptase enzyme. Protease inhibitors prevent maturation of virus protein by competitively inhibiting HIV protease (an enzyme essential for viral protein cleavage). Blockage of this enzyme leads to immature, noninfectious virus particles being produced.[22] **PIs along with NRTIs can reduce plasma viral load to undetectable levels for prolonged periods.**

NOTE: Although unique considerations associated with pregnancy should be discussed, pregnancy is not a reason to defer ARV treatment.

While the NRTI zidovudine (ZDV) is no longer considered a preferred medication for treatment in the nonpregnant woman, it continues as a first-line agent used during pregnancy because of its extensive safety profile and use experience in pregnant women. ZDV has shown efficacy in decreasing perinatal transmission of HIV by rapidly crossing the placenta and providing protective serum levels of medication in the fetus. Efavirenz, a nonnucleoside reverse-transcriptase inhibitor, is contraindicated in the first 8 weeks of pregnancy due to risk of teratogenicity, although it's a first-line ARV for treatment naïve women who are not pregnant. Because of potential hepatotoxicity and fatal rash, nevirapine (another NNRTI) should not be routinely used in treatment naïve women with CD4 cell counts greater than 250 cells/mm.[3]

Providers experienced in ARV drug therapy should assist in development of the drug regimen for all HIV-infected women who become pregnant. These providers will take into account treatment naivety, tolerance, history of ARV drug exposure, prior resistance testing, virologic response, level of viral suppression, patient drug adherence, pregnancy-related changes that can affect medication choice, risk of side effects, and potential short- and long-term effects of the medications on babies born to women with HIV. Other factors considered are tolerability, convenience, and individual drug interactions. Monitoring for complications of ARV drugs is based upon the known adverse effects of each drug. Women may require monitoring of hematologic markers, renal function, or liver function tests during their pregnancy. There are conflicting results in studies looking at the contribution of ARV medications to fetal teratogenicity, gestational diabetes mellitus, fetal growth, low birth weight, and preterm birth. Standard assessments and prenatal screening should aid the treatment team in the identification of any complications of pregnancy that may be a result of antiretroviral therapies. The pregnancy risks must always be weighed against the risks of loss of virologic control and subsequent perinatal transmission if antiretroviral medications are changed.

TABLE 12.6	SIDE EFFECTS OF ANTIRETROVIRAL THERAPY
Nucleoside analogs	The most concerning adverse effect of this category of drugs is mitochondrial toxicity manifested as lactic acidosis or symptomatic hyperlactatemia.[35] Symptoms of these effects include weight loss, nausea, vomiting, right upper quadrant pain, abdominal bloating, myalgias, and fatigue. Zidovudine commonly causes these effects of mitochondrial toxicity.
NNRTIs	Most of the side effects seen with this category of antiretrovirals are from nevirapine. Rash and hepatotoxicity are the most concerning effects.
Protease Inhibitors	Common side effects with PIs include rash, gastrointestinal symptoms, dry eyes and mouth, nephrolithiasis and headache. **Protease inhibitors** have also been reported to cause hyperglycemia, new-onset diabetes mellitus, exacerbation of existing diabetes mellitus, and diabetic ketoacidosis. Because pregnancy can also cause hyperglycemia (as seen with gestational diabetes), pregnant women receiving protease inhibitor drugs should be monitored closely for hyperglycemia.[36]

- **Are there serious side effects of ARV therapy?**

Drug intolerance is the leading reason necessitating a change in ARV therapy. See Table 12.6 for common side effect of ARV therapy.

NOTE: Providers who are treating HIV-infected pregnant women and their newborns are advised to report cases of prenatal exposure to ARV drugs to the Antiretroviral Pregnancy Registry (APR).

- **What is the Antiretroviral Pregnancy Registry?[37]**

The APR is an epidemiologic project to collect observational, non experimental data on ARV drug exposure during pregnancy for the purpose of assessing the potential teratogenicity of these drugs. Registry data will be used to supplement animal toxicology studies and assist clinicians in weighing the potential risks and benefits of treatment for individual patients. The registry is a collaborative project of the pharmaceutical manufacturers with an advisory committee of obstetric and pediatric practitioners. It is strongly recommended that healthcare providers who are treating HIV-infected pregnant women and their newborns report cases of prenatal exposure to ARV drugs (either alone or in combination) to the APR. The registry does not use patient names and birth outcome follow-up is obtained from the reporting physician by registry staff. *Referrals should be directed to: Telephone: 1–800–258–4263, Fax: 1–800–800–1052.*

Prenatal Care in the HIV-Infected Pregnant Woman

Favorable maternal outcomes and low incidence of perinatal HIV transmission are associated with comprehensive prenatal care of HIV-infected women.

Fetal Assessment

Early ultrasonography is important for accurate dating in the event of incomplete viral suppression requires early birth. Additionally, a detailed second-trimester ultrasound evaluation of fetal anatomy should be done in women who were on a combination of ARV medications during their first trimester. Although there has not been data to suggest an increase in congenital birth defects while taking these medications, there are limited data on new ARVs being administered. Regular assessment of fundal height will aid in the assessment for poor fetal growth, which has been associated with ARV use in some studies, particularly protease inhibitors.[38] When amniocentesis or any other invasive procedure is indicated, limited data do not show an additional risk for in utero transmission of HIV in those on an effective ARV regimen with undetectable plasma viral loads.

Laboratory Testing

- Hematocrit: Maternal anemia has been associated with increased risk of perinatal HIV transmission.[39] Complete blood count should be done every 3 months.

- HIV RNA: Viral load should be assessed at the initial prenatal visit, 2 to 4 weeks after initiating or changing ARV regimens, monthly until undetectable, and at least every 3 months during pregnancy, depending on the amount of viral suppression present. If adherence to the medication regimen is a concern, more frequent monitoring should be done because of the increased risk of perinatal HIV transmission associated with HIV viremia during pregnancy. At 34 to 36 weeks' gestation, HIV RNA levels should be assessed to determine mode of birth.

- CD4 cell count: CD4 cell count should be monitored at the initial prenatal visit and at least every 3 months until delivered. In women who are clinically stable with consistently suppressed viral loads on an ARV regimen that has increased their CD4 count well above the threshold for opportunistic infections, CD4 testing can be done every 6 months. While a decline in absolute CD4 count is seen during pregnancy due to hemodilution, there is usually no effect on the CD4 cell percentage.[40,41] The CD4 cell criteria for treatment are the same as in nonpregnant HIV-infected patient.

- Serum chemistry panel will screen for adverse effects of some drug therapies.

- Gestational diabetes mellitus screening: Women on protease inhibitors may require screening for gestational diabetes mellitus earlier than usual, as these agents have been associated with glucose intolerance in the HIV-infected population.

- Hepatitis: Co-infection with viral hepatitis is common in HIV-infected patients, so pregnant HIV-infected women should be screened for both hepatitis B and C. Women with chronic hepatitis B or C infection should be screened for antibodies to hepatitis A virus.

Immunizations

Necessary immunizations should be given as early as possible in the course of HIV infection because the ability to form specific antibodies after immunizations becomes progressively impaired as the disease advances. (Remember that immune system function declines as the disease advances.) Live pathogen vaccines, such as the MMR (measles–mumps–rubella), are contraindicated, but killed or inactivated vaccines are considered safe.[22] In addition to routine immunizations administered during pregnancy, HIV-infected women should also receive the pneumococcal vaccine and hepatitis A and B, if not infected in the past.

A thorough history and physical examination should be performed to identify health concerns in the mother that may also affect fetal well-being. Along with an initial social, emotional, and nutritional assessment, the initial medical assessment of the HIV-infected woman should address any history of opportunistic infections, tuberculosis, STDs, medications, immunizations, substance abuse, fevers, and weight loss (indicating underlying opportunistic infection). In addition to the usual physical assessments, these women should also be evaluated for any signs or symptoms of advanced HIV infection, concomitant STDs, viral hepatitis, and history of prior and current ARV medications.

Intrapartum Management

Mode of Birth

In women on effective ARV regimens whose plasma HIV RNA <1,000 copies/mL, overall incidence of HIV transmission is low whether delivered vaginally or by cesarean birth. Additionally, duration of rupture of membranes does not increase transmission incidence.[42–45] Based on these data, cesarean births should only be carried out for obstetrical indications. Conversely, pre labor cesarean birth at 38 weeks' gestation (before onset of labor and rupture of membranes) significantly decreases the risk of perinatal transmission in women with HIV and viral loads >1,000 copies/mL. This may include women not on an ARV regimen, those presenting late in pregnancy, or those who are not responding to their current ARV regimen.[46] An HIV-infected woman who presents in labor or with ruptured membranes prior to a scheduled cesarean birth must receive individualized management. The current HIV RNA level, duration of membrane rupture, and current ARV regimen are all taken into account when planning the safest mode of birth for these women.

Duration of rupture of membranes was associated with a risk of perinatal HIV transmission prior to the widespread administration of combination ARV medications. Outcomes have improved with the current regimens. In a prospective study published in 2012,[46] there were no cases of HIV transmission in 144 women with HIV RNA <1,000 copies/mL who had rupture of membranes more than 4 hours prior to birth. In the same study in women with >1,000 copies/mL HIV RNA receiving combination ARV therapy, perinatal transmission was 3.8% if duration of rupture of membranes was less than 4 hours, compared with 4.9% if 4 or more hours. These data included women who delivered via cesarean as well as vaginally, and the difference noted was not statistically significant. The only independent risk factor for perinatal transmission was a viral load greater than 10,000 copies/mL.[46]

Preterm Premature Rupture of Membranes

The presence of HIV infection in a pregnant woman should not alter management in the presence of preterm premature rupture of membranes. Decisions regarding birth timing should be based on obstetrical best practice considering the prematurity risks for the newborn. There is no data to suggest that a course of antenatal corticosteroids to enhance fetal lung maturity should be omitted in women with HIV and preterm premature rupture of membranes.

Antiretrovirals

Administration of ARVs should continue throughout labor or cesarean birth. Additional ZDV administration may be indicated to decrease mother-to-child transmission, depending on viral load. Intravenous ZDV is an NRTI recommended for women with HIV RNA greater than 1,000 copies/mL near birth, unknown HIV RNA levels and those with possible poor adherence to their medication regimen. Intravenous ZDV should be administered 3 hours before cesarean birth in those with HIV RNA >1,000 copies/mL. If an HIV-infected woman presents in labor with no history of an ARV regimen, she should be given intravenous ZDV immediately to minimize the risk of perinatal transmission. Conversely, if an HIV-infected woman is adhering to her combination ARV therapy, and has a viral load less than 1,000 copies/mL consistently in late pregnancy, intravenous ZDV is not recommended, as it has not been shown to further decrease the risk of perinatal transmission.[34,47,48]

Other Interventions

Because most infants born to HIV-positive women are not infected with HIV, care must be taken to protect and prevent further exposure of these infants to the virus. Avoiding procedures that increase risk for infection is an important element in reducing the risk. Procedures that increase risk of HIV infection in the fetus include invasive procedures and extended exposure to potentially infected body fluids. *The following should generally be avoided because of a potential increased risk of transmission, unless there are clear obstetric indications:*

- **Artificial rupture of membranes**
  - **Internal fetal heart rate monitoring**—The spiral electrode pierces the scalp of the fetus and permits exposure to maternal amniotic fluid, so it should be avoided.
  - **Fetal pH scalp sampling**—Fetal scalp sampling involves breaks in the skin surface of the fetus to obtain a small blood sample for analysis. It can increase the potential for inoculation with HIV. Unless an urgent medical reason exists for performing this procedure, it is not recommended in the HIV-infected woman.
- **Operative vaginal birth**—With the use of forceps and vacuum extractors, there's a risk of breaking the skin, exposing the fetus to maternal body fluids.
  - **Episiotomy**—Newborns can also be infected during the birth process by exposure to the woman's infected body fluids.
- **Cutting the cord with contaminated instruments**—Sterile instruments should be used to cut and clamp the cord after birth. This reduces the risk of cross-contamination from instruments that have been in contact with maternal tissues and body fluids.

Overall obstetric management should be aimed at minimizing the duration of fetal exposure to maternal blood and body fluids.

Treatment of the Newborn

- Dry the newborn immediately after the birth to remove all maternal blood and amniotic fluid.
- Gently remove excess fluid and blood from the nares and oropharynx with a bulb syringe, mucus extractor, or meconium aspirator with wall suction set on low setting. Because of the operator's risk of exposure to body fluids, do not use a suction device that requires the operator to provide suction by placing one end of the device in his or her mouth.

- Bathe the newborn under a radiant warmer as soon as the newborn is stable and before eye prophylaxis, injections, or blood draws. Thorough cleansing with a mild, non medicated soap removes amniotic fluid and blood from the body surface, which is essential in reducing the chance of infection. Thoroughly clean the eye area before applying antibiotic prophylaxis. Failure to remove the maternal fluids from the ocular area before prophylaxis placement can result in exposure of the mucous membranes to the virus. Alcohol should be used to prepare an injection site. The alcohol should be allowed to dry completely before the puncture is made to prevent possible skin contamination and body fluids from being transmitted into the tissues.
- *Prophylaxis:* To decrease the risk for acquiring HIV, the newborn of an HIV-infected woman should be administered prophylaxis after birth, appropriately dosed for gestational age. The goal is to protect the newborn from any virus that may have entered fetal circulation during labor, or through exposure that occurred during vaginal birth.[34]

Recommendations for newborn medications:
- *Women taking antepartum ARVs with viral suppression at birth*
  - Administration of ZDV for 6 weeks remains the standard of care. This may be decreased to 4 weeks if the woman's viral load has been suppressed throughout her pregnancy, and she has adhered to her regimen.
  - ZDV, at gestational age-appropriate doses, should be initiated as close to the time of birth as possible, preferably within 6 to 12 hours of delivery.
- *Women taking antepartum ARVs without viral suppression at birth*
  - These newborns should receive prophylactic ZDV for 6 weeks. There should be consideration for adding nevirapine to the regimen for those whose mothers have a high viral load.
- *Women without antepartum ARV therapy*
  - The newborns at highest risk for acquiring HIV are those born to women who initiated care for their disease late in pregnancy, not on ARV therapy and those diagnosed with HIV at the time of birth. Newborns who are born to women who have not received ARV medications during pregnancy require 6 weeks of ZDV prophylaxis as well as 3 doses of nevirapine—at birth, 48 hours later, and 96 hours after the second dose.
- *Women with unknown HIV status*
  - When an infant is born to a woman whose HIV status is unknown postpartum, rapid HIV antibody testing should be done on either the woman or infant as soon as possible. Newborn ARV prophylaxis with ZDV and nevirapine should be initiated immediately if the rapid test is positive, while awaiting confirmatory HIV test results.

NOTE: In the United States., the use of ARV drugs other than ZDV and nevirapine cannot be recommended as prophylaxis to prevent HIV transmission because of lack of dosing and safety data.[34]

Breastfeeding

Due to risk of mother-to-child transmission, HIV-infected women should be educated that breastfeeding is not recommended. Although therapy with combination ARV medications significantly decreases transmission incidence, the risk is not completely eliminated. Although drug levels are consistent in maternal plasma, they can vary widely in breast milk. Some medications lead to high concentrations in breast milk, while others lead to drug levels significantly less than those in the maternal bloodstream.[49–51] Another concern is the effect of chronic ARV therapy exposure of the newborn via breast milk. Given the safety, availability and affordability of alternative feeding options in the United States, HIV-infected women should not breastfeed their newborns.

Postpartum Management

- **What about care of the postpartum HIV-infected woman?**

Postpartum Antiretrovirals

Administration of ARV medications in the postpartum period should be managed as in all nonpregnant individuals with HIV. Modification of the regimen may be indicated if agents were used during pregnancy which are not ideal for long-term administration. Some women discontinue their ARV medications after delivery, or only take them episodically during pregnancies. It is unknown if discontinuation of these medications after birth by women with high CD4 cell counts affects disease progression.

NOTE: If ARV therapy is discontinued for any reason, all agents should be stopped and restarted simultaneously to prevent the development of drug resistance.[33]

Education, counseling regarding viral suppression with the regimen, and social support are important in the postpartum period to maximize adherence.

Preventing Postpartum Hemorrhage

Methergine should not be co-administered to women receiving PIs. Concomitant use of ergotamines and PIs has been associated with exaggerated vasoconstrictive responses. When uterine atony results in excessive postpartum bleeding in women receiving PIs, alternate uterotonics should be administered. In contrast, administration of additional uterotonic agents may be needed when other ARV drugs that are CYP3A4 inducers (e.g., nevirapine, efavirenz, etravirine) are used because of the potential for decreased Methergine levels and inadequate treatment effect.[34]

Special Considerations

> • **Are there special issues to consider in the inpatient management of HIV-infected women?**

The following factors must be addressed so that an effective, individualized plan of care can be developed and implemented:

Infection Control

Infection control measures must be a primary concern when providing care for the pregnant HIV-positive patient. The potential for infection of hospital personnel is certainly important; however, it is not the only consideration in the labor management of these patients. Obvious concerns are for fetal infection with HIV and for maternal infection because of potential immunocompromise and anemia. The following procedures are meant to help protect the HIV-positive woman from infection:

- **Reduce exposure to opportunistic organisms**—Limit vaginal examinations, avoid invasive procedures, avoid episiotomies and lacerations, and attend to aseptic and sterile technique when performing procedures.
- **Monitor the woman closely for signs of infection**—Check vital signs and be especially alert for increasing temperature and pulse. Perform respiratory auscultation at regular intervals. Closely review laboratory results.
- **Monitor the woman closely for signs of infection**—Check vital signs and be especially alert for increasing temperature and pulse. Perform respiratory auscultation at regular intervals. Closely review laboratory results.
- **Be alert for signs of chorioamnionitis**—The higher incidence of STIs combined with the potential for immunocompromise in HIV-positive women places the woman at risk for ascending infection. These infections have been implicated as possible causes of premature rupture of the membranes. These women require close monitoring of maternal vital signs (especially elevations of temperature and pulse), and continuous external intensive fetal surveillance to detect any signs of infection (e.g., increasing baseline rate, tachycardia, or decreasing variability).

Additional guidelines for the birth of a mother at high risk or infected with HIV include the following:

- Follow universal precautions carefully to protect *yourself* from accidental needlesticks, splatter, or contact with body fluids.
- Carefully maintain patient hygiene. Keep the skin and perineum as clean and dry as possible. Change disposable underpads frequently. Closely follow institutional guidelines for care of urinary catheters and intravenous lines.

- Review the woman's chart for evidence of normal or abnormal fetal growth (ultrasound reports, maternal weight gain, and fundal height measurements). Many factors associated with HIV infection, such as drug use, poverty, and inadequate prenatal care, have an impact on the weight and condition of the newborn at birth.
- Observe the patient and laboratory values for signs of thrombocytopenia and anemia (common side effects of ZDV therapy).
- Handle blood- and body-fluid–stained linen according to institutional infection control guidelines. Dispose of soiled linens promptly after use to reduce the chance of accidental contact with personnel.
- Follow recommended guidelines of the institution for sterilization, disinfection, and housekeeping.
- Inform the nursery staff of the woman's HIV status.
- Use universal precautions when caring for the newborn.

Psychosocial Needs

For most people, the birth of a baby is a time of happiness, joy, and celebration. **However, the HIV-positive woman *might* have ambivalent feelings about the birth process.** She might feel happy about motherhood, *but* at the same time be worried about her health and her newborn's health. This can interfere with bonding and can contribute to the development of postpartum blues or depression. The following actions can help promote maternal–infant bonding.

- Encourage the new mother to hold her newborn as soon as possible after birth.
- Personalize the newborn. Reinforce positive qualities of the newborn (e.g., pretty eyes, hair; has all her fingers and toes) and call the newborn by name.
- Encourage maternal–infant interaction. Encourage the woman to touch, talk to, and examine the newborn.
- Promote family involvement in the birth process by allowing family attendance. Encourage participation in the labor, birth, and postpartum period.

Many emotional and psychological adjustments are also occurring during this critical time. The following actions can help to promote psychological adjustment:

- If a psychiatric professional or a social worker has followed the woman, with her permission, notify that person of her status.
- Allow the woman to verbalize her feelings. Listening to her concerns will often help to reduce her anxiety and assist her in coming to terms with issues she must face.
- Do not avoid the woman because of her HIV status. Your time with her is therapeutic because women like her often feel isolated and are commonly ostracized by others.
- Avoid judgmental behavior and attitudes when providing care.
- Keep the new mother informed of both her status and that of her newborn (before and after birth). Counsel the woman regarding necessary health screenings for her newborn and herself.

NOTE: Remember that HIV is a family disease. It affects every family member, regardless of whether they are infected.

Ethical Issues

The care of the HIV-positive woman includes many emotionally charged issues for both patients and staff. These issues demand recognition and consideration to ensure that optimal care is provided to patients. The following are some of the key issues that affect both the patient and staff in the care of HIV-positive patients.

- **Confidentiality**—It is a central issue in the treatment of HIV/AIDS patients. Unauthorized disclosure of a woman's HIV status by healthcare workers is not only unethical but can cause irreparable damage to the woman by affecting social, occupational, and personal relationships. Fear of disclosure can keep women from seeking early prenatal care, receiving any prenatal care, and consenting to testing for HIV. Organizations must have well-established policies and procedures for handling and maintaining HIV-related confidential information that conform to state and federal laws.

If a breach of confidentiality occurs, it can serve as grounds for legal action.

- **Right to medical care**—This means that each individual has a right to expect the best possible health care regardless of his or her disease state.

- **Consent and coercion issues**—These include the fact that each patient has the right to full information regarding treatment options available. Decisions made by HIV-positive patients about their care should be with the full knowledge of the potential benefits, risks, indications, and side effects for both her and her unborn or newborn baby. Threat, coercion, and incomplete information have no place in patient care. Healthcare professionals have the opportunity and responsibility to help the woman to understand options for and implications of treatment.

Patient and Family Education

The HIV-positive woman, in labor, might not be able to fully concentrate on complex or lengthy explanations; therefore, effective education during this period can be difficult. In addition to information related to the labor and birth process, the following should be presented in a thorough, but concise, manner:
- Risks and benefits of medication therapy
- Contraindications to breastfeeding
- Immediate care of the newborn
- Immediate care of the woman during the postpartum period

As long as the woman and newborn are stable, the primary focus in the immediate postpartum period should be on the promotion of bonding. Extensive information concerning self-care, newborn care, contraception, lifestyle, nutrition, and transmission of HIV should be covered later.

HIV infection continues to occur in women of childbearing age with many learning of their HIV status when they become pregnant. Recent advances in both ARV and obstetric interventions can aid in reducing perinatal transmission. This involves comprehensive planning of care for the HIV-infected woman who is planning on becoming pregnant or who is already pregnant. Healthcare providers can have a major positive influence on these women and their ability to access and maintain care, as well as on both maternal and newborn outcomes.

Resources for Current HIV Information

- APR: apregistry.com
- AIDSinfo; Information on AIDS Treatment, Prevention and Research: aidsinfo.nih.gov

A U.S. Department of Health and Human Services project providing information on HIV/AIDS clinical trials and treatment.
- AIDS Education Global Information System (AGEiS): actgnetwork.org
- HIV/AIDS Treatment Info Service: hivatis.org, 800–448–0440
- Association of Nurses in AIDS Care (ANAC): nursesinaidscare.org, 800–260–6780

Professional association that provides information and advises members about clinical and policy issues related to nursing and HIV care.
- The Body: thebodypro.com

A comprehensive website of HIV information and resources for healthcare professionals.
- Centers for Disease Control and Prevention National Prevention Information Network: cdcnpin.org, 800–458–5231

Offers up-to-date epidemiologic information, daily updates on HIV/AIDS, and patient-oriented information.
- National Perinatal HIV Hotline: 888–448–8765
- CDC National AIDS Hotline: 800–232–4636

(See Table 12.2.)

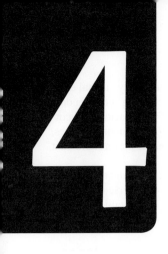

Sexually Transmitted Infections

CYNTHIA F. KRENING AND
ANNE MOORE

Introduction

STDs or STIs can complicate pregnancy and pose multiple threats to both the woman and her fetus. Maternal infection with an STD is often associated with miscarriage, fetal anomalies, stillbirth, PTL, and low birth weight, as well as increased neonatal morbidity and mortality and long-term adverse health consequences in childhood.

Most of the diseases discussed here are defined as STDs. Although not currently categorized as such, bacterial vaginosis (BV) and candidiasis (monilia) are included because of the potential adverse perinatal events associated with each of them. Infections with HIV, hepatitis B virus (HBV), hepatitis C virus (HCV), herpes simplex virus 1 and 2 (HSV-1 and HSV-2, respectively), and human papilloma virus (HPV) have no associated cures or vaccines. A vaccine for the prevention of the four most common types of HPV is available but it is currently not recommended for use in pregnancy.

During admission of the laboring woman, careful attention to her prenatal history, physical examination, and laboratory workup can identify the presence of an unresolved, untreated, or undertreated STD or the potential for such. When such risk is diagnosed, therapies and preventive strategies for labor, birth, and postpartum can be integrated into the mother's nursing and medical management. Newborn evaluation and appropriate therapy can be instituted immediately. The challenge is to identify the risk! Subsequent education during the postpartum period will affect the mother's understanding of the infection, self-care, and prevention. It is especially important that the mother appreciates any need for special newborn care, including early symptoms and the need for prompt medical attention.

Bacterial Vaginosis

BV is a change in vaginal flora in which normal hydrogen peroxide–producing (H_2O_2) lactobacillus, predominant in the healthy vagina, are replaced with an overgrowth of anaerobic bacteria, mostly anaerobic gram-negative rods. Although not considered a definitive STD, BV has epidemiologic elements consistent with those of an STD.

Epidemiology

BV is the most common cause of vaginitis in women of childbearing age. The prevalence of BV in pregnant women is similar to that in the general population, about 29%.[1] In the United States, BV is found in approximately 50% of African-American women, 32% of Hispanic women, and 23% of Caucasian women.[1] Risk factors consistently associated with BV (and other STIs) include smoking (this may simply be a marker for sexual behavior, however), douching, and multiple or new sexual partners.[2,3] BV is seen somewhat more frequently in conjunction with other STIs such as HSV type 2, gonorrhea, chlamydia, and trichomonas infections, and occurs more often in women who are sexually active than in women who are not.[1] BV is more strongly associated with age greater than 25 years. This is contrary to most STIs, whose highest rates are almost always in women younger than 25.[1,2] The presence of BV increases a woman's susceptibility to HIV infection.[4]

- **What are the clinical features of BV?**

The vagina harbors both gram-positive and gram-negative bacteria. However, only relatively few different types of bacteria are found in large numbers in the healthy vaginal environment.

Lactobacilli are dominant bacteria and contribute to the maintenance of a healthy vaginal environment with a pH of 3.8 to less than 4.5. The absence of normally occurring (endogenous) vaginal lactobacilli is important in the acquisition of BV. The absence of these lactobacilli correlates with a loss of vaginal acidity (pH greater than 4.5) seen in BV.[2] Hormonal changes, specifically estrogen loss, (e.g., during menstruation and pregnancy) appear to play a significant role in decreasing colonization of lactobacilli.[2]

Many women and their newborns who harbor anaerobic bacteria such as *G. vaginalis*, *Mobiluncus* species, and *Mycoplasmas* never manifest any signs of infection or adverse outcomes.[1] Additionally, some women do not normally colonize H_2O_2-producing lactobacilli. Common complaints are an off-white, thin vaginal discharge and/or a fishy vaginal odor, although 50% to 75% of women with BV are asymptomatic.

• What are potential perinatal consequences of BV?

Research in pregnant and nonpregnant women suggests that BV in the lower genital tract is associated with an increased risk of infection in the upper genital tract; upper genital tract involvement may be one mechanism by which infection leads to inflammation, uterine contractions, and subsequent PTL and birth.[5] In addition, pregnant women with BV are at an increased risk for PPROM, chorioamnionitis, and postpartum endometritis.[4] The increased risk for preterm birth attributable to BV correlates with PTL from chorioamnionitis. The pathogenesis associated with BV (and other vaginal infections) is believed to result, in part, from enzymes and endotoxins that weaken the amniotic membrane, leading to bacterial penetration of the intrauterine environment and subsequent infection and labor stimulation.[2,5] There are no known risks to the newborn from maternal BV.

• How are women screened and diagnosed?

ACOG and the CDC do not support routine screening for BV in all pregnant women or in women with a previous preterm birth. However, women with symptoms should be tested and treated during pregnancy according to CDC recommendations.[4] Gram stain is the gold standard for diagnosis of BV. Clinical diagnosis made according to Amsel criteria correlates well with gram stain results. Three of the following four elements must be present to make the diagnosis. The four criteria are the following:
1. Thin homogeneous white discharge coating the vaginal walls
2. A vaginal pH of greater than 4.5
3. A positive "whiff" test (fishy odor)
4. The presence of "clue" cells under microscopic examination

Vaginal cultures are unreliable and generally not used. Half of all women who meet the current criteria for the diagnosis of BV are asymptomatic. Adverse perinatal outcomes with BV appear to be much more significant when infection is present before 20 weeks' gestation.

• How is BV treated?

All pregnant women who have symptomatic BV require treatment to decrease the symptoms of vaginal infection.[4] Treatment of asymptomatic BV during pregnancy does not decrease the incidence of PTL birth.[4] Recommended treatment regimens during pregnancy are:
- Metronidazole 250 mg orally, three times daily for 7 days OR
- Metronidazole 500 mg orally, twice daily for 7 days OR
- Clindamycin 300 mg orally, twice daily for 7 days (In breastfeeding women, clindamycin has been associated with colitis in the infant.)

NOTE: *Oral doses of medication are preferred since vaginal administration has less systemic efficacy for the treatment of upper genital infection.*

Candidiasis vaginalis (Monilia)

Candidal vulvovaginal infection is a common fungal infection usually caused by one of three *Candida* species: *C. albicans*, *C. glabrata*, or *C. tropicalis*. *C. albicans* is the causative agent in 80% to 90% of infections, but the other two species are increasingly being associated with infection.[4]

Epidemiology

Candidiasis is the second most common vaginal infection in women (BV being the most common).[4] Approximately 75% of women have at least one infection in their lifetime, and 40% to 45% will experience two or more episodes.[4] Candida is generally not considered an STD; however, it appears to be sexually associated because there is increased frequency of the infection at the time women become sexually active.

Risk for acquiring vulvovaginal candidal infection is associated with uncontrolled diabetes, use of certain antibiotics, pregnancy, and immunosuppression.[6] Epidemiologic data on the disease are incomplete. It is not reportable, and often self-treated or self-diagnosed without the benefit of microscopy or culture.

• **What are the clinical features of candidiasis?**

The most prevalent symptom of candidiasis is vulvar pruritus. Other symptoms include abnormal vaginal discharge, vaginal soreness, vulvar burning, painful intercourse (dyspareunia), and dysuria. Erythema in the vulvovaginal area; thick, white patches adhering to the vaginal walls; or a thick, curdy, odorless vaginal discharge may be observed on inspection.

• **Are there perinatal consequences of candidiasis?**

Pregnancy may predispose some women to candidiasis due to significant increases in estrogen, which alter glycogen content in the vagina. Although various species of Candida normally inhabit the vagina, any change in vaginal homeostasis may permit an overgrowth of fungi, resulting in infection. Vulvovaginal candidiasis commonly occurs during pregnancy. The organism can be cultured from the vagina in approximately 25% of women nearing term. Maternal vaginal infection does not appear to have any association with adverse pregnancy outcomes. However, *Candida* species may be transmitted to the newborn from the vagina during birth resulting in clinical manifestations in the newborn varies depending on the location and extent of the infection. Thrush is an infection of the buccal mucosa, gingiva, and tongue. *Candida* also can appear as diaper dermatitis.[7] Newborns and especially infants with very low birth weight (VLBW) have qualitative and quantitative deficiencies in humoral and cellular immunity. This can allow *Candida* to penetrate lymphatics, blood vessels, and other tissues, resulting in disseminated infection.[7]

• **How are women screened and diagnosed with candidiasis?**

Maternal diagnosis is most frequently done by microscopic examination of vaginal discharge to visualize yeasts, hyphae, or pseudohyphae. A Gram stain and culture can also be done. *Note that a positive culture in the absence of symptoms should not lead to treatment.* As has been stated, *Candida* species are a part of many women's vaginal flora.[4] Newborn evaluation *of local infection* can be done by microscopic examination (wet prep) of the local site. Newborn disseminated *candidiasis* is diagnosed by blood culture.

• **What is the treatment for candidiasis?**

Maternal Treatment

Treatment is indicated for the relief of symptoms. A number of over-the-counter (OTC) treatments are available to women to relieve symptoms and provide greater than 80% cure rates with uncomplicated infection. In pregnancy, the CDC recommends 7-day topical azole therapies.[4]

Examples of OTC vaginal creams include the following:
- Clotrimazole (Gyne-Lotrimin, Mycelex) 1% cream, 5 g per vagina at bedtime for 7 days
- Miconazole (Monistat), 2% cream, 5 g per vagina for 7 days

NOTE: *Oral fluconazole (Diflucan) is contraindicated in the first trimester of pregnancy due to an association with birth defects.*

Systemic absorption after maternal vaginal administration of azoles is minimal, so topical use of these agents is fine for the breastfeeding woman.

Newborn Treatment

Treatment varies with the location and extent of infection and the infant's age.

- *Thrush* is usually treated with nystatin (Mycostatin) suspension, 1 mL given orally four to six times a day for 5 to 10 days.
- Candida *diaper dermatitis* is treated with nystatin ointment, miconazole cream, or clotrimazole cream three times a day for 7 to 10 days. Nystatin with a corticosteroid (mycology ointment) is used in severe cases.
- Systemic or disseminated candidal infection is treated with amphotericin B. This is the mainstay of therapy for the newborn and is well tolerated by the VLBW infant.

Chlamydia

Chlamydia is a small, gram-negative bacterium whose most common strains infect the mucosal epithelium (preferentially infects the squamocolumnar junction of the cervix) of the genital tract, causing infection of the cervix, destruction of the host cell, and, when untreated, infection of the upper genital tract.

Epidemiology

Chlamydia is the most common bacterial STI in the United States and is common in pregnant women. Infection in pregnancy can have serious maternal and newborn consequences.[8] Infection is significantly underreported because most women are asymptomatic. In addition, simple, cost-effective screening tests are not available.[9,10]

Risk factors for chlamydia are the presence or history of other STIs, multiple sexual partners, or a new partner within the last 3 months, inconsistent barrier contraception, unmarried status, African-American race, and low socioeconomic class.[10] The highest rates are seen in adolescent women and young adults.[10] Undiagnosed, untreated infection may lead to pelvic inflammatory disease (PID), a major cause of infertility among women, and ectopic pregnancy.

• What are the clinical features of chlamydia?

Epithelial tissues of the urethra, rectum, conjunctiva, and the nasopharynx are susceptible to infection. In women, chlamydia most commonly infects the cervical epithelial tissue and may extend to the endometrium, salpinx, and peritoneum causing PID. Women with symptoms report vaginal discharge, abnormal vaginal bleeding, purulent endocervical discharge, and itching or burning when voiding. Urethral infection frequently accompanies cervicitis, and causes symptoms of a urinary tract infection. Some studies have documented an association with acquiring HIV when chlamydia infection is present.[10]

• What are the potential perinatal consequences of chlamydia?

Effective prenatal screening and maternal treatment would prevent neonatal infection. However, reinfection during pregnancy is not uncommon, especially among adolescents and inner-city minority young women. Chlamydial infection during pregnancy increases the risk for preterm rupture of membranes, preterm birth, and low–birth-weight infants.[10] Perinatal transmission may be transplacental, transmembrane, or through exposure to maternal secretions such as breast milk; however, transmission most commonly occurs through exposure to maternal blood and vaginal secretions at the time of vaginal birth.

Despite effective therapy, many infants are born to infected mothers annually. Untreated partners, noncompliance in treatment, reinfection, and lack of prenatal care all play a role.

Genitourinary infection at 24 weeks' gestation has been found to be associated with a twofold to threefold increased risk of subsequent preterm birth.[11] If the mother is undiagnosed or untreated, 20% to 50% of infants delivered vaginally will develop conjunctivitis, and 5% to 30% will develop pneumonia.[12] Afebrile pneumonia in infants up to 3 months of age is often caused by maternally transmitted chlamydial infection. The infection often occurs weeks after hospital discharge.

• **How do you screen for and diagnose chlamydia?**

The diagnostic test of choice for chlamydial infection of the genitourinary tract is nucleic acid amplification testing (NAAT) of vaginal swabs. The CDC recommends screening all pregnant women at the first prenatal visit, and rescreening in the third trimester if younger than 25 years of age or high risk. When screening/testing for chlamydia, one should also test for gonorrhea in susceptible adults and neonates.

• **What is the treatment for chlamydia?**

Maternal Treatment

Appropriate completed treatment during pregnancy prevents transmission to sex partners and the newborn during birth.

NOTE: Treatment of the infected individual and partner should be done at the same time. Both partners should abstain from intercourse until treatment is completed.

Recommended treatment regimens are the following[13]:
- Azithromycin, 1 g orally in a single dose

OR

- Amoxicillin, 500 mg orally three times a day for 7 days (cure of chlamydia in pregnancy is lower than in nonpregnant women, especially when the treatment is with amoxicillin).
- Reculture in 3 weeks, preferably with NAAT to ensure therapeutic cure.

NOTE: Doxycycline, levofloxacin, erythromycin estolate, and ofloxacin are contraindicated in pregnancy and lactation.

Neonatal Treatment[13]

The recommended regimen for ophthalmia neonatorum caused by *C. trachomatis* is:
- erythromycin base or ethylsuccinate, 50 mg/kg per day, orally, divided into 4 doses daily, for 14 days. Topical treatment is ineffective and not recommended. Erythromycin is only 80% effective in treatment, so follow-up is recommended to determine if a second course of therapy is necessary.

Gonorrhea

Gonorrhea is a bacterial infection of the mucous membranes of the genitourinary tract; it is caused by the gram-negative bacterium *Neisseria gonorrhoeae.*

Epidemiology

It is estimated that there are 700,000 new cases of gonorrhea annually in the United States, making it the second most common bacterial STD diagnosis.[13] The disease is transmitted almost exclusively by sexual contact. The risk of a woman being infected by an infected male partner is approximately 50% per episode of vaginal intercourse. The risk of a male being infected by an infected female is 20% per episode of vaginal intercourse. The presence of gonorrhea is a marker for the possibility of concomitant chlamydial infection, owing to the clinical similarities.

Risk factors include adolescence, drug abuse, prostitution, poverty, multiple sex partners, as well as being single or having other STDs. Adolescents experience some of the highest rates. Immunity is not conferred by infection. Most cases either resolve spontaneously or are treated and resolved within a few weeks. Newborns may acquire the infection during birth through an infected birth canal. Disseminated gonococcal infection results from gonococcal bacteremia and has been cited as occurring in 0.5% to 3.0% of infected individuals.

• **What are the clinical features of gonorrhea?**

The most commonly infected site in women is the cervix and most are asymptomatic. When symptoms are present, signs and symptoms include painful urination (dysuria), usually without frequency or urgency; purulent cervical discharge; friable cervical mucosa; and cervical, uterine, or adnexal tenderness. In the majority of women with gonococcal cervicitis, the bacteria can also be found in the urethra.[14]

• What are the potential perinatal consequences of gonorrhea?

Maternal

Gonococcal infection may result in adverse pregnancy outcomes in any of the trimesters and include the following[14]:
- Miscarriage
- Preterm birth
- Premature rupture of membranes
- Chorioamnionitis—if infection present at the time of birth

Newborn

In an untreated infected mother, vertical transmission to her baby during birth may occur 30% to 50% of the time. Infants born to infected mothers may have:
- lower mean birth weight,
- conjunctivitis,
- pharyngitis,
- gonococcemia, and
- arthritis.

Ophthalmia neonatorum is the most common form of gonorrhea in newborns. Without prompt treatment, blindness can occur as a result of corneal ulceration and perforation. Isolation of an infected newborn is recommended until after 24 hours of treatment.

• How do you screen for and diagnose gonorrhea?

Laboratory diagnosis depends on identification of *N. gonorrhoeae* at an infected site. A screening test for gonorrhea is recommended at the first prenatal visit, and a repeat test should be done after 28 weeks' gestation in women with risk factors.[15] Repeat testing in the third trimester is recommended in any pregnant woman who tested positive at an earlier workup because reinfection is common. NAAT is the preferred test for an accurate diagnosis.[14]

NOTE: *Syphilis, HIV, and chlamydia screening and treatment are strongly recommended in any individual who has tested positive for gonorrhea because these infections are commonly found concomitantly with gonorrheal infection.*

• What is the treatment for gonorrhea?

Treatment of gonorrhea has been complicated by the development of antimicrobial resistance. Because of this resistance, oral cephalosporins are no longer recommended for effective treatment.[16]
- For uncomplicated gonococcal infections during pregnancy, recommended treatment is ceftriaxone, 250 mg intramuscularly (IM; single dose) plus azithromycin 1 g (PO; single dose) due to its low rates of resistance.
- A test of cure is recommended after treatment of a pregnant woman.
- In the presence of PID during pregnancy, parenteral antibiotics should be administered to prevent adverse pregnancy outcomes.[17]
- Intrapartum prophylaxis for the newborn is instituted by the instillation of a 1% aqueous solution of silver nitrate onto the conjunctiva soon after birth. Topical application of erythromycin or tetracycline ointment can also be used.

Herpes Simplex Virus Infection

The HSV invades sensory or autonomic nervous system ganglia and is expressed as an infection of mucosal surfaces such as the oropharynx, cervix, and vulva. Acute infection (often asymptomatic) is followed by a remission period. It is essentially a chronic infection with frequent or rare exacerbations. Two types of the virus, HSV-1 and HSV-2, differ to some degree in biologic, biochemical, and antigenic properties. Up to 50% of first cases of genital herpes are caused by HSV-1.

Epidemiology

Genital herpes is the second most prevalent STI in the world, with at least 50 million people with HSV-2 genital herpes in the United States.[18] The true prevalence rate is much higher than that reported because the infection is often subclinical.[18] Most cases of recurring genital herpes are caused by HSV-2, although the incidence of anogenital infections from HSV-1 is increasing and is estimated to be the cause of most new genital HSV in the United States.[18,19]

The virus can be transmitted through intimate contact and sexual activity, as well as during vaginal birth. The majority of genital herpes infections are transmitted by those who are asymptomatic during a period of subclinical viral shedding or if unaware that they have the infection. Individuals with genital HSV-2 experience more recurrences and subclinical viral shedding than those with genital HSV-1. Women are more easily infected with HSV-2 than men.[20] Risk factors are age, duration of sexual activity, race, previous genital infections, and number of sexual partners. Clinical designations of genital HSV include primary, first-episode genital nonprimary, and recurrent infection.

• What are the clinical features of HSV?

Symptoms of HSV vary widely depending on whether the infection is primary, nonprimary, or recurrent. Lesions of HSV are often multiple, causing local pain and itching, and have the appearance of wet blisters or crusted vesicles. Genital ulcerative lesions are vulnerable to infection with other STDs (e.g., syphilis, HIV).

- **Primary genital infection** is the first occurrence of HSV. Clinical confirmation depends on the absence of **HSV-1** and **HSV-2** antibodies at the time the individual acquires the genital infection due to **HSV-1** or **HSV-2.**
  - The primary lesions can be severe, with painful genital ulcers, pruritus, dysuria, fever, tender inguinal lymphadenopathy, and headache, or the patient can be asymptomatic.
  - When systemic symptoms (malaise, fever, and myalgia) occur with herpetic infections, it is generally thought to be a primary infection reflecting a high viremic load.
  - Symptoms usually peak in 4 to 5 days and can last as long as 2 to 3 weeks.
  - Shedding of the virus from the cervix occurs intermittently in infected women, regardless of whether symptoms are present.
- **First-episode genital nonprimary HSV** is diagnosed when the development of genital herpes infection/lesion(s) occurs in an individual who has pre-existing antibodies that are different from the HSV type of the current lesion.
  - The woman may be symptomatic or asymptomatic.
  - Prior HSV-1 infection provides *some* protection from an HSV-2 infection.
  - Signs and symptoms of the first-episode genital nonprimary infections are usually milder than primary infection.
- **Recurrent genital infection** is genital HSV infection in a person who is seropositive for the HSV type recovered from the lesion.
  - Symptoms tend to be mild and localized or the patient may have no symptoms at all.
  - Many individuals experience *prodromal symptoms* of tingling, burning, itching, tenderness, or a swelling sensation followed by the herpes outbreak of lesions in about 24 hours.[21]
  - Over time, symptoms are usually less acute and frequency of outbreaks is reduced.
  - Usually, herpetic blisters or ulcers are confined to the genital region. They are less tender, and may be atypical in appearance.
  - The duration of lesions and viral shedding are shorter than during the primary infection.
  - After an initial infection, recurrences can be frequent and triggered by menstruation, stress, trauma, and ultraviolet light rays (sun exposure).
  - Genital HSV recurrence is higher in those infected with HSV-2 than with HSV-1.[22]
  - Shedding of the virus from the genital tract is intermittent, occurring in both symptomatic and asymptomatic individuals.
  - Viral quantity tends to be lower when no lesion is present, but a susceptible partner can be infected. This is what makes this STI so difficult to prevent.

• What are the potential perinatal consequences of HSV?

During pregnancy, transmission to the newborn is the major complication of maternal HSV infection, and can result in serious morbidity and mortality. Viral shedding can occur in the absence of lesions or symptoms. Transmission can occur from direct contact with virus shed from the cervix, vagina, vulva, or perineum. Maternal–fetal (vertical) transmission appears to be related to gestational age. The rate of vertical transmission is reduced in the presence of pre-existing maternal HSV-2 antibodies. However, having HSV-1 antibodies does not appear to reduce vertical transmission.

NOTE: When maternal infection is primary but asymptomatic, cervical shedding of the virus also incurs a risk of preterm birth and possible HSV transmission to the newborn.

- There is a 30% to 56% transmission rate of genital herpes to the neonate from an infected mother when the infection is acquired near the time of birth.[22,23] This high rate of infection is due to the absence of anti-HSV antibodies and greatest viral exposure during primary infection.
- The rate of transmission is low (less than 3%) after a vaginal birth among women with recurrent infections or if the infection is acquired during the first half of pregnancy.[23]
- Vaginal birth should be avoided if the woman has signs and symptoms of an outbreak; the potential for transmission to the neonate as high as 80% to 90%.[8]
- Cesarean birth can decrease but not eliminate the risk of neonatal HSV infection.[23,24]
- Other risk factors for neonatal infection include preterm birth, application of fetal spiral electrodes (FSEs), and vacuum or forceps application.
- When genital lesions are present, transcervical procedures should be avoided, although transabdominal procedures are not contraindicated.
- In the setting of PPROM and active HSV infection, management must balance the risks of prematurity versus the risk of fetal or neonatal infection.
- Mothers with active lesions should use caution when handling their newborns.
- Breastfeeding is contraindicated only if an obvious herpetic lesion is on the breast.

Neonatal infections can develop as three different entities[25]:
1. Localized to the skin, eye, or mouth (SEM disease)
2. Systemic, causing encephalitis with or without skin lesions
3. Disseminated in organs such as the lungs, liver, adrenal glands, skin, or central nervous system (CNS)

When infection is localized to the skin, eyes, or mouth, neonatal mortality is rare. With CNS involvement and disseminated disease, mortality is 50% to 85%.[26]

NOTE: The herpes virus is acquired by direct contact. Family members with oral lesions can infect the newborn by hand/mouth contact.

• How is the woman screened and diagnosed with HSV?

Routine HSV screening during pregnancy and weekly late third trimester screening are **not** recommended for women with a history of herpes. Many, if not most, newborns develop HSV infection in the absence of a maternal history of the disease.
- A herpes diagnosis should be made by polymerase chain reaction (PCR) or viral culture in the presence of active genital lesions.
- Type-specific serologic tests are preferred in those without active disease.
- Real-time PCR assays for HSV DNA are more sensitive (and costly) than viral cell cultures of the lesion(s), can differentiate between HSV-1 and HSV-2, and are also helpful in detection of asymptomatic HSV shedding.[23,27]
- When cultures are performed, a Dacron swab is generally used for collection. The vesicles should be scraped (unroofed) to sample the fluid within; moist ulcers and crusts are scraped well. Specimens are placed in viral transport media.[27] The sensitivity of viral culture of genital lesions is the greatest when lesions are vesicular. Overall sensitivity of cultures is approximately 50%.[27]
- The availability of reliable, type-specific serologic test for HSV-1 or HSV-2 antibodies has increased detection of asymptomatic individuals. Results reflect the presence/absence of IGG antibodies, indicating past infection/exposure. IGM testing is NOT recommended as the information regarding CURRENT infection status should be determined by culture/PCR.

Many recommend routine serologic tests in conjunction with routine prenatal laboratory testing to provide insurance that transmission to the neonate by an asymptomatic mother is reduced. If results are HSV-2 IGG positive, suppressive antiviral therapy can be introduced in late gestation, further minimizing the risk of exposure. Serologic testing should be offered to pregnant women whose partner(s) have a history of genital HSV infection (as should) counseling to discordant couples to reduce the risk of transmission during pregnancy.[27]

• What is the treatment for HSV?

The goal of management is to reduce or prevent neonatal risk of exposure to HSV during the latter half of pregnancy and during birth.

All women with a history of HSV should be questioned about prodromal symptoms, and examined for visual lesions when presenting for evaluation in labor and delivery. Studies demonstrate that antiviral therapy (oral or parenteral) shortens the course and morbidity of infection and the duration of viral shedding, but does not eliminate latent HSV.

The ACOG treatment recommendations are summarized as follows[23]:

Based on limited or inconsistent scientific evidence (Level B):

- Women with primary or first-episode genital nonprimary HSV during pregnancy should be treated with antiviral therapy. Acyclovir 400 mg orally three times daily for 7 to 10 days will decrease the duration of symptoms and viral shedding.
- Intravenous antiviral therapy may be administered to pregnant women with severe genital HSV or disseminated herpetic infections.
- Women with active recurrent genital herpes lesions at or beyond 36 weeks' gestation should be offered suppressive viral therapy. Acyclovir (400 mg orally three times daily) decreases the risk of clinical recurrence as well as asymptomatic viral shedding at delivery.
- Cesarean birth should be performed on women with the first-episode or recurrent HSV infection who have active genital lesions or prodromal symptoms at the onset of labor.

Based on consensus and expert opinion[23]:

- There is no consensus on the gestational age at which the risks of prematurity outweigh the risks of HSV in women with preterm rupture of membranes. For women at or beyond 36 weeks' gestation who are at risk for recurrent HSV, antiviral therapy also may be considered.

NOTE: In women with no active lesions or prodromal symptoms during labor, cesarean birth should not be performed on the basis of a history or recurrent disease. In addition, nongenital herpetic lesions (e.g., on the thigh or buttocks) should be covered with an occlusive dressing. The woman can then deliver vaginally.

- Avoiding the use of FSEs in fetal monitoring, forceps- or vacuum-assisted births, and artificial rupture of membranes during labor may minimize the risk of transmission.
- The CDC recommends using oral acyclovir (class C) during pregnancy if the first episode of HSV infection occurs. Acyclovir given in late pregnancy reduces the incidence of cesarean birth in women with recurrent outbreaks by reducing the frequency of recurrences at term.[25]
- Two class B antiherpetic drugs, famciclovir (Famvir) and valacyclovir (Valtrex), with their increased bioavailability, involve less frequent dosing to achieve the same therapeutic results as acyclovir. However, currently only acyclovir is FDA approved for use during pregnancy. The CDC has maintained a drug registry for women treated with acyclovir during pregnancy. To date, no increase in fetal abnormalities has been shown with the use of Acyclovir in all trimesters of pregnancy.[28]

Human Papillomavirus Infection

Human papillomavirus (HPV) is an infection of the skin and mucous membranes. Genital HPV is the most common STD in the United States, with approximately 14 million new infections diagnosed each year. There are more than 150 types of HPV, with 40 of them infecting the genital area. Most infections cause no symptoms and are self-limiting, although persistent HPV infection can cause cervical cancer as well as other anogenital cancers, genital warts, and oropharyngeal cancer.

Epidemiology

Approximately 50% of the sexually active population is infected with HPV at least once in their lifetime. The most consistent risk factor for genital HPV infection is sexual activity.[29,30] Studies repeatedly show high levels of infection in women, with the highest levels among young women (age 15 to 24).[29-31] Data on actual prevalence are difficult to gather because reporting of HPV is based on visible lesions and some testing measures (e.g., Pap smears and subsequent workup) but many women have no symptoms and remain undiagnosed.

• What are the clinical features of HPV?

HPV infections are transmitted primarily by sexual contact with an infected partner. The asymptomatic lesions are highly contagious. Nonsexual transmission may occur, but is uncommon; the virus has been detected on underwear, sex toys, tanning salon benches, and wet towels, and has been cultured from gloves, instruments, and specula. The inability to culture HPV eliminates the possibility of documenting infectability. The incubation period ranges from 3 weeks to 8 months, with an average of 3 months.

- HPV viral strains 6 and 11 result in visible external genital warts, or *condylomata acuminata.* Most appear as small cauliflower-like clusters that may itch or burn. An estimated 1% of the sexually active population in the United States may have genital warts at any one time.[31]
- Persistent high-risk HPV types 16 and 18 are the biggest risk factors for cervical cancer.[31,32]
- *Strong risk factors for cervical cancer and its precursors* include age at first intercourse (16 years or younger), a history of multiple sexual partners, history of genital HPV infection or another STI, the presence of other genital tract neoplasia, and prior cervical tissue changes such as a squamous intraepithelial lesion. Additional risk factors include active or passive smoking, immunodeficiency (as in HIV infection), poor nutrition, and a current or past sexual partner with risk factors for STIs.[32]
- The diagnostic spectrum of HPV infection ranges from clinically visible lesions to subclinical infection as seen by colposcopy to latent infection in which HPV DNA is diagnosed with tissue evaluation.
- The majority of HPV infections are transient, subclinical, or asymptomatic. In symptomatic cases, irritation, bleeding, pruritus, and often, fleshy, pink, warty raised lesions are present singularly or in clusters on affected areas, such as the surface of the perineum, introitus, vagina, cervix, and anus.
- Most HPV infections appear to be temporary and are probably cleared by an active cell-mediated immune response. Ninety percent of new infections clear within 2 years. However, reactivation to reinfection is possible.[31]
- Evidence suggests the following[31]:
  - Barrier methods of contraception lower the incidence of cervical neoplasia, probably because of lessened exposure to HPV.
  - Exposure to cigarette smoking is associated with increased risk.
  - Increased intake of micronutrients and other dietary factors such as carotenoids and folic acid are associated with decreased risk.
  - Education about risk factors for cervical cancer may lead to behavioral modification, resulting in diminished exposure.

• What are the potential perinatal consequences of HPV?

Genital warts, symptoms of HPV infection that can be seen, tend to grow more rapidly in number and size, and become more friable during pregnancy. Rarely, viral transmission of HPV types 6 or 11 can cause respiratory papillomatosis in infants and children. It's not clear if the route of transmission is transplacental, perinatal, or postnatal. It's also unclear if cesarean birth prevents respiratory papillomatosis in infants, so it should not be the mode of birth solely to prevent transmission of HPV infection to the newborn.[31] Cesarean birth may be necessary for women with genital warts obstructing the pelvic outlet, or if vaginal birth could result in excessive bleeding.

• How is HPV prevented, screened, and diagnosed?

HPV vaccines are approved for use in females aged 9 to 26 to prevent HPV genital infection. The bivalent vaccine provides immunity to HPV types 16 and 18. The quadrivalent vaccine is effective against HPV types 6 and 11 which cause 90% of genital warts, as well as types 16 and 18 which cause 70% of cervical cancers. Clinical trial data have shown vaccine efficacy through declines in incidence and persistence of cervical and vulvovaginal infection.[33] Although the vaccine is currently listed as pregnancy category B, it is not recommended for use during pregnancy due to the limited amount of data.

NOTE: *Although condylomata acuminata are easily seen on external surfaces with the naked eye, HPV disease on the cervix usually requires magnification (colposcopy) and the application of acetic acid for identification.*

- **How is HPV treated?**

Maternal Treatment

- Subclinical genital HPV infection usually clears spontaneously; so specific antiviral therapy is not recommended to eradicate the infection. No evidence exists that treatments eradicate or affect the natural course of HPV infection.
- Visible genital warts may resolve on their own, remain unchanged, or increase in the number or size. Treatment should take into consideration the preference of the woman and available resources as no definitive evidence indicates that any of the current treatments are superior to any other.[31] Treatment options include topical solutions, creams, gels, and ointments, as well as cryotherapy or surgical removal of the warts.
- Cervical intraepithelial neoplasia (CIN) is premalignancy of the uterine cervix. Women with CIN 1 resulting from high-risk HPV should not have excision or ablation during pregnancy. Reevaluation 6 weeks postpartum should direct the management plan. In pregnant women with CIN 2 and 3, without evidence of invasive disease, the two management recommendations are the following[34]:
  - Defer reevaluation to 6 weeks postpartum as high-grade lesions noted during pregnancy frequently regress postpartum.
  - Repeat evaluation with cytology and colposcopy, no more often than every 12 weeks. Biopsy should only be repeated if the lesion appears worse, or invasive disease is suggested by cytology. There is substantial morbidity with cervical conization in pregnancy.

Newborn Treatment

- Both medical and surgical approaches may be used in treating laryngeal papillomatosis in the newborn.

Syphilis

Syphilis is a complex STD caused by the spirochete *Treponema pallidum.* Approximately 30% of individuals acquire the disease during the first sexual exposure to a partner with a primary lesion. Maternal infection may be transmitted vertically to the fetus and result in congenital syphilis.

Epidemiology

In the United States, in 2013, there were 5.3 cases of syphilis per 100,000.[35] Racial, ethnic, and geographic disparities in the incidence of syphilis persist. For the first time, western states experience the highest rates.[35] It disproportionately affects populations living near or below the poverty level, as well as those involved in high-risk activities such as prostitution, illicit drug use, and multiple sexual partners. The number of cases of primary and secondary syphilis increased in the United States from 2005 to 2013, with a total of more than 16,000 reported cases.[35]

- **What are the clinical features of syphilis?[36]**

The disease is divided into primary, secondary, and latent phases.

Primary Syphilis

- The incubation period for primary syphilis ranges from 10 to 90 days. A chancre usually develops 3 to 4 weeks after exposure.

- The chancre of *primary syphilis* occurs at the site of inoculation and appears as a red, painless ulcer with raised edges and a granulation base (button appearance). Cervical chancres are common in exposed pregnant women, most likely due to the friable cervix, which is easily infected. The highly infectious chancre persists for 1 to 6 weeks and spontaneously heals. Often, nontender, enlarged inguinal lymph nodes can be palpated.

Secondary Syphilis

- *Secondary syphilis* occurs several weeks after the primary chancre appears. In approximately 15% of women, a chancre may still be present. This secondary stage involves more widespread dissemination of the *T. pallidum* and is, therefore, characterized by symptoms of systemic involvement:
  - Low-grade fever
  - Sore throat
  - Headache
  - Malaise
  - Adenopathy
  - Rashes on mucosal and skin surfaces.
  - Alopecia, mild hepatitis, and kidney involvement may develop
- The lesions of secondary syphilis may be mild and even go unnoticed. Some women develop characteristic genital lesions of secondary syphilis called *condylomata lata*. They appear as white, raised, and moist lesions and are highly infectious. These lesions resolve in 3 to 12 weeks, and the disease enters the latent phase. Syphilis titers are usually highest during secondary syphilis.

Latent Syphilis

- *Latent syphilis* refers to infection in individuals who have reactive serologic tests but no clinical manifestations.
- *Latency* is divided into the following:
  - *Early*—1 year or less from the beginning of infection
  - *Late*—more than 1 year from the beginning of infection
- Infectiousness continues throughout early latency, but transmission is unlikely in late latency.

Tertiary Syphilis

- *Tertiary syphilis* develops after years of untreated disease. The skeletal, central nervous, and cardiovascular systems may be seriously affected.

- **What are the potential perinatal consequences of syphilis?**

The clinical course of syphilis is not altered by pregnancy, although pregnancy outcomes are drastically affected by syphilis. Transmission of the disease largely depends on the duration of maternal disease. The most affected infants are those conceived in women with primary or secondary syphilis. Infants conceived in women with early–late or late-stage disease are less affected.[36] Syphilis can cause infection in both the unborn and newborn. The infection can be transmitted to the fetus in utero during any trimester of pregnancy and at any stage of the disease, presumably transplacentally or during delivery by newborn contact with a genital lesion. As gestation advances, the frequency of vertical transmission increases, but fetal infection is less severe later in pregnancy.

- Untreated maternal infection can result in perinatal death in up to 40% of cases.
- If syphilis is acquired before pregnancy, up to 80% of fetuses may be infected.[37]
- Pregnancy outcomes in the presence of untreated syphilis include spontaneous pregnancy loss during the second or third trimester, intrauterine growth restriction, stillbirth, nonimmune hydrops, preterm birth, and perinatal death. Congenital deafness, neurologic impairment, and bone deformities can occur in surviving infants.
- In spite of the risks, *most newborns born to women with untreated syphilis, irrespective of disease stage or duration, do not have clinical or laboratory evidence of infection at birth. If left untreated, these infants may develop clinical signs and symptoms months or years later.*[38]
- The infection *is not* transmitted via breastfeeding *unless* an infectious lesion is present on the breast.

• How are women screened for and diagnosed with syphilis?

Diagnostic workup and treatment of syphilis infection in the pregnant woman require a thorough understanding of the natural history of the disease and how it relates to stages (primary, secondary, and latency), clinical progressions and relapse, and the proper evaluation of therapeutic results. Establishing the diagnosis in a pregnant woman is essentially the same as that for a nonpregnant woman. Dark-field microscopic examination to identify spirochetes is the most accurate method of diagnosing syphilis. However, serology is the most common method of confirming infection.

Two basic types of serology are used: the specific treponemal test and the nontreponemal antibody test (VDRL, RPR).

- The nontreponemal antibody tests rapid plasma reagin (RPR) and Venereal Disease Research Laboratory (VDRL) are reported as reactive or nonreactive. A positive test is reported as reactive with a titer.
- These tests are positive in the majority of women with primary syphilitic lesions and in all women with secondary syphilis. However, it should be noted that most will be positive only after 4 to 6 weeks of initial infection.
- These tests are not highly specific; therefore, a second confirmatory test is performed on anyone with an initial positive test.

The CDC recommends screening all pregnant women at the first prenatal visit, and retesting in the third trimester if the woman is at high risk, living in an area with a high incidence, was not previously tested, or had a positive test in the first trimester. Diagnosis of syphilis in the pregnant woman is most often made by serologic screening at the first visit and repeated at 28 to 32 weeks' gestation. Most states have statutes that require antepartum testing for syphilis. When there is not a documented history of adequate treatment, a negative VDRL/RPR or EIA result does not mean that treatment is not needed. Inadequate treatment may lead to nonresolution of infection and relapses that can result in congenital infection.

NOTE: Approximately 15% of individuals with primary syphilis will be seronegative at initial testing.[7] This is due to the prozone phenomenon, which is the result of an excess amount of anticardiolipin antibody present in a patient's serum, which interferes with the test chemically. Therefore, repeat testing should be performed on anyone at risk of recent infection.

• How is fetal syphilis diagnosed?

Syphilis readily crosses the placenta resulting in fetal infection. Transplacental transmission can occur at any gestational age. As gestation advances, the frequency of vertical transmission increases, but the severity of fetal infection decreases with infection later in the pregnancy. Fetal infections acquired in the first trimester can result in miscarriage, stillbirth, intrauterine growth restriction, hydrops fetalis, preterm birth, and neonatal death. Prenatal diagnosis is possible using ultrasonography, which can identify fetal hydrops and hepatosplenomegaly when maternal syphilis is diagnosed after 20 weeks' gestation. There may be ultrasound evidence of other fetal complications from syphilis including encephalitis, bone deformities, endocarditis, and chorioretinitis.

Infection in the fetus is indicated by placental involvement and results in hepatic dysfunction followed by chorioamnionitis, ascites, hydrops, thrombocytopenia, and anemia. Most often, the diagnosis depends on testing the newborn after birth, at which time serology testing, physical examination, and laboratory testing are used. Detection of spirochetes in amniotic fluid and in fetal blood through cordocentesis can also be done.

• How is congenital syphilis diagnosed?

- The incidence of congenital syphilis relates to the incidence of disease in women. Lack of prenatal care or late care in women with syphilis contributes to most cases of congenital syphilis.
- Syphilis is confirmed by the demonstration of spirochetes in lesions, body fluids, or tissue using dark-field microscopy, immunofluorescence, or histologic examination.
- PCR technique is highly specific for detecting *T. pallidum* in amniotic fluid and neonatal serum and spinal fluid.
- A large, edematous placenta is usually seen.

- The two most common clinical findings are hepatosplenomegaly and jaundice. Other evidence of congenital syphilis includes nonimmune hydrops, jaundice, rhinitis, skin rash, and pseudoparalysis of an extremity.[18]
- Serologic testing of maternal serum is preferable to testing the neonate's serum or umbilical cord blood because a low maternal titer owing to late infection may result in a negative test on the neonate when, in fact, the infection exists in an early stage.[18]
- Infants born to mothers who have reactive treponemal and nontreponemal tests must be evaluated with a quantitative nontreponemal serologic test on infant serum.[18]

• What is the recommended treatment for syphilis?

Maternal Therapy

Maternal syphilis treatment decreases congenital infection risk in the fetus. Treatment of early maternal syphilis, a minimum of 30 days before birth, is the most important factor in decreasing the risk of congenital syphilis in the neonate.

- Benzathine penicillin is the drug with documented efficacy during pregnancy for both acquired and congenital syphilis. Penicillin administration effectively treats maternal disease, prevents transmission to the fetus and treats fetal disease as well.
- There are no proven alternatives to penicillin treatment during pregnancy.
- Penicillin desensitization is recommended for pregnant women with a severe penicillin allergy, by exposing the patient to small amounts of oral penicillin and gradually increasing the dose until an effective level is attained. Then the appropriate penicillin regimen can be administered. This requires hospitalization and careful monitoring, but is usually successful. Desensitization produces a temporary tolerance of penicillin, but does not prevent future allergic reactions.
- Erythromycin may affect a maternal cure but not prevent congenital syphilis. Currently, it is not recommended for infected pregnant women.
- Recommended treatment according to CDC guidelines is as follows[18]:

Primary:	Benzathine penicillin G 2.4 million units IM
Secondary:	Benzathine penicillin G 2.4 million units IM
Early latent (1 year or less):	Benzathine penicillin G 2.4 million units IM
Late latent (more than 1 year), unknown duration, or tertiary syphilis	Benzathine penicillin G 7.2 million units IM total: 3 doses of 2.4 million units at 1 week intervals.

- A treatment reaction occurring in up to 60% of patients treated for early syphilis in pregnancy is called the Jarisch–Herxheimer reaction. Manifestations include fever, chills, hypotension, headache, rash, and myalgia, which occur within 1 to 2 hours of treatment and resolve by 24 to 48 hours. Pregnant women may experience frequent uterine contractions, premature labor, concerning fetal heart rate patterns, and decreased fetal activity. The reaction usually occurs when abundant spirochetes are dying and it is self-limited.[18]
- Antipyretics can be used to relieve symptoms.
- Six and 12 months after treatment, patients should be clinically and serologically reexamined. Nontreponemal titers should decrease by fourfold by 6 months after therapy, and become nonreactive by 12 to 24 months.
- In the presence of treatment failure, patients should receive another course of benzathine penicillin.
- All sexual partners should be treated.

Congenital Syphilis

The CDC recommends that every infant with suspected or proven congenital syphilis has a cerebrospinal examination before treatment.[18]

Infants	Benzathine penicillin G 50,000

Trichomonas (Trichomoniasis)

Trichomonas vaginalis is a common vaginal infection caused by a flagellated protozoan and is spread through sexual activity. Co-infection with other STDs and BV is common.

Epidemiology

Trichomonas is one of the most common, curable STDs, with the highest incidence in African-American women. It is estimated that there are close to four million people with trichomonas in the United States, and more than one million new cases each year.[39] Associated risk factors include multiple sex partners, low socioeconomic status, history of STDs, and no condom use.

• What are the clinical features of trichomonas?

Symptoms vary widely in women with trichomonas. Women may be asymptomatic. Common symptoms include foul-smelling or frothy green (yellow/green) vaginal discharge, pruritus, vulvar irritation and redness. Occasionally, abdominal pain, dysuria, and dyspareunia are experienced.[39]

• What are the potential perinatal consequences of trichomonas?

Vaginal trichomoniasis has been associated with adverse pregnancy outcomes such as PPROM, preterm birth, and low birth weight.[39] Unfortunately, treatment has not been shown to decrease the incidence of perinatal morbidity. Rarely, a female newborn can acquire the infection during vaginal birth and exhibit vaginal discharge after birth. Breastfeeding women taking metronidazole should pump and dump for 24 hours after their one-time dose to allow for drug excretion.[40]

• How do you screen for and diagnose trichomonas?

Routine screening is not indicated in all pregnancies. Testing should be performed when a woman seeks care for vaginal discharge.
- Wet mount preparation for microscope examination is the most common diagnostic technique. This can be done immediately in an office setting, but sensitivity is only approximately 60% to 70%.
- FDA-approved tests to diagnose trichomonas include the following[4]:
  - The OSOM Trichomonas Rapid Test—an immunochromatographic capillary flow dipstick technology
  - The Affirm VP III—nucleic acid probe test
- Both are performed on vaginal discharge samples and have a sensitivity of more than 83% and a specificity of more than 97%. Both point-of-care tests provide information in less than 1 hour.
- Availability of liquid-based cultures is another sensitive and highly specific commercially available method of diagnosis.

• How is trichomonas treated?

During pregnancy, asymptomatic infections do not require treatment, as data have shown that treatment can increase the risk of preterm birth. Some providers may choose to treat asymptomatic trichomonas near term to prevent perinatal transmission. All symptomatic pregnant women should receive treatment, regardless of gestational age.
- Metronidazole 2 g PO single dose (category B in pregnancy) is the drug of choice for symptomatic trichomonas in all trimesters of pregnancy as it has not demonstrated teratogenicity. 500 mg orally may be given twice daily for 5 to 7 days for less side effects.[40]
- Sexual partners should be treated, and sexual intercourse should be avoided until both partners have completed treatment.
- Trichomonas infection in neonates is treated with metronidazole.

PART 5

Hepatitis

SUZANNE McMURTRY BAIRD AND
BETSY BABB KENNEDY

Introduction

• What is hepatitis infection?

Hepatitis is an acute or chronic infection of the liver. There are several types of hepatitis based on the viral cause, transmission, symptoms, and chronicity. Perinatal effects depend on the type of hepatitis infection. Diagnosis of type is by specific antibody testing. The types of hepatitis, transmission, epidemiology, and other key features regarding are listed in Table 12.7.

Because of transmission risks, Hepatitis B is the focus of the remainder of this section.

Hepatitis B

Hepatitis B infection is a preventable acute or chronic liver disease caused by the HBV. HBV enters the body of a nonimmune person and is found in liver cells (hepatocytes), where it replicates (reproduces itself). The virus also travels to the bloodstream. There are three antigens associated with the HBV[1,2]:

- HBsAg—surface antigen; part of the HBV that is found in the blood of someone who is infected. If this test is positive, HBV is present and the woman is infectious.
- HBcAg—core antigen associated with viral nucleic acid.
- HBeAg—protein secreted from infected cells; a marker for high levels of viral replication; indicates a highly infectious state.

HBV has been found in body fluids such as saliva, menstrual and vaginal discharge, semen, colostrum, breast milk, and serous exudates. These fluids have been implicated as vehicles of infection transmission. The incubation period averages 90 days (ranges from 60 to 150 days). However, HBV may be detected within 30 to 60 days after infection.[1,2]

When individuals develop *active* disease, whether symptomatic or not, there are two possible outcome pathways: (1) they experience complete resolution or (2) the virus remains in the body in a chronic state. Individuals who retain the virus in a ***chronic*** state are at risk for two potential situations[2]:

1. Becoming a chronic active hepatitis carrier who can transmit the disease to others under certain conditions
2. Developing chronic liver disease and/or primary hepatocellular carcinoma (cancer of the liver)

In the United States, there has been a dramatic decrease in acute hepatitis B due to effective vaccination programs and early detection in at risk individuals.[2] The most common risk factors are outlined in Table 12.8.

Screening

Identifying the antigens and antibodies for HBV in the blood of infected individuals confirms that the individual is either in the active disease state, a carrier, or immune. During pregnancy, every woman should be screened for hepatitis B at the first prenatal visit by testing for the following antigen and antibody markers[2]:

TABLE 12.7	HEPATITIS		
TYPE	**CHRONIC VS. ACUTE**	**TRANSMISSION**	**KEY FEATURES**
A	Acute	Oral–fecal	Second most common form of hepatitis in the United States Infection in adults is usually asymptomatic Perinatal transmission is extremely rare
B	Acute and chronic	Sexual Parenteral	85–90% of individuals acutely infected effectively clear the virus, 10–15% develop into a chronic carrier state, less than 1% develop fulminant hepatitis HBeAg presence indicates a highly infections acute state Estimated that 1 million people are chronic viral carriers Incidence in pregnancy: 1–2 per 1,000 pregnancies (acute) and 5–15 per 1,000 pregnancies (chronic) If the woman is seropositive for hepatitis B AND HBeAg, the risk of vertical perinatal transmission is 70–90% if immunoprophylaxis is not given to the newborn within 12 hrs after birth Transmission due to exposure of newborn to maternal blood and body fluids during birth
C	Chronic	Sexual Parenteral Perinatal	Infection is usually asymptomatic Risk of perinatal transmission is low in those with lower serum concentration and no co-existing HIV Higher rate of transmission (up to 25%) in those with high serum concentration and/or HIV infection Elective cesarean for those with high titers prior to labor and rupture of membranes to reduce transmission risk Vaginal birth for those with undetectable serum concentrations Breastfeeding does not pose risk of transmission to neonate
D	Chronic	Previous hepatitis B infection Sexual Parenteral Perinatal	Epidemiology similar to hepatitis B Dependent upon co-infection with hepatitis B Perinatal transmission can occur but is uncommon due to immunoprophylaxis for hepatitis B
E	Acute	Contaminated water	Similar to hepatitis A Rare in United States High mortality rate in developing countries Clinical presentation similar to hepatitis A Perinatal transmission is extremely rare.
G	Chronic	Sexual Parenteral Perinatal	More common than hepatitis C, but less virulent Usually asymptomatic Co-infection with hepatitis A, B, C and HIV is common Documented perinatal transmission, but minimal clinical effect in woman and newborn

From World Health Organization. (2015). Hepatitis B. Retrieved from: http://www.who.int/mediacentre/factsheets/fs204/en/; Centers for Disease Control and Prevention. Viral hepatitis–hepatitis B information. http://www.cdc.gov/hepatitis/hbv/hbvfaq.htm#overview; Bernstein, H. B. (2012). Maternal and perinatal infection–viral. In Gabbe, S. G., Niebyl, J. R., Simpson, J. L., et al. (Eds.), *Obstetrics: Normal and problem pregnancies* (6th ed., pp. 1108–1139). Philadelphia, PA: Saunders.

TABLE 12.8	RISK FACTORS FOR HBV

Sex partner or household contact who is positive for HBsAg
Recent or current use of IV drugs
Co-infection with HCV or HIV
History of evaluation or treatment for a sexually transmitted infection
Inmate at a correctional facility
In need of immunosuppressive therapy
More than one sex partner in previous 6 mo
Patient or parents born in regions with high hepatitis B virus rate and patient not vaccinated as an infant
Undergoing hemodialysis

From World Health Organization. (2015). Hepatitis B. Retrieved from: http://www.who.int/mediacentre/factsheets/fs204/en/; Centers for Disease Control and Prevention. Viral hepatitis–hepatitis B information. http://www.cdc.gov/hepatitis/hbv/hbvfaq.htm#overview; Bernstein, H. B. (2012). Maternal and perinatal infection–viral. In Gabbe, S. G., Niebyl, J. R., Simpson, J. L., et al. (Eds.), *Obstetrics: Normal and problem pregnancies* (6th ed., pp. 1108–1139). Philadelphia, PA: Saunders.

- Hepatitis B surface antigen (HBsAg).
- Hepatitis B surface antibody (HBsAB or anti-HBc)—antibody formed in response to HBV; antibody present if vaccinated or recovered from hepatitis B infection.
- Hepatitis B core antibody (HBcAB or anti-HBc)—a positive test may indicate exposure to HBV.

The presence of HBsAg in serum (positive result) identifies any infected person in either an acute or carrier state. *The test does not differentiate between an acute or chronic state.*

NOTE: *More than 90% of women found to be HBsAg positive on routine screening will be hepatitis B carriers.*[2]

If HBsAg is present, additional tests are needed to identify the degree of infectivity and whether the woman is in the acute or chronic carrier state. Recommended additional testing for a positive screen includes the following[2–5]:

- HBeAg
- Hepatitis B e antibody (anti-HBe)
- HBV DNA
- Aminotransferase level

Sometimes women completely recover from the disease, and when tested, HBsAg and HBeAg are not present. These women are not carriers and will not transmit the disease. The mother-to-infant transmission process in the perinatal is known as ***vertical transmission.*** Vertical transmission most likely occurs in the following ways[2]:

- Transplacental infection
- Infant ingestion of infected maternal fluids (blood, amniotic fluid, or breast milk) during the process of birth and postpartum

Risk of transmission is most likely when infection occurs during the third trimester and if the woman is in an especially acute infectious state, with her blood testing positive for both HBsAg and HBeAg serologic markers.[2–5]

NOTE*: The CDC Immunization Practices Advisory Committee recommends routine screening of all pregnant women as the only strategy that will provide control of perinatal transmission of HBV infection in the United States.*[2,6]

Screening mothers also means that families of infected or carrier patients can then be tested and immunized as a component of hepatitis B transmission prevention. Women who present with no prenatal care or without documentation of prenatal care and laboratory testing results should have a hepatitis B screen done immediately. Women who have incomplete documentation of their hepatitis B status should have the remaining serologic markers evaluated to determine their infectious and/or carrier state.[2–6]

- Is HBeAg present?
- Has the HBsAg marker cleared and is anti-HBs present, denoting immune status?
- Has the HBsAg marker persisted for more than 6 months, indicating a carrier state?

• What are the clinical features of HBV infection?

Many infected patients are asymptomatic during the acute phase of infection. However, acute illness symptoms may occur and is often misdiagnosed as "the flu," especially if no jaundice is present. Symptoms may last for several weeks and include the following[1–3]:

- Anorexia
- Malaise
- Nausea
- Vomiting
- Abdominal pain
- Jaundice
- Extrahepatic symptoms—skin rashes, arthralgias, and arthritis

Hepatitis B infection is the most common cause of jaundice in pregnancy and generally runs its course over a 3- to 4-week period, but symptoms can remain for as long as 6 months.[7]

• How is hepatitis B managed during pregnancy?

Maternal complications from HBV are not common and pregnancy is *not* thought to aggravate the course of the disease in developed countries. Management is focused on supportive measures during an acute infection in women with symptoms and in women with chronic disease. In addition, preparation for birth and newborn care is necessary to decrease risk of perinatal transmission. The following list outlines pregnancy specific recommendations:

- All women should be screened at the first prenatal visit.[2]
- Women who are HBsAg negative but at high risk of contracting HBV infection need to be counseled that vaccination is recommended during pregnancy.[2,5]
- Amniocentesis may be performed for genetic testing and/or fetal lung maturity using a 22-gauge needle under ultrasound guidance.[2,3]
- Liver enzymes and prothrombin time (PT) should be monitored if the woman is symptomatic.[2,3,8]
- Antiviral therapy has been used to treat acute and chronic HBV infection in pregnancy and prevent perinatal transmission, especially in the woman with a high viral load.[9]
  - Lamivudine 150 mg PO starting at 34 weeks' gestation to decrease perinatal HBV transmission in high-risk women.[9]
  - Telbivudine 600 mg PO daily during weeks 24 through 32 weeks' gestation.[10]
  - Consideration should be given to duration of therapy, potential adverse effects to the fetus, efficacy, and the risk of drug resistance.[2,8–11]
  - Alternative medications are tenofovir, adefovir dipivoxil, interferon α-2b, peginterferon α-2b, and entecavir.[2,11]
- Consult with a hepatologist if the woman has a high HBV DNA level, liver involvement, or a positive HBcAg.[2,3]
- Vaccination against hepatitis A should be encouraged to prevent further liver damage.[2]
- Women rarely need hospitalization during pregnancy unless dehydration or marked liver damage has occurred.
- No special dietary prescriptions are needed. Management of nausea and vomiting may be necessary to improve nutrition.[2]
- In the event of severe symptoms of anorexia, nausea, vomiting, and diarrhea, hospitalization is recommended and the goals of treatment are to[2,3]:
  - correct fluid and electrolyte imbalance
  - assess for liver damage
  - promote rest
  - minimize infection transmission
- There is conflicting data regarding management of women with PPROM. Therefore, care planning should include disease chronicity and individualized for each woman (Table 12.9).

Prevention of Perinatal Transmission

Perinatal transmission from HBsAg-positive women can occur in utero (transplacental transfer during a threatened abortion), at birth, or after birth. The rate of transmission approaches 90% without active and passive immunity.[2] Perinatal transmission is associated with maternal predelivery HBV DNA levels (viral load).[12–14] Because of this risk, some providers may assess measurements of the viral load between 30 and 34 weeks' gestation.[3]

NOTE: Studies do not demonstrate that cesarean birth lowers the risk of neonatal hepatitis B infection if the woman has a viral load less than 1,000,000 IU/mL. Therefore, this route of birth should be reserved for obstetric indications and in women with high viral loads.[12,13]

Transmission is greatly reduced with universal vaccination of **all newborns** within 12 hours of birth.[2,15] In addition, the newborn of an HBsAg-positive woman should receive hepatitis B immune globulin as well. The primary goal in treating the newborn is prevention of the infant becoming a carrier of hepatitis B. Ninety percent of infected newborns become chronic carriers of HBsAg.[2] Approximately 25% of these infants will die from cirrhosis of the liver or liver cancer.[2]

Postpartum Care

In the immediate postpartum period, there is no reason to separate mother and baby due to disease. Liver enzymes may increase during the postpartum period in women with chronic

TABLE 12.9	INTRAPARTUM CARE PLANNING
MATERNAL HBsAg STATUS	**INTRAPARTUM PLAN OF CARE**
Woman not previously tested and/or status unknown	**Care of the Woman** • Obtain maternal serum HBsAg on admission. **Care of the Newborn** • If woman is positive, obtain informed consent and administer hepatitis B immune globulin (HBIg) immediately and within 7 d of birth.
Negative screen	**Care of the Newborn** • Obtain informed consent and administer hepatitis B vaccine prior to discharge. • If birth weight is <4 lb, 6 oz (2,000 g), postpone first dose of vaccine until 1 mo of age.
Positive screen	**Care of the Woman** • Obtain appropriate referrals and consultations as indicated. • Avoid invasive procedures. These should be performed only after careful assessment of risks versus benefits. Examples include the following: 　○ Internal scalp electrode monitoring 　○ Internal uterine pressure monitoring 　○ Vaginal examination after rupture of membranes 　○ Vacuum extraction 　○ Forceps birth • Breast feeding not contraindicated. • Encourage vaccination against hepatitis A to prevent further liver injury. • Provide information concerning hepatitis B that discusses the following: 　○ Mode of transmission 　○ Perinatal concerns 　○ Prevention of HBV transmission to contacts 　○ Substance abuse treatment, as indicated 　○ Medical evaluation and treatment for chronic hepatitis B **Care of the Newborn** • Dry the newborn immediately after birth to remove maternal blood and amniotic fluid. • Gently remove excess fluid and blood from the nares and oropharynx as indicated. Take care to avoid traumatizing the mucous membranes. • Bathe the newborn early and thoroughly with a mild, nonmedicated soap under radiant heat as soon as possible. • Obtain informed consent for administration of immune globulin (100 IU HBIg) and vaccine prior to birth if possible. • Administer HBIg and hepatitis B vaccine within 12 hrs of birth. • If birth weight is less than 4 lb, 6 oz: give birth dose, but do not count as part of the 3-dose series, and give next dose at 1 mo of age (will receive four total doses) • Delay administration of vitamin K until after the initial bath. • Remove potentially infectious maternal blood and secretions before any application of eye medications. • If the infant is born with additional problems, any life-threatening situation takes priority. • Instruct re. follow-up care, screening, and CDC immunization recommendations.

From World Health Organization. (2015). Hepatitis B. Retrieved from: http://www.who.int/mediacentre/factsheets/fs204/en/; Centers for Disease Control and Prevention. Viral hepatitis–hepatitis B information. http://www.cdc.gov/hepatitis/hbv/hbvfaq.htm#overview; Bernstein, H. B. (2012). Maternal and perinatal infection–viral. In Gabbe, S. G., Niebyl, J. R., Simpson, J. L., et al. (Eds.), *Obstetrics: Normal and problem pregnancies* (6th ed., pp. 1108–1139). Philadelphia, PA: Saunders; Mast, E. E., Margolis, H. S., Flore, A. E., et al. A comprehensive immunization strategy to eliminate transmission of hepatitis B virus infection in the United States. National Center for Infectious Diseases. Retrieved from: http://www.cdc.gov/mmwr/preview/mmwrhtml/rr5416a1.htm?s_cid = rr5416a1_e US Preventative Services; Han, G. R., Xu, C. L., Zhao, W., et al. (2012). Management of chronic hepatitis B in pregnancy. World Journal of Gastroenterology, *18*(33), 4517–4521.

HBV. Even though uncommon, "immunologic flares" in chronic HBV (acute hepatic failure) can occur in the postpartum period. There are no predictors of flares and may be related to an immunologic adjustment after birth—similar to withdrawal from corticosteroids.[16]

Breastfeeding

The CDC states that the infant of a hepatitis B-infected or carrier woman is not likely to be at risk for contracting the disease through breastfeeding, even though HBV DNA has been detected in the colostrum of HBsAg-positive women. Data suggests that benefits of breastfeeding outweigh risk of transmission.[2] Education of the woman should include proper techniques for nipple care, inspection of the breasts for cracks and skin breaks, and to stop breastfeeding on the affected breast (but continue to express milk to prevent engorgement) if she experiences any of the above. *The woman does not have to stop breastfeeding.*[2]

Patient and Family Education

Education of the woman and her family includes the following:
- Her hepatitis status
- The potential for transmission
- Methods to prevent transmission
- The need for complete immunization for the baby over the next 6 months

PRACTICE/REVIEW QUESTIONS

After reviewing this module, answer the following questions.

1. What are the three phases of HIV infection?

   a. _____

   b. _____

   c. _____

2. If a woman has not been tested for HIV during pregnancy, a rapid test may be done on admission to labor and delivery with expected results within _____.

3. The medication _____ has shown efficacy in decreasing perinatal transmission of HIV by rapidly crossing the placenta and providing protective serum levels of medication in the fetus.

4. In women on effective ARV regimens with a low viral load, duration of rupture of membranes does not increase transmission incidence.

   a. True

   b. False

5. Two intrapartum interventions that should generally be avoided because of a potential increased risk of transmission, unless there are clear obstetric indications include:

   a. _____

   b. _____

6. Methergine should not be co-administered to women receiving protease inhibitors.

   a. True

   b. False

7. A newborn of HIV-infected women should receive prophylactic _____.

8. State three ways in which newborns can acquire HIV from their mothers.

   a. _____

   b. _____

   c. _____

9. List six steps you should take while caring for the newly delivered baby that can reduce the risk of HIV transmission to the newborn.

   a. _____

   b. _____

   c. _____

   d. _____

   e. _____

   f. _____

10. Isolation is not necessary for the HIV-infected mother or mother with AIDS.

    a. True

    b. False

11. **Early** clinical signs and symptoms of chorioamnionitis are:

    a. _____

    b. _____

    c. _____

12. Funisitis is the inflammation of the _____.

13. Women with ruptured fetal membranes should have hourly cervical exams to check for the progress of labor.

    a. True

    b. False

14. You are caring for a woman who comes into Labor and Delivery complaining of ruptured membranes 24 hours ago. On examination, you assess purulent, malodorous amniotic fluid leaking from the vagina. Her vital signs are temperature 101, heart rate 113, respiratory rate 24, and BP 152/100. You would suspect _____.

15. Vaginal and rectal GBS cultures should be performed between _____ to _____ weeks' gestation on all women.

16. List four indications for intrapartum GBS prophylaxis antibiotic administration during labor.

    a. _____

    b. _____

    c. _____

    d. _____

17. When obtaining a GBS culture, the nurse should swab first swab the _____ and then insert the swab into the woman's _____.

18. Gonococcal infection may result in adverse pregnancy outcomes in any of the trimesters including:

    a. _____

    b. _____

    c. _____

    d. _____

19. Without prompt treatment of newborns of women with _____, neonatal blindness can occur as a result of corneal ulceration and perforation.

20. To minimize risk of HSV transmission during labor, the following should be avoided:

    a. _____

    b. _____

    c. _____

21. What is the most important factor in decreasing the risk of congenital syphilis in the neonate?

    a. _____

22. Transmission of hepatitis B virus from an infected or carrier mother to the newborn is most likely to occur as the baby comes into contact with infected amniotic fluid or blood during the birth process.

    a. True

    b. False

23. List five areas of education that should be addressed with the newly delivered hepatitis B carrier woman and her family.

    a. _____

    b. _____

    c. _____

    d. _____

    e. _____

PRACTICE/REVIEW ANSWER KEY

1. a. Acute infection and seroconversion
   b. Asymptomatic infection
   c. AIDS
2. 1 hour
3. Zidovudine
4. a. True
5. Any two of the following:
   AROM, application of FSE, scalp pH sampling, forceps, vacuum, episiotomy, cutting the cord with a contaminated instrument
6. a. True
7. Zidovudine
8. a. Vertical transmission during pregnancy
   b. Through contact with infected blood and bodily fluids during birth
   c. Breastfeeding
9. a. Assign one nurse to attend to the newborn after birth.
   b. Dry the newborn immediately after birth to remove all maternal blood and amniotic fluid.
   c. Gently remove excess fluid and blood from the nares and oropharynx.
   d. Aspirate stomach contents using a bulb syringe, mucus extractor, or meconium aspirator with wall suction on a low setting.
   e. Delay administration of vitamin K until after the newborn is bathed.
   f. Bathe the newborn early and thoroughly with a mild, nonmedicated soap under radiant heat as soon as the infant is stable.
10. a. True
11. a. Maternal fever >100.4°F
    b. Maternal tachycardia (>100 bpm)
    c. Fetal tachycardia
12. Umbilical cord
13. False; frequent cervical exams increases the likelihood for the development of chorioamnionitis due to vertical transmission from the vagina and rectal areas.
14. Chorioamnionitis
15. 35 and 37 weeks' gestation

16. a. Previous infant with invasive GBS disease
    b. GBS bacteriuria during any trimester of the current pregnancy
    c. Positive GBS vaginal-rectal screening culture in late gestation during current pregnancy
    d. Unknown GBS status at the onset of labor (culture not done, incomplete, or results unknown) and any of the following:
       • Delivery at <37 weeks' gestation
       • Amniotic membrane rupture ≥18 hours
       • Intrapartum temperature ≥100.4°F (≥38.0°C)
       • Intrapartum Nucleic acid amplification test (NAAT) positive for GBS
17. Vagina; rectum
18. a. Miscarriage
    b. Preterm birth
    c. Premature rupture of membranes
    d. Chorioamnionitis—if infection present at time of birth.
19. gonorrhea
20. a. the use of FSEs in fetal monitoring
    b. forceps- or vacuum-assisted births
    c. artificial rupture of membranes
21. a. treatment of early maternal syphilis for a minimum of 30 days before birth
22. a. True
23. a. How hepatitis B could be transmitted to the infant and the importance of proper handwashing after handling blood-soiled materials (e.g., in changing the mother's perineal pads before handling the baby)
    b. The potential for saliva causing transmission of the infection
    c. The risks the mother's hepatitis carrier status poses for the infant
    d. The risks and benefits of immunization for the infant
    e. The need for complete immunization plans for the baby over the next 6 months

R E F E R E N C E S

Part 1

1. Duff, P. (2012). Maternal and perinatal infection–bacterial. In Gabbe, S. G., Niebyl, J. R., Simpson, J. L., et al. (Eds.), *Obstetrics: Normal and problem pregnancies* (6th ed., pp. 1140–1155). Philadelphia, PA: Saunders.
2. Yoon, B. H., Romero, R., Moon, J. B., et al. (2001). Clinical significance of intra-amniotic inflammation in patients with preterm labor and intact membranes. *American Journal of Obstetrics & Gynecology, 185*, 1130–1136.
3. Tita, A. T., & Andrews, W. W. (2010). Diagnosis and management of clinical chorioamnionitis. *Clinical Perinatology, 37*(2), 339–354.
4. Rickert, V. I., Wiemann, C. M., Hankins, G. D., et al. (1998). Prevalence and risk factors of chorioamnionitis among adolescents. *Obstetrics & Gynecology, 92*(2), 254–257.
5. Seaward, P. G., Hannah, M. E., Myhr, T. L., et al. (1997). International Multicentre Term Prelabor Rupture of Membranes Study: Evaluation of predictors of clinical chorioamnionitis and postpartum fever in patients with prelabor rupture of membranes at term. *American Journal of Obstetrics & Gynecology, 177*(5), 1024–1029.

6. Eschenbach, D. A. (1993). Ureaplasma urealyticum and premature birth. *Clinical Infectious Disease, 17*(suppl 1), S100–S106.
7. Dashe, J. S., Rogers, B. B., McIntire, D. D., et al. (1999). Epidural analgesia and intrapartum fever: Placental findings. *Obstetrics & Gynecology, 93*(3), 341–344.
8. Lau, J., Magee, F., Qiu, Z., et al. (2005). Chorioamnionitis with a fetal inflammatory response is associated with higher neonatal mortality, morbidity, and resource use than chorioamnionitis displaying a maternal inflammatory response only. *American Journal of Obstetrics and Gynecology, 193*, 708–713.
9. Holcroft, C. J., Askin, F. B., Patra, A., et al. (2004). Are histopathologic chorioamnionitis and funisitis associated with metabolic acidosis in the preterm fetus? *American Journal of Obstetrics & Gynecology, 191*(6), 2010–2015.
10. American Academy of Pediatrics. (2011). Policy statement—recommendations for the prevention of perinatal group B streptococcal (GBS) disease. *Pediatrics, 128*(3), 611–616.

Part 2

1. Verani, J. R., McGee, L., & Schrag, S. J. (2010). Prevention of perinatal group B streptococcal disease-revised guidelines from CDC, 2010. *Recommendations and Reports: Morbidity and Mortality Weekly Report, 59*(RR-10), 1–23. Retrieved from: http://www.cdc.gov/mmwr/preview/mmwrhtml/rr5910a1.htm?s_cid = rr5910a1_w
2. American College of Obstetricians and Gynecologists. (2011). Prevention of early-onset group B streptococcal disease in newborns. Committee Opinion No. 485. *Obstetrics & Gynecology, 117*. Retrieved from: http://www.acog.org/Resources_And_Publications/Committee_Opinions/Committee_on_O
3. Centers for Disease Control and Prevention. (2010). Prevention of perinatal group B streptococcal disease. *Morbidity and Mortality Weekly Report, 59*(RR-10). Retrieved from: http://www.cdc.gov/mmwr/preview/mmwrhtml/rr5910a1.htm?s_cid = rr5910a1_w
4. American Academy of Pediatrics. (2011). Policy statement—recommendations for the prevention of perinatal group B streptococcal (GBS) disease. *Pediatrics, 128*(3), 611–616.
5. Randis, T. M., & Polin, R. A. (2012). Early-onset group B streptococcal sepsis: New recommendations from the Centres for Disease Control and Prevention. *Archives of Disease in Childhood, Fetal and Newborn Education, 97*(4), F291–F294.

Part 3

1. Bennet, N. J., & Gilroy, S. A. (2014). *HIV disease* [Online]. Retrieved from: medscape.com
2. CDC. (1993). Revised classification system for HIV infection and expanded surveillance case definition for AIDS among adolescents and adults. *Morbidity and Mortality Weekly Report 1992, 41* (no. RR-17).
3. Panel on Opportunistic Infections in HIV-Infected Adults and Adolescents: Recommendations from the Centers for disease Control and Prevention, the National Institutes of Health and the HIV Medicine Association of the Infectious Diseases Society of America. (2013). *Guidelines for the prevention and treatment of opportunistic infections in HIV-infected adults and adolescents.* https://aidsinfo.nih.gov/guidelines/html/4/adult-and-adolescent-oi-prevention-and-treatment-guidelines/0. Accessed Jan 30, 2016.
4. COHIS. (2000). *AIDS/HIV opportunistic infections* [Online]. Retrieved from: www.medvalet.com/index.html
5. UNAIDS. (2013). *2013 report on the global AIDS epidemic.* Geneva: Author.
6. Quinn, T. C., Bartlett, J. A., & Bloom, A. (2014). *The global human immunodeficiency virus pandemic.* Retrieved from: UpToDate.com

7. Centers for Disease Control and Prevention. (2013). *HIV in the United States: At a glance.* Atlanta, GA.

8. Centers for Disease Control and Prevention. (2013). *HIV and AIDS in the United States by geographic distribution.* Atlanta, GA.

9. Centers for Disease Control and Prevention. (2014). *HIV among women.* Atlanta, GA.

10. Centers for Disease Control and Prevention. (2014). *HIV among pregnant women, infants and children in the United States.* Atlanta, GA.

11. Centers for Disease Control and Prevention. (2014). *HIV transmission risk.* Atlanta, GA.

12. Piot, P. (2006). AIDS: From crisis management to sustained strategic response. *Lancet, 368,* 526–530.

13. Centers for Disease Control and Prevention. (1987). Recommendations for prevention of HIV transmission in health-care settings. *Morbidity and Mortality Weekly Report, 36*(SU02), 1–19.

14. Chin, J. (1994). The growing impact of HIV/AIDS pandemic on children born to HIV-infected women. *Clinics in Perinatology, 21*(1), 111–114.

15. Barkowsky, W., Krasinski, K., Pollack, H., et al. (1992). Early diagnosis of human immunodeficiency virus infection in children less than 6 months of age: Comparison of polymerase chain reaction, culture, and plasma antigen captive techniques. *Journal of Infectious Diseases, 166*(3), 616–619.

16. Centers for Disease Control and Prevention. (2014). *HIV testing.* Atlanta, GA.

17. Centers for Disease Control and Prevention. (2014). *Laboratory testing for the diagnosis of HIV infection: Updated recommendations.* Atlanta, GA.

18. Centers for Disease Control and Prevention. (2006). *Revised recommendations for HIV testing of adults, adolescents and pregnant women in health-care settings.* Atlanta, GA.

19. Watts, D. H. (2002). Management of human immunodeficiency virus infection in pregnancy. *New England Journal of Medicine, 346*(24), 1879–1891.

20. French, R., & Brocklehurst, P. (1998). The effect of pregnancy on survival in women infected with HIV a systematic review of the literature and meta-analysis. *British Journal of Obstetrics and Gynaecology, 105*(8), 827–835.

21. Minkoff, H. (2003). Human immunodeficiency virus infection in pregnancy. *Obstetrics and Gynecology, 101,* 797–810.

22. Anderson, J. (Ed.). (2006). *A guide to the clinical care of women with HIV: 2005 edition* [Online]. Rockville, MD : U.S. Dept. of Health and Human Services, Health Resources and Services Administration, HIV/AIDS Bureau, 2005.

23. Truong, H. M., Sim, M. S., Dillon, M., et al. (2010). Correlation of immune activation during late pregnancy and early postpartum with increases in plasma HIV RNA, CD4/CD8 T cells, and serum activation markers. *Clinical and Vaccine Immunology, 17*(12), 2024–2028.

24. Watts, D. H., Lambert, J., Stiehm, E. R., et al. (2003). Progression of HIV disease among women following delivery. *Journal of Acquired Immune Deficiency Syndromes, 33,* 585–593.

25. Mofenson, L. M., Centers for Disease Control and Prevention, U.S. Public Health Service Task Force. (2002). U.S. Public Health Service task force recommendations for use of antiretroviral drugs in pregnant HIV-1–infected women for maternal health and interventions to reduce perinatal HIV-1 transmission in the United States. *Morbidity and Mortality Weekly Report Recommendations and reports, 51*(RR-18), 1–38.

26. Lambert, J. S., Watts, D. H., Mofenson, L., et al. (2000). Risk factors for preterm birth, low birth weight, and intrauterine growth retardation in infants born to HIV-infected pregnant women receiving zidovudine. *AIDS, 14*(10), 1389–1399.

27. Anderson, B. A., & Cu-Uvin, S. (2014). Use of antiretroviral medications in pregnancy HIV-infected patients and their infants in resource-rich settings. UpToDate.

28. Centers for Disease Control and Prevention. (2001). Revised recommendations for HIV screening of pregnant women. *Morbidity and Mortality Weekly Report, 50*(RR19), 59–86. Retrieved from: http://www.cdc.gov/mmwr/preview/mmwrhtml/rr5019a2.htm. Accessed Jan 30, 2016.

29. Cooper, E. R., Charurat, M., Mofenson, L., et al. (2002). Combination antiretroviral strategies for the treatment of pregnant HIV-1-infected women and prevention of perinatal HIV-1 transmission. *Journal of Acquired Immune Deficiency Syndromes, 29,* 484–494.

30. Siegfred, N., van der Merwe, L., Brocklehurst, P., et al. (2011). Antiretrovirals for reducing the risk of mother-to-child transmission of HIV infection. *Cochrane Database System Review, 6,* CD003510.

31. Hoffman, R. M., Black, V., Technau, K., et al. (2010). Effects of highly active antiretroviral therapy duration and regimen on risk for mother-to-child transmission of HIV in Johannesburg, South Africa. *Journal of Acquired Immune Deficiency Syndromes, 54,* 35–41.

32. Read, P. J., Mandalia, S., Khan, P., et al. (2012). When should HAART be initiated in pregnancy to achieve an undetectable HIV viral load by delivery? *AIDS, 26,* 1095–1103.

33. Public Health Service Task Force. (2006). *Public Health Service Task Force recommendations for the use of antiretroviral drugs in pregnant HIV-1 infected women for maternal health and interventions to reduce perinatal HIV-1 transmission in the United States* [Online]. Retrieved from: https://aidsinfo.nih.gov/ContentFiles/PerinatalGL07062006051.pdf. Accessed Jan 30, 2016.

34. Panel on Treatment of HIV-Infected Pregnant Women and Prevention of Perinatal Transmission. (2014). *Recommendations for use of antiretroviral drugs in pregnant HIV-1-infected women for maternal health and interventions to reduce perinatal HIV transmission in the United States* [Online]. Retrieved from: aidsinfo.nih.gov

35. Bartlett, J. G. (2014). Counseling HIV-infected patients regarding potential side effects of antiretroviral therapy. UpToDate.

36. ATIS. (2006). *Guidelines for the use of antiretroviral agents in HIV-infected adults and adolescents* [Online]. Retrieved from: www.thebody.com/hivatis/

37. Glaxo Wellcome Inc. (2000). *Antiretroviral pregnancy registry* [Online]. Retrieved from: www.glaxowellcome.com/preg_reg/antiretroviral.html

38. Anderson, B. A., & Cu-Uvin, S. (2014). Prenatal evaluation and intrapartum management of the HIV-infected patient in resource-rich settings. UpToDate.

39. Mehta, S., Manji, K. P., Young, A. M., et al. (2008). Nutritional indicators of adverse pregnancy outcomes and mother-to-child transmission of HIV among HIV-infected women. *The American Journal Of Clinical Nutrition, 87,* 1639–1649.

40. Tuomala, R. E., Kalish, L. A., Zorilla, C., et al. (1997). Changes in total, CD4+, and CD8+ lymphocytes during pregnancy and 1 year postpartum in human immunodeficiency virus-infected women. The Women and Infants Transmission Study. *Obstetrics and Gynecology, 89,* 967–974.

41. Miotti, P. G., Liomba, G., Dallabetta, G. A., et al. (1992). T lymphocyte subsets during and after pregnancy: Analysis in human immunodeficiency virus type 1-infected and uninfected Malawian mothers. *The Journal of Infectious Diseases, 185,* 1116–1119.

42. European Collaborative Study. (2005). Mother-to-child transmission of HIV infection in the era of highly active antiretroviral therapy. *Clinical Infectious Diseases, 40,* 458–465.

43. Townsend, C. L., Cortina-Borja, M., Peckham, C. S., et al. (2008). Low rates of mother-to-child transmission of HIV following effective pregnancy interventions in the United Kingdom and Ireland, 2000–2006. *AIDS, 22*, 973–981.

44. Forbes, J. C., Alimenti, A. M., Singer, J., et al. (2012). A national review of vertical HIV transmission. *AIDS, 26*, 757–763.

45. Cotter, A. M., Brookfield, K. F., Duthely, L. M., et al. (2012). Duration of membrane rupture and risk of perinatal transmission of HIV-1 in the era of combination antiretroviral therapy. *American Journal of Obstetrics and Gynecology, 207*, 482.e1–e5.

46. International Perinatal HIV Group. (1999). The mode of delivery and the risk for vertical transmission of human immunodeficiency virus type 1—a meta-analysis of 15 prospective cohort studies. *New England Journal of Medicine, 340*, 977–987.

47. Briand, N., Warszawsi, J., Mandelbrot, L., et al. (2013). Is intrapartum intravenous zidovudine for prevention of mother-to-child HIV-1 transmission still useful in the combination antiretroviral therapy era? *Clinical Infectious Diseases, 57*, 903–914.

48. Wong, V. V. (2011). Is peripartum zidovudine absolutely necessary for patients with a viral load less than 1,000 copies/ml? *Journal Obstetrics and Gynecology, 31*, 740–742.

49. Colebunders, R., Hodossy, B., Burger, D., et al. (2005). The effect of highly active antiretroviral treatment on viral load and antiretroviral drug levels in breast milk. *AIDS, 19*, 1912–1915.

50. Schneider, S., Peltier, A., Gras, A., et al. (2008). Efavirenz in human breast milk, mothers', and newborns' plasma. *Journal of Acquired Immune Deficiency Syndromes, 48*, 450–454.

51. Rezk, N. L., White, N., Bridges, A. S., et al. (2008). Studies on antiretroviral drug concentrations in breast milk: Validation of a liquid chromatography-tandem mass spectrometric method for the determination of 7 anti-human immunodeficiency virus medications. *Therapeutic Drug Monitoring, 30*, 611–619.

Part 4

1. Allsworth, J. E., & Peipert, J. F. (2007). Prevalence of bacterial vaginosis: 2001–2004 National Health and Nutrition Examination Survey Data. *Obstetrics and Gynecology, 109*(1), 114–120.

2. Morris, M., Nicoll, A., Simms, I., et al. (2001). Bacterial vaginosis: A public health review. *British Journal of Obstetrics and Gynaecology, 108*, 439–450.

3. Bradshaw, C. S., Walker, S. M., Vodstrcil, L. A., et al. (2014). The influence of behaviors and relationships on the vaginal microbiota of women and their female partners: the WOW Health Study. *The Journal of Infectious Diseases, 209*, 1562–1572.

4. Centers for Disease Control and Prevention. (2015). *Sexually transmitted diseases treatment guidelines, 2015*. Atlanta, GA: Center for Surveillance, Epidemiology, and Laboratory Services, Centers for Disease Control and Prevention (CDC), U.S. Department of Health and Human Services. Retrived from: http://www.cdc.gov/std/tg2015/tg-2015-print.pdf. Accessed on Jan 30, 2016.

5. Riggs, M. A., & Klebanoff, M. A. (2004). Vaginal infections and preterm birth. *Clinical Obstetrics and Gynecology, 47*(4), 796–807.

6. Sobel, J. D. (2014). Candida vulvovaginitis. UpToDate. Retrieved from: uptodate.com

7. Edwards, M. S. (2002). The immune system. Part 3: Fungal and protozoal infections. In Fanaroff, A. A., & Martin, R. J. (Eds.), *Neonatal-perinatal medicine: Diseases of the fetus and infant* (Vol. 2, 7th ed., pp. 745–748). St. Louis, MO: Mosby.

8. Centers for Disease Control and Prevention. (2013). Sexually transmitted diseases. In *STDs & pregnancy – CDC fact sheet*. Atlanta, GA.

9. Weinstock, H., Berman, S., & Cates, W., Jr. (2004). Sexually transmitted diseases among American youth: Incidence and prevalence estimates, 2000. *Perspectives in Sexual Reproductive Health, 36*, 6–10.

10. Zenilman, J. M. (2012). Genital chlamydia trachomatis infections in women. UpTo Date. Retrieved from: uptodate.com

11. Andrews, W. W., Goldenberg, R. L., Mercer, B., et al. (2000). The Preterm Prediction Study: Association of second-trimester genitourinary chlamydia infection with subsequent spontaneous preterm birth. *American Journal of Obstetrics and Gynecology, 183*(3), 662–668.

12. Pammi, H., & Hammerschlag, M. R. (2013). Chlamydia trachomatis infections in the newborn. UpToDate. Retrieved from: uptodate.com

13. Centers for Disease Control and Prevention. (2010). 2010 sexually transmitted diseases treatment guidelines. *Morbidity and Mortality Weekly Report, 59*(No. RR-12).

14. Ghanem, K. G. (2014). Clinical manifestations and diagnosis of Neisseria gonorrhoeae infection in adults and adolescents. UpToDate. Retrieved from: uptodate.com

15. Miller, J. M., Maupin, R. T., Mestad, R. E., et al. (2003). Initial and repeated screening for gonorrhea during pregnancy. *Sexually Transmitted Diseases, 30*(9), 728–730.

16. Centers for Disease Control and Prevention. (2012). Update to CDCs sexually transmitted diseases treatment guidelines, 2010: Oral cephalosporins no longer a recommended treatment for gonococcal infections. *Morbidity and Mortality Weekly Report, 61*(31), 590–594.

17. Swygard, H., Sena, A. C., & Cohen, M. S. (2013). Treatment of uncomplicated gonococcal infections. UpToDate. Retrieved from: uptodate.com

18. Centers for Disease Control and Prevention. (2010). 2010 sexually transmitted diseases treatment guidelines: Diseases characterized by genital, anal, or perianal ulcers. *Morbidity and Mortality Weekly Report, 59*(No. RR-12).

19. Bernstein, K. I., Bellamy, A. R., Hook, E. W., 3rd, et al. (2013). Epidemiology, clinical presentation, and antibody response to primary infection with herpes simplex virus type 1 and type 2 in young women. *Clinical Infectious Diseases, 56*, 344–351.

20. Centers for Disease Control and Prevention. (2010). Seroprevalence of herpes simplex virus type 2 among persons aged 14–49 years—United States, 2005–2008. *Morbidity and Mortality Weekly Report, 59*, 456–459.

21. Riley, L. E., & Wald, A. (2013). Genital herpes simplex virus infection and pregnancy. UpToDate. Retrieved from: uptodate.com

22. Albrecht, M. A. (2014). Treatment of genital herpes simplex virus infection. UpToDate. Retrieved from: uptodate.com

23. ACOG practice bulletin. (2007). Clinical management guidelines for obstetrician-gynecologists. No. 82 June 2007. Management of herpes in pregnancy. *Obstetrics and Gynecology, 109*(6), 1489–1498.

24. Brown, Z. A., Wald, A., Morrow, A., et al. (2003). Effect of serologic status and cesarean delivery on transmission rates of herpes simplex virus from mother to infant. *Journal of the American Medical Association, 289*, 203–209.

25. Baker, D. (2007). HSV in pregnancy. *Current Opinion in Infectious Diseases, 20*, 73–76.

26. Handsfield, H. H., Waldo, B., Brown, Z. A., et al. (2005). Neonatal herpes should be a reportable diease. *Sexually Transmitted Diseases, 32*(9), 521–525.

27. Albrecht, M. A. (2014). Epidemiology, clinical manifesations, and diagnosis of genital herpes simplex virus infection. UpToDate. Retrieved from: uptodate.com

28. Briggs, G. G., Freeman, R. K., & Yaffe, S. J. (2013). Acyclovir. In *Drugs in pregnancy and lactation* (8th, e-book).

29. Centers for Disease Control and Prevention. (2014). Human papillomavirus vaccination: Recommendations of the Advisory Committee on Immunization Practices. *Morbidity and Mortality Weekly Report, 63*(RR05), 1–30.

30. Palefsky, J. M. (2014). Epidemiology of human papillomavirus infections. UpToDate. Retrieved from: uptodate.com

31. Centers for Disease Control and Prevention. (2013). Genital human papillomavirus (HPV) module. In *STD prevention program and training branch.* Atlanta, GA.

32. Centers for Disease Control and Prevention. (2010). Human papillomavirus (HPV) infection. In *Sexually transmitted diseases treatment guidelines, 2010.* Atlanta, GA.

33. Paavonen, J., Naud, P., Salmerón, J., et al. (2009). Efficacy of human papillomavirus (HPV)-16/18 AS04-adjuvanted vaccine against cervical infection and precancer caused by oncogenic HPV types (PATRICIA): Final analysis of a double-blind, randomised study in young women. *Lancet, 374,* 301–314.

34. Massad, L. S., Einstein, M. H., Huh, W. K., et al. (2012). 2012 updated consensus guidelines for the management of abnormal cervical cancer screening tests and cancer precursors. *Journal of Lower Genital Tract Disease, 17,* S1–S27.

35. Centers for Disease Control and Prevention. (2014). Primary and secondary syphilis—United States, 2005–2013. *Morbidity and Mortality Weekly Report, 63*(18), 402–406.

36. Centers for Disease Control and Prevention. (2013). Self-study STD modules for clinicians—syphilis. In *Division of STD prevention.* Atlanta, GA.

37. Centers for Disease Control and Prevention. (2012). 2012 sexually transmitted diseases surveillance. In *Division of STD prevention.* Atlanta, GA.

38. Hicks, C. B., & Sparling, P. F. (2013). Pathogenesis, clinical manifestations, and treatment of early syphilis. UpToDate. Retrieved from: uptodate.com

39. Centers for Disease Control and Prevention. (2013). Self-study STD modules for clinicians—vaginitis. In *Division of STD prevention.* Atlanta, GA.

40. Sobel, J. D. (2015). Trichomoniasis. In UpToDate. Waltham, MA. Retrived from: http://www.uptodate.com/contents/trichomoniasis. Accessed August 23, 2015.

Part 5

1. World Health Organization. (2015). Hepatitis B. Retrieved from: http://www.who.int/mediacentre/factsheets/fs204/en/

2. Centers for Disease Control and Prevention. (2015). Viral hepatitis—hepatitis B information. http://www.cdc.gov/hepatitis/hbv/hbvfaq.htm#overview

3. Bernstein, H. B. (2012). Maternal and perinatal infection—viral. In Gabbe, S. G., Niebyl, J. R., Simpson, J. L., et al. (Eds.), *Obstetrics: Normal and problem pregnancies* (6th ed., pp. 1108–1139). Philadelphia, PA: Saunders.

4. Jonas, M. M. (2009). Hepatitis B and pregnancy: An underestimated issue. *Liver International, 29*(suppl 1), 133–139.

5. Chen, H. L., Lin, L. H., Hu, F. C., et al. (2012). Effects of maternal screening and universal immunization to prevent mother-to-infant transmission of HBV. *Gastroenterology, 142,* 773–781.

6. Mast, E. E., Margolis, H. S., Flore, A. E., et al. A comprehensive immunization strategy to eliminate transmission of hepatitis B virus infection in the United States. National Center for Infectious Diseases. Retrieved from: http://www.cdc.gov/mmwr/preview/mmwrhtml/rr5416a1.htm?s_cid = rr5416a1_e US Preventative Services

7. Sookolan, S. (2006). Liver disease during pregnancy: Acute viral hepatitis. *Annals of Hepatology, 5,* 231–236.

8. Han, G. R., Xu, C. L., Zhao, W., et al. (2012). Management of chronic hepatitis B in pregnancy. *World Journal of Gastroenterology, 18*(33), 4517–4521.

9. Tran, T. T. (2013). Hepatitis B virus in pregnancy. *Clinical Liver Disease, 2*(1), 29–33.

10. Wu, Q., Huang, H., Xiaowen, S., et al. (2015). Telbivudine prevents vertical transmission of hepatitis B virus from women with high viral loads: A prospective long-term study. *Clinical Gastroenterology and Hepatology, 13*(6), 1170–1178.

11. Wang, L., Kourtis, A. P., Ellington, S., et al. (2013). Safety of tenofovir during pregnancy for the mother and fetus: A systematic review. *Clinical Infectious Disease, 57,* 1773–1181.

12. Pan, C. Q., Zou, H. B., Chen, Y., et al. (2013). Cesarean section reduces perinatal transmission of hepatitis B virus infection from hepatitis B surface antigen-positive women to their infants. *Clinical Gastroenterology and Hepatology, 11*(10), 1349–1355.

13. Yang, J., Zeng, X. M., Men, Y. L., et al. (2008). Elective caesarean section versus vaginal delivery for preventing mother to child transmission of hepatitis B virus: A systematic review. *Virology Journal, 5,* 100.

14. Kubo, A., Shlager, L., Marks, A. R., et al. (2014). Prevention of vertical transmission of hepatitis B: An observational study. *Annals of Internal Medicine, 160,* 828–835.

15. Schillie, S., Walker, T., Veselsky, S., et al. (2015). Outcomes of infants born to women infected with hepatitis B. *Pediatrics, 135,* e1141–e1147.

16. Elefsiniotis, I., Vezali, E., Vrachatis, D., et al. (2015). Postpartum reactivation of chronic hepatitis B virus infection among hepatitis B e-antigen-negative women. *World Journal of Gastroenertology, 21*(4), 1261–1267.

Care of the Laboring Woman with Diabetes

MARIBETH INTURRISI

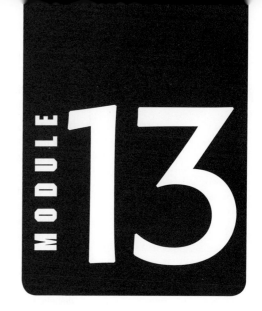

MODULE 13

When you have completed this module, you should be able to recall the meaning of the following terms and abbreviations.

blood glucose (BG)
body mass index (BMI)
continuous glucose monitoring system (CGMS)
diabetes
type 1 diabetes mellitus (T1DM)
type 2 diabetes mellitus (T2DM)
gestational diabetes mellitus controlled with diet
  and exercise (GDMA1)
gestational diabetes mellitus controlled with
  diet, exercise, and requiring the addition of
  oral meds and/or insulin (GDMA2)
diabetic ketoacidosis (DKA)
diabetogenic
endogenous insulin
exogenous insulin
euglycemia
hyperglycemia
hyperinsulinemia
hypoglycemia unawareness

insulin sensitivity
insulin resistance
leptin
nephropathy
neuropathy
organogenesis
polycystic ovary syndrome (PCOS)
polydipsia
polyphagia
polyuria
postprandial
pre-existing/overt diabetes
retinopathy
registered dietitian (RD)
subcutaneous (SC)
self-monitoring of blood glucose (SMBG)
total daily dose (of insulin) (TDD)
tumor necrosis factor alpha (TNF-α)

Epidemiology of Diabetes

Diabetes is a significant public health challenge for the United States. According to the 2014 report from the Centers for Disease Control (CDC), in the United States[1]:

- 29.1 million (9.3% of the US population) has diabetes
  - 21.0 million are diagnosed
  - 8.1 million (28% of people) with diabetes are undiagnosed
- 86 million (37% of US adults aged 20 years and older) have prediabetes
- 13.4 million adult women have diabetes

Like diabetes, obesity is a national epidemic with an increase in both prevalence and incidence. Rates of obesity and diabetes parallel each other. In states where obesity is >29%, diabetes is >9%. In 2013, these rates existed in 45 states.[2] Obesity is one of the highest risk factors for the development of T2DM.[3] Age, gender, and race also affect the prevalence of diabetes. Diabetes is increased in pregnant women >25 years of age and in non-Hispanic Blacks, Hispanic/Latino Americans, American Indians, East Indians, Alaska Natives, Asian Americans, and Native Hawaiian and Pacific Islanders (Table 13.1).[1,4]

TABLE 13.1 RISK FACTORS FOR TYPE 2 DIABETES AND GESTATIONAL DIABETES
BMI ≥25 kg/m² or ≥23 kg/m² in Asian Americans *and* have additional risk factors
Previous history of: GDM, macrosomia, unexplained stillbirth, malformed infant
Family history of overt diabetes among first-degree relatives
High-risk ethnic groups: African American, American Indian, Hispanic/Latina, Asian/Pacific Islander, South-East Asian, East Indian
Chronic use of medications which adversely affect normoglycemia (steroids, betamimetics, atypical antipsychotics)
History of prediabetes, polycystic ovarian syndrome, coronary vascular disease, hypertension, hyperlipidemia, acanthosis nigricans
Glucosuria
Family history of overt diabetes among first-degree relatives
Physical inactivity

From American Diabetes Association. (2015). Management of diabetes in pregnancy. Sec. 12. In *Standards of medical care in diabetes–2015. Diabetes Care, 38*(s1), S77–S79.

During pregnancy, 90% of all cases of diabetes are women with gestational diabetes mellitus (GDM). Approximately 9.2% of pregnant women in the United States are diagnosed with GDM.[5] Depending on race and ethnicity of the population, and upon method of diagnosis, the prevalence may range from 2% to 18%.[1,5] Within the postpartum period 5% to 10% of women with GDM are found to have diabetes, usually type 2.[6]

Women with a history of GDM have a 35% to 60% chance of developing T2DM within the 10 to 20 years of the index pregnancy. GDM represents one of the highest risk factors for developing T2DM.[3]

Classification of Diabetes

In 1997, the Expert Committee on the Diagnosis and Classification of Diabetes Mellitus eliminated the old categories of insulin-dependent diabetes mellitus (IDDM) and non–insulin-dependent diabetes mellitus (NIDDM) and established new terminology based on pathophysiology and not on use of insulin (Table 13.2).

TABLE 13.2	CRITERIA FOR THE DIAGNOSIS OF DIABETES (T1DM, T2DM) IN THE NONPREGNANT POPULATION

HbA1C ≥6.5%. The test should be performed in a laboratory using a method that is NGSP-certified and standardized to the DCCT assay.[a]

OR

FPG ≥126 mg/dL. Fasting is defined as no caloric intake for at least 8 hrs.[a]

OR

2-hr plasma glucose ≥200 mg/dL during an OGTT. The test should be performed as described by the WHO, using a glucose load containing the equivalent of 75 g anhydrous glucose dissolved in water.[a]

OR

In a woman with classic symptoms of hyperglycemia or hyperglycemic crisis, a random plasma glucose ≥200 mg/dL.

[a]In the absence of unequivocal hyperglycemia, result should be confirmed by repeat testing.

From American Diabetes Association. (2015). Management of diabetes in pregnancy. Sec. 12. In *Standards of medical care in diabetes–2015. Diabetes Care, 38*(s1), S77–S79.

NOTE: *Our current terminology uses the Arabic 1 and 2 (type 1 and type 2) instead of the Roman numerals I and II.*

In 2003, the committee recognized two categories in which glucose metabolism is defective—impaired fasting glucose (IFG) and impaired glucose tolerance (IGT). IFG and IGT are risk factors for future diabetes and cardiovascular disease. Blood glucose values indicative of prediabetes are values above the normal range but not in the range of overt diabetes. This category is important because these BG values are associated with other metabolic disorders such as obesity, hyperlipidemia, cardiovascular disease, and polycystic ovarian syndrome. Prediabetes (preDM) is similar to gestational diabetes. They both share the pathophysiology of T2DM and they are both primarily treated with lifestyle interventions: healthy eating and being active. Each condition has a conversion rate to T2DM of about 50% over the subsequent 10 years after diagnosis. In the Diabetes Prevention Program, people with prediabetes who are treated with diet, exercise and/or, metformin delayed T2DM beyond 5 years.[7–9] (See Table 13.3 for the categories associated with an increased risk for diabetes.)

TABLE 13.3	CATEGORIES OF INCREASED RISK FOR DIABETES (PREDIABETES)
Impaired fasting glucose (IFG)	FPG 100 to 125 mg/dL
Impaired glucose tolerance (IGT)	2-hr plasma glucose after a 75-g glucose load (OGTT): 140 to 199 mg/dL
	HbA1C
	5.7–6.4%

From American Diabetes Association. (2015). Management of diabetes in pregnancy. Sec. 12. In *Standards of medical care in diabetes–2015. Diabetes Care, 38*(s1), S77–S79.

The primary categories of diabetes include T1DM and T2DM with GDM and prediabetes as high-risk conditions leading to T2DM. While there are other less common categories of diabetes, the following table will summarize the characteristics of T1DM, T2DM, PreDM, and GDM. See Table 13.4: characteristics of diabetes, prediabetes, and gestational diabetes. Understanding the differences and similarities between these categories is essential to the optimum care of women with diabetes during pregnancy. The common denominator among all categories of diabetes is hyperglycemia and its adverse effects.

TABLE 13.4 CHARACTERISTICS OF T1DM, T2DM, PreDM, GDM

CONDITION	TYPE 1DM	TYPE 2DM	PreDM	GDM
Incidence	**5–10%**	**90–95%**	**30%**	**2–18%**
Pathophysiology	• Autoimmune destruction of pancreas • Reduces the facilitation of glucose into cells • Over time, very little to no insulin is produced • Results in hyperglycemia • High levels of glucose destroy blood vessels resulting in end-organ disease	• Abnormal insulin secretion and/or liver, muscle, and fat cell resistance to insulin • Increases the demand on the pancreas to produce more insulin • Beta cell exhaustion occurs • Results in hyperglycemia/end-organ disease	• Mild–moderate insulin resistance and decreased insulin effectiveness • BG higher than normal, not in range of overt diabetes • Due to risk factors 50% develop T2DM in 10 y	• Mild–moderate insulin resistance and decreased insulin effectiveness • BG higher than normal, not in range of overt diabetes • Due to severe placenta-mediated insulin resistance
Etiology	• Genetic susceptibility and a triggering environmental insult • A virus or "toxin" activates gene expression, turning antibodies on to the insulin-secreting cells of the pancreas	• Genetic or environmental (obesity/lifestyle) • One third of individuals with T2DM are under or at normal BMI	Same as T2DM	Same as T2DM
Symptoms	• Weight loss • Hyperphagia • Polyuria • Polydipsia • Hyperglycemia • Dehydration • Ketoacidosis • Coma	• Chronic fatigue • Frequent infections such as UTIs, vaginal yeast, slow healing sores • May present with vascular complications (HTN, MI, stroke, microalbuminuria, visual changes) • Ketoacidosis is relatively rare	• May be asymptomatic or similar to T2DM • Ketoacidosis is absent	• May be asymptomatic or similar to T2DM • Ketoacidosis is absent
Markers	• C-peptide low or absent • Glutamic decarboxylase 65(GAD-65) • Other anti-insulin antibodies • Sensitive to exogenous insulin	• C peptide initially high or normal • Autoantibodies usually absent • Acanthosis nigricans • Relatively resistant to insulin	• C-peptide normal or elevated • Autoantibodies usually absent • Acanthosis nigricans • Relatively resistant to insulin	• C-peptide normal or elevated • Autoantibodies usually absent • Acanthosis nigricans • Relatively resistant to insulin
Onset	• Most diagnosed in childhood • Almost half of T1DM is diagnosed after age 20 as latent autoimmune diabetes of the adult (LADA)	• Most diagnosed in adulthood • When combined with obesity, may be seen in children and teens	• May be diagnosed at puberty in high-risk children • Only one third are diagnosed, most remain undiagnosed	• Diagnosed during pregnancy • Incidence related to population and method of diagnosis
Ethnicity	Highest in non-Hispanic whites	Highest in non-White ethnic groups	Highest in non-White ethnic groups	Highest in non-White ethnic groups

table continues on page 373

CONDITION	TYPE 1DM	TYPE 2DM	PreDM	GDM
Insulin use	• MUST have exogenous insulin • "Sensitive" to insulin requiring relatively low doses except during pregnancy when insulin resistance mediated by the placenta • Multiple daily injections (MDI) or continuous subcutaneous infusion of insulin (CSII)	• Can be controlled with healthy lifestyle habits, with weight loss or weight-loss surgery • May use oral agents alone or in combination with insulin or (MDI or CSII)	• No insulin but may benefit from Metformin	• Most achieve normo-glycemia with diet and exercise alone (GDMA1) • About 30–40% require medication either oral or insulin (GDMA2)
Predisposing risk factors	• First-degree relative with DM • Non-Hispanic white ancestry • Age <20 yrs but increasing adult onset • Baby >4 Kg • Presence of other autoim-mune diseases such as thy-roiditis, celiac, cystic fibrosis, rheumatoid arthritis, lupus	• First-degree relative with DM • Non-White ethnicity ancestry • Age >45 yrs but increasing in teens and young adults • BMI >25 • Previous history of abnormal glucose tolerance, i.e., GDM • Acanthosis nigricans • Baby >9 lb • Sedentary lifestyle • Hypertension ≥140/90 mm Hg. • Chronic use glycogenic medi-cations, i.e., Steroids, atypical anti psychotics	• Same as type 2	• Same as type 2

From Centers for Disease Control and Prevention. (2014). *National diabetes report.* http://www.cdc.gov/diabetes/pubs/statsreport14/national-diabetes-report-web.pdf. Accessed May 1, 2015; Centers for Disease Control and Prevention. (2011). *National diabetes fact sheet.* Atlanta, GA: United States Department of Health and Human Services; American Diabetes Association. (2015). Management of diabetes in pregnancy. Sec. 12. In *Standards of medical care in diabetes—2015. Diabetes Care, 38*(s1), S77–S79; Committee on Practice Bulletins–Obstetrics. (2013). Practice Bulletin No.137: Gestational diabetes mellitus. *Obstetrics & Gynecology, 122,* 406–416; Daley, J. (2014). Diabetes in pregnancy. In Simpson, K., & Creehan, P. (Eds.), *Perinatal nursing* (4th ed., pp. 203–223); Barbour, L. A., McCurdy, C. E., Hernandez, T. L., et al. (2007). Cellular mechanisms for insulin resistance in normal pregnancy and gestational diabetes. *Diabetes Care, 30* (suppl 2), S112–S119.

Adverse Perinatal Outcomes of Hyperglycemia During Pregnancy

Effects of diabetes on women are unique because hyperglycemia can affect not only the wom-an's health but also that of her unborn child and that child's lifelong health. During pregnancy, women with pre-existing diabetes, type 1 (T1DM) and type 2 (T2DM), have the most risk for perinatal morbidity and mortality. Risks to the fetus depend on the level and severity of maternal hyperglycemia prior to pregnancy, during the time of conception, and throughout gestation.[12,13] If glycemic control is poor (HbA1C >7%) during conception and in the first trimester during *organogenesis* (first 8 weeks' gestation, when major organs are developing), congenital anoma-lies or miscarriage can occur. Miscarriage rates for women with pre-existing diabetes are as high as 30%. Cardiac and neural tube defects are the most common malformations.[14]

Hyperglycemia during the second and third trimesters of pregnancy can result in exces-sively large babies posing short- and long-term risks to both mother and child. These risks affect women with T1DM, T2DM, and GDM.[15–17]

This is the result of elevated maternal blood glucose freely crossing the placenta while insulin cannot. The fetus then produces its own insulin resulting in hyperinsulinemia. High levels of insulin combined with high levels of glucose in the fetus result in storage of excess fat in the abdomen of the fetus leading to macrosomia.[18,19] The third trimester is the time of rapid weight gain, development of muscle mass and fat stores for the newborn.

Congenital malformations are not common in GDM. Maternal hyperglycemia generally develops at the end of the second trimester when placental hormones increase maternal insulin resistance. Maternal insulin secretion must double to maintain normoglycemia.[11] Insulin resistance will continue to rise through the third trimester, often tripling the requirement for insulin secre-tion from the pancreas. Women with normal carbohydrate metabolism are able to produce enough endogenous insulin to maintain normoglycemia. Women with defective carbohydrate metabolism have mild–severe hyperglycemia depending on the severity of their defect. For this reason, screen-ing for GDM is recommended at 24 to 28 weeks' gestation for all pregnant women who have not

TABLE 13.5 ADVERSE PERINATAL AND FUTURE OUTCOMES RELATED TO HYPERGLYCEMIA DURING THE SECOND HALF OF PREGNANCY[5,22,23]	
FOR THE BABY	**FOR THE MOTHER**
• Palsies (birth injuries)	• Polyhydramnios
• Polycythemia–jaundice	• Preeclampsia
• Poor feeding	• Preterm birth
• Pulmonary immaturity	• Pyelonephritis
• Prolonged nursery stay	• Dystocia (abnormal labor)
• Rarely–stillborn	• Cesarean birth
INCREASED FUTURE RISKS	
Insulin resistance	Type 1 and 2: worsening of retinopathy
Diabetes	Type 1 and 2: Worsening of nephropathy
Hypertension	GDM: metabolic syndrome
Metabolic Syndrome	GDM: type 2 diabetes
Obesity	GDM: HTN

already been diagnosed with diabetes or hyperglycemia.[20,21] See Table 13.5 that outlines adverse effects of hyperglycemia on pregnancy outcomes during the second half of pregnancy.

Diagnosing Gestational Diabetes

For over 50 years in the United States, the diagnosis of diagnosing gestational diabetes (GDM) has been based on criteria that predict the future risk of the mother for developing T2DM. O'Sullivan and Mahan focused on subsequent maternal disease in 1,700 women using a 100-g OGTT at 28 weeks' gestation.[24] Diagnosing GDM has been based on identifying women at risk for type 2 diabetes in their future and not on perinatal outcomes. Blood glucose cutoffs for the 3-hour, 100-g OGTT were based on a statistical calculation and **not** on levels of glycemia with increasing risks for adverse outcomes. The 3-hour OGTT cutoffs have been adjusted as blood glucose laboratory determination has changed. The last adjustment was made by Carpenter and Coustan in 1982 and was adopted by ACOG and ADA.

Countries in most of the world have used a 2-hour, 75-g OGTT using various blood glucose cut points derived in various ways. Inconsistent diagnosing criteria across the world preclude any accurate study of GDM; therefore we cannot apply study findings universally limiting the development of best practices.

Overt diabetes, characterized by moderate to severe hyperglycemia, clearly increases the risk of adverse pregnancy outcome. In order to know who and when to treat mild hyperglycemia (AKA GDM), one must know what level of glucose intolerance during pregnancy, short of diabetes, is associated with the risk of adverse perinatal outcomes. This information could help to develop a global, evidence-based method of diagnosing GDM. The Hyperglycemia and Adverse Pregnancy Outcomes (HAPO) study published in 2008 focused on fetal effects of maternal hyperglycemia in 25,505 pregnant women at 15 centers in 9 countries using a 2-hour, 75-g OGTT at 24 to 28 weeks' gestation. The HAPO epidemiologic study was the first to conclusively establish a relationship between maternal glucose concentrations and undesirable perinatal outcomes (macrosomia, neonatal hyperinsulinemia, neonatal hypoglycemia, and preeclampsia) in women not previously diagnosed with diabetes. There was a continuous, positive, independent relationship between maternal BG and percent newborn body fat and between cord C-peptide concentrations and percent newborn fat. This suggests that the relationship between maternal glycemia and fetal fat deposition is mediated by fetal insulin production.[25]

The International Association of Diabetes in Pregnancy Study Group (IADPSG) convened a group of experts to translate the findings of the HAPO study to a method of diagnosing GDM that could be used globally. In 2010, the recommendations suggested BG cut points which represented an odds ratio of 1.75 of risk to experience the adverse outcomes. A one-step, 2-hour Oral Glucose Tolerance Test (using 75 g of Glucola) was recommended to be administered to all pregnant women, not previously diagnosed with diabetes at 24 to 28 weeks' gestation. Blood glucose cut points were as follows: fasting ≥92 mg/dL, 1 hour, ≥180 mg/dL, and 2 hour ≥153 mg/dL. GDM

TABLE 13.6 COMPARISON OF THE TWO STEP (ACOG/ADA) AND THE ONE STEP (ADA, WHO) METHODS OF DIAGNOSING GDM

DIFFERENCES	CARPENTER AND COUSTAN (TWO-STEP)	IADPSG (ONE-STEP)
Research basis	Predicts future risk of maternal T2DM	Predicts adverse perinatal outcomes for mother and newborn
Administered at 24–28 weeks' gestation	Uses 2 steps: Nonfasting 1-hr 50-g Glucola GLT; if >129 or 139 mg/dL, then administer fasting 3-hr 100-g Glucola OGTT	Uses one step: Eliminates 1-hr GLT. All women are tested with fasting 2-hr 75-g Glucola OGTT
Cut points for abnormal values	Fasting 95; 1 hr 180; 2 hr 155; 3 hr 140	Fasting 92; 1 hr 180; 2 hr 153
Diagnosis requirements	2 abnormal values	1 abnormal value
Prevalence of GDM in USA	2–14%	~18%

From American Diabetes Association. (2015). Management of diabetesin pregnancy. Sec. 12. In *Standards of medical care in diabetes–2015. Diabetes Care, 38*(s1), S77–S79; Committee on Practice Bulletins–Obstetrics. (2013). Practice Bulletin No.137: Gestational diabetes mellitus. *Obstetrics & Gynecology, 122*, 406–416; International Association of Diabetes and Pregnancy Study Groups Consensus Panel, Metzger, B. E., Gabbe, S. G., Persson, B., et al. (2010). International association of diabetes and pregnancy study groups recommendations on the diagnosis and classification of hyperglycemia in pregnancy. *Diabetes Care, 33*(3), 672–682; World Health Organization. (2013). *Diagnostic criteria and classification of hyperglycemia first detected in pregnancy*. Geneva: World Health Org., (WHO/NMH/MND/13.2).

is diagnosed if **1 value is abnormal**. The ADA adopted the one-step method in 2011 but ACOG chose to stay with the two-step method (Table 13.6).

The IADPSG criteria will identify approximately 18% of all pregnant women in the United States as having GDM.[26] This was thought to place an undue demand on the provider, healthcare system, and the woman's pregnancy. The controversy continues until more data can be supplied which supports the identification and treatment of this high-risk group of woman and their offspring. Currently, the World Health Organization, American Diabetes Association, ACE, and many countries in Europe and Asia have adopted the IADPSG guidelines.

The ADA and ACOG agree that women with high risk factors for T2DM should be tested for undiagnosed type 2 diabetes at the first prenatal visit using one of the methods of diagnosing diabetes in the nonpregnant population (see Table 13.2 for diagnosing diabetes in the nonpregnant population). This recommendation makes it possible to diagnose T2DM (and rarely T1DM) in pregnancy so that aggressive treatment can begin early and women with undiagnosed overt diabetes can be identified and appropriately followed up postpartum.[26]

Normal Glucose Metabolism

The nutritive substance used in the greatest quantities by humans is carbohydrate. Carbohydrates (CHO) are ingested with the food we eat or produced by our liver. After being converted into glucose, CHO is utilized by all our cells, especially by our muscles, which should constitute nearly half our body mass.

Production and consumption of CHO is so well regulated that a constant BG level is maintained between approximately 70 and 110 mg/dL. The constancy of the BG level is controlled by a complex physiological homeostatic mechanism because BG level is such an important factor in many chemical and physiological processes.

Normal glucose metabolism involves the following pathways
1. While eating, carbohydrates are broken down by the stomach into **glucose**.
2. **Glucose** is absorbed into the blood via the intestine.
3. **Glucose** in the blood stimulates the pancreas to release insulin.
4. **Insulin** is released in two phases from the pancreatic β cells in the islets of Langerhans:
   • First phase of insulin response refers to the change in insulin concentration relative to the elevation in glucose concentration within the first 5 minutes after glucose is sensed.

- Second phase of insulin response refers to the rate of insulin release relative to the glucose concentration 5 to 60 minutes after glucose is sensed. This gradual release of insulin is under the feedback control of the blood glucose. Hyperglycemia increases the secretion of insulin and hypoglycemia diminishes or completely inhibits it.

5. **Insulin** causes the following actions:
   - Stimulates entry of glucose into cells for utilization as energy
   - Promotes the storage of glucose as glycogen in muscles and liver cells
   - Inhibits release of glucose from the liver or from muscle glycogen
   - Stimulates entry of amino acids into cells
   - Enhances fat storage and prevents the mobilization of fat for energy
   - Inhibits the formation of glucose from noncarbohydrates (e.g., amino acids)

6. Glucagon **is secreted from the alpha cells of the pancreas**:
   - Stops the production of insulin when BG drops below 70 mg/dL
   - Causes the release of glucose from glycogen (liver)
   - Releases fatty acids from stored triglycerides (fat)

The balance between these two hormones (**insulin and glucagon**) holds metabolism "on the line," promoting a stable homeostasis of glucose in the blood.

• How is glucose metabolism changed during pregnancy?

Many metabolic changes occur during pregnancy to optimize the growth of the fetus. Because the fetus depends entirely on the mother for its supply of energy, maternal adaptations must occur to increase glucose supply to the fetus. Initially human chorionic gonadotropin (HCG) stimulates the corpus luteum (the part of the follicle left behind in the ovary during ovulation) to produce estrogen and progesterone in the first 10 weeks after conception, until the placental cells can do so by themselves. By approximately 8 to 15 weeks' gestation glucose homeostasis is altered by the increases in estrogen and progesterone that cause pancreatic β-cell hyperplasia (multiplication of cells), with subsequent increased insulin secretion. Since insulin resistance has not yet developed, women with pre-existing diabetes often experience hypoglycemia as a result of the following factors:
- Increased glucose utilization (developing fetus) causes approximately a 10% reduction in maternal BG
- Increased insulin secretion (pancreatic hyperplasia) results in increased glycogen stores and decreased hepatic glucose production causing the fasting BG to lower (Fig. 13.1)

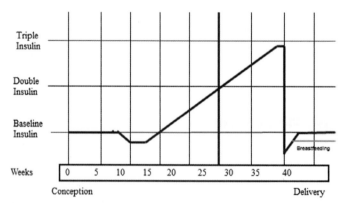

FIGURE 13.1 Insulin requirements in pregnancy. (From California Department of Public Health. *California Diabetes and Pregnancy Program.* Retrieved from: https://www.cdph.ca.gov/programs/cdapp)

In the second and third trimesters, levels of human placental lactogen (HPL), human placental growth hormone (hPGH), progesterone, estrogen, tumor necrosis factor alpha (TNF-α), leptin, and cortisol increase progressively and cause increasing tissue resistance to insulin action.[11]

Maternal cells are "blinded" by placental hormones inhibiting recognition of insulin. As hormone levels rise, insulin resistance increases and the maternal pancreas secretes more insulin. Maternal hyperinsulinemia provides the fetus with adequate substrate to grow (Glucose). Normal pregnancy can be viewed as a progressive condition of insulin resistance, hyperinsulinemia, and mild postprandial hyperglycemia. The mild postprandial hyperglycemia serves to increase the amount of time that maternal glucose levels are elevated above the basal after a meal, thereby increasing the flux of ingested nutrients from mother to the fetus and enhancing fetal growth.

Maternal hyperglycemia (diabetes during pregnancy) results when the mother's cells already have trouble recognizing insulin (insulin resistance) as in T2DM, prediabetes, polycystic ovarian syndrome, metabolic syndrome, obesity, or a pre-existing inherited tissue defect. Insufficient insulin secretion may also be a factor in maternal hyperglycemia when the woman's pancreas cannot produce the extra insulin needed to meet increasing pregnancy demands.

Accelerated Starvation of Pregnancy

Throughout pregnancy, there is an increased risk for fasting ketosis due to the following metabolic factors during pregnancy that allow energy to come from sources other than carbohydrates such as fats and protein (protects fetus from lack of carbohydrate):

- Increased levels of fatty acids
- Increased triglycerides
- Increased ketones (pregnant women form ketones within a few hours of not eating—for this reason small frequent meals every 2 to 3 hours are recommended during pregnancy)

These metabolic factors cause increased fat breakdown, and decreased maternal glucose production in the fasting state. This allows for increased utilization of fat stores for maternal energy, therefore protecting muscle mass from breakdown.

Antepartum Management for Women with Hyperglycemia during Pregnancy

Healthy Eating

By far the most important way to control BG is to eat a healthy diet. The three cornerstones in the treatment of **all types** of diabetes during pregnancy include the following:

- Balanced meal plan
- Carbohydrate control
- Weight management

NOTE: A registered dietitian (RD) who is knowledgeable concerning pregnancy and diabetes should be consulted to create an individualized, culturally appropriate meal plan.

Being Active

Just as healthy eating is essential to the management of hyperglycemia for all types of diabetes, exercise must also be incorporated into the plan of care. Being active for 30 to 60 minutes per day is encouraged because muscle activity does the following:

- Increases insulin sensitivity lowering blood glucose levels[3]
- Increases utilization of glucose, especially after a meal[3]
- Improves blood glucose control and may eliminate the need for insulin therapy[28]
- Reduces risk of excessive weight gain[29,30]
- Decreases risk of preeclampsia[31]
- Reduced the weight of the newborn by approximately 150 g.[32] A woman with T1DM should check her BG before, during, and after exercise. If the BG is <100 mg/dL, she should consume 15 to 30 g CHO to prevent hypoglycemia. She should always carry her meter and glucose tabs or a snack. If the BG >200 mg/dL, she should not exercise until BG is less than 180 mg/dL. If there are urine ketones present she should give an insulin correction and drink several glasses of water and wait to exercise until the ketones have cleared. Physical activity does not always improve BG control especially in an insulin deficient state. BG will continue to rise. For women with T1DM exercise can only lower BG if adequate insulin is available.[33]

Self-Monitoring of Blood Glucose

The goal of antepartum management is to achieve BG values as close to normal as is safe to reduce the risk of adverse perinatal outcomes. The BG values, which have the most significant effect on fetal macrosomia and cesarean birth are the fasting and the peak BG after a meal.[34,35]

The HAPO study found that 11.9% of pregnant women had a fasting BG greater than 90 mg/dL in the beginning of the third trimester. This cutoff detected 22.1% of LGA neonates and 15.1% of primary cesarean deliveries.[19] Nondiabetic, pregnant women wearing a continuous glucose monitoring system (CGMS) were shown to have a peak postprandial time (min) 70 ± 13.[36] In diabetic and nondiabetic pregnancies, maximal postprandial glucose excursions occur between 60 and 90 minutes after meal ingestion and correlate more closely with 1- than 2-hour postprandial measurements.[36] Some authors suggest that 60 minutes is a reasonable time to identify the peak postprandial since it is easier for women to remember and is closest to the average time from first bite of carbohydrate to peak BG.[35,37] Therefore, checking the 1-hour BG after the first bite of carbohydrate has been selected to represent the peak for most diabetes in pregnancy programs.

In an earlier study Langer found that when the mean daily BG value was 87 to 100 mg/dL, the rate of large for gestational age (LGA) and macrosomia was comparable to that in the general population, which is approximately 10%. Of importance to note is that fasting hyperglycemia greater than 105 mg/dL is associated with an increased risk of intrauterine fetal death (IUFD) in the last 4 to 8 weeks' gestation.[38] When the mean BG was greater than 105 mg/dL the incidence of LGA increased more than twofold. The HbA1c had no relationship in the third trimester to these outcomes and could not be used to evaluate thresholds for improving outcomes in terms of macrosomia.[39]

Establishing target BG has been challenging. While the fasting BG target of less than 90 mg/dL is somewhat evidenced based[26] there are no studies that show how close to "normal" the peak postprandial should be to show a significant improvement in outcomes (see Table 13.7).

TABLE 13.7 BLOOD GLUCOSE (BG) VALUES IN NORMAL PREGNANT WOMEN IN THE THIRD TRIMESTER	
BLOOD GLUCOSE (BG)	**mg/dL**
Mean	**83.7** $\pm$ 8
Fasting	**75** $\pm$ 12
Preprandial	**78** $\pm$ 11
Peak postprandial	**110** $\pm$ 16
Peak postprandial time (min)	**70** $\pm$ 13
1-hr postprandial	**105** $\pm$ 13
2-hr postprandial	**97** $\pm$ 11
Mean blood glucose at nighttime (mg/dL)	**68** $\pm$ 10

From Hod, M., & Yogev, Y. (2007). Goals of metabolic management of gestational diabetes. *Diabetes Care, 30*(suppl 2), S180–S187.

NOTE: During pregnancy, a 1-hour postprandial glucose value is more predictive of macrosomia than fasting values.[35]

Until consensus on these guidelines is achieved, the ADA recommends setting targets based on clinical experience and individualizing care. Table 13.8 summarizes several national organizations' suggested BG targets for women with diabetes during pregnancy.

Frequency of SMBG

• **How often should women check their BG level during pregnancy?**

Women should be taught to check their BG using a home meter. The frequency of testing is determined by how well the BG is controlled and whether or not insulin is being used premeal. In general, women following dietary therapy alone (GDMA1) or taking oral medications (GDMA2)

TABLE 13.8	BLOOD GLUCOSE TARGETS DURING PREGNANCY						
BG (mg/dL)	ADA 2008 T1 & T2DM	ADA 2015 T1 & T2 DM FOR HYPOGLYCEMIA UNAWARENESS	ACOG 2005 T1 & T2DM	ACOG 2001 GDM	ACOG 2013 GDM	ADA 2015 GDM
Fasting/premeal	60–99	<105	<95/<100	<90	<95	<92 (IADPSG)
1 hr PP	100–129	<155	<140	<130–140	<140	<140
2hr PP		<130	<120	<120	<120	<120
Mean daily	<110	Not specified	>87	<100	>87	<100
Bedtime/3 AM	60–99	<105	>60		Not specified	Not specified
HbA1C	<6%	<7%	<6%	NA	NA	NA

From American Diabetes Association. (2015). Management of diabetes in pregnancy. Sec. 12. In *Standards of medical care in diabetes–2015*. *Diabetes Care, 38*(s1), S77–S79; Committee on Practice Bulletins–Obstetrics. (2013). Practice Bulletin No.137: Gestational diabetes mellitus. *Obstetrics & Gynecology, 122*, 406–416; Kitzmiller, J. L., Block, J. M., Brown, F. M., et al. (2008). Managing pre-existing diabetes for pregnancy: Summary of evidence and consensus recommendations for care. *Diabetes Care, 31*, 1060–1079; International Association of Diabetes and Pregnancy Study Groups Consensus Panel, Metzger, B. E., Gabbe, S. G., Persson, B., et al. (2010). International association of diabetes and pregnancy study groups recommendations on the diagnosis and classification of hyperglycemia in pregnancy. *Diabetes Care, 33*(3), 672–682.

obtain fasting and postprandial BG values. The postprandial value allows women to observe how their blood glucose responded to the CHO content of the meal. During pregnancy, a 1-hour postprandial glucose value is more predictive of macrosomia than premeal values.[34,35] In addition, women with GDM, who checked their fasting and post meal peak blood sugar daily (4 BG checks per day), had less macrosomia than those who had their BG checked in clinic once a week.[40]

Women with pre-existing diabetes (T1DM and T2DM) may be accustomed to checking fasting BG and before meals to decide how much insulin they may need to use to cover CHO in the meal while accounting for the premeal BG. They do not generally check post meal BG when not pregnant; therefore, checking their post meal peak may be challenging but necessary. When using insulin to control fasting BG, bedtime, and occasional 3 AM BG may be needed to fine tune insulin dosing. Suggested frequencies for testing are listed in Table 13.9 and can be modified depending on the woman's circumstances.

TABLE 13.9	DAILY SELF-MONITORING BLOOD GLUCOSE (SMBG) SUGGESTED FREQUENCIES		
	T1DM/T2DM	GDMA2	GDMA1
Fasting	X	X	X–checks may be reduced according to BG control
Premeal	X	X–when starting premeal insulin–may DC if WNL	
Peak postprandial	X	X	X–as above
Before and after snacks	Using insulin pump		
Bedtime	X	As needed	
3 AM	When change in basal bedtime dose	When starting basal insulin at bedtime	

From Committee on Practice Bulletins–Obstetrics. (2013). Practice Bulletin No.137: Gestational diabetes mellitus. *Obstetrics & Gynecology, 122*, 406–416; Kitzmiller, J. L., Block, J. M., Brown, F. M., et al. (2008). Managing preexisting diabetes for pregnancy: Summary of evidence and consensus recommendations for care. *Diabetes Care, 31*, 1060–1079.

Continuous Glucose Monitoring System

The use of CGMS has become more common—especially among women with T1DM. However, CGMS cannot replace fingerstick (capillary) BG measurement since there is a lag time of 10 to 15 minutes for the glucose in the blood to reach the interstitial space. Therefore, accuracy maybe compromised.[41]

Recent advances in technology have improved algorithms that attempt to eliminate the discordance between the values. A CGM may be worn for 7 days or more and can give real-time information to the wearer. The CGM must be calibrated several times a day by obtaining a fingerstick BG and setting the CGM to the capillary BG. BG readings from the CGM must be checked with a fingerstick if any action is to be taken on the results. CGM has been particularly useful in alerting the patient to rapidly rising or falling BG using a system of up and down arrows. A randomized control trial found improved glycemic control in the third trimester, lower birth weight, and reduced risk of macrosomia with CGM use during pregnancy with T1DM.[42] More research is needed to support these findings.

HbA1C

Another measure of glucose control is the HbA1C. As red blood cells circulate in the blood stream glucose attaches to the hemoglobin. The rate of attachment is determined by the glucose concentration of the blood. Because the lifespan of red blood cells averages 120 days the predictability of HbA1C ranges from 6 to 12 weeks. However, a reduction in the HbA1C is seen throughout pregnancy due to a more rapid turnover of red cells, which occurs every 2 to 6 weeks. Thus glycosylated hemoglobin does not correlate well with SMBG. This is especially true in patients who have gestational diabetes whose BG is mildly elevated in comparison to type 1 and type 2 diabetes patients. Using HbA1C as a tool for monitoring glycemic goals and treatment adjustment in managing GDM is not effective.[36] In addition, by the end of the first trimester the fasting BG drops approximately 10%, contributing to the lowering of HbA1C.[43,44] Another contribution to a lower HbA1C occurs when frequent hypoglycemia combines with high postprandial elevations. The fetal insulin response is to the highest BG not to the average BG. It is important to note that iron deficiency anemia and hypertriglyceridemia falsely increases the HbA1C.[45]

Correlations have been made between first trimester HbA1C and the rate of congenital malformations and miscarriage.[14,46] Rowan and associates noted that HbA1C equal to or greater than 5.9% obtained close to 8 weeks' gestation, identified all women with undiagnosed overt diabetes (T2DM) and a group of women with GDM at significantly increased risk of adverse pregnancy outcome.[47] During the third trimester there are no significant correlations between HbA1C and adverse outcomes such as macrosomia.[48] The use of HbA1C to follow glycemic control is limited to women with T1DM and T2DM who have more variation in their BG and for whom the goal of HbA1C <6% has been recommended.[1,12]

Ketone Testing

Daily fasting urine ketone testing is also controversial and lacking strong evidence of benefit.[12,49,50] Fasting starvation ketones (associated with a low BG or normal BG) are not uncommon in pregnant women because of pregnancy's accelerated starvation after just a few hours of no carbohydrate intake. In addition, urine ketones do not correlate well with serum ketones. It is recommended to measure urine ketones during pregnancy when the pregnant woman with T1DM becomes ill (nausea and vomiting, fever, inability to eat or drink) and exhibits persistent hyperglycemia >200 mg/dL. Women with T1DM are prone to diabetic ketoacidosis at lower levels of BG than outside pregnancy. If ketones measure moderate or large, and BG persists >200 mg/dL, women with T1DM should contact the provider.

Medication (T1DM, T2DM, and GDMA2)

While all women with T1DM and most women with T2DM require insulin during pregnancy, most women with GDM achieve BG control with diet and exercise alone (GDMA1). If more than 3 fasting BG **or** more than 6 post meal BG values are above target after diet and exercise have been optimized, pharmacologic treatment should be initiated. Approximately 30% to 40% of women require pharmacologic treatment.[51] In the past decade, oral medications have been used to treat mild hyperglycemia in pregnancy.[52,53] Reducing the maternal BG levels in GDM has been shown to reduce macrosomia, and preeclampsia.[54,55]

Types of Insulin

Insulin analogs and NPH are currently the most used and effective insulins during pregnancy (see Table 13.10).[56,57]

- **Rapid-acting Insulin analogs** are used via multiple daily injections (MDI) or in SC insulin pumps.

TABLE 13.10	INSULINS MOST USED DURING PREGNANCY				
TYPE OF INSULIN	**EXAMPLES**	**CATEGORY**	**ONSET**	**PEAK**	**DURATION**
Mealtime or BOLUS	Humalog (lispro) *Eli Lilly*	B	15 mins	30–90 mins	3–4 hrs
Rapid-acting	NovoLog (aspart) *Novo Nordisk*	B		40–50 mins	3–5 hrs
Analog	Glulisine (Apidra) *Aventis*	C		55 mins	3–5 hrs
BASAL Intermediate-acting (NPH)	Humulin N *Eli Lilly*	B	1–2 hrs	6–8 hrs	10–20 hrs
	Novolin N *Novo Nordisk*	B			
Long-acting analogs	Levemir (Detemir) *Novo*	B	1–2 hrs	None	12–20 hrs
	Glargine (Lantus)	C			24 hrs

From Trujillo, A. (2007). Insulin analogs and pregnancy. *Diabetes Spectrum, 20*(2), 94–101.

- **Short-acting regular human insulin** is used in intravenous drips but not for MDI or insulin pumps because the peak of its action does not match the peak of carbohydrate after a meal.
- **Intermediate-acting Insulin NPH** begins to work in 2 to 4 hours and peaks at about 6 to 8 hours.
- **Long-acting analogs** begin to work in 1 to 2 hours, have a more consistent action, no real peak, less hypoglycemia.

Insulin Dosing

Insulin dosing regimens differ depending on the type of diabetes, current maternal weight, blood glucose levels, gestational age, and individual response to therapy. (See Table 13.11 for insulin dosing calculation.)

TABLE 13.11	INSULIN DOSE CALCULATIONS DURING PREGNANCY	
WEEKS OF GESTATION	**TOTAL DAILY INSULIN T1DM**	**TOTAL DAILY INSULIN T2DM OR OBESE GDMA2, T1DM**
Weeks 1–18	0.4–0.5 units/kg	0.7–0.9 units/kg
Weeks 18–26	0.6–0.7 units/kg	0.8–1.0 units/kg
Weeks 26–36	0.8–0.9 units/kg	0.9–1.1 units/kg
Weeks 36–40	0.9–1.0 units/kg	1.0–2.0 units/kg
Calculate total daily dose (TDD) X current maternal weight in kg.		

Divide total daily dose (TDD) into 50% basal insulin (NPH, Lantus, or Levemir) and 50% bolus/premeal insulin (See rapid-acting analogs in Table 13.13.) After the first trimester, the ratio of basal to bolus insulin may change to 40% basal and 60% bolus due to the increasing postprandial insulin resistance to CHO intake.

From California Department of Public Health. *California diabetes and pregnancy program.* Available at: https://www.cdph.ca.gov/programs/cdapp

---

KEY POINTS
- Insulin requirements for women with T1DM who are <u>sensitive to insulin</u> are generally less than women with T2DM or GDM who are insulin resistant.
- Obesity (high maternal weight) increases insulin requirements because fat cells increase <u>insulin resistance.</u>
- Glucotoxicity, chronic high blood sugar, increases <u>insulin resistance</u> requiring more insulin to bring the glucose down to normal ranges.
- Pregnancy is a state of increasing <u>insulin resistance</u> which peaks around 32 to 34 weeks and drops abruptly with the delivery of the placenta.
- Insulin requirements in all women double to triple by term.

Insulin is not a stand-alone tool. Insulin dose adjustments are necessarily based on carbohydrate consumption, exercise, and current BG. Sliding scales arbitrarily suggest an insulin dose for a certain BG value without regard to other factors. Sliding scales are obsolete and should not be used in lieu of scheduled insulin.[60] Instead, a premeal correction algorithm is used to adjust insulin when the premeal BG is not in target. A premeal algorithm directs extra insulin or less insulin needed to reach a post meal BG in the target for pregnancy (see Table 13.12).[60]

TABLE 13.12 PREMEAL CORRECTION ALGORITHM		
<70 mg/dL	2 units less	Eat right away, inject insulin after the meal
70–99 mg/dL	Give basic dose	Inject, eat CHO right away
100–129 mg/dL	1 unit more	Inject, eat in 15 mins
130–159 mg/dL	2 units more	Inject, check BG in 30 mins, eat when <130
160–189 mg/dL	3 units more	Inject, check BG in 60 mins, eat when <130
>190 mg/dL	4 more units, notify provider	Inject, check in 60 mins, eat per provider orders

From California Department of Public Health. *California diabetes and pregnancy program.* Available at: https://www.cdph.ca.gov/programs/cdapp

NOTE: Algorithms prevent hyperglycemia while sliding scales chase hyperglycemia, often stacking insulin and causing iatrogenic hypoglycemia which then is over treated causing a cycle of hyper–hypoglycemia.

Insulin Administration

During pregnancy, it is suggested that insulin be administered in the abdomen to insure consistency of absorption. As the uterus grows it may be necessary to select subcutaneous sites at the back upper hip since the stretched skin in the front of the abdomen may be tender.
- Sites within the abdomen should be rotated. Rotation of the injection site is critical to prevent lipohypertrophy, which reduces absorption by 25%.[61] Insulin should be injected when it is in room temperature. It does not need refrigeration unless the temperature is above 80 or below 40 where it is stored.[61]
- Insulin in vials must be discarded 30 days after first puncture. Insulin pens have varying lengths of use before expiring (See manufacturer).
- Alcohol wipes are avoided (unless in the hospital setting) as they tend to dry out the skin and leave cracks where microorganisms can enter.[61]

Glucose Lowering Oral Medications

Oral agents have been reintroduced in the management of diabetes during pregnancy. There are several reviews of sulfonylureas (glyburide) and biguanides (metformin) used primarily in pregnancies complicated by gestational diabetes. Oral glucose lowering agents (OGLA) were once thought to be associated with an increased incidence of congenital malformations. However, the issue of malformations has been shown to be related to hyperglycemia (a known teratogen) from poor glucose control rather than teratogenicity from the oral medication. A meta-analysis of the safety of oral agents (metformin and glyburide) in the first trimester supports this contention.[62]

Many women with GDM can safely achieve acceptable glycemic control with glyburide or Metformin.[63] However, insulin remains the optimum first-line treatment for hyperglycemia during pregnancy because it does not cross the placenta and can more reliably achieve tight glycemic control. Most of the published data that concern utilization of oral agents in pregnancy is in the GDM population.[52,53] OGLA alone is unlikely to be effective in women with type 2 unless the degree of beta cell impairment is minimal. OGLA may be indicated when:
- Mild hyperglycemia persists during GDM (fasting <110 mg/dL; postprandial <180)
- The woman refuses to take insulin or is needle phobic
- The woman expresses a strong desire to take OGLA

For women with PCOS, metformin may be used in the preconception treatment plan and continued through pregnancy. As an adjunct to insulin, metformin may be used to enhance sensitivity to insulin and reduce the therapeutic dose.[53] Some providers consider oral medications to be first line for treatment.

Problem Solving

Problem solving is an orderly way of finding solutions to problems. Women with diabetes during pregnancy must draw on their problem-solving skills to self-manage the challenge of glucose control. Diabetes is a complex process that involves personal perspective and individual coping skills. Problem recognition is the first step in successful problem solving.

• What are the Signs and Symptoms of Hyperglycemia?

All women with diabetes during pregnancy should recognize hyperglycemia and attempt to identify the cause. One important strategy is reviewing daily food and BG records in order to analyze associations between CHO consumed and subsequent BG levels. For example, a woman consuming milk with breakfast might notice that it makes her BG rise above target but if consumed at dinner it does not. She can decide to eliminate milk from breakfast and have it later in the day instead. Another important association one can make is that activity right after the meal can lower the BG significantly. These lessons learned may help women to stay healthy after pregnancy. Table 13.13 outlines the symptoms of hyperglycemia.

TABLE 13.13 EDUCATION IN RECOGNIZING AND TREATING HYPERGLYCEMIA
RECOGNITION
Increased thirst (polydipsia)
Excessive urination (polyuria)
Increased hunger (polyphagia)
Blurred vision
Headaches
Extreme fatigue
TREATMENT
Check BG
If greater than 200 mg/dL give a correction dose of insulin and check BG in 30 mins
Drink a full 8-ounce glass of water every 15 mins
Check urine ketones—if moderate to large, call provider for further instructions
If BG remains greater than 200 for 2 hrs, call provider for further instructions
Do not exercise while BG is over 200 mg/dL

• What are the Signs and Symptoms of Hypoglycemia?

Hypoglycemia presents another problem solving opportunity. Women who take medication that directly lowers BG (insulin and/or glyburide) must be taught the symptoms of hypoglycemia and how to treat it. It is important to identify what may have contributed to the low BG so it could be prevented in the future. For example, a meal or snack may have been delayed or skipped; or exercise may have coincided with the peak action of an insulin bolus. Women taking insulin or glyburide should carry glucose tabs (or 15-g CHO snack or juice) at all times. Glucose tabs are preferred by providers because they are pure glucose and when taken with water work rapidly. Women using premeal insulin should have a BG of greater than 90 to 100 at 1 hour post meal. The BG may be driven lower since the insulin action is still working. A cup of milk or a fruit (15 g) should be taken to prevent a subsequent low. Table 13.14 outlines the treatment of hypoglycemia.

TABLE 13.14	TREATMENT OF HYPOGLYCEMIA: RULE OF 15

Causes of Hypoglycemia:

Delay a meal or snack	Take too much insulin or glyburide
Skip a meal or snack	Exercise more than usual
Eat too little	

Symptoms of Hypoglycemia:

Headache	Pounding heart
Dizziness	Difficulty talking
Drowsiness	Tingling of mouth
Cold sweat	Irritability
Difficulty concentrating	Extreme hunger

If BG >50 mg/dL <70 mg/dL:
   1. Give 15 g liquid Carbohydrate: 8-oz nonfat milk or 4-oz juice or 4 glucose tabs with water
   2. Recheck BG in 15 mins
   3. Repeat no.1 if still <70 mg/dL
   4. Repeat BG check every 15 mins until BG >70 × 2

If BG <50 mg/dL:
   1. Give 30 g liquid carbohydrate: 8-oz juice or 8 glucose tabs with H_2O
   2. Recheck BG in 15 mins
   3. If <70 mg/dL, repeat no.1
   4. Repeat BG, check every 15 mins until BG >70 × 2
   If found unconscious: Give GLUCAGON 0.5 to 1 mg SC or IM stat. Call 911.

From California Department of Public Health. *California diabetes and pregnancy program.* Available at: https://www.cdph.ca.gov/programs/cdapp

Reducing Risks

Antenatal Maternal–Fetal Surveillance

The risks of hyperglycemia to the mother and fetus have been well described earlier in the module. Women who have persistent hyperglycemia require insulin or oral medication to keep BG controlled. Therefore women with T1DM, T2DM, and GDMA2 will undergo additional tests of fetal and maternal well-being to anticipate and prevent possible adverse outcomes before they occur.

The most common occurrence of perinatal morbidity in addition to macrosomia is preeclampsia. Women with GDM have a 14% risk of developing preeclampsia compared with ~7% risk for women without diabetes.[64] Overweight and obesity contribute strongly to the risk of hypertensive disorders during pregnancy.[64] Several studies have demonstrated that when BG is in target range, the rate of preeclampsia is cut in half.[19]

Perhaps the most influential consequence of uncontrolled BG during pregnancy is the risk for stillbirth (death of fetus after 20 weeks' gestation), and it is increased in the last 4 weeks of pregnancy.[65] Before the discovery of insulin in 1922, a woman T1DM had almost no chance of a healthy baby and women were told not to attempt pregnancy. In the 1950s, fetal death rates were reported as high as 20/1,000 births in women with T1DM.[66]

Rates of stillbirths differ according to the type of diabetes. Women with T2DM appear to have higher rates than women with T1DM for a variety of reasons. T2DM is currently more common in pregnancy than T1DM because of an earlier age at which T2DM is diagnosed; it is often associated with obesity; it occurs more frequently in non-Caucasians and in socioeconomically challenged individuals. All of these characteristics have a higher risk of stillbirth by themselves. Langer and associates found that women who had untreated GDM had a stillbirth rate of 5.4/1,000, whereas nondiabetic control patients had a stillbirth rate of 1.8/1,000. Pregnant women who have diabetes appear to have improved outcomes with some form of antepartum surveillance. However, the best methods, the best timing interval for testing, the optimal gestational age to begin testing, and the more accurate interpretations of the testing lack significant data.

Antepartum fetal **surveillance along with maternal glycemic control** seems to improve perinatal outcome to a modest to significant degree (see Table 13.15).[39,66]

TABLE 13.15 TESTS OF FETAL–MATERNAL WELL-BEING

TEST		FIRST TRIMESTER	SECOND TRIMESTER	THIRD TRIMESTER
HbA1C	To assess risk for anomalies in the first trimester, to verify BG control in the second and third trimesters	T1DM, T2DM	T1DM, T2DM	T1DM, T2DM
Retinal exam (repeat each trimester if retinopathy)	Retinopathy present at the beginning of pregnancy can worsen as pregnancy advances	T1DM, T2DM		
Micro albumin and 24-hr urine for total protein, creatinine clearance, serum creatinine	Identify nephropathy, establish baseline renal function	T1DM, T2DM	T1DM, T2DM	T1DM, T2DM
TSH/FT4 (repeat as indicated by results) thyroxine-stimulating hormone/free thyroxine 4	Thyroiditis (hyper or hypo) can be an auto-immune disease. Women with T1DM have a 40% risk and 20% in T2DM Abnormal maternal thyroid function can adversely affect pregnancy outcomes	T1DM, T2DM, GDMA2 (early dx)		
Ultrasound–dates	Accurate dates are important to limit adverse outcomes from less than 39 wks' births	T1DM, T2DM, GDMA2 (early dx)		
Ultrasound for fetal anatomy—detecting anomalies: 18 wks	Women with T1DM, T2DM, and with obesity (with or without diabetes) are at increased risk for malformations which can be identified as early as 18 wks		T1DM, T2DM, All pregnant women	
Ultrasound for fetal growth. Comparison of head circumference (which is usually consistent with GA) to abdominal circumference (which is ahead of the GA in a fetus with macrosomia and hyperinsulinemia) AC >75% suggests increased risk for fetal hyperinsulinemia/ macrosomia (Kjos 2007)	Macrosomia has the potential of complicating pregnancy in all women with hyperglycemia except in women with vasculopathy. Diminished blood flow to end organs may diminish blood flow to the uterus resulting in a growth restricted fetus		28 wks T1DM, T2DM,	32,36 wks T1DM, T2DM, GDMA2 (PRN)
Fetal heart echo: 20–24 wks	Women with T1DM, T2DM are at increased risk for fetal cardiac malformations which can be identified more in detail by a fetal echo, not all cardiac anomalies are found but those which are most serious can be found		T1DM, T2DM	
Kick counts: 28 wks	A well-oxygenated fetus moves frequently, a slowing down or absence of fetal movement can alert the mother to call her provider and gain reassurance through an NST			T1DM, T2DM, GDM A2, GDMA1
[a]NST/AFI	A reactive nonstress test and amniotic fluid index >8 can be reassuring of adequate oxygenation for 5–7 d.			T1DM, T2DM, GDM A2
EKG: age >35; or any T2DM; T1DMx 10 yrs	Increased risk for macrovascular disease	T1DM, T2DM		

[a]T1DM, T2DM with vasculopathy (retinopathy, nephropathy, and hypertension) begin weekly @ 28 weeks.
T1DM, T2DM: Begin twice weekly @ 32 weeks.
GDMA2: Once weekly begin @ 32 weeks then twice weekly @ 36 weeks.
From Kitzmiller, J. L., Block, J. M., Brown, F. M., et al. (2008). Managing preexisting diabetes for pregnancy: Summary of evidence and consensus recommendations for care. *Diabetes Care, 31*, 1060–1079; California Department of Public Health. *California diabetes and pregnancy program.* Available at: https://www.cdph.ca.gov/programs/cdapp; Stagnaro-Green, A., Abalovich, M., Alexander, E., et al.(2011). Guidelines of the American Thyroid Association for the diagnosis and management of thyroid disease during pregnancy and postpartum. *Thyroid, 21*, 1081–1125.

Intrapartum Management for Women with Hyperglycemia During Pregnancy

Timing of Birth

The timing of birth should be based on maternal BG control, maternal health, and fetal status. ACOG and ADA recommend that women with T1DM, T2DM, and GDMA2 be delivered between 39 and 40 weeks. If a medically indicated birth is planned before 39 weeks, an amniocentesis must be performed to confirm lung maturity. A cesarean birth should be an option for women if the EFW is greater than 4,500 g to avoid trauma to the newborn.

Women with GDMA1 with excellent glucose control and normal fetal growth delivery may be managed expectantly until 41 weeks is reached. The risk of expectant management is lower than the risk of delivery at 36 weeks, (17.4 vs. 19.3 per 10,000), but at 39 weeks, the risk of expectant management exceeds that of delivery (RR 1.8, 95% CI: 1.2 to 2.6).[65] Women going beyond 40 weeks' gestation should have twice weekly NST/AFI. Table 13.16 lists indications to induce prior to 39 weeks' gestation.

TABLE 13.16 INDICATIONS FOR DELIVERY PRIOR TO 39 WEEKS GESTATION WITH DIABETES
Vasculopathy restricting fetal growth (IUGR)
Worsening nephropathy
Prior stillbirth
Preeclampsia with severe features
Poor blood glucose control

NOTE: *Early induction of labor for suspected macrosomia is not endorsed by ACOG but accelerated fetal size* **with poor BG control** *qualifies.*[23]

Specific Goals of Intrapartum Management for All Types of Diabetes

Some interventions during labor are dependent on the TYPE of diabetes the woman has. It is imperative that the provider is knowledgeable of the precise type of diabetes in order to provide appropriate interventions (see Table 13.17). Women with T1DM must always have an external source of insulin as they cannot use any source of glucose (from their liver or from oral or IV intake) without insulin.

Maintain BG: 70 to 110 mg/dL in order to prevent:
- **maternal** hyperglycemia/acidosis and compromised
- **fetal** hyperinsulinemia
- **neonatal** hypoglycemia

Women with T2DM and GDMA2 may achieve the blood glucose target of 70 to 110 mg/dL by avoiding dextrose intravenous fluids and thus may not need insulin when NPO and in active labor. It is extremely unlikely that women with GDMA1 will require insulin in labor. Continuous intravenous (IV) insulin infusion may begin for a woman with T1DM when her BG is 70 or greater. It is important to determine when the last dose of insulin was and how long it is expected to last when preparing to start IV insulin. The activity of the uterine muscle during labor will use maternal glucose to contract and levels in the blood stream will lower. In rare cases, women with type 1 diabetes may need little to no insulin during labor especially if they have previously taken insulin which is effective for the duration of the labor. See Table 13.18 for an example IV insulin algorithm.

Potential Complications of Labor

The risk of complications increases with increasing levels of maternal BG and include the following:
- Fetal macrosomia (AC > HC)
- Undiagnosed fetal anomalies (T1DM, T2DM, obesity)
- Preeclampsia (all DM types)

TABLE 13.17	GENERAL GUIDELINES TO NURSING CARE OF WOMEN IN LABOR WITH DIABETES COMPLICATING PREGNANCY

Maintain Target BG 70–110 mg/dL to Optimize Fetal Oxygenation during Labor and Prevent Newborn Hypoglycemia

DM TYPE	GDMA1 (DIET/EXERCISE ONLY)	GDMA2 (TAKING ORALS OR INSULIN)	TYPE 2 DM (INSULIN ALONE OR WITH METFORMIN)	TYPE 1 DM—ALWAYS NEEDS INSULIN
Admission	D/C all previous orders Obtain POC Glucose Check specimen to lab POC/lab w/i 15% Time and description of last oral intake	D/C all previous orders Obtain POC Glucose Check specimen to lab POC/lab w/i 15% Time of last basal insulin dose or oral medication Time of last bolus insulin dose Time and description of last oral intake	D/C all previous orders Obtain POC Glucose Check specimen to lab POC/lab w/i 15% Time of last basal insulin dose or oral dose Time of last bolus insulin dose Time and description of last oral intake	D/C all previous orders Obtain POC Glucose Check specimen to lab POC/lab w/i 15% Time of last basal insulin dose Time of last bolus insulin dose Time and description of last oral intake
Diet WHEN TAKING MEALS BG TARGET IS <90 FASTING PREMEAL; <130 1 HR AFTER MEAL	If taking meals use prenatal DAPP diet If epidural or in labor clear noncaloric liquids or NPO per OB and anesthesia	If taking meals use prenatal DAPP diet If epidural or in labor Clear noncaloric liquids or NPO per OB and anesthesia	If taking meals use prenatal DAPP diet If epidural or in labor Clear noncaloric liquids or NPO per OB and anesthesia	If taking meals use prenatal DAPP diet If epidural or in labor clear noncaloric liquids or NPO per OB and anesthesia
IV therapy	Main Line: LR @125 mL/hr IVPB D5LR@100 mL/hr with LR @ 50 mL/hr as needed for: • when NPO and BG less than 70 >50 mg/dL • D/C D5 when BG ≥100	Main Line: LR @125 mL/hr IVPB D5LR@100 mL/hr with LR @ 50 mL/hr as needed for: • NPO and BG less than 80 >70 • D/C D5 when BG ≥100	Main Line: LR @125 mL/hr IVPB D5LR@100 mL/hr with LR @ 50 mL/hr as needed for: • NPO and BG less than 80 >70 • D/C D5 when BG ≥100	Main Line: LR @125 mL/hr IVPB D5LR@100 mL/hr with LR @ 50 mL/hr as needed for: • NPO and BG less than 80 >70 • D/C D5 when BG ≥100
Activity	Unrestricted until epidural	Unrestricted until epidural	Unrestricted until epidural	Unrestricted until epidural
POC glucose checks during labor	Every 4 hrs during labor except when BG is >110 mg/dL, then check in 60 mins, if remains >110 and IV insulin algorithm is initiated then check hourly	Every 2 hrs during labor except when BG is >110 mg/dL then check every 30 mins until ≤110 × 2 or insulin drip algorithm is initiated, then check hourly	Every 1 hr during labor except when BG is >110 mg/dL then check every 30 mins until ≤110 × 2 or insulin drip algorithm is initiated, then check hourly	Every 1 hr during labor/induction and/or IV insulin or SC insulin pump is infusing. Check every 30 mins when BG is >110 mg until ≤110 mg/dL × 2
Hypoglycemia (see treating protocol for L&D)	Implement orders at BG less than 50 mg/dL	Implement orders at BG less than 70 mg/dL	Implement orders at BG less than 70 mg/dL	Implement orders at BG less than 70 mg/dL
Managing hyperglycemia	Call provider to consider IV insulin drip algorithm when BG is greater than 110 × 2	Call provider to consider IV insulin drip algorithm when BG is greater than 110 × 2	Call provider to consider IV insulin drip algorithm when BG is greater than 100 × 2. Report any other insulin on board	Implement IV insulin infusion algorithm when BG is greater than 70 × 2 and no other SC insulin is on board
IV insulin algorithm in units	111–140 mg/dL = 2 141–170 mg/dL = 3 171–200 mg/dL = 4 If >180 × 2 call provider (rare)	111–140 mg/dL = 2 141–170 mg/dL = 3 171–200 mg/dL = 4 If >180 × 2 call provider	90–110 mg/dL = 1 111–140 mg/dL = 2 141–170 mg/dL = 3 171–200 mg/dL = 4 If >180 × 2 call provider	70–90 mg/dL = 0.5 90–110 mg/dL = 1 111–140 mg/dL = 2 141–170 mg/dL = 3 171–200 mg/dL = 4 If >180 × 2 call provider
Initial postpartum target BG: GDMA1 and GDMA2: <100 fasting <140 1 hr after the meal T1DM and T2DM <110 fasting/premeal <160 1 hr post meal	D/C IV insulin drip/D5 (if any) after delivery of placenta Check BG once before transfer to PP. If greater than targets report to postpartum to continue BG checks fasting and post meals until they are in the target range If NPO check every 6 hrs until less than 100	D/C IV insulin drip after delivery of placenta Check BG once before transfer to PP. If greater than targets report to postpartum to continue BG checks fasting and post meals until they are in the target range If NPO check every 6 hrs until less than 100	D/C IV insulin drip after delivery of placenta Check BG q2h before transfer to PP If NPO check every 6 hrs until taking food When taking food check pre- and post meals bedtime and 3 AM if taking bedtime basal insulin	Cut IV insulin drip algorithm in half after placenta 70–90 mg/dL = 0 90–111 mg/dL = 0.5 111–140 mg/dL = 1 141–170 mg/dL = 2 171–200 mg/dL = 3 If > 200 × 2 call provider – Check BG q1h before transfer. D/C IV insulin when about to have food and fluid by mouth.

table continues on page 388

387

DM TYPE	GDMA1 (DIET/EXERCISE ONLY)	GDMA2 (TAKING ORALS OR INSULIN)	TYPE 2 DM (INSULIN ALONE OR WITH METFORMIN)	TYPE 1 DM—ALWAYS NEEDS INSULIN
				Use 1/3 to 1/2 last SC basal/bolus insulin regimen before labor. Check BG premeal, post meal, 3 AM, before and after Breastfeeding—risk of hypoglycemia is high in the first 24–48 hr after birth
Activity	Unrestricted until epidural	Unrestricted until epidural	Unrestricted until epidural	Unrestricted until epidural
POC glucose checks during labor	Every 4 hrs during labor except when BG is >110 mg/dL, then check in 60 mins, If remains > 110 and IV Insulin algorithm is initiated then check hourly	Every 2 hrs during labor except when BG is >110 mg/dL then check every 30 mins until ≤110 × 2 or Insulin drip algorithm is initiated, then check hourly	Every 1 hr during labor except when BG is >110 mg/dL then check every 30 mins until ≤110 × 2 or Insulin drip algorithm is initiated, then check hourly	Every 1 hr during labor/induction and/or IV insulin or SC insulin pump is infusing. Check every 30 mins when BG is >110 mg until ≤110 mg/dL × 2
Hypoglycemia (see treating protocol for L&D)	Implement orders at BG less than 50 mg/dL	Implement orders at BG less than 70 mg/dL	Implement orders at BG less than 70 mg/dL	Implement orders at BG less than 70 mg/dL
Managing hyperglycemia	Call MD to consider IV insulin drip algorithm when BG is greater than 110 × 2	Call MD to consider IV insulin drip algorithm when BG is greater than 110 × 2	Call provider to consider IV insulin drip algorithm when BG is greater than 100 × 2. Report any other insulin on board	Implement IV insulin infusion algorithm when BG is greater than 70 × 2 and no other SC insulin is on board
IV insulin algorithm in units	111–140 mg/dL = 2 141–170 mg/dL = 3 171–200 mg/dL = 4 If >180 × 2 call provider (rare)	111–140 mg/dL = 2 141–170 mg/dL = 3 171–200 mg/dL = 4 171–200 mg/dL = 4 171–200 mg/dL = 4 171–200 mg/dL = 4 If >180 × 2 call provider	90–110 mg/dL = 1 111–140 mg/dL = 2 141–170 mg/dL = 3 171–200 mg/dL = 4 If >180 × 2 call provider	70–90 mg/dL = 0.5 90–110 mg/dL = 1 111–140 mg/dL = 2 141–170 mg/dL = 3 171–200 mg/dL = 4 If >180 × 2 call provider
Initial postpartum target BG: GDMA1 and GDMA2: <100 fasting <140 1 hr after the meal T1DM and T2DM <110 fasting/premeal <160 1 hr post meal	D/C IV insulin drip/D5 (if any) after delivery of placenta Check BG once before transfer to PP. If greater than targets report to postpartum to continue BG checks fasting and post meals until they are in the target range If NPO check every 6 hrs until less than 100	D/C IV insulin drip after delivery of placenta Check BG once before transfer to PP. If greater than targets report to postpartum to continue BG checks fasting and post meals until they are in the target range If NPO check every 6 hrs until less than 100	D/C IV insulin drip after delivery of placenta Check BG q2h before transfer to PP If NPO check every 6 hr until taking food When taking food check pre- and post meals bedtime and 3 AM if taking bedtime basal insulin	Cut IV insulin drip algorithm in half after placenta 70–90 mg/dL = 0 90–111 mg/dL = 0.5 111–140 mg/dL = 1 141–170 mg/dL = 2 171–200 mg/dL = 3 If > 200 × 2 call provider – Check BG q1h before transfer. D/C IV insulin when about to have food and fluid by mouth. Use 1/3 to 1/2 last SC basal/bolus insulin regimen before labor. Check BG pre- and post meal, 3 AM, before and after breakfast as risk of hypoglycemia is high in the first 24–48 hr after birth

- Abnormal FHR tracing—fetal hypoxemia from maternal hyperglycemia—(more likely with T1DM or T2DM)
- Abnormal labor: Active phase arrest, failure to descend, cephalopelvic disproportion, shoulder dystocia, slow slope active phase (all types DM who have a macrosomic fetus)
- Emergency cesarean birth

Causes of Hyperglycemia during Labor

Despite the fact that women are NPO or taking clear noncarbohydrate liquids during active labor, they can develop hyperglycemia. The greater the islet cell damage the more likely these

TABLE 13.18 CONTINUOUS INTRAPARTUM INTRAVENOUS
INSULIN ALGORITHM

BLOOD GLUCOSE (mg/dL)	INSULIN (Units/hr)
<70	0.0
71–90	0.5 (start DM1 here)
91–110	1 (start DM2 here)
111–130	2 (start GDMA2 here)
131–150	3
151–170	4
171–190	5
>190	Call provider, check ketones

stressors will increase the BG. Therefore, women with T1DM and T2DM are at greater risk for hyperglycemia. In addition, other causes of hyperglycemia in labor include the following:
- Infection/fever: avoid prolonged ruptured membranes (>24 hours)
- Betamimetics: terbutaline, ephedrine, epinephrine
- Steroids: Betamethasone (effects will last about 5 days)
- Stress: pain, fear, anxiety—consider early epidural if desired
- Too much IV D5 (greater than 150 mL/hr)
- Not enough insulin

It is important to check the BG with different frequencies for women with different types of diabetes. Checking BG frequently is critical to keeping BG in target. Continuous fetal monitoring should be used during labor to monitor closely for signs of fetal compromise in women with T1DM, T2DM, and GDMA2. Women with GDMA1 may have intermittent monitoring.

NOTE: Anticipate shoulder dystocia whether or not the estimated fetal weight is high because the distribution of fetal fat is in the shoulders and abdomen in the infant of a mother with diabetes.

Indications of shoulder dystocia include, an EFW >4,000 g and the "turtle" sign occurring with the birth of the head (the head is extremely tight against the perineum) (refer to Module 16 for more information on shoulder dystocia). Nursing management of women with DM in the intrapartum period is summarized in Table 13.17.

Immediate Postpartum Interventions for all Types of DM

If the baby's Apgars are normal, and there are no signs of hypoglycemia, the baby should be dried and placed skin to skin on the mother's abdomen/chest. Signs of newborn hypoglycemia include the following:
- Jitteriness
- Cyanosis
- Apnea
- Hypothermia
- Poor tone
- Poor feeding
- Lethargy
- Seizures

The mother should be strongly encouraged to breast feed to help reverse the over stimulation of the newborn pancreas experienced in utero. In addition to the significant benefits of breastfeeding for all mothers and infants, breastfeeding after pregnancy with DM may have additional benefits including[68,69]:
- Reduced risk of obesity in the child (with breastfeeding for a duration of at least 6 months)
- Improved weight control as well as improved lipid and glucose panels for the woman in the first 3 months after birth

The asymptomatic newborn should have his/her first BG taken 30 minutes after the feeding. If the BG is taken at birth it may be closer to maternal BG. Within an hour after birth the newborn capillary BG should reflect his or her own BG. The newborn with symptoms of hypoglycemia should have a BG check immediately. See Module 18 for further discussion of blood glucose screening and hypoglycemia in the newborn.

Postpartum Management of the Women with Hyperglycemia during Pregnancy

The management issues during the postpartum period include insulin adjustment, breastfeeding, and balancing of self-care needs of the mother with the needs of her newborn.

Medication Adjustment (T1DM, T2DM)

After the delivery, insulin requirements decrease dramatically. Very little or no insulin is required for the first 24 to 72 hours primarily for type 2 but may also happen infrequently for women with type 1. The total daily insulin dose should be readjusted to one third of the pregnancy pre labor dose for women with T1DM and at one half for women with T2DM. Women with T2DM may prefer to return to oral medication use rather than insulin.

Breastfeeding (T1DM, T2DM)

Oral agents such as metformin or glyburide have been found to be safe during lactation.[3] Breastfeeding removes glucose from the maternal blood stream to make lactose in the mother's milk. Thus breastfeeding can lower blood glucose enough that hypoglycemia may occur during a nursing session. Women with pre-existing diabetes on insulin postpartum should check BG pre- and post breastfeeding a few times to establish how much they drop from a breastfeeding session. If BG <100 mg/dL before a session the mother should take 15 g of carbohydrate without insulin (i.e., 8-oz milk). Frequent hypoglycemia can reduce breast milk production. The newborn should be monitored for signs of hypoglycemia.

NOTE: There is some evidence that metformin (a galactorrheic) may be useful in maintaining milk supply.

Breasts should be examined and patient should be taught signs and symptoms of mastitis. Women with hyperglycemia will be at greater risk for infections such as mastitis, wound infection, and endometritis.

Self-care (T1DM, T2DM)

A 2-week postpartum visit is useful to assess glucose control and insulin needs as they may change frequently during this time. Assurance must be made that the woman has a healthcare provider to monitor and assist her with diabetes care during the first 6 weeks postpartum and between pregnancies.

At the 6-week postpartum visit a depression screen should be administered as lack of sleep, newborn care, and self-care can be overwhelming. Preconception counseling regarding future pregnancies and methods to space pregnancies should be discussed. An HbA1c should be ordered for >12 weeks postpartum when pregnancy effects on the HbA1c are diminished. Weight loss and normal BMI goals are be discussed.

Medication Adjustment (GDMA2)

With the delivery of the fetal–placental unit, the diabetogenic (diabetic-causing) effects of placental hormones are diminished. If insulin is infusing it should be immediately discontinued. Women with gestational diabetes usually regain glycemic control. To ensure that this occurs, blood glucose values should be assessed in the immediate postpartum period by checking at least one fasting and a postprandial BG before the woman leaves the hospital.

Self-care (GDMA1, GDMA2)

Assessment of maternal glycemic status should be reevaluated with a 2-hour OGTT with 75 g of glucose at approximately 6 weeks.

Of great significance is the risk for the mother to develop T2DM or metabolic syndrome later in life. Estimates vary on the risks of T2DM after gestational diabetes. Estimates range from 17% to 63% within 5 to 16 years after pregnancy[70] and an 8-year cumulative risk of postpartum diabetes was 52.7%.[71] Insulin use, ethnicity, elevated body mass index, detection of islet autoantibodies, and age at birth are all predictors for the long-term development of T2DM; however, insulin use during pregnancy is the strongest predictor.[72] The long-term implications for the offspring are an increased risk for obesity and IGT or diabetes later in life.[73]

Breastfeeding can lower the mother's BG. Therefore, the woman should not breast feed just before testing, during the 2-hours after ingesting 75 grams of Glucola, and until the blood test is drawn. Breastfeeding is encouraged for at least 6 months. Upon testing, the woman should be reclassified as diabetic, IFG, IGT, or normoglycemic (normal BG). After delivery, approximately 15% of patients will have the diagnosis of IFG, IGT, or diabetes.[38] All women should also be educated regarding lifestyle modifications such as exercise and diet. Exercise, proper diet, and breastfeeding help the mother to maintain normal body weight, which helps to decrease insulin resistance. Symptoms of hyperglycemia should be reviewed with her. If these symptoms occur later in life, medical attention should be obtained. Assessment of glucose control should be recommended at a minimum of 3-year intervals.[3] Future pregnancy plans and contraceptive methods should also be discussed. Future pregnancy plans should be reviewed, with emphasis on ensuring optimal glycemic control before the next conception. Data reveal a recurrence rate of GDM between 30% and 84%.[74]

In a sample of low-income women with pregestational diabetes and GDM compared with those without diabetes had nearly double the odds of experiencing depression during the perinatal period. ACOG suggests screening all women for depression during and after pregnancy.[75]

Ketoacidosis Identification and Management

DKA is a life-threatening emergency seen in 1% to 2% of pregnancies complicated by diabetes, usually T1DM. Maternal mortality is rare, but fetal mortality ranges from 5% to 15%.[76] A higher incidence is seen during pregnancy because DKA develops more rapidly (accelerated starvation) and at less severe levels of hyperglycemia (<200 mg/dL).[50] The most common precipitating event is emesis from any cause, followed by b-sympathomimetics (terbutaline), and combined with antenatal corticosteroids (betamethasone). Other contributing variables included infection, poor patient compliance, insulin pump failure, undiagnosed T1 or T2 DM diabetes, and provider management errors (not enough insulin).[76] The most common symptoms in pregnancy include vomiting, dehydration, and polyuria. An arterial blood gas can confirm DKA with a pH ≤7.3, elevated base deficit, and an anion gap. Urine and serum ketones are present. Blood urea nitrogen and serum creatinine may be elevated due to dehydration. Treatment should be prompt: intravenous insulin therapy and normal saline fluid replacement to correct insulin deficiency and severe dehydration (see Table 13.19).

TABLE 13.19	TREATMENT OF DIABETIC KETOACIDOSIS IN PREGNANCY
Admission	• Admit to a critical care unit • Insert two large bore IV lines • Insert an arterial line • Insert Foley catheter • NPO
Assessment	• Daily weight • Frequent vital signs until values are within defined limits; follow with vital signs every hour until DKA is resolved • Continuous pulse oximetry • Consider arterial line placement • Strict hourly intake and output • Continuous fetal monitoring for greater than 23 weeks' gestation. If less than 24 weeks' gestation obtain FHR every 4 hrs • Maternal EKG • Continuous ECG
Stat labs	• Arterial blood gas (ABG), initial serum glucose then fingerstick glucose, serum betahydroxybutyrate, (serum ketones) serum electrolytes, anion gap. Obtain on admission and every 1–2 hrs until anion gap is resolved
Other labs	• Urinalysis (including urine ketones), urine culture, chest x-ray to rule out infection
Fluid therapy	• Use normal saline alone for initial fluid • Estimate 100 mL/kg bodyweight (if patient weighs 70 kg = 7 L need to be replaced) • Provide total replacement over the first 24–48 hrs with ~75% on the first day. Infuse initial 1–2 L of NS (without added electrolytes) by rapid infusion over 1–2 hrs. Reduce IV rate to 500 mL/hr in the third hour, and then **infuse ½ NS** @ 250 mL/hr until the woman has received all calculated fluid replacement. This should infuse in the first IV site
Insulin therapy	• Use a solution of 500 units of regular insulin **(R)** in 500 units NS (1 mL = 1 unit) • Prime IV tubing for ~20 mL (insulin binds to plastic). This solution should be IVPB to a liter of NS in the second IV site • Begin insulin therapy with an IV bolus of 0.1 unit insulin per kg ◦ Example: (70 kg = 7 units) then infuse 0.1 unit per kg continuously until ketones clear from the blood and urine and the anion gap is resolved. Add D51/2 NS @125 mL/hr to the second IV when BG is 200 mg/dL

Electrolytes	• Potassium chloride (KCl) is most often needed because K binds with ketones and is excreted in the urine; anticipate a deficit of 5–10 mEq/kg
	  ◦ Maintain serum K^+ level at 4–5 mEq/L
	  ◦ If normal kidney function (normal serum creatinine in pregnancy is less than 1.0 mg/dL) all women in DKA should have replacement
	  ◦ With replacement, maintain adequate urine output (0.5 mL/kg/hr)
	  ◦ Suggested protocol using serum K^+:
	    ▪ *5 mEq/L:* No treatment
	    ▪ *4–5 mEq/L:* Add 20 mEq/L KCl in 1,000 mL 0.9% NS and infuse at 150 mL/hr
	    ▪ *3–4 mEq/L:* Add 30 mEq/L KCl in 1,000 mL 0.9% NS and infuse at 150 mL/hr
	    ▪ *<3 mEq/L:* Add 40 mEq/L KCl in 1,000 mL 0.9% NS and infuse at 150 mL/hr
	• Phosphate replacement not normally required. If serum phosphate less than 1 mg/dL or if evidence of cardiac dysfunction, replace using potassium phosphate
	• Bicarbonate is not used because it could potentially elevate fetal PCO_2

From Guo, R. X., Yang, L. Z., Li, L. X., et al. (2008). Diabetic ketoacidosis in pregnancy tends to occur at lower blood glucose levels: Case-control study and a case report of euglycemic diabetic ketoacidosis in pregnancy. *The Journal of Obstetrics and Gynaecology Research, 34*(3), 324–330; Parker, J., & Conway, D. (2007). Diabetic ketoacidosis in pregnancy. *Obstetrics and Gynecology Clinics of North America, 34*(3), 533–543, xii; Kamalakannan, D., Baskar, V., Barton, D., et al. (2003). Diabetic ketoacidosis in pregnancy. *Postgraduate Medical Journal, 79*(934), 454–457.

PRACTICE/REVIEW QUESTIONS

After reviewing this module, answer the following questions.

1. How is diabetes diagnosed?

   a. _____

   b. _____

   c. _____

2. What are the characteristics of type 1 diabetes?

   a. _____

   b. _____

   c. _____

   d. _____

   e. _____

3. What are the characteristics of T2DM?

   a. _____

   b. _____

   c. _____

   d. _____

   e. _____

   f. _____

   g. _____

   h. _____

4. What is *gestational diabetes*?

   _____

5. At what gestational age should laboratory screening for gestational diabetes be performed?

   _____

6. What are premeal blood glucose goals during pregnancy?

   _____

7. What are 1-hour postprandial blood glucose goals during pregnancy?

   _____

8. What does the HbA1c measure?

   _____

9. What is *hypoglycemia?*

   _____

10. How many carbohydrate grams per day should women with diabetes consume in the second and third trimesters?

    _____

11. What is the major complication of insulin therapy?

    _____

    _____

12. What is the action of glyburide?

    _____

13. What is the action of metformin?

    _____

14. What changes in insulin requirements occur during the first, second, and third trimesters?

    _____

    _____

15. How does pregnancy affect pre-existing diabetes?

    a. _____

    b. _____

    c. _____

    d. _____

    e. _____

    f. _____

16. When does the fetal pancreas begin to function?

    _____

17. When and how often should NSTs begin in pregestational diabetes?

    _____

18. Can oral diabetic medications be used while breastfeeding?

    _____

19. Describe the two methods of diagnosing GDM.

    _____

    _____

    _____

20. Describe when and with whom preconception counseling begins for women with pre-existing diabetes:

    _____

PRACTICE/REVIEW ANSWER KEY

1. Diabetes can be diagnosed using any of the following three methods and must be confirmed on a subsequent day:

   a. Acute symptoms of diabetes plus a casual plasma glucose concentration that is greater than or equal to 200 mg/dL

   b. Fasting plasma glucose that is greater than or equal to 126 mg/dL

   c. 2-hour plasma glucose that is greater than or equal to 200 mg/dL during an oral GTT

2. a. It develops at any age, but two thirds of all cases are diagnosed before age 18.

   b. Symptoms include significant weight loss, polyuria, and polydipsia with hyperglycemia.

   c. DKA is possible.

   d. The woman is dependent on exogenous insulin.

e. Coma and death can result if diagnosis and/or treatment are delayed.

3. a. It accounts for 90% to 95% of all diabetes in the United States.

   b. It is usually diagnosed after the age of 30, but can occur at any age.

   c. Often, women are asymptomatic at the time of diagnosis. Because T2DM frequently goes undiagnosed for years, many women have end-organ complications such as retinopathy, neuropathy, or nephropathy at the time of diagnosis.

   d. Endogenous insulin levels may be increased, normal, or decreased. The need for exogenous insulin is variable.

   e. Insulin resistance with impaired glucose tolerance is usually seen in the first stages.

   f. Risks of developing T2DM increases with age, obesity, and lack of physical activity.

   g. HHNS may develop.

   h. Most women are obese or have an increased percentage of body fat distributed mainly in the abdominal region.

4. Glucose intolerance develops or is first discovered during pregnancy; insulin resistance and diminished insulin secretion is usually seen.

5. 24 to 28 weeks' gestation

6. 60 to 95 mg/dL

7. <130 to 140 mg/dL

8. The HbA1c reflects the weighted mean of blood glucose over the past 4 to 6 weeks.

9. Blood glucose level of 70 mg/dL or lower

10. 258 pounds = 117 kg

    117 × 25 kcal/kg per day = 2,925

    Her requirements are 2,925 calories each day.

11. a. Before initiating an exercise program, all women should have a medical evaluation, be educated on benefits and risks of exercise, and understand the potential effects of exercise on glucose levels.

    b. Obtain metabolic control before exercising. Exercise is safe when glucose levels are between 90 and 140 mg/dL. If blood glucose is above 250 mg/dL, the urine should be checked for ketones. If positive for ketones, exercise should be delayed until glycemic control is obtained and ketones are resolved. If ketones are negative but blood glucose is above 300 mg/dL, be cautious with exercise.

    c. Exercise programs should last less than 45 minutes.

    d. Meals should be consumed 1 to 3 hours before the exercise program.

    e. Insulin should be given in the abdomen and not injected into active muscles. Decrease the bolus insulin if its peak coincides with the exercise period.

    f. Monitor blood glucose before and after exercise. Identify when changes in the insulin regimen or diet are necessary. Learn the way the body responds to different types of exercise.

    g. Monitor necessary food intake. Eat extra carbohydrates as needed to prevent hypoglycemia and always have carbohydrates available during and after exercise.

    h. Include a warm-up an cool-down period with each exercise session.

    i. Avoid exercising in the supine position after the first trimester to prevent aortocaval compression and hypotension.

12. Hypoglycemia

13. No. Although research has been done to compare the use of glyburide with insulin use among women with gestational diabetes, its use during pregnancy has *not* been approved by the U.S. Food and Drug Administration.

14. Usually in the first trimester, insulin requirements are slightly decreased, but they increase in the second and third trimesters. They again decrease during the immediate postpartum period.

15. a. Insulin requirements

    b. Retinopathy

    c. Nephropathy

    d. Coronary artery disease

    e. Neuropathy

    f. DKA

16. Approximately 13 weeks

17. Usually begin NSTs at 32 weeks' gestation on a weekly basis and increase to twice a week at 36 weeks' gestation

18. No. The oral medications are secreted through the breast milk and may affect the infant.

19. Gestational diabetes is diagnosed by an elevated 1-hour screening glucose challenge test of 140 mg/dL or greater, which is followed by a diagnostic 3-hour glucose challenge test. The patient is diagnosed with gestational diabetes if two or more values exceed the following: NDDG criteria: fasting, 105 mg/dL; 1 hour, 190 mg/dL; 2 hour, 165 mg/dL; and 3 hour, 145 mg/dL; Carpenter and Coustan criteria: fasting, 95 mg/dL; 1 hour, 180 mg/dL; 2 hour, 155 mg/dL; and 3 hour, 140 mg/dL.

20. All women of childbearing age who are planning a pregnancy

REFERENCES

1. Centers for Disease Control and Prevention. (2014). *National diabetes report.* http://www.cdc.gov/diabetes/pubs/statsreport14/national-diabetes-report-web.pdf. Accessed May 1, 2015.

2. Centers for Disease Control and Prevention. (2011). *National diabetes fact sheet.* Atlanta, GA: United States Department of Health and Human Services.

3. American Diabetes Association. (2015). Management of diabetes in pregnancy. Sec. 12. In *Standards of medical care in diabetes—2015. Diabetes Care, 38*(s1), S77–S79.

4. Committee on Practice Bulletins—Obstetrics. (2013). Practice Bulletin No.504: Gestational diabetes mellitus. *Obstetrics & Gynecology, 122,* 406–416.

5. DeSisto, C. L., Kim, S. Y., & Sharma, A. J. (2014). Prevalence estimates of gestational diabetes mellitus in the United States, pregnancy risk assessment monitoring system (PRAMS), 2007–2010. *Prev Chronic Disease, 11:*E104.

6. American College of Obstetricians & Gynecologists. (2001). *Gestational diabetes (Practice Bulletin No. 30).* Washington, DC: Author.

7. Tuomilehto, J., Lindstrom, J., Eriksson, J. G., et al. (2001). Prevention of type 2 diabetes mellitus by changes in lifestyle among subjects with glucose intolerance. *New England Journal of Medicine, 344*(18), 1343–1350.

8. Ratner, R. E., Christophi, C. A., Metzger, B. E., et al. (2008). Diabetes Prevention Program Research Group. Prevention of diabetes in women with a history of gestational diabetes: Effects of metformin and lifestyle interventions. *Journal of Clinical Endocrinology & Metabolism, 93*, 4774–4779.

9. Tobias, D. K., Hu, F. B., Chavarro, J., et al. (2012). Healthful dietary patterns and type 2 diabetes mellitus risk among women with a history of gestational diabetes mellitus. *Archives of Internal Medicine, 177*, 1566–1572.

10. Daley, J. (2014). Diabetes in pregnancy. In Simpson, K., & Creehan, P. (Eds.), *Perinatal nursing* (4th ed., pp. 203–223). Philadelphia, PA: Lippincott and Williams and Wilkins.

11. Barbour, L. A., McCurdy, C. E., Hernandez, T. L., et al. (2007). Cellular mechanisms for insulin resistance in normal pregnancy and gestational diabetes. *Diabetes Care, 30* (suppl 2), S112–S119.

12. Kitzmiller, J. L., Block, J. M., Brown, F. M., et al. (2008). Managing preexisting diabetes for pregnancy: Summary of evidence and consensus recommendations for care. *Diabetes Care, 31*, 1060–1079.

13. Metzger, B. E., Lowe, L. P., Dyer, A. R., et al. (2008). HAPO Study Cooperative Research Group. Hyperglycemia and adverse pregnancy outcomes. *New England Journal of Medicine, 358*, 1991–2002.

14. Jensen, D. M., Korsholm, L., Ovesen, P., et al. (2009). Periconceptional A1C and risk of serious adverse pregnancy outcome in 933 women with type 1 diabetes. *Diabetes Care, 32*, 1046–1048.

15. Crume, T. L., Ogden, L., Daniels, S., et al. (2011). The impact of in utero exposure to diabetes on childhood body mass index growth trajectories: The EPOCH study. *Journal of Pediatrics, 158*(6), 941–946.

16. Dabelea, D., Hanson, R. L., Lindsay, R. S., et al. (2000). Intrauterine exposure to diabetes conveys risks for type 2 diabetes and obesity: A study of discordant sibships. *Diabetes, 49*, 2208–2211.

17. Ehrlich, S. F., Crites, Y. M., Hedderson, M. M., et al. (2011). The risk of large for gestational age across increasing categories of pregnancy glycemia. *American Journal of Obstetrics and Gynecology, 204*(3), 240.e1–e6.

18. Landon, M., Catalano, P., & Gabbe, S. (2012). Diabetes mellitus complicating pregnancy. In *Obstetrics: Normal and problem pregnancies* (6th ed., pp. 887–922). Philadelphia, PA: Elsevier Saunders.

19. Moore, T., Hauguel-De Mouzon, S., & Catalano, P. (2014). Diabetes in pregnancy. In Creasy, R. K., & Resnick, R. (Eds.), *Maternal fetal medicine: Principles and practice* (7th ed., pp. 988–1022). Philadelphia, PA: Elsevier Saunders.

20. Hartling, L., Dryden, D. M., Guthrie, A., et al. (2013). Benefits and harms of treating gestational diabetes mellitus: A systematic review and meta-analysis for the U.S. Preventive Services Task Force and the National Institutes of Health Office of Medical Applications of Research. *Annals of Internal Medicine, 159*, 123–129.

21. Moyer, V. (2014). Screening for gestational diabetes mellitus: US Preventative Services Task Force Recommendations Statement. *Annals of Internal Medicine, 160*(6), 414–420.

22. Beucher, G., Viaris de Lesegno, B., & Dreyfus, M. (2010). Maternal outcome of gestational diabetes mellitus. *Diabetes & Metabolism, 36*(6 pt 2), 522–537.

23. ACOG Practice Bulletin. (2005). Clinical management guidelines for obstetrician-gynecologists. Number 60, March 2005.

24. O'Sullivan, J. B., Mahan, C. M., Charles, D., et al. (1973). Screening criteria for high-risk gestational diabetic patients. *American Journal of Obstetrics & Gynecology, 116*, 895–900.

25. Cowett, R. (1991). *Principles of perinatal-neonatal metabolism.* New York: Springer.

26. International Association of Diabetes and Pregnancy Study Groups Consensus Panel, Metzger, B. E., Gabbe, S. G., Persson, B., et al. (2010). International association of diabetes and pregnancy study groups recommendations on the diagnosis and classification of hyperglycemia in pregnancy. *Diabetes Care, 33*(3), 672–682.

27. World Health Organization. (2013). *Diagnostic criteria and classification of hyperglycemia first detected in pregnancy.* Geneva: World Health Org., (WHO/NMH/MND/13.2).

28. deBarros, M., Lopes, M., Francisco, R., et al. (2010). Resistance exercise and glycemic control in women with gestational diabetes mellitus. *American Journal of Obstetrics & Gynecology, 203*(6), 556.e1–e6.

29. Artal, R., Catanzaro, R., Gavard, J. A., et al. (2007). A lifestyle intervention of weight-gain restriction: Diet and exercise in obese women with gestational diabetes mellitus. *Applied Physiology, Nutrition, and Metabolism Physiologie Appliquée, Nutrition Et Métabolisme, 32*(3), 596–601.

30. Snapp, C., & Donaldson, S. (2008). Gestational diabetes mellitus: Physical exercise and health outcomes. *Biological Research for Nursing, 10*(2), 145–155.

31. Weissgerber, T., Wolfe, L., Davies, G., et al. (2006). Exercise in the prevention and treatment of maternal-fetal disease: A review of the literature. *Applied Physiology, Nutrition, and Metabolism, 31*(6), 661–674.

32. Hopkins, S. A., Baldi, J. C., Cutfield, W. S., et al. (2010). Exercise training in pregnancy reduces offspring size without changes in maternal insulin sensitivity. *Journal of Clinical Endocrinology & Metabolism, 95*, 2080–2088.

33. Perkins, B., & Riddell, M. (2006). Diabetes and exercise: Using the insulin pump to maximum advantage. *Canadian Journal of Diabetes, 30*(1), 72–79.

34. DeVeciana, M., Major, C. A., Morgan, M. A., et al. (1995). Postprandial versus preprandial blood glucose monitoring in women with gestational diabetes mellitus requiring insulin therapy. *New England Journal of Medicine, 333*, 1237–1241.

35. Combs, C. A., Gavin, L. A., Gunderson, E., et al. (1992). Relationship of fetal macrosomia to maternal postprandial glucose control during pregnancy. *Diabetes Care, 15*, 1251–1257.

36. Hod, M., & Yogev, Y. (2007). Goals of metabolic management of gestational diabetes. *Diabetes Care, 30*(suppl 2), S180–S187.

37. Buhling, K. J., Winkel, T., Wolf, C., et al. (2005). Optimal timing for postprandial glucose measurement in pregnant women with diabetes and a non-diabetic pregnant population evaluated by the Continuous Glucose Monitoring System (CGMS). *Journal of Perinatal Medicine, 33*(2), 125–131.

38. Gabbe, S. G., & Graves, C. R. (2007). Management of diabetes mellitus complicating pregnancy. In Queenan, J. (Ed.), *High-risk pregnancy* (pp. 98–109). Washington, DC: American College of Obstetricians and Gynecologists.

39. Langer, O., Yogev, Y., Most, O., et al. (2005). Gestational diabetes: The consequences of not treating. *American Journal Obstetrics Gynecology, 192*, 989–997.

40. Hawkins, J. S., Casey, B. M., Lo, J. Y., et al. (2009). Weekly compared with daily blood glucose monitoring in women with diet-treated gestational diabetes. *Obstetrics and Gynecology, 113*(6), 1307–1312.

41. Chitayat, L., Zisser, H., & Jovanovic, L. (2009). Continuous glucose monitoring during pregnancy. *Diabetes, Technology & Therapeutics, 11*(suppl 1), S105–S111.

42. Murphy, H. R., Rayman, G., Lewis, K., et al. (2008). Effectiveness of continuous glucose monitoring in pregnant women with diabetes: Randomised clinical trial. *British Medical Journal, 337*, a1680.

43. Mills, J. L., Jovanovic, Y., Knopp, R., et al. (1998). Physiological reduction in fasting plasma glucose concentration in the first trimester of pregnancy: The Diabetes in Early Pregnancy Study. *Metabolism, 47*, 1140–1144.

44. Nielsen, L., Ekbom, P., Damm, P., et al. (2004). HbA1c levels are significantly lower in early and late pregnancy. *Diabetes Care, 27*(5), 1200–1201.

45. Sacks, D. B. (2011). A1C versus glucose testing: A comparison. *Diabetes Care, 34*(2), 518–523.

46. Miller, E., Hare, J. W., Cloherty, J. P., et al. (1981). Elevated maternal hemoglobin A1c in early pregnancy and congenital anomalies in infants of diabetic mothers. *New England Journal of Medicine, 304*, 1331–1334.

47. Rowan, J. (2011). Metformin in pregnancy the offspring follow up. *Diabetes Care, 34*, 2279–2284.

48. Weissmann-Brenner, A., O'Reilly-Green, C., Ferber, A., et al. (2004). Does the availability of maternal HbA1c results improve the accuracy of sonographic diagnosis of macrosomia? *Ultrasound in Obstetrics & Gynecology, 23*(5), 466–471.

49. Jovanovic- Peterson, L., & Peterson, C. (1991). Sweet success, but an acid aftertaste? *New England Journal of Medicine, 325*, 959–960.

50. Guo, R. X., Yang, L. Z., Li, L. X., et al. (2008). Diabetic ketoacidosis in pregnancy tends to occur at lower blood glucose levels: Case-control study and a case report of euglycemic diabetic ketoacidosis in pregnancy. *The Journal of Obstetrics and Gynaecology Research, 34*(3), 324–330.

51. Durnwald, C. P., & Landon, M. B. (2008). A comparison of lispro and regular insulin for the management of type 1 and type 2 diabetes in pregnancy. *The Journal of Maternal-Fetal & Neonatal Medicine: The Official Journal of the European Association of Perinatal Medicine, the Federation of Asia and Oceania Perinatal Societies, the International Society of Perinatal Obstetricians, 21*(5), 309–313.

52. Langer, O., Conway, D. L., Berkus, M. D., et al. (2000). A comparison of glyburide and insulin in women with gestational diabetes mellitus. *New England Journal of Medicine, 343*, 1134–1138.

53. Rowan, J. A., Hague, W. M., Gao, W., et al. (2008). Metformin versus insulin for the treatment of gestational diabetes. *New England Journal of Medicine, 358*(19), 2003–2015.

54. Crowther, C. A., Hiller, J. E., Moss, J. R., et al. (2005). Effect of treatment of gestational diabetes mellitus on pregnancy outcomes. *New England Journal of Medicine, 352*(24), 2477–2486.

55. Landon, M. B., Spong, C., Thom, E., et al. (2009). A multicenter, randomized trial of treatment for mild gestational diabetes. *New England Journal of Medicine, 361*(14), 1339–1348.

56. Pollex, E., Moretti, M. E., Koren, G., et al. (2011). Safety of insulin glargine use in pregnancy: A systematic review and meta-analysis. *Annals of Pharmacotherapy, 45*(1), 9–16.

57. Mathiesen, E. R., Hod, M., Ivanisevic, M., et al., Detemir in Pregnancy Study Group. (2012). Maternal efficacy and safety outcomes in a randomized, controlled trial comparing insulin detemir with NPH insulin in 310 pregnant women with type 1 diabetes. *Diabetes care, 35*(10), 2012–2017.

58. Trujillo, A. (2007). Insulin analogs and pregnancy. *Diabetes Spectrum, 20*(2), 94–101.

59. California Department of Public Health. *California diabetes and pregnancy program.* Available at: https://www.cdph.ca.gov/programs/cdapp

60. Hirsch, I., & Farkas-Hirsch, R. (2001). Sliding scale or sliding scare: It's all sliding nonsense. *Diabetes Spectrum, 14*(2), 81.

61. Siminerio, L., Kulkarni, K., Meece, J., et al. (2011) .Strategies for insulin injection therapy in diabetes self-management. *American Association of Diabetes Educators, 37*(6), 1–10.

62. Gutzin, S. J., Kozer, E., Magee, L. A., et al. (2003). The safety of oral hypoglycemic agents in the first trimester of pregnancy: A meta-analysis. *Canadian Journal of Clinical Pharmacology, 10*, 179–183.

63. Dhulkotia, J. S., Ola, B., Fraser, R., et al. (2010). Oral hypoglycemic agents vs insulin in management of gestational diabetes: A systematic review and metaanalysis. *American Journal of Obstetrics & Gynecology, 203*, 457.e1–e9.

64. Yogev, Y., Xenakis, E., Langer, O. (2004). The association between preeclampsia and the severity of gestational diabetes: The impact of glycemic control. *American Journal of Obstetrics and Gynecology, 191*, 1655–1660.

65. Rosenstein, M. G., Cheng, Y. W., Snowden, J. M., et al. (2012). The risk of stillbirth and infant death stratified by gestational age in women with gestational diabetes. *American Journal of Obstetrics and Gynecology, 206*(4), 309.e1–e7.

66. Dudley, D. (2007). Diabetic-associated stillbirth: Incidence, pathophysiology, and prevention. *Obstetrics & Gynecology Clinics of North America, 34*(2), 293–307, ix.

67. Stagnaro-Green, A., Abalovich, M., Alexander, E., et al. (2011). Guidelines of the American Thyroid Association for the diagnosis and management of thyroid disease during pregnancy and postpartum. *Thyroid, 21*, 1081–1125.

68. Pereira, P. F., Alfenas Rde, C., & Araújo, R. M. (2014). Does breastfeeding influence the risk of developing diabetes mellitus in children? A review of current evidence. *Journal of Pediatrics (Rio J), 90*, 7–15.

69. Stuebe, A. M., Rich-Edwards, J. W., Willett, W. C., et al. (2005). Duration of lactation and incidence of type 2 diabetes. *Journal of the American Medical Association, 294*, 2601–2610.

70. Ben-Haroush, A., Yogev, Y., & Hod, M. (2004). Epidemiology of gestational diabetes mellitus and its association with type 2 diabetes. *Diabetes Medicine, 21*, 103–113.

71. Lobner, K., Knopff, A., Baumgarten, A., et al. (2006). Predictors of postpartum diabetes in women with gestational diabetes mellitus. *Diabetes, 55*, 792–797.

72. Lee, A. J., Hiscock, R. J., Wein, P., et al. (2007). Gestational diabetes mellitus: Clinical predictors and long-term risk of developing type 2 diabetes. *Diabetes Care, 30*, 878–883.

73. Perkins, J. M., Dunn, J. P., & Jagasia, S. M. (2007). Perspectives in gestational diabetes mellitus: A review of screening, diagnosis, and treatment. *Clinical Diabetes, 25*, 57–62.

74. Kim, C., Berger, D. K., & Chamany, S. (2007). Recurrence of gestational diabetes mellitus. *Diabetes Care, 30*, 1314–1319.

75. American College of Obstetricians & Gynecologists. (2015). *Screening for perinatal depression. Committee Opinion No. 630.* Washington, DC: Author.

76. Parker, J., & Conway, D. (2007). Diabetic ketoacidosis in pregnancy. *Obstetrics and Gynecology Clinics of North America, 34*(3), 533–543, xii.

77. Kamalakannan, D., Baskar, V., Barton, D., et al. (2003). Diabetic ketoacidosis in pregnancy. *Postgraduate Medical Journal, 79*(934), 454–457.

Special Considerations for Individualized Care of the Laboring Woman

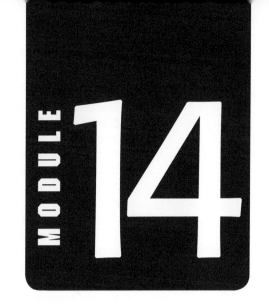

MODULE 14

SUZANNE McMURTRY BAIRD,
BETSY BABB KENNEDY, AND JENNIFER DALTON

As you complete this module you will learn:

1. Potential age-related issues and complications during pregnancy
2. Selected intrapartum care principles for women with disabilities
3. Associated risks of pregnancy in obese women
4. Nursing considerations for obese women during labor, birth, and the immediate postpartum period
5. Maternal and fetal complications associated with substance use in pregnancy
6. Nursing management for women with substance use in pregnancy
7. Direct and indirect effects of intimate partner violence against pregnant women
8. Healthcare provider's role in screening for pregnant victims of intimate partner violence
9. Possible interventions and resources for pregnant victims of intimate partner violence

body mass index

pannus

obstructive sleep apnea

opioid

neonatal abstinence syndrome

intimate partner violence

cycle of violence

Some women who present for care during pregnancy do not fit the "typical" picture associated with pregnancy—young and healthy. They may require special consideration owing to a variety of circumstances related to age, physical disabilities, obesity, or substance abuse. These women present unique challenges—but also opportunities for healthcare providers to assist them in having a positive birth experience. Nonjudgmental, nonbiased, and supportive individualized care should be provided.

PART 1

Age-Related Pregnancy Considerations

Teen Pregnancy

• What factors contribute to and influence teen pregnancy?

Teen pregnancy is a multifactorial issue that is not, unfortunately, a new phenomenon. The birth rate for 15- to 19-year-olds is 26.5 per 100,000 teenagers aged 15 to 19 years—down 10% from 2012 for all races and the lowest ever reported in the United States.[1] However, the United States teen pregnancy rate remains significantly higher than other Western industrialized nations. In addition, social and racial disparities exist with higher pregnancy rates in non-Hispanic black, Hispanic/Latino, American Indian/Alaskan Native, and the socioeconomically disadvantaged of any race.[1] Many factors contribute to the rate of teen pregnancy, who are psychologically and physiologically vulnerable. Some of these influential factors include[2]:

- Education
- Low socioeconomic status
- Low income
- Underemployment
- Neighborhood—physical disorder, income level

The teen who becomes pregnant must accomplish both the developmental tasks of adolescence as well as pregnancy. Assuming adult roles (having a baby) before completing the work of adolescence can have significant long-term consequences that include:

- Prolonged dependence on parents/family/society
- Education: only 50% graduate high school by age 22 and less than 2% graduate college by the age of 30[3]
- Higher rates of depression and low self-esteem
- Higher rates of child abuse and neglect
- More likely to be incarcerated[4]
- More likely to become teen parents themselves (repeating the cycle)

• What are the risks of teen pregnancy?

Teen pregnancy is a risk of poor perinatal outcomes, which may be related to nutrition, lack of prenatal care, or the ability to access health care and social services.[5] These risks include:

- Iron deficiency anemia: exacerbated in pregnancy; prenatal vitamins and increased intake of iron-rich foods should be encouraged.
- Preterm labor and birth: during prenatal care discuss the subtle signs and symptoms of preterm labor and when to contact provider.
- Low–birth-weight infants: closely tied to preterm birth and maternal weight gain.
- Preeclampsia: one of the most common complications of teen pregnancy.
- Higher rates of cephalopelvic disproportion: more common in younger teens who have not completed their physical growth.[6]

Physical care for the teen during labor does not differ from other labor patients. However, the teen may require additional support and encouragement from family and the healthcare team. Social work should be consulted when the teen is admitted in order to begin the process for activation of community supportive services and fulfill any state reporting requirements.

Referrals to well-baby clinics, programs for school-aged mothers, community organizations, and state social service organizations may provide needed support.

• What should the nurse include in postpartum education for the teen mother?

Extensive teaching occurs during the postpartum period (for an in-depth discussion on postpartum education, refer to *Module 17*). Education should be "teen friendly" and include the mother's family/support members since they will be involved in care and future health decisions. After birth, careful assessment of the teen mother should be done to determine her knowledge regarding infant and self-care. As the nurse, you may need to spend additional time observing the mother's interactions with her infant. Teens may have unrealistic views of the reactions of their infants, and get frustrated easily. Early return to their obstetric provider may be of benefit for assessment of complications and to reinforce teaching concepts. Teen-specific education areas are listed below.

Breastfeeding

Teen mothers are less likely to initiate and sustain breastfeeding. Focused education during the prenatal and postpartum periods should include not only nutritional and immunologic benefits of breastfeeding, but also financial, decreased interpregnancy rates, and improved mother–infant bonding.[5]

Depression

Even though postpartum depression screening is routine, obstetric providers should be aware that teen mothers experience higher rates of depression. There are several published screening tools that may be utilized.

Birth Control

The Centers for Disease Control (CDC) has set prevention of teen pregnancy as one of their public health priorities.[7] It is estimated that 35% of recently pregnant adolescents experience a rapid repeat pregnancy increasing the risk of preterm birth, low birth weight, and small for gestational age.[8] Repeat pregnancy within 2 years may also impact the mother's ability to finish education and pursue job opportunities.[8] Since the vast majority of teen pregnancies are unintended, there should be an education focus on methods of birth control and prevention of sexually transmitted infections. Long-acting reversible contraceptive methods, such as intrauterine devices and contraceptive implants, are effective and are recommended for adolescent women.[9]

Advanced Maternal Age (35 Years or Older)

• What factors contribute to the increase in mothers giving birth over the age of 35 years?

Even though the overall number of births each year has declined, the number of women over age 35 years who give birth and the mean age at which women give birth have risen steadily since 2000.[7] There are several factors that have contributed to this trend, such as:
- Availability of effective birth control options
- Increased number of women pursuing advanced education and delaying parenthood until they are professionally established
- The increase in later marriage and second marriages
- The increased availability of assisted reproductive techniques

---

• What are the risks associated with advanced maternal age?[10–14]

Adverse pregnancy outcomes are associated with advanced maternal age. With the exception of pre-existing health issues such as hypertension, obesity, or diabetes, the pathogenesis of adverse outcomes is not well understood. In addition, it is unclear at what age after 35 that risk increases. In general, it is thought that after age 35, risks continue to increase with age.
- Fetal chromosomal abnormalities
- Fetal congenital malformations

- Ectopic pregnancy
- Spontaneous abortion
- Stillbirth
- Placenta previa
- Maternal mortality
- Pre-existing medical conditions, such as chronic hypertension or diabetes
- Cesarean birth (elective and emergent)
- Preeclampsia
- Gestational diabetes
- Preterm birth

- **Are there differences in intrapartum and postpartum care for the mother over age 35 years?**

Care of the woman over 40 years in labor does not differ physically from care of other laboring women. If the woman has other medical conditions, such as diabetes or hypertension, care needs are modified to include interventions related to these conditions.

In the postpartum period, the provider should be aware that the older woman may find the childbirth experience and care of a newborn more exhausting than anticipated. The postpartum period may be a time of social isolation as well. The woman who gives birth after age 40 years may find that her peers are more likely to be the parents of adolescents and young adults and removed from the concerns of a new mother. Another concern for the older woman who gives birth is that she may be part of the "sandwich generation." These are women who are caring for elderly parents as well as children, which may be emotionally, physically, and financially draining.

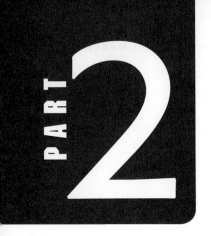

Women with a Physical Disability

The woman with a physical disability who presents for care during pregnancy may need specific modifications related to her condition. Care should be designed so that needs are planned and potential problems are addressed. Prejudices may exist regarding the ability of the disabled to give birth and parent successfully, and the care provided should be positive and supportive. Care for the woman with a disability needs to be comprehensive and interdisciplinary. When the needs related to the pregnancy and the woman's disability is fully met, her ability to have a positive birth experience is facilitated.

• When should care planning begin?[1]

At the first prenatal visit, it is important to explore support, assistance, or modifications the woman feels are necessary. A complete and open discussion is essential so that any requests can be initiated. In anticipatory planning, it is also important to discuss any assistance she feels she will need to care for her infant after birth. The provider should be careful not to convey the message that because she is disabled she is not competent. However, if assistance will be required, it is best to know ahead of time and make plans. Some women require assistance, some may require modifications to their homes, some require adaptive equipment, and some do not require anything different from every other new mother.

Known disease specific complications or limitations, such as decreased balance, spasticity and muscle weakness, altered gait, reduced bone density, osteoporosis, comorbidities, certain medications, and dietary imbalances place the woman with a disability at higher risk for falls.[1] Pregnancy further enhances risk for falls as the woman's body habitus changes from the enlarging uterus, and the center of gravity shifts. Assistive devices, such as a wheelchair, braces, or a walker may be needed to decrease fall risk. Avoiding excessive gestational weight gain, continuing with range of motion and stretching exercises may improve mobility during pregnancy.[2] When the woman is admitted to the hospital setting, an environmental assessment is recommended in order to improve safety. Remove any unnecessary equipment in the room and map out best paths within the hospital room for mobilization. The bed should be kept in the lowest position with wheels locked and call lights placed within the woman's reach at all times. Signage placed outside and/or within the woman's room to indicate that she is at high risk for a fall is indicated according to defined hospital practices.[2]

NOTE: *Dietary deficiencies are common in women with physical disabilities—access to healthy foods, difficulty in chewing, dysphagia, or gastric absorption delays. Pregnancy may compound these deficiencies and result in physiologic anemia or fetal growth issues.*[1]

• How is mode of delivery decided upon?[1]

Decisions regarding mode of delivery should be made based on obstetric indications. The woman, her provider, and her disability specialist should collaborate to discuss any issues that might impact the mode of delivery. Vaginal delivery is possible for many disabled women and is the preferred mode of delivery whenever possible. *Cesarean birth should never be done arbitrarily because of a disability.* Anesthesia may be a concern, especially in women with spinal cord injuries or other neurologic conditions. A consultation with an anesthesiology provider before labor is suggested so that a comprehensive plan for pain management can be developed.

During labor and/or regional anesthesia, monitor the woman's bladder status and prevent overdistention. Consider "laboring down" for second stage management to prevent fatigue and anticipate the potential need for operative vaginal birth. Depending on physical limitations, positioning for birth may require modifications.[2]

Needs during the postpartum period vary based on changes that may have occurred during pregnancy and birth. A more prolonged recovery and hospitalization may be necessary and should be assessed on a case-by-case basis. Breastfeeding should be encouraged, although some modifications and adaptive equipment may be required, especially if the disability involves the upper extremities. Lactation consultants are helpful in identifying positions and adaptive equipment needs that will facilitate successful breastfeeding. Consider consultation with an occupational therapist for a home visit as indicated to identify equipment that can be used in the home environment for infant and self-care. Such equipment may include cribs that are low or that attach to wheelchairs. Also consider the need for home health follow-up and make the referral, if needed. Include the woman and her family in all discussions. Table 14.1 outlines an example care plan.

TABLE 14.1	PLAN OF CARE FOR WOMEN WITH A PHYSICAL DISABILITY IN PREGNANCY

Goals:
- Management of symptoms
- Prevention of complications
- Optimization of function
- Understanding of self-care and demonstrates necessary psychomotor skills for care after discharge

Preconception	• Family planning • Counsel regarding risks • Determine medication dosing based on disease symptoms and remission • Physical and cognitive assessment
Antepartum	• Monitor for progression of symptoms or effects of disease on physical and mental abilities • Determine modifications in medications (as indicated) • Collaborate with physical therapy to develop plan for care needs • Fall risk teaching with physical changes of pregnancy • Assess for asymptomatic bacteruria • Plan labor and birth care needs (may require preadmission care conference) • Preadmission assessment with anesthesiology
Labor and Birth	• "Labor down"/passive descent during second stage of labor to decrease energy utilization and likelihood of fatigue • Assist with positioning to facilitate vaginal birth • Prepare for possible operative vaginal birth (as indicated based on physical needs) • Pain management as indicated and desired • Cesarean birth for obstetrical needs

Postpartum	• Fall risk in women with physical symptoms and fatigue
	  ◦ Assist with ambulation until demonstrated ability
	  ◦ Utilize adaptive aids as necessary
	  ◦ Fall precautions implemented
	• Evaluate safe environment
	• Infection control precautions
	• VTE prophylaxis as indicated
	• Anticipate need for assistance with care of woman and newborn
	• Space care activities over time to decrease fatigue
	• Breastfeeding is encouraged
	  ◦ Evaluate safety of medications
	• Monitor for progression of symptoms
	• Prevent overdistention of bladder
	  ◦ Utilize bladder scanner as indicated
	• Physical therapy consult as indicated
	• Occupational therapy consult as indicated
	• Nutritional consult as indicated
	• Dietary modifications with swallowing difficulties

From Baird, S. M., Dalton, J. (2013). Multiple sclerosis in pregnancy. *Journal of Perinatal and Neonatal Nursing, 27*(3), 232–241.

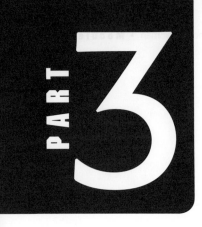

PART 3

Obesity

Since 1980, the prevalence of obesity has more than doubled worldwide. The World Health Organization considers obesity one of the most serious global health problems of the 21st century.[1] Obesity is defined as a body mass index (BMI) of greater than or equal to 30. In 2014, 34.9% of the adult population in the United States was obese.[1] Table 14.2 outlines the WHO classification of weight based on BMI.

TABLE 14.2 WORLD HEALTH ORGANIZATION CLASSIFICATION OF WEIGHT

WORLD HEALTH ORGANIZATION CLASSIFICATION OF WEIGHT

Normal weight	BMI 18.5–24.9
Overweight	BMI 25–29.9
Obese	BMI 30–39.9
Morbidly obese	BMI 40 or more

From World Health Organization. (2015). *Obesity and overweight.* WHO. http://www.who.int/mediacentre/factsheets/fs311/en/. Accessed January 23, 2015.

NOTE: *To calculate BMI:*

$$\frac{\text{Prepregnancy Weight (kg)}}{\text{Height (m)}^2}$$

Recent data describe obesity as it occurs in women:
- Prevalence of women with BMI >25 has more than doubled in the last 20 years.[2]
- A total of 56% of women of child-bearing age are overweight, 30% are obese, and 8% morbidly obese.[3,4]
- Pregnancy is associated with permanent weight increase in every BMI category.[5]

Prenatal Care

Each visit to an obstetric provider should include a head-to-toe assessment, with special attention to weight gain/loss trends. For morbidly obese women, a bariatric scale may be required for weight assessment. In 2009, the Institute of Medicine[6] published guidelines for recommended gestational weight gain based on prepregnancy BMI (Table 14.3). Since 2009, when the recommendations were published, additional research has been conducted which indicates that <u>no weight gain</u> or even <u>weight loss</u> in obese or morbidly obese patients decreases rates of

TABLE 14.3 IOM GUIDELINES

Institute of Medicine guidelines for recommended gestational weight gain based on prepregnancy body mass index (2009)

PREPREGNANCY BODY MASS INDEX	TOTAL WEIGHT GAIN RANGE (lb)
Underweight (less than 18.5 kg/m²)	28–40
Normal weight (18.5–24.9 kg/m²)	25–35
Overweight (25–29.9 kg/m²)	15–25
Obese (greater than 30 kg/m²)	11–20

preeclampsia, macrosomia, cesarean and operative vaginal births, neonatal admissions to the NICU, and improves APGAR scores.[7]

• What are the risks of pregnancy in the presence of obesity?

Obese women are at increased risk of complications and often enter pregnancy with pre-existing comorbidities such as chronic hypertension, type 2 diabetes, obstructive sleep apnea, and/or hypercholesterolemia.[4,8]

NOTE: *The higher the mother's BMI, the higher her risk of developing complications during or after pregnancy.*[4]

TABLE 14.4 MATERNAL RISKS	
Gestational diabetes	• 3–8 times higher risk of developing gestational diabetes vs. normal weight women due to insulin resistance[9]
Hypertension	• 50% will develop preeclampsia[5] • For accurate assessment of blood pressure, make sure the appropriate sized cuff is used—cuff that is too small gives a falsely elevated reading
Prolonged or dysfunctional labor	• Prolonged labor as BMI increases • Decreased uterine contraction intensity[10] • High cholesterol levels may prolong or cause dysfunctional labor[11] • Rate of failed induction is two times that of normal weight women[11]
Operative vaginal and cesarean birth	• Due to macrosomia and dysfunctional labor patterns[11]
Anesthesia	• Difficult due to positioning, obscure landmarks, adipose tissue[12] • May impair pain management during labor[12] • Difficult airway risk[12] • Higher risk of aspiration if general anesthesia used[12]
Postoperative	• Wound breakdown[4] • Dehiscence[4]
Infections	• Increased risk of surgical site infections[4] • Endometriosis rates increased[4]
Venous thromboembolism (VTE)	• Obesity and pregnancy both increase risk of VTE[8] • Early use of sequential compression devices and early ambulation decrease the risk of venous thrombus formation
Sleep disordered breathing	• Physiologic changes of pregnancy that increase risk • Nasopharyngeal edema • Decreased functional residual capacity • Increased waking at night • Weight gain[13]
Maternal death	• Associated with aspiration, failed intubation, hemorrhage, thromboembolism, and stroke • Cesarean section also increases mortality due to prolonged operative time, wound infection, dehiscence, endometritis, atelectasis, and pneumonia[14]

• What are the nursing considerations for labor, birth, and the postpartum period?

When obese women are admitted for delivery, it may be necessary to use special bariatric equipment including beds, wheelchairs, bedside commodes, and operating room table extensions. Lifts and other devices for repositioning and transport of obese women should be available for safe patient handling and prevention of work related injury to care providers. Table 14.6 is an example care plan for the obese woman.

TABLE 14.5 FETAL/NEWBORN RISKS	
Spontaneous miscarriage	• 2–3-fold increase in early miscarriage[15]
Congenital anomalies	• Twice as likely to have a fetus with a neural tube defect compared to a woman of normal weight[15] • Higher rates if combined with diabetes
Stillbirth	• Rate double that of normal weight women[16]
Prematurity	• Data shows higher incidence • Indicated birth due to other risk factors[17]
Macrosomia	• Twice as common in obese women due to gestational diabetes • Greater risk of hypoglycemia[7]
Birth injury	Due to macrosomia[7]

Breastfeeding	• Obese women are less likely to breastfeed due to:
	  ◦ Mechanical issues of positioning
	  ◦ Maternal issues from birth such as prolonged labor, cesarean delivery, or postpartum complications

Childhood obesity	• Babies born to obese mothers are more likely to develop obesity by the time they reach the age of 4[18]

Admission

Obese women are less likely to have spontaneous labor.[4] When the woman is admitted for birth (spontaneous or induced), complete a full risk assessment that includes medical disease and surgical history, complications associated with previous and current pregnancy. Assessment regarding symptoms or a previous diagnosis of obstructive sleep apnea is also recommended on all obese women due to a predisposition of right-sided heart failure and secondary pulmonary hypertension.[19] The use of a pulse oximeter may be helpful to alert the provider to any signs of maternal hypoxemia, especially in women with sleep apnea or those who have received medications associated with respiratory depression.[5] The following screening questions in Table 14.7 are helpful in screening.

Determining fetal position may be difficult depending on the body habitus of the woman. By palpating the abdomen, try to determine the outline of the uterus and establish fundus first. Ask where she feels fetal movement and use information to establish fetal contours. If unable to determine fetal position, an ultrasound examination may be necessary—which may also be difficult.

Morbidly obese mothers are two times more likely to deliver a baby weighing greater than 4,500 g, and more likely to be admitted to the neonatal intensive care unit due to low APGAR scores.[7] These risks in combination with medical complications (diabetes) consider having the neonatal team at birth.

Labor

The class II and III obese woman is a high-risk patient. Nurse-to-patient ratio during active labor is recommended 1:1 per AWHONN staffing guidelines.[22] There may be need for 2:1 staffing during procedures such as positioning for epidural, holding legs in vaginal birth, position changes or holding the pannus away from the field in vaginal birth or cesarean section.

In the absence of other comorbidities or complications, obesity alone is not an indication for elective birth prior to 39 weeks.[8] However, more frequent induction of labor is related to comorbidities and higher incidence of post-dates pregnancy. If labor is induced, there is a higher incidence of failed induction with slower and less productive labor progression due to adipose tissue production of leptin, which can inhibit contractions. In combination with difficulty in monitoring uterine contractions, higher doses of oxytocin may be utilized. If the woman is attempting a vaginal birth after cesarean (VBAC), trial of labor failure rates reach as high as 39%.[4]

Positioning for comfort and optimizing physiologic status may be difficult due to diminished lung capacity, chest wall compliance, gas exchange, functional residual capacity, and an

TABLE 14.6 PLANNING FOR CARE OF THE OBESE WOMAN DURING LABOR

Goals:
- *Effective fetal and uterine monitoring with ability to monitor progress of labor and fetal status*
- *Adequate pain control during labor, birth, and postpartum*
- *Expected labor progress*
- *Vaginal birth*

Prior to Admission	• Determine facility capabilities
	  • What is the toilet weight limit?
	  • Can the woman get into the shower?
	• Determine equipment needs for labor and birth
	• Preanesthesiology evaluation
	  • Informed consent
	  • Airway (e.g., fiberoptic intubation capability)
	  • Equipment/supply needs (e.g., epidural needles)
	  • Comorbidities
	  • Cardiac and respiratory evaluation
	• Emergency preparedness—conduct drills to determine needs
	  • Does the bed move through the doorway if emergent transport to the OR is indicated?
	  • How many staff members will it take to transport patient in an emergency?
	• Informed consent by provider
		Bariatric equipment needs (on site or rental)
		• Scales
		• Examination table
		• Bed
		• OR table or extenders
		• Stirrups
		• Wheelchair
		• Commode
		• BP cuff (up to 60 cm arm circumference)
		• Lifting/transfer equipment (e.g., air assisted lateral transfer, power transport gurney, sit to stand, lifts)
		• Hospital gowns
		<u>Instruments</u>
		• Speculum—extra long
		• Retractors—extra long
		• Difficult intubation

Admission	• Complete a risk assessment
	• Notify anesthesiology team and develop plan of care for pain management and emergency needs
	• Determine staffing needs
	  • 1:1 RN to patient ratio recommended if continuous EFM required
	  • Extra staff for positioning, transfer, and/or transport assigned
	  • OR staff for retraction during vaginal birth assigned
	• Obtain needed equipment and supplies
	• If cesarean section is required:
	  • Aspiration prophylaxis
	  • Antibiotic dose increase
	  • Thromboprophylaxis: Sequential compression devices placed prior to surgery; risk assessment for heparin therapy depending on anesthesia type and duration
	  • Extra scrub personnel for retraction
	  • Appropriately sized instruments

Postpartum	• Evaluate fall risk and implement necessary precautions • Early ambulation according to patient's condition and provider orders; sequential compression devices remain on until ambulation • Evaluate vaginal bleeding frequently since uterine position/tone assessment and massage may be difficult • Assist with breastfeeding positioning • Lactation consultation as needed • Observe for signs and symptoms of infection • Educate woman/support regarding signs and symptoms of pulmonary embolus • Dietary consult as indicated • Occupational therapy consult as indicated • Assess discharge needs • If patient has suspicion or confirmed diagnosis of sleep apnea, monitor with pulse oximetry post-op and consider continuous positive airway pressure (CPAP) as indicated • Respiratory therapy consult as indicated

From Gunatilake, R. P., Perlow, J. H. (2011). Obesity and pregnancy: Clinical management of the obese gravida. *American Journal of Obstetrics & Gynecology, 204*(2), 106–119; James, D. C., Maher, M. A. (2009). Caring for the extremely obese woman during pregnancy and birth. *Maternal Child Nursing, 34*(1), 24–30; Kribs, J. M. (2014). Obesity in pregnancy: Addressing risks to improve outcomes. *Journal of Perinatal and Neonatal Nursing, 28*(1), 32–40.

TABLE 14.7 SCREENING QUESTIONS

Screening Questions for Obstructive Sleep Apnea
- Do you snore?
- Do you wake up tired after a full night's sleep?
- Do you fall asleep during the day?
- Have you been told you stop breathing at night while you are sleeping?
- Do you have a history of hypertension?

Note: If "yes" to 2 or more questions, refer to a Sleep Specialist

increased work of breathing in obese patients.[19] An upright or semi-Fowler's position facilitates lung expansion, maternal comfort, and labor progress. As with all pregnant women, it is especially important to avoid a supine position to prevent pressure on the uterus and venacaval syndrome.[19]

External fetal monitoring is challenging in obese women due to maternal body habitus and may require a nurse to remain at the bedside in order to hold the monitor in place for continuous monitoring. Evaluation of uterine activity by palpation may also be difficult or impossible due to abdominal adipose tissue. Internal monitoring, when possible, may give the most accurate information regarding fetal heart rate and uterine activity. There are available adjunct fetal monitoring devices available to assist with continuous and more accurate fetal and uterine monitoring.

Because obese women are at increased risk for labor dystocia and prolonged labor, accurate assessment is very important.[10] The benefit of internal monitoring during active labor once membranes are rupture may be considered. However, artificial rupture of membranes in early labor for the purpose of internal monitoring is not recommended.

Progress of labor should be carefully monitored, as obese women may have prolonged labor, a dysfunctional labor pattern, and failure of descent (refer to *Module 6* for a review of labor management issues).[10] All of these factors increase the risk of a cesarean and operative vaginal birth. Be prepared and educate the woman and family for this potential outcome.

Anesthesia

Anesthesia poses risks for obese women due to[12]:
- Airway complications
- Cardiopulmonary dysfunction
- Perioperative morbidity
- Technical challenges
- Pain management challenges

It is recommended that a woman who is obese obtain a consult with an anesthesiology provider during the prenatal period, especially if she has a diagnosis of sleep apnea.[21,23] If consultation cannot be accomplished during that time, interview and assessment by an anesthesia provider should be done as soon as possible after admission to the labor and delivery unit. Obese women are at increased risk for cesarean birth, so early consultation allows for development of a comprehensive plan of care and plan for emergent birth due to the potential for difficult intubation. Airway complications are the most common cause of anesthesia-related maternal death.[12] The woman's plan of care may consider early placement of neuraxial anesthesia for comfort and to decrease oxygen consumption in labor. However, up to 74% of women weighing greater than 300 lb will require more than one attempt for placement and may become displaced with movement. In addition, there is a high incidence of failure (up to 42% reported).[12] With increased incidence of obstructive sleep apnea, close assessment of pulse oximetry trends should be provided post-op or if analgesics cause drowsiness.[23]

Abnormalities of second stage of labor may also increase the risk for the obese woman. Often, it is more difficult to continuously monitor the fetal heart rate. Positioning may require the assistance of additional staff. The obese woman has a higher incidence of operative vaginal birth due to soft tissue dystocia and poor maternal pushing efforts as compared to normal weight women. If vacuum extraction is attempted, there is a 40% failure rate.[8,19] If shoulder dystocia occurs, the team should be prepared due to the difficulty in performing maneuvers.[19]

TABLE 14.8 RISK OF CESAREAN BIRTH IN THE PRESENCE OF OBESITY			
	BMI < 30	**BMI 30–34.9**	**BMI ≥ 35**
Cesarean n = 16,102	20.7%	33.8%	47.4%

Cesarean Birth

There is a higher risk of cesarean birth in obese women.[24,25] See Table 14.8.

If a cesarean birth is required, there is an increase in blood loss, longer incision to delivery time (increased surgery time), increased risk of infection, and increased risk of venous thromboembolism (VTE).[4] Antibiotic dosing for cesarean birth may be adjusted to enhance antimicrobial coverage. Future births are impacted once an obese woman has a cesarean birth. VBAC success rates are poor in the morbidly obese woman and few providers would recommend a trial of labor after cesarean with the risks of needing to do an emergent cesarean birth with a very high-risk patient.[19]

Postpartum

The obese postpartum woman has a higher risk for postpartum hemorrhage due to prolonged labor, an increased induction rate, incidence of a macrosomic infant, and the difficulty in finding the fundus for effective fundal massage.[19] Postpartum infection is also higher with an increased incidence of wound infection, delayed healing, and endometritis.[24] Dosing of antibiotics may need adjustment to effectively treat the infection.[19]

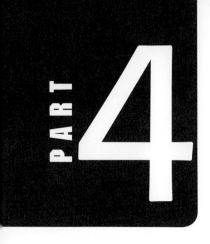

PART 4

Substance Use and Abuse

Substance use in the United States is at its highest point in a decade and misuse and overdose deaths have become a public health crisis. Women comprise 30% of the addicted population and the majority are of childbearing age.[1] In 2012, the use rate of illicit substances during pregnancy was 5.9%—up from 4.4% in 2010—increasing the risk for complications in both the woman and baby.[1]

NOTE: *These alarming data do not include the use of legally available alcohol, prescription drugs, or tobacco.*

Healthcare providers encountering women with substance abuse issues have responsibility for:
- Screening and identification
- Education
- Know local, community resources
- Referral for treatment
- Adhering to safe prescribing practices

Effects

Drug use, including prescription medications, can directly affect the woman and result in a direct or indirect affect on the fetus.[2]

Maternal and fetal/newborn effects of specific drugs are outlined in Table 14.9.

Screening

Universal screening for substance use and abuse is done easily and quickly, increases identification of pregnant women for intervention and referral. Substance use is prevalent in all populations so providers should never make assumptions based on age, race, or socioeconomic status. Many users will not show physical signs or symptoms. Universal screening is nonbiased, supportive, and non-stigmatizing. Substance use may be unknown unless self reported, through screening, or if biological testing is done. There are many verbal screening tools available and should be utilized during the first prenatal visit and routinely throughout pregnancy. Ensure privacy for the patient, and continue with nonjudgmental language.[3,4] Examples of Screening questions are presented in Display 14.1.

Urine toxicology is not recommended for universal screening, but may be used as a follow-up screening method, if indicated. If drug testing is used, honest communication about testing and reporting with the woman is required. Information should include the planned testing, purpose of the test, management based on results, and benefits or consequences of testing. The woman may refuse consent, but testing of the newborn may occur as indicated.

• What are the potential signs of maternal substance abuse?

The nurse should also be aware of potential signs of maternal substance abuse because of the increased risk of complications. Clinical observation including medical history, behaviors, physical signs, and laboratory findings may be cues for potential substance use and abuse:
- Late entry to prenatal care or does not seek prenatal care
- Failure to keep appointments or leaving without being seen
- Noncompliance with recommended treatments

TABLE 14.9 EFFECT ON THE MOTHER, FETUS, AND INFANT OF COMMONLY ABUSED DRUGS

DRUG	POTENTIAL EFFECTS ON MOTHER	POTENTIAL EFFECTS ON FETUS/INFANT
1. Cocaine and crack: may be smoked, inhaled, or injected	• Increased heart rate, and respiratory rate • Vasoconstriction • Decreased blood flow to placenta • Abruption • First trimester miscarriages	• IUGR and small for gestational age (Gouin) • Preterm birth (Gouin) • Cardiac development abnormalities • Arrhythmia • Stillbirth • SIDS • Failure of infant to respond to consoling, irritable behavior • Questionable long term–learning disabilities
2. Marijuana: smoked or consumed in food	• Increased number of mothers with anemia • Loss of short-term memory • Increased maternal heart rate	• Increased fine tremors • Irritability • Sleep disturbances • Unknown long-term effects
3. Amphetamines and meth-amphetamines: smoked, oral, injected	• Increased heart rate and respiratory rate • Vasoconstriction • Decreased blood flow to the placenta • Increased abruption	• Irritability • Poor feeding • Questionable long-term effects
4. Narcotics and opiates: oral, smoked, and injected	• Poor nutritional status • Increased rate of preterm labor and birth • If mother is IV user, may be HIV, hepatitis B positive, and at risk for subacute bacterial endocarditis and STDs	• Increased rates of IUGR • Withdrawal symptoms in the newborn (usually within 72 hours) • Restless, high-pitched shrill cry, inconsolable, seizures

HIV, human immunodeficiency virus; IV, intravenous; IUGR, intrauterine growth restriction; SIDS, sudden infant death syndrome; STD, sexually transmitted disease.

DISPLAY 14.1 SUBSTANCE USE SCREENING TOOL EXAMPLES

CRAFFT[5]

[a]For use with adolescents and young adults

C: Have you ever ridden in a **CAR** driven by someone (including yourself) who was high or had been using alcohol or drugs?

R: Do you ever use alcohol or drugs to **RELAX**, feel better about yourself or fit in?

A: Do you ever use alcohol or drugs while you are by yourself or **ALONE**?

F: Do you ever FORGET things you did while using alcohol or drugs?

F: Do your **FAMILY** or **FRIENDS** ever tell you that you should cut down on your drinking or drug use?

T: Have you ever gotten in **TROUBLE** while you were using alcohol or drugs?

[a]Two or more positive answers trigger further assessment

4Ps[6]

1. **P**arents: Did any of your parents have a problem with alcohol or other drug use?
2. **P**artner: Does your partner have a problem with alcohol or drug use?
3. **P**ast: In the past, have you had difficulties in your life because of alcohol or other drugs, including prescription medications?
4. **P**resent: In the past month, have you consumed any alcohol or used other drugs?

[a]Any yes answers trigger further questions

- Inadequate weight gain and/or malnourished appearance
- Defensive or hostile behavior
- Frequent accidents or falls
- Signs of depression
- Signs of agitation or euphoria
- Dilated or constricted pupils
- Needle marks, thrombosed veins, and cellulitis
- Neonatal withdrawal symptoms

Management of the woman with substance abuse must be collaborative and should include dieticians (nutrition counseling), social workers, nurses, physicians, and addiction specialists. To provide effective care and gain a trusting relationship with the woman, healthcare team members should be nonjudgmental and nonpunitive. However, some state laws may require reporting and criminal charges for endangerment and/or fetal harm. Discussions regarding treatment options should be explored. Pregnancy may represent a period when the woman recognizes the need for care and intervention. Referrals to addiction specialists, inpatient treatment programs, 12-step programs, and individual counseling should be considered and tailored to the woman's needs. The management of substance abuse may require hospitalization, as withdrawal may have negative effects on both maternal and fetal health depending upon the substance.

Tobacco

Smoking during pregnancy is one of the most preventable causes of infant morbidity and mortality. In 2012, over 18% of pregnant women used tobacco, resulting in the cost of smoking-related pregnancy complications greater than $300 million.[7] Women who are more likely to use tobacco in pregnancy are single, Caucasian, high school education or less, low socioeconomic status, concerned about weight gain, and use of other substances. Tobacco use has the potential for adverse events in the fetus/newborn and mother. Most data reflect a correlation between the number of cigarettes smoked per day and complication rates.

- **Fetal/Newborn Complications**

- Accounts for 20% to 30% of low–birth-weight infants
- Preterm birth and premature rupture of membranes
- Infant death
- Risk of sudden infant death syndrome (SIDS)—increases threefold with prenatal and postnatal exposure
- Higher hyperactivity/inattention scores
- Childhood asthma

Maternal Complications

- Placental abnormalities due to vasoconstriction and vasospasm
  - Abruption
  - Previa

Alcohol

An estimated 20% to 30% of women report drinking during pregnancy. In addition, 7.6% (or 1 in 13) report drinking within the last month and 1.4% report binge drinking (4 or more drinks on an occasion) within the last month.[8,9] Data show that the highest estimates of pregnant women who drink are age 35 to 44 years, white, college graduates, and employed.[8,9] Alcohol easily crosses the placental barrier and has well-established teratogenic properties. Exposure during pregnancy, in any amount and at any gestational age, can cause developmental, cognitive, and behavior issues during childhood. Fetal alcohol spectrum disorder (FASD) is a broad diagnosis with several diagnostic subcategories based on symptoms/effects. Fetal alcohol syndrome (FAS) is the most serious complication and requires three criteria for diagnosis:

1. Growth problems: prenatal and postnatal height, weight, or both less than the 10th percentile.

2. Facial dysmorphia: smooth philtrum, thin vermillion border, small palpebral fissures
3. Central nervous system abnormalities: structural abnormalities, neurologic problems, below normal functional performance

   Screening tools for alcohol use have been validated for utilization during pregnancy. One example is the TACE questionnaire.

Tolerance: How many drinks does it take for you to feel high?
Annoyed: Do you feel annoyed by people complaining about your drinking?
Cut Down: Have you ever felt the need to cut down on your drinking?
Eye-opener: Have you ever had a drink first think in the morning?

Marijuana

Cannabis sativa (marijuana) is the most commonly used illicit drug in the United States, with self-reported prevalence of 2% to 5% during pregnancy. Currently, there is no clear evidence of poor perinatal effects of marijuana use during pregnancy and some states are legalizing marijuana for recreational use.[7,10,11] Maternal effects of marijuana may include central nervous system depression, respiratory infections (bronchitis, sinusitis, pharyngitis), and learning or social behavior changes in attention, memory, and information processing. THC (9-tetrahydrocannabiol) is one of the most potent compounds in marijuana and has been shown to cross the placenta producing fetal plasma levels, and pass to the newborn in breast milk. It is important to remind women that although marijuana is legalized for use in some states, it may pose risks, as do alcohol and tobacco because there are no known safe limits in pregnancy. Providers must be prepared to have conversations with women and families because of the possible implications for care.

Opiates

Heroin, codeine, fentanyl, morphine, opium, methadone, oxycodone, meperidine, hydro-morphone, hydrocodone, propoxyphene, buprenorphine[12-14]

Opiate use can involve illegal drugs or medications often prescribed for pain management. Prescription narcotic use is second only to marijuana in the number of current users. Prescriptions for "pain killers" have increased 400% in the last decade. Opiate-related deaths have tripled and are responsible for more deaths than all illicit substances combined. Death due to opiate use is usually associated with respiratory depression. Heroin is a rapid-acting opiate with a short half-life and use of this highly addictive drug is on the rise. Physical addiction to opiates will result in tolerance and a need for higher and more frequent dosing to prevent withdrawal, which may begin within 4 to 6 hours of use. Withdrawal during pregnancy is not recommended since it may cause maternal hypertension, agitation, respiratory depression, somnolence, and death. Fetal compromise is also associated with maternal withdrawal.

   To prevent maternal withdrawal from opiates, maintenance therapy with methadone has been utilized in pregnancy for over 30 years. The intent of maintenance therapy is to:
   • prevent withdrawal
   • prevent illegal, unsupervised opiate use
   • encourage prenatal care and substance treatment programs
   • decrease criminal activity

Methadone is a synthetic, long-acting opioid that does not provide euphoria or interference in the woman's daily activities, and is not associated with birth defects. **Buprenorphine** (subutex, suboxone) is a newer alternative to methadone and is tapered gradually to reduce the craving for opiates and maternal withdrawal symptoms.[13] An expected disadvantage of methadone or buprenorphine treatment is neonatal abstinence syndrome (NAS) (withdrawal in the neonate).[15] NAS should be anticipated and managed by the neonatal team.

NOTE: Many women using opiates will not be identified through biological screening as oxycodone and hydrocodone do not show up with some routine screening tests.

Cocaine

Cocaine is a highly addictive, rapid-acting drug that causes acute sympathetic nervous system stimulation resulting in vasoconstriction, which is intensified if used with alcohol.[16] Potential maternal effects include tachycardia, hypertension, cardiac arrhythmias, coronary artery vasospasm, seizures, and stroke. In addition, the pregnant woman is at an even higher risk of thrombus formation due to platelet activation and thromboxane production.[16,17] Crack is a pure form of cocaine that when smoked can cause acute lung injury, pulmonary edema, and impaired gas exchange. Pregnancy-related adverse outcomes during labor include preterm birth, abruption, fetal compromise, hypertensive crisis, and meconium-stained fluid.[18]

NOTE: Maternal signs and symptoms of cocaine use may be confused as symptoms of preeclampsia/eclampsia.

With stimulant abuse (see methamphetamine, also), there is significant risk of placental abruption, and continuous electronic fetal monitoring is recommended to observe and assess for uterine hypertonus.[19]

Methamphetamine

Meth, Speed, Ice, Crystal, Chalk, Crank, Glass, Black Beauties, Biker's Coffee

Methamphetamine is a powerful stimulant made from over-the-counter medication (pseudoephedrine) and household products.[20] Because of its inexpensive street value, long half-life (12 hours), increased energy and weight loss association, methamphetamine use has been on the rise in the United States since the 1980s.

Short-Term Effects	**Long-Term Effects**
• Hypertension	• Anxiety and depression
• Cardiac arrhythmias	• Confusion and memory loss
• Seizures	• Insomnia
• Hyperthermia	• Weight loss
	• Dental problems ("meth mouth")
	• Violent behavior
	• Psychotic behavior (visual and auditory hallucinations)
	• Skin sensations (described as bugs crawling under the skin)

Withdrawal symptoms from methamphetamine include depression, anxiety, fatigue, and profound drug cravings. If used during pregnancy, there is a risk of small for gestation age (SGA) and low–birth-weight infants. Since methamphetamines are passed through breast milk and result in higher concentrations in the newborn, women who are using them should not breastfeed.

Labor Considerations

• **What should the nurses consider in planning intrapartum and postpartum care for the woman with substance abuse issues?**

Labor management is not significantly changed from routine intrapartum care with route of birth dependent upon obstetric factors. A thorough history including recent drug use is important and a serology screening for hepatitis and HIV may be completed if the woman's status is unknown. The neonatal resuscitation team may need to be alerted to be present for delivery, and social services should be consulted. Attention is also required around issues of replacement opioids, labor analgesia, and monitoring. Opioid replacements should be continued in labor and taken on the day of a scheduled cesarean birth.[21] If a woman presents without prenatal care and is experiencing opioid withdrawal, Methadone or buprenorphine may be initiated.[21] Pain control during labor and birth may be challenging for some addicted women, particularly those who are addicted to narcotics and opiates. If the woman presents in labor while still using drugs, determining the type, amount, or combination of drugs used is important, as the illicit drugs used may interact with other medications administered. For example, methadone interacts with several medications and should not be given with narcotic agonist–antagonist (butorphanol, nalbuphine, pentazocine)—which may cause acute withdrawal.[14] If buprenorphine is used, opioids for pain management must not be given until therapeutic levels are reached.[21] If determined safe, pain medications should never be withheld because of concerns they may contribute to further addiction. If the woman has been using opiates, higher doses to achieve pain management should be anticipated. Regional and local anesthetics may be used for pain management during labor and birth. Nonpharmacologic methods of pain management should be explored, including back rubs, hot or cold compresses, sacral pressure, deep breathing and relaxation, and guided imagery. Support and encouragement from the healthcare team may decrease fear and anxiety that can heighten the perception of pain. Continuous electronic fetal monitoring is indicated with stimulant use (cocaine and methamphetamine) due to risk of placental abruption.

Immediate postpartum pain management can be accomplished with nonopioids in women experiencing vaginal birth. Postoperative birth pain management may be managed in a routine manner. It is important to remember that women with opioid dependency may require higher doses of opioid analgesics for pain management; therefore, individualized care in consultation with anesthesiology providers is important. Breastfeeding guidance is needed in women with substance abuse issues to determine an appropriate plan based on the risks/benefits of breast milk exposure, but breastfeeding can lessen symptoms of NAS, increase bonding, and be a motivating factor in abstinence from substance abuse. The postpartum period is also a time when many mothers are very highly motivated to make healthy life changes, yet it is also a time of high risk for relapse. If the woman is actively using drugs at the time of her birth, she may be counseled to consider addiction treatment options with referrals. Some states require reporting a drug-addicted mother to child protective services. Providers need to be familiar with policies and laws in the state where they practice. Addiction is powerful and women must be supported in any effort to abstain or reduce substance abuse. Withdrawal is difficult and is associated with risks to both the woman and fetus. Abstinence is the goal, but any steps toward the goal are promising steps.

Withdrawal Effects in the Newborn

When a fetus is exposed in-utero due to maternal use or abuse of certain substances, congenital anomalies, fetal growth restriction, increased risk for preterm birth, impaired neural development, and/or withdrawal symptoms or toxicity in the newborn, may occur.[22] Symptoms seen in the neonate may be the result of withdrawal or acute toxicity. Neonatal symptoms worsen in withdrawal as drug levels decrease, while neonatal symptoms from toxicity decrease as drug levels decrease. The most commonly encountered withdrawal in neonates is from opioid exposure, called NAS. Presentation of NAS can vary depending upon the history of maternal use, timing of last dose prior to delivery, maternal/neonate metabolism, birth weight and gestational age, and other factors. Symptoms include:

- CNS irritability/neurologic excitability (high-pitched crying, wakefulness, hyperactive deep tendon reflexes, exaggerated Moro reflex)
- GI tract dysfunction (vomiting, diarrhea, poor feeding and weight gain, fever, temperature instability, uncoordinated sucking, dehydration)

Most neonates exposed to opioids will display some symptoms, but a smaller number will need pharmacologic treatment. Symptoms of withdrawal may not be recognized in the immediate newborn period, as they may not begin until hours or days after birth depending upon the substance involved.

The intrapartum nurse should be aware of and document the woman's history of substance use. Maternal urine screening may be useful and umbilical cord sampling may also be used to reflect in utero exposure. Supportive measures for the neonate, including minimizing external stimuli, further screening, and/or pharmacologic treatment, if appropriate, are usually initiated in the nursery.

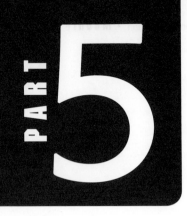

PART 5

Intimate Partner Violence

• What is intimate partner violence (IPV)?

Intimate partner violence (IPV), or abuse of a woman by a known perpetrator, has reached epidemic proportions. There are many myths and misconceptions about IPV, but the intrapartum nurse must be aware of truth surrounding this public health issue. Inevitably, an intrapartum nurse will care for women who are being abused at the hands of their partners. This type of violence may be known by other terms, such as woman battering, and domestic violence, but it is important to recognize that an intimate partner can be a current or former spouse, partner, boyfriend, or girlfriend.[1] The violence characterized by IPV may be physical, sexual, emotional, or threatened in nature. See Display 14.2 for examples of the types of violence.

DISPLAY 14.2 PRIMARY TYPES OF INTIMATE PARTNER VIOLENCE

Physical violence is an intentional use of force (actual or threatened) and may include:
- Pushing
- Slapping
- Punching
- Kicking
- Choking
- Beating
- Burning
- Biting
- Shaking
- Scratching
- Assault with a weapon (knife, gun, or other)
- Tying down or restraining
- Refusal to allow access to medical care when needed
- Leaving the woman in a dangerous place

Sexual violence includes acts such as:
- Degrading sexual comments
- Threatened force to compel the woman to engage in sexual acts against her will
- Sabotaging efforts at contraception, refusal to practice safe sex
- Intentionally hurting the woman during sex (including the use of objects intravaginally, orally, or anally)
- Pursuing sex with the woman when she is unable to avoid participation, unable to communicate unwillingness, or to understand the nature of the act
- Rape

Emotional, psychological, or verbal *abuse* refers to acts of:
- Humiliation
- "Name calling"
- Intimidation
- Belittling
- Insulting
- Ridiculing
- Deliberately embarrassing (especially in public)
- Social isolation
- Withholding of finances or resources
- Controlling of activities

NOTE: This is not a complete list. Abuse may include anything the victim perceives as threatening. The victim feels that she must comply with the abuser's wishes or things that are important to her, such as persons or objects, may be harmed.

• How often does IPV occur?

More than one in three women have experienced physical or sexual violence, or stalking by an intimate partner in their lifetime with approximately 4.8 million incidents of physical or sexual violence occurring annually.[2] A common misconception is that IPV affects only a small percentage of pregnant women. Although the prevalence of abuse varies depending on the source, true prevalence is difficult to establish due to nondisclosure and underreporting. It is estimated that 324,000 women per year are pregnant when violence occurs, with homicide contributing to the maternal mortality rate.[3–5] Although some practitioners and lay people may believe that pregnancy offers protection for a woman who has previously been abused, changes in the pattern of violence during pregnancy remain unclear. Many women who experience IPV before pregnancy continue to be abused during pregnancy and violence may actually increase. In addition, pregnancy may increase the frequency of sexual victimization of the woman.[6]

Risk Factors

• Who is at risk for violence during pregnancy?

Victims of violence come from every age group, religion, ethnic and racial group, socioeconomic level, educational background, and sexual orientation. No groups are immune.[7,8] However, research has demonstrated a higher prevalence of violence during pregnancy in some groups of pregnant women. Factors that have been associated with an increased incidence of violence include: younger women, lower income and education levels, unmarried and minority status.[8]

Cycle of Violence

• What is the cycle of violence?

Walker described a cycle of violence that can be divided into three phases (Fig. 14.1).[9] The nurse may see the pregnant victim in the tension-building phase or the reconciliation phase in the intrapartum period. It is rare, but not impossible, that an acute episode of violence would take place in an intrapartum setting. The pattern can last for a long or a short period of time, with the violence typically becoming more intense with each cycle.[9]

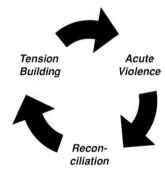

FIGURE 14.1   Cycle of Violence

Tension-building phase—Victim is compliant, but the abuser becomes angry with increasing frequency and intensity, with frequent threats of harm, humiliation, and intimidation.
Acute violence phase—Intentional use of force, including the behaviors listed previously, as well as sexual abuse, possibly increasing in severity with each cycle.
Honeymoon or reconciliation phase—Victim is showered with apologies and affection by the abuser, abuser gives assurances that the behavior will never happen again, makes excuses for the behavior, or denies that violence occurred.

Effects of Violence in Pregnancy

Violence against a pregnant woman may result in harm to both the woman and the fetus.[8,10] The direct effects of violence in pregnancy can be severe. Women may present with acute injuries to the head, face, breasts, abdomen, genitalia, and reproductive system. Maternal abdominal trauma can cause acute fetal injury from placental abruption, fetal fractures, rupture of the uterus, miscarriage (spontaneous abortion), hemorrhage, and fetal death. Indirect effects of violence can include: delayed or inadequate prenatal care, exacerbation of chronic illnesses, poor maternal weight gain, infection, anemia, increased tobacco and/or substance use, chronic maternal anxiety and/or depression, low birth weight, still birth, and preterm delivery, and result in poor neonatal outcomes.

Screening for Violence

Screening was once reserved until warning signs were observed, but recognition that violence may be occurring with no visible signs with active attempts at concealment has led to recommendations for universal screening at regular and routine intervals.[10–13] During pregnancy, there is a unique opportunity for identification of violence against women as they engage in frequent visits with healthcare providers throughout the pregnancy. Pregnancy may also be a powerful motivator for women to change their situations and hope for a better future with a new baby. Women are in the intrapartum setting for a relatively short period of time, yet there is a rapport, fostering a sense of advocacy, trust, and care that may make the woman feel comfortable enough to disclose abuse. Upon admission to the birth setting, ask the woman questions appropriate for screening during the initial assessment. Questions should be asked when the woman is apart from her partner, family, or friends, which may create challenges in the intrapartum setting.

• **What kind of questions should the nurse ask the woman about IPV?**

Appropriate phrasing allows for comprehensive, specific questions. Examples of phrases used for various aspects of screening are given in Display 14.3.[10,11,14–18] Ensure privacy and frame questions as universal, not due to suspicion. Explain to the mother about confidentiality and the laws regarding reporting of abuse in the state. Ask questions and listen to the responses in a nonjudgmental manner.

Interventions

• **What should the nurse do if the mother discloses abuse?**

Follow specific steps if the woman discloses abuse.

Step One—Acknowledge the Abuse

If the woman discloses abuse, the most important thing to do is to validate her concerns.

NOTE: If the woman discloses abuse, DO NOT respond with questions such as "Why don't you leave?" or "Why do you stay with him/her?" This may make her feel that she is responsible for the violence.[14]

The woman may feel alone and ashamed. It is important to respond to the disclosure appropriately. Use supportive statements such as:
  • "You are not alone."
  • "I'm glad you told me, we see lots of women in similar situations."
  • "You don't deserve this; we can help."
  • "It is not your fault."
  • "There are resources available to help you."
  • "I am concerned for your safety."
  • "We can help you with information and resources."

DISPLAY 14.3 SCREENING EXAMPLES FOR IPV

Framing Statements:
- "Because violence is so common in many women's lives and because there is help available for women being abused, I now ask every patient about domestic abuse."
- "I am so concerned about family violence that I now ask all of my patients about it, just like I ask about other health issues."
- "I would like to ask you a few questions about physical or emotional trauma because we know that these are common and affect women's health."

Confidentiality:
- "Know that everything we talk about is confidential. I won't talk about it with anyone else unless you tell me... (application of state laws regarding mandatory reporting)."

Sample Questions:
- HITS–Has your partner or any family member:
  - Physically HURT you?
  - INSULTED or talked down to you?
  - THREATENED you with harm?
  - SCREAMED or cursed at you during the pregnancy?
- "Does your partner ever humiliate you, put you down, or shame you?"
- "Has someone made you worry about your safety or the safety of your child (children)?"
- "Since you've been pregnant, have you been kicked, hit, slapped, forced into sexual activities, or otherwise physically hurt by someone?"
- "Has your partner ever forced you to do something sexually that you didn't want to do?"
- "Does your partner support your decision about being pregnant?"

From Centers for Disease Control, Division of Reproductive Health, National Center for Chronic Disease Prevention and Health Promotion. (n.d.). *Intimate partner violence, a guide for clinicians.* Atlanta, GA. www.cdc.gov/reproductivehealth/violence/IntimatePartnerViolence/index. htm. Accessed July 19, 2015; Walker, L. E. (1984). *The battered woman syndrome.* New York, NY: Springer; Author. (2012). Intimate partner violence. ACOG Committee Opinion No. 518. *Obstetrics and Gynecology, 119*(2 pt 1), 412–417; Association of Women's Health, Obstetric, and Neonatal Nurses. (2015). AWHONN Position Statement. Intimate partner violence. *Journal of Obstetric, Gynecologic, and Neonatal Nursing, 44*(3), 405–408; Brigham and Women's Hospital. (2004). *Domestic violence: A guide to screening and intervention.* Boston, MA: Author; Griffin, M. P., & Koss, M. P. (2002, January 31). Clinical screening and intervention in cases of partner violence. *Online Journal of Issues in Nursing, 7*(1), manuscript 2. Retrieved from: www.nursingworld.org/ojin/topic17/tpc17_2.htm; Sherin, K. M., Sinacore, J. M., Li, X. Q., et al. (1998). HITS: A short domestic screening tool for use in a family practice setting. Family Medicine, 30,508–512; Soeken, K. L., McFarlane, J., Parker, B., et al. (1998). The abuse assessment screen: A clinical instrument to measure frequency, severity, and perpetrator of abuse against women. In Campbell, J. C., (Ed.): *Empowering survivors of abuse: Health care for battered women and their children* (pp. 195–203).

Step Two–Evaluate and Facilitate Treatment of Physical Complaints Related to Abuse

Notify the primary care provider and collaboratively complete a physical assessment and facilitate treatment of current and/or past injuries from abuse.

Step Three–Assess Immediate Threat to the Woman

It is important to determine if there is an immediate threat to the woman.
- Is the abuser present at the birth setting?
- Does the woman require hospitalization?
- If the woman is to be discharged, does she feel that the abuser will harm her that day?
- Are there weapons in the household?
- Are the woman's other children or loved ones in danger?
- Does the woman feel safe enough to go home?
- Does the woman need immediate counseling?
- Does the woman want immediate police assistance?

Step Four–Assist With the Development of a Safety Plan

If there is an immediate threat of harm to the woman, a safety plan should be developed. The plan provides steps to follow if in a dangerous situation. It should include detailed information about defensive measures such as the following[7,14]:
- Finding easy access to an exit
- Practicing how to get away safely
- Having a bag packed and keys ready to leave
- Using code words for calling the police

- Having a planned destination if she needs to leave suddenly
- Having access to keys, money, and important documents

There are many resources and pamphlets available for assistance in development of a safety plan.

Step Five—Provide Information, Resources, and Referrals

Identify for the woman any available support systems at the birth setting. A staff social worker may be contacted to help with consultation. Resources in the community, support groups, shelters, legal aid, child protective services, hotline phone numbers, law enforcement, clergy, or other victim advocates should be described, including national resources. Try to recognize any specific and unique needs when making referrals.

NOTE: Having brochures available and visible in the birth setting area lets the woman know that it is a safe place, even if she is not yet ready to disclose abuse.[15]

Step Six—Document Assessments, Findings, and Actions

- **What should the nurse document?**

Accurate and appropriate documentation of findings in situations of IPV are of the utmost importance. The woman's medical records are frequently used in court and relied upon to be objective and legible.[7,14] The language used should be nonjudgmental, specific, and not leave room for misinterpretation or undermine the woman's credibility. Use quotation marks in charting to document in the woman's own words. Recommendations for information to be included in the documentation can be found in Table 14.10.

TABLE 14.10 DOCUMENTATION OF INTIMATE PARTNER VIOLENCE	
PORTION OF ASSESSMENT	**RECOMMENDING INFORMATION TO RECORD**
Relevant history	• Chief complaint • Medical problems related to the abuse • Detailed account of abusive situation including name and relationship of abuser, date, time, location, weapon used, nature of threats and witnesses • Statements made by the woman about the abuse • Past history of abuse • Relationship of past or current abuse to chief complaint
Results of assessment and laboratory or diagnostic procedures	• Specific gynecologic, neurologic, psychologic findings related to IPV • Description of injuries in detailed manner (use a body map for location) • Relationship of diagnostic procedure to current or past abuse • Photograph injuries
Photograph injuries	• Document consent for photographs • Label and date any photographs
Interventions	• Information provided • Resources identified • Options discussed • Safety assessment and planning • Referrals made • Mandatory reporting if applicable • Follow-up arrangements

From Centers for Disease Control, Division of Reproductive Health, National Center for Chronic Disease Prevention and Health Promotion. (n.d.). *Intimate partner violence, a guide for clinicians.* Atlanta, GA. www.cdc.gov/reproductivehealth/violence/IntimatePartnerViolence/index.htm. Accessed July 19, 2015; Brigham and Women's Hospital. (2004). *Domestic violence: A guide to screening and intervention.* Boston, MA: Author.

- **What does the nurse do if the woman denies abuse, but the nurse still suspects it?**

If the woman denies abuse but it is strongly suspected, her "no" response should still be documented.[7] Respect her autonomy and review the available resources with her. Even though it may be frustrating, every time the woman is asked, she may come closer to disclosing her abuse. If the woman's account of an injury and the clinical findings are in conflict, note the difference in a narrative.

Mandatory Reporting

Mandatory reporting remains controversial as women may feel threatened by possible retaliation if the healthcare provider reports the abuse.[10] Few states have mandatory reporting for IPV, but many have laws regarding mandatory reporting of gunshot or knife wounds, as well as abuse of children or individuals with disabilities. *Become familiar with and follow the state laws regarding reporting requirements.*

Overcoming Barriers to Care

Women who are experiencing IPV may have several reasons for not disclosing (fear of judgment, shame, uncertainty, cultural differences, lost hope) and nurses cite many reasons for discomfort with screening (personal history, attitudes, fear of offending). Yet, intrapartum nurses are an essential part of a collaborative team in identifying and assisting victims of IPV. The acronym "RADAR" can help nurses remember their responsibilities as it relates to IPV in any setting.[18]

ROUTINELY ask women about IPV.
ASK the woman direct and specific questions in screening for IPV.
DOCUMENT the woman's injuries.
ASSESS the woman's safety.
REVIEW with the woman all possible options.

SUGGESTED RESOURCES

- Futures Without Violence (previously known as Family Violence Prevention Fund)
  www.futureswithoutviolence.org
- National Coalition Against Domestic Violence
  www.ncadv.org
- National Network to End Domestic Violence
  www.nnedv.org
- National Resource Center on Domestic Violence
  www.nrcdv.org
- Office on Violence Against Women (U.S. Department of Justice)
  www.usdoj.gov/ovw

PRACTICE/REVIEW QUESTIONS

1. List potential pregnancy complications for a teen mother:
   a. _____
   b. _____
   c. _____
   d. _____
   e. _____

2. When doing postpartum teaching for a teen mother, which components would you highlight and why?

3. List some of the potential pregnancy complications for women with advanced maternal age:

4. List some of the nursing care considerations to prevent falls in women with a physical disability:

5. Labor and birth considerations for a woman with a physical disability include "Labor down"/passive descent during second stage of labor to decrease energy

421

utilization and likelihood of fatigue, _____ preparing for possible operative vaginal birth (as indicated based on physical needs), _____ and cesarean birth for obstetrical needs.

6. List the BMI for the following weight categories of obesity:

   Normal _____

   Overweight _____

   Obese _____

   Morbidly obese _____

7. In planning for the morbidly obese woman for labor, list some of the equipment needs.

   _____

   _____

   _____

   _____

   _____

8. What are some of the risk factors for the obese pregnant woman?

   _____

   _____

   _____

   _____

   _____

9. List five potential signs of maternal substance abuse.

   a. _____

   b. _____

   c. _____

   d. _____

   e. _____

10. To coordinate care for the woman with substance abuse, some of the disciplines to include in planning include:

    a. _____

    b. _____

    c. _____

    d. _____

11. The intent of opiate maintenance therapy with methadone or buprenorphine is:

    a. _____

    b. _____

    c. _____

    d. _____

12. State two reasons why pregnancy is a unique opportunity IPV screening.

a. _____

b. _____

13. State two appropriate responses from the nurse in response to a woman's disclosure of abuse.

   a. _____

   _____

   _____

   b. _____

   _____

   _____

14. Consent should be obtained and documented for any photographs taken of the victim's injuries.

    a. True

    b. False

PRACTICE/REVIEW ANSWER KEY

1. Iron deficiency anemia, preterm labor and birth, low–birth-weight infant, preeclampsia, and higher rates of cephalopelvic disproportion
2. Breastfeeding:
   Depression:
   Birth Control:
3. Fetal chromosomal abnormalities, fetal congenital malformations, ectopic pregnancy, spontaneous abortion, stillbirth, placenta previa, maternal mortality, pre-existing medical conditions, such as chronic hypertension or diabetes, cesarean birth (elective and emergent), preeclampsia, gestational diabetes, preterm birth
4. Assist with ambulation until demonstrated ability, utilize adaptive aids as necessary, implement hospital fall precautions
5. Assist with positioning; pain management
6. Normal weight BMI 18.5 to 24.9
   Overweight BMI 25 to 29.9
   Obese BMI 30 to 39.9
   Morbidly Obese BMI >40
7. Bariatric bed, wheelchair, stretcher, OR table extensions, operative instruments, epidural needles, stirrups, lifts, sliding mats
8. Increased risk of VTE, hypertension, diabetes, falls, failed induction of labor, cesarean birth
9. Late entry to prenatal care or does not seek prenatal care, failure to keep appointments or leaving without being seen, noncompliance with recommended treatments, inadequate weight gain and/or malnourished appearance, defensive or hostile behavior, frequent accidents or falls, signs of depression, signs of agitation or euphoria, dilated or constricted pupils, needle marks, thrombosed veins, and cellulitis, neonatal withdrawal symptoms.
10. Dieticians (nutrition counseling), social workers, nurses, physicians, and addiction specialists
11. Prevent withdrawal, prevent illegal, unsupervised opiate use, encourage prenatal care and substance treatment programs, decrease criminal activity

12. a. Most women seek prenatal care when they are pregnant.
    b. Pregnancy is a powerful motivator for change.
13. Any two of the following:
    a. "You are not alone."
    b. "I'm glad you told me; we see lots of women in similar situations."
    c. "You don't deserve this; we can help."
    d. "It is not your fault."
    e. "There are resources available to help you."
    f. "I am concerned for your safety."
    g. "We can help you with information and resources."
14. a. True

REFERENCES

Part I

1. Martin, J. A., Hamilton, B. E., Osterman, M. J. K., et al. (2015). Birth: Final data for 2013. *National Vital Statistics Report, 64*(1), 1–69, 72. Retrieved from: http://www.cdc.gov/nchs/data/nvsr/nvsr62/nvsr62_09.pdf#table02
2. Penman-Aguilar, A., Carter, M., Snead, M. C., et al. (2013). Socioeconomic disadvantage as a social determinant of teen childbearing in the U.S. *Public Health Reports, 128*(suppl 1), 5–22.
3. Shuger, L. (2012). *Teen pregnancy and high school dropout: What communities are doing to address these issues.* Washington, DC: The National Campaign to Prevent Teen and Unplanned Pregnancy and America's Promise Alliance; Pregnancy and America's Promise Alliance.
4. Hoffman, S. D. (2008). *Kids having kids: Economic costs and social consequences of teen pregnancy.* Washington, DC: The Urban Institute Press.
5. McCracken, K. A., & Loveless, M. (2014). Teen pregnancy: An update. *Current Opinions in Obstetrics and Gynecology, 26,* 355–359.
6. Malabarey, O. T., Balayla, J., & Abenhaim, H. A. (2012). The effect of pelvic size on cesarean delivery rates: Using adolescent maternal age as an unbiased proxy for pelvic size. *Journal of Pediatric and Adolescent Gynecology, 25*(3), 190–194.
7. National Campaign to Prevent Teen and Unplanned Pregnancy. (2014). Counting it up: The public costs of teen childbearing. Retrieved from: http://www.cdc.gov/teenpregnancy/aboutteen-preg.htm#_edn3
8. Baldwin, M. K., & Edelman, A. B. (2013). The effect of long-acting reversible contraception on rapid repeat pregnancy in adolescents: A review. *Journal of Adolescent Health, 52,* S47–S52.
9. Committee on Adolescent Healthcare Long-Acting Reversible Contraception Working Group, The American College of Obstetricians and Gynecologists. (2012). Committee opinion no. 539: Adolescents and long-acting reversible contraception: Implants and intrauterine devices. *Obstetrics and Gynecology, 120,* 983–988.
10. Ludford, I., Scheil, W., Tucker, G., et al. (2012). Pregnancy outcomes for nulliparous women of advanced maternal age in South Australia, 1998–2008. *Australian and New Zealand Journal of Obstetrics and Gynecology, 52,* 235–241.
11. Kenny, L. C., Lavender, T., McNamee, R., et al. (2013). Advanced maternal age and adverse pregnancy outcome: Evidence from a large contemporary cohort. *PLOS One, 8*(2), e56583. Retrieved from: http://www.ncbi.nlm.nih.gov/pmc/articles/PMC3577849/
12. Laopaiboon, M., Lumbiganon, P., Intarut, N., et al. (2014). Advanced maternal age and pregnancy outcomes: A multicountry assessment. *BJOG, 121,* 49–56.
13. Wang, Y., Tanbo, T., Abyholm, T., et al. (2011). The impact of advanced maternal age on obstetric and perinatal outcomes in singleton gestations. *Achieves of Gynecology and Obstetrics, 284*(1), 31–37.
14. Bayrampour, H., & Heaman, M. (2010). Advanced maternal age and risk of cesarean birth: A systematic review. *Birth, 37*(3), 219–226.

Part II

1. Signore, C., Spong, C. Y., Krotoski, D., et al. (2011). Pregnancy in women with physical disabilities. *Obstetrics and Gynecology, 117*(4), 935–947.
2. Baird, S. M., & Dalton, J. (2013). Multiple sclerosis in pregnancy. *Journal of Perinatal and Neonatal Nursing, 27*(3), 232–241.

Part III

1. World Health Organization. (2015). *Obesity and overweight.* WHO. http://www.who.int/mediacentre/factsheets/fs311/en/. Accessed January 23, 2015.
2. Ogden, C. L., Carroll, M. D., Kit, B. K., et al. (2014). Prevalence of childhood and adult obesity in the United States, 2011–2012. *Journal of the American Medical Association, 311*(8), 806–814.
3. Artal, R., & Flick, A. (2013). Obesity and weight gain in pregnancy. *Contemporary OB/GYN.* http://contemporaryobgyn.modernmedicine.com/. Accessed December 15, 2014.
4. The American College of Obstetricians and Gynecologists. (2013). ACOG Committee opinion no. 549: Obesity in pregnancy. *Obstetrics & Gynecology, 121,* 213–217.
5. Heavey, E. (2011). Obesity in pregnancy: Deliver sensitive care. *Nursing, 41*(10), 43–50.
6. Institute of Medicine of the National Academies. (2009). *Weight gain during pregnancy: Reexamining the guidelines.* Washington, DC: National Academies Press.
7. Blomberg, M. (2011). Maternal and neonatal outcomes among obese women with weight gain below the new Institute of Medicine recommendations. *Obstetrics and Gynecology, 117,* 1065–1070.
8. The American College of Obstetricians and Gynecologists. (2014). Challenges for overweight and obese women. Committee Opinion 591. *Obstetrics & Gynecology, 123,* 726–730.
9. Chu, S. Y., Kim, S. Y., Schmid, C. H., et al. (2007). Maternal obesity and risk of cesarean delivery: A meta-analysis. *Obstetrics Review, 8,* 385–394.
10. Kominiarek, M. A., Zhang, J., Vanveldhuisen, P., et al. (2011). Contemporary labor patterns: The impact of maternal body mass index. *American Journal of Obstetrics and Gynecology, 205*(3), 244.e1–e8.
11. Wolfe, K. B., Rossi, R. A., & Warshak, C. R. (2011). The effect of maternal obesity on the rate of failed induction of labor. *American Journal of Obstetrics & Gynecology, 205*(2), 128.e1–e7.
12. Badve, M. H., Golfeiz, C., & Vallejo, M. C. (2014). Anesthetic considerations for the morbid obese parturient. *International Anesthesiology Clinics, 52*(3), 132–147.
13. Balserak, B. I., & Pien, G. W. (2010). Sleep-disordered breathing and pregnancy: Potential mechanisms and evidence for maternal and fetal morbidity. *Current Opinion in Pulmonary Medicine, 16*(6), 574–582.
14. Stamilio, D. M., & Scifres, C. M. (2014). Extreme obesity and postcesarean maternal complications. *Obstetrics & Gynecology, 124*(2), 227–232.
15. Jungheim, E. S., Travieso, J. L., Carson, K. R., et al. (2012). Obesity and reproductive function. *Obstetrics & Gynecology Clinics of North America, 39*(4), 479–493.

16. Cnattingius, S., Bergstrom, R., Lipworth, L., et al. (1998). Pre-pregnancy weight and the risk of adverse pregnancy outcomes. *New England Journal of Medicine, 338*, 147–52.

17. Baeten, J. M., Bukusi, E. A., & Lambe, M. (2001). Pregnancy complications and outcomes among overweight and nulliparous women. *American Journal of Public Health, 91*, 436–440.

18. Stothard, K. J., Tennant, P. W., Bell, R., et al. (2009). Maternal over-weight and obesity and the risk of congenital anomalies. A systematic review and meta-analysis. *Journal of the American Medical Association, 301*(6), 636–650.

19. Gunatilake, R. P., & Perlow, J. H. (2011). Obesity and pregnancy: Clinical management of the obese gravida. *American Journal of Obstetrics & Gynecology, 204*(2), 106–119.

20. James, D. C., & Maher, M. A. (2009). Caring for the extremely obese woman during pregnancy and birth. *Maternal Child Nursing, 34*(1), 24–30.

21. Kribs, J. M. (2014). Obesity in pregnancy: Addressing risks to improve outcomes. *Journal of Perinatal and Neonatal Nursing, 28*(1), 32–40.

22. Association of Women's Health, Neonatal, and Obstetric Nursing. (2015). Guidelines for professional registered nurse staffing for perinatal units. Washington, DC.

23. Fung, A., Wilson, D., Barnes, M., et al. (2012). Obstructive sleep apnea and pregnancy: The effect on perinatal outcomes. *Journal of Perinatology, 32*, 399–406.

24. Magriples, U., Kershaw, T. S., Rising, S. S., et al. (2009). The effects of obesity and weight gain in young women on obstetric outcomes. *American Journal of Perinatology, 26*, 365–371.

25. Fyfe, E. M., Anderson, N. H., North, R. A., et al. (2011). Risk of first-stage and second-stage cesarean delivery by maternal body mass index among nulliparous women in labor at term. *Obstetrics & Gynecology, 117*, 1315–1322.

Part IV

1. U.S. Department of Health and Human Services Substance Abuse and Mental Health Services Administration Center for Behavioral Health Statistics and Quality. (2013). Results from the 2012 national survey of drug use and health: summary of national findings. Rockville, MD.

2. Behnke, M., & Smith, V. C., Committee on Substance Abuse & Committee on Fetus and Newborn. (2013). Prenatal substance abuse: Short and long-term effects on the exposed fetus. *Pediatrics, 131*, e1009–e1024.

3. The American College of Obstetrics and Gynecology. (2008). At risk drinking and illicit drug use: Ethical issues in obstetric and gynecologic practice. Committee Opinion no. 422. *Obstetrics and Gynecology, 112*(6), 1449–1460.

4. American College of Obstetricians and Gynecologists Committee on Health Care for Underserved Women. (2006). psychosocial risk factors: Perinatal screening and intervention. Committee Opinion No. 343. *Obstetrics and Gynecology, 108*(2), 469–477.

5. Center for Adolescent Substance Abuse Research, Children's Hospital Boston. (2009). The CRAFFT screening interview. Boston, MA: CeASAR. Retrieved from: www.ceasar.org/CRAFFT/pdf/ CRAFFT_English.pdf

6. Ewing, H. A. (1990). *Practical guide to intervention in health and social services with pregnant and postpartum addicts and alcoholics: Theoretical framework, brief screening tool, key interview questions, and strategies for referral to recovery resources.* Martinez, CA: Born Free Project, Contra Costa County Department of Health Services.

7. Brown, H. L., & Graves, C. R. (2013). Smoking and marijuana use in pregnancy. *Clinical Obstetrics and Gynecology, 56*(1), 107–113.

8. American College of Obstetricians and Gynecologists Committee on Health Care for Underserved Women. (2011). At-risk drinking and alcohol dependence: Obstetric and gynecologic implications. Committee Opinion No. 496. *Obstetrics and Gynecology, 118*(2 pt 1), 383–388.

9. Centers for Disease Control. (2012). Alcohol use and binge drinking among women of childbearing age–United States, 2006–2010. *Morbidity and Mortality Weekly, 61*(28), 534–538.

10. Desai, A., Mark, K., & Terplan, M. (2014). Marijuana use and pregnancy: Prevalence, associated behaviors, and birth outcomes. *Obstetrics and Gynecology, 123*(1), 46s.

11. American College of Obstetricians and Gynecologists Committee on Obstetric Practice. (2015). Marijuana use during pregnancy and lactation. Committee Opinion No. 637. *Obstetrics and Gynecology, 126*(1), 234–238

12. Savage, C., & Platt, O. (2014). Care of women who use opioids during pregnancy and the immediate postpartum period. *Journal of Addictions Nursing, 25*(1), 56–59.

13. Jones, H. E., Deppen, K., Hudak, M. L., et al. (2013). Clinical care for the opioid using pregnant and postpartum women: The role of obstetric providers. *American Journal of Obstetrics and Gynecology,* (13), 1058–1052.

14. American College of Obstetricians and Gynecologists, Committee on Health care of Underserved Women and the American Society of Addiction Medicine. (2012). Committee opinion: Opioid abuse, dependence and addiction in pregnancy. *Obstetrics and Gynecology, 119*(5), 1070–1076.

15. Jones, H. E., Kaltenbach, K., Heil, S. H., et al. (2010). Neonatal abstinence syndrome after methadone or buprenorphine exposure. *New England Journal of Medicine, 363*, 2320–2331.

16. Cain, M. A., Bornick, P., & Whiteman, P. (2013). The maternal, fetal and neonatal effects of cocaine exposure in pregnancy. *Clinical Obstetrics and Gynecology, 56*(1), 124–132.

17. Gouin, K., Murphy, K., & Shah, P. S. (2011). Effects of cocaine use during pregnancy on low birth weight and preterm birth: Systematic review and meta-analysis. *American Journal of Obstetrics and Gynecology, 204*(4), 340.e1–e12.

18. Chasnoff, I. J., Burns, K. A., & Burns, W. J. (1987). Cocaine use in pregnancy: Perinatal morbidity and mortality. *Neurotoxicol Teratol, 9*, 291–293.

19. Izquierdo, L., & Yonke, N. (2014). Fetal surveillance in late pregnancy and during labor. *North American Clinics in Obstetrics & Gynecology, 41*, 307–315.

20. American College of Obstetricians and Gynecologists. (2011/Reaffirmed 2013). Methamphetamine abuse in women of reproductive age. Committee Opinion 479. *Obstetrics and Gynecology, 117*, 751–755.

21. Gopman, S. (2014). Prenatal and postpartum care of women with substance abuse disorders. *North American Clinics in Obstetrics & Gynecology, 41*, 213–228.

22. Hudak, M., & Tan, R., Committee on Fetus and Newborn. (2012). Neonatal drug withdrawal. *Pediatrics, 129*(2), e540–e560.

Part V

1. Saltzman, L. E., Fanslow, J. L., McMahon, P. M., et al. (1999). *Intimate partner violence surveillance: Uniform definitions and recommended data elements, version 1.0.* Atlanta, GA: National Center for Injury Prevention and Control, Centers for Disease Control and Prevention.

2. Black, M., Basile, K., Breidig, M., et al. (2011). *The National Intimate Partner and Sexual Violence Survey (NISVS): 2010 summary report.* Atlanta, GA: National Center for Injury Prevention and Control, Centers for Disease Control and Prevention.

3. Family Violence Prevention Fund. (2010). *Reproductive health and partner violence guidelines: An integrated response to intimate partner violence and reproductive coercion.* San Francisco, CA: FVPF.

4. Gazmararian, J. A., Lazorick, S., Spitz, A. M., et al. (2006). Violence and reproductive health: Current knowledge and future research directions. *Journal of the American Medical Association, 275,* 1915–1920.

5. McFarlane, J., Campbell, J. C., Sharps, P., et al. (2002). Abuse during pregnancy and femicide: Urgent implications for women's health. *Obstetrics and Gynecology, 100*(1), 27–36.

6. Martin, S. L., Harris-Britt, A., Li, Y., et al. (2004). Changes in intimate partner violence during pregnancy. *Journal of Family Violence, 19*(4), 201–210.

7. Centers for Disease Control, Division of Reproductive Health, National Center for Chronic Disease Prevention and Health Promotion. (n.d.). *Intimate partner violence, a guide for clinicians.* Atlanta, GA. www.cdc.gov/reproductivehealth/violence/IntimatePartnerViolence/index.htm. Accessed July 19, 2015.

8. Bailey, B. (2010). Partner violence during pregnancy: Prevalence, effects, screening and management. *International Journal of Women's Health, 2,* 183–197.

9. Walker, L. E. (1984). *The battered woman syndrome.* New York, NY: Springer.

10. Author. (2012). Intimate partner violence. ACOG Committee Opinion No. 518. *Obstetrics and Gynecology, 119*(2 pt 1), 412–417.

11. Desphande, N., & Lewis-O'Connor, A. (2013). Screening for intimate partner violence during pregnancy. *Reviews in Obstetrics & Gynecology, 6*(3–4), 141–148.

12. Association of Women's Health, Obstetric, and Neonatal Nurses. (2015). AWHONN Position Statement. Intimate partner violence. *Journal of Obstetric, Gynecologic, and Neonatal Nursing, 44*(3), 405–408.

13. American College of Nurse Midwives. (2013). Violence against women. *Position statement.* Washington, DC.

14. Brigham and Women's Hospital. (2004). *Domestic violence: A guide to screening and intervention.* Boston, MA: Author.

15. Griffin, M. P., & Koss, M. P. (2002, January 31). Clinical screening and intervention in cases of partner violence. *Online Journal of Issues in Nursing, 7*(1), manuscript 2. Retrieved from: www.nursingworld.org/ojin/topic17/tpc17_2.htm

16. Sherin, K. M., Sinacore, J. M., Li, X. Q., et al. (1998). HITS: A short domestic screening tool for use in a family practice setting. *Family Medicine, 30,* 508–512.

17. Soeken, K. L., McFarlane, J., Parker, B., et al. (1998). The abuse assessment screen: A clinical instrument to measure frequency, severity, and perpetrator of abuse against women. In Campbell, J. C. (Ed.), *Empowering survivors of abuse: Health care for battered women and their children* (pp. 195–203). Thousand Oaks, CA: Sage Publications.

18. Alpert, E. J., Freud, K. M., Park, C. C., et al. (1992). *Partner violence: How to recognize and treat victims of abuse.* Waltham: Massachusetts Medical Society.

Care of the Woman Experiencing Operative Vaginal and Cesarean Birth

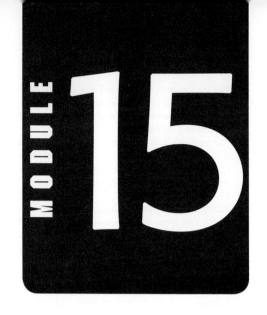

MODULE 15

DONNA R. FRYE AND SARAH BRANAN

Part 1

Operative Vaginal Birth

Part 2

Cesarean Birth

Objectives *As you complete this module, you will learn:*

1. Indications for operative vaginal and cesarean birth
2. Indications and contraindications for operative vaginal birth (vacuum-assisted and forceps-assisted)
3. Risks and benefits of vacuum-assisted and forceps-assisted birth
4. Nursing considerations for operative vaginal and cesarean birth
5. The most common types of forceps and their uses
6. Types of cesarean births
7. Guidelines for identifying appropriate VBAC candidates
8. Indications for and risks of cesarean birth
9. Roles of the nurse during the preoperative, intraoperative, and postoperative period
10. Ways to promote family-centered care for the woman experiencing operative birth

Key Terms *When you have completed this module, you should be able to recall the meaning of the following terms. You should also be able to use the terms when consulting with other health professionals. Terms are defined in this module or in the glossary at the end of this book.*

cephalopelvic disproportion (CPD)
cesarean birth
cesarean delivery upon maternal request
cesarean hysterectomy
classic incision
dystocia
emergency cesarean birth
elective birth
forceps-assisted birth
low-segment transverse incision

low-segment vertical incision
neuraxial anesthesia
operative vaginal birth
primary cesarean birth
repeat cesarean birth
shoulder dystocia
trial of labor (TOL) or trial of labor after cesarean (TOLAC)
vacuum-assisted birth (vacuum extraction)
vaginal birth after cesarean (VBAC)

426

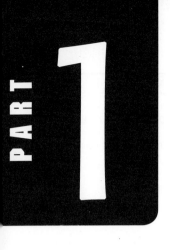

PART 1

Operative Vaginal Birth

Although most women desire and set a goal for spontaneous vaginal birth, complications may arise, necessitating consideration of other options to facilitate birth such as application of forceps or vacuum, or cesarean section. Operative vaginal birth, assisted by vacuum or forceps, is a modification in the mode of delivery implemented by the primary care provider in certain circumstances in order to reduce maternal or fetal risk. While the overall rate of operative vaginal birth has decreased (3.5% of all births), vacuum-assisted births have increased. Vacuum-assisted births account for 4% of all vaginal births, while forceps-assisted births represent 1%.[1]

Vacuum-Assisted Birth (Vacuum Extraction)

Vacuum-assisted birth is achieved by the use of a vacuum cup attached to the fetal head (occiput). Suction is used to create negative pressure developing an artificial caput (chignon), and ensuring a snug fit of the cap onto the head (Fig. 15.1). The birth attendant uses *gentle traction* while the woman actively pushes with contractions to help the fetal head descend and shorten the second stage of labor.

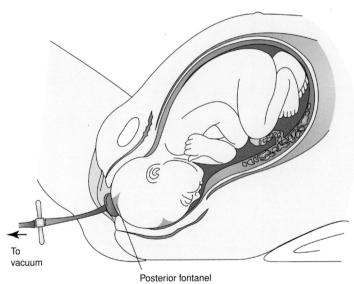

To vacuum

Posterior fontanel

FIGURE 15.1 Vacuum extraction. (From Pillitteri, A. (2007). *Maternal & child health nursing: Care of the childbearing & childrearing family* (5th ed.). Philadelphia, PA: Lippincott Williams & Wilkins.)

- **Why is vacuum used to assist birth?**

Vacuum may be used in a variety of situations. Some of the most common scenarios are summarized in Display 15.1.

For vacuum-assisted birth to be successful[1–3]:
- The fetus must be in a vertex (cephalic) presentation, engaged, with the head position known

---

DISPLAY 15.1 INDICATIONS FOR OPERATIVE VAGINAL BIRTH

Prolonged second stage of labor:
- Nulliparous women—lack of continuous progress for 3 hrs with neuraxial anesthesia or 2 hrs without neuraxial anesthesia
- Multiparous women—lack of continuous progress for 2 hrs with neuraxial anesthesia or 1 hr without neuraxial anesthesia

Fetal compromise
- Immediate or potential which may include, but is not limited to, abruption, category III EFM pattern

Maternal benefit
- Poor pushing effort (secondary to exhaustion, neuraxial anesthesia)
- Cardiac, pulmonary, cerebrovascular, or neurologic disease

From American College of Obstetrics and Gynecologists. (2002; reaffirmed 2012). Practice Bulletin No. 17. Operative vaginal delivery. *Obstetrics & Gynecology, 95*(6).

- The membranes must be ruptured to ensure proper placement
- The woman's cervix should be completely dilated to avoid potential lacerations

Contraindications to vacuum use include[1–3]:
- face or breech presentation
- evidence of CPD as determined by the obstetric provider
- fetal osteogenesis imperfecta
- gestational age less than 34 weeks
- estimated fetal weight less than 2,500 g or greater than 4,000 g
- live fetus with a known bleeding disorder

- **What are the risks of vacuum-assisted birth?**

The newborn commonly experiences cup marks, bruising, and minor lacerations (Fig. 15.2). *These effects are lessened with the use of a soft cup.*[3,4]

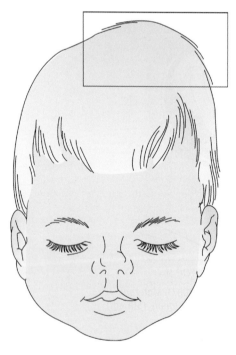

FIGURE 15.2 Caput succedaneum. (From Pillitteri, A. (2007). *Maternal & child health nursing: Care of the childbearing & childrearing family* (5th ed.). Philadelphia, PA: Lippincott Williams & Wilkins.)

Other risks include[1,3]:
- cephalohematoma
- subgaleal hematoma
- retinal hemorrhage
- intracranial hemorrhage
- skull fractures

NOTE: Scalp avulsions, abrasions, blistering, bruising, and other trauma are more likely to occur when the vacuum is applied for a prolonged period of time (longer than 20 minutes) or with excessive suction (maximum pressure force should not be longer than 10 minutes).[5,6]

BE PREPARED: Shoulder dystocia may be more frequently encountered with mid pelvic vacuum extraction and has a higher risk of brachial plexus injury than forceps-assisted or cesarean births.[1]

Maternal complications are rare, but may include pain, bladder trauma, perineal lacerations, and soft tissue injuries to the vulva, vagina, cervix, and anal sphincter.[2,5] Perineal wound infections, vaginal bleeding, uterine atony, and anemia may also result from vacuum-assisted birth.[1,7]

• **What is the nurse's responsibility in a vacuum-assisted birth?**

The nurse's role in a vacuum-assisted birth is twofold: educating the woman and family about the procedure and assisting the provider. Nursing actions are summarized in Display 15.2.

DISPLAY 15.2 NURSING ACTIONS: OPERATIVE VAGINAL BIRTH

1. **Provide the woman and her support person(s) with education about the procedure and prepare her for vaginal birth.**
   • Verify informed consent for instrument use (vacuum, forceps).
   • Place the woman in lithotomy position to provide for optimal traction.
   • Empty the woman's bladder to decrease risk of trauma.
   • Instruct the woman that she will actively push with uterine contractions.
   • Explain to the woman that the baby will probably have a finding of caput succedaneum (Fig. 15.2). This is considered a normal finding and generally resolves within 24 hrs of birth).
2. **Prepare the room for the procedure and assemble necessary equipment and team members.**
   • Assure equipment for neonatal resuscitation is available and in working order.
   • Assure that the provider's preferred instrument is available.
   • Anticipate the need for pain management and have the anesthesiology provider at birth.
   • Alert the neonatal resuscitation team for attendance at birth.
3. **Perform a Time Out**
   • Interprofessional participation to confirm informed consent, provider roles, and fetal positioning.
4. **Attempt assessment of the fetal heart rate (FHR) throughout the procedure and document findings.**
   • Remove internal monitoring devices (fetal scalp electrode, IUPC).
   • If continuous EFM is not used or the tracing is uninterpretable, the FHR should be auscultated and documented every 5 min.
   • Alert the provider to abnormal FHR characteristics.
5. **Be prepared and have a contingency plan for a failed operative vaginal birth.**
   • Alert the charge nurse that the physician is attempting an operative vaginal birth.
   • Determine the capability to perform a cesarean section, if necessary.
6. **Note and document the time of the first application of the vacuum/forceps.**
   • While cup detachment may occur, best practice recommendations state a maximum of 2–3 detachments before the procedure is abandoned.
   • The maximum total time of vacuum application should not exceed 20 minutes, the time of maximum pressure force should not be longer than 10 minutes, and manufacturer's recommendations should be observed.
   • Help the provider maintain situational awareness of time elapsed with discrete prompts regarding time.
   • Steady traction should only be applied during contractions while the woman is actively pushing. The birth should be accomplished without rocking or torque movements by the provider.
7. **Assess the neonate after birth for signs of trauma at the site of the device application.**
   • Continue to observe the infant during the newborn transition period for signs of trauma.
8. **Assess the immediate postpartum woman for signs of perineal trauma, lacerations, or increased bleeding.**
9. **Document all nursing interventions during the birth. (See Module 20 for additional information regarding documentation)**

From American College of Obstetrics and Gynecologists. (2002; reaffirmed 2012). Practice Bulletin No. 17. *Operative vaginal delivery. Obstetrics & Gynecology, 95*(6); Nichols, C. M., Pendlebury, L. C., Jennell, J. (2006). Chart documentation of informed consent for operative vaginal delivery: Is it adequate? *Southern Medical Journal, 99*(12), 1337–1339.

• **What are the advantages of vacuum-assisted birth?**

Vacuum is generally preferred to forceps for operative vaginal birth because it is easier to apply and there is less associated maternal trauma. Provider preference training and frequency of use are also considerations.[5,6]

Forceps-Assisted Birth

Obstetrical forceps are metal blades designed to curve around the fetal head and help to facilitate birth. Forceps are shaped to fit the fetal head and maternal pelvis using blades that are curved to provide the best traction in a variety of situations. The blades are joined with a locking pin, screw, or groove to limit compression of the fetal skull.[2,7,8]

Incidence of forceps-assisted birth varies according to birthing facility and the skill and experience of the provider. The incidence has decreased in the last few decades as providers opt for the use of the vacuum or cesarean section.[7,9]

• Why are forceps used?

Forceps are used for a variety of situations, similar to the indications for use of the vacuum (Display 15.1). Forceps may also be used in cases of malpresentation for rotation of the fetal head. Other indications for use of forceps instead of the vacuum are listed in Display 15.3. Under these conditions, forceps are considered safer than vacuum-assisted birth.[2,6,10,11]

DISPLAY 15.3 SPECIFIC INDICATIONS FOR FORCEPS-ASSISTED BIRTH

- Assisted delivery of the head in a breech delivery
- Face presentation
- Maternal conditions (e.g., cardiac, cerebrovascular, or neurologic conditions)
- Instrumented birth with the woman under general anesthetic
- Cord prolapse in the second stage of labor

From American College of Obstetrics and Gynecologists. (2002; reaffirmed 2012). Practice Bulletin No. 17. *Operative vaginal delivery. Obstetrics & Gynecology, 95*(6).

• What are the advantages of forceps-assisted birth?[1,3,6,7]

Although vacuum-assisted birth is now more common, forceps have some advantages, including:
- decreased failure rate
- expedites vaginal birth at a more rapid rate
- allows the provider to rotate the fetal head to an occiput anterior position to facilitate birth

• What are the classifications of forceps?[1,7]

There are different classifications of forceps applications for use in various situations and are dependent on fetal station.
- *Outlet forceps* are used when the fetal head is visible at the vaginal introitus without separating the labia to guide and control the birth.
- *Low forceps* are used when the leading part of the fetal head is at least +2 station.
- In *midforceps* application, the fetal head is engaged but above +2 station.

Figure 15.3 illustrates the application of outlet forceps on the fetal head. Midforceps application is not frequently done except in emergent situations due to increased maternal and newborn morbidity. However, it may be considered by the physician if it is determined to be a more rapid approach to birth than a cesarean section in an emergent situation.

NOTE: High forceps applications are no longer a part of current obstetric practice due to the incidence of maternal and fetal injury.[2,12]

There are a variety of forceps in use today. The more common types and their uses are found in Display 15.4. As with vacuum-assisted birth, for forceps to be safely attempted, the provider should be knowledgeable and experienced with the type of forceps and credentialed to perform the procedure and a cesarean birth if there is a failed attempt. In addition, the physician must verify the following:
- membranes are ruptured
- cervix is completely dilated
- the fetal head is engaged (Note: this may be difficult if excessive caput is present)
- the fetal head position is known

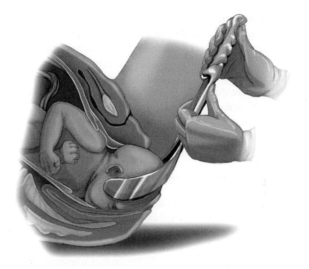

FIGURE 15.3 Forceps-assisted delivery: application of the forceps to the fetal head. (From Orshan, S. A. (2008). *Maternity, newborn, & women's health nursing.* Philadelphia, PA: Lippincott Williams & Wilkins.)

DISPLAY 15.4 TYPE AND USE OF FORCEPS

- Simpson or Elliot forceps are used for outlet vaginal deliveries and are designed for application to the molded fetal head.
- Kielland or Tucker-McLane forceps are used for rotational deliveries and are appropriate for application to the fetal head with little or no molding.
- Piper forceps which have a reverse pelvic curve are used for breech deliveries.

From Wegner, K. A., & Bernstein, I. M. (2014). *Operative vaginal delivery.* Retrieved from: www.uptodate.com; Incerpi, M. (2010). Operative vaginal delivery. In Goodwin, T. A., Montoro, M. N., Muderspach, L., et al. (Eds.), *Management of common problems in obstetric and gynecology* (pp. 41–44). Blackwell Publishing; Simms, R., & Hayman, R. (2013). Instrumented vaginal delivery. *Obstetrics, Gynaecology, and Reproductive Medicine, 23*(9), 270–278.

- the fetal presenting part is vertex (if face presentation, chin should be anterior)
- cephalopelvic disproportion should **not** be suspected by the provider

In preparation for a forceps birth, the nurse should make sure the woman's bladder is empty and she has adequate pain management/anesthesia. If the physician anticipates a potentially difficult attempt, an anesthesiology provider, surgical team, and individuals capable of neonatal resuscitation should be readily available.[1,7,12,13] Nursing considerations in care of the woman undergoing a forceps-assisted birth are similar to those of vacuum-assisted birth. They are summarized in Display 15.2.

Morbidity after forceps-assisted birth is associated with fetal station and the degree of rotation required to effect birth (the higher the station and degree of rotation increases maternal and fetal morbidity). Risks include:
- Fetal/newborn
  - facial nerve palsy
  - intracranial hemorrhage
- Maternal
  - lacerations—vagina, cervix, perineum
  - episiotomy extension
  - uterine atony and postpartum hemorrhage
  - hematoma formation
  - bladder dysfunction and urinary retention
  - fecal incontinence

NOTE: *Notify the primary care provider if the woman develops complications from operative vaginal birth.*[5]

The woman may require more analgesia in the postpartum period and a longer hospital stay than with a spontaneous or vacuum-assisted birth. For additional information regarding immediate postpartum care, review *Module 17.*

Clinical Considerations of Operative Vaginal Birth

If forceps birth is attempted but not achieved, then a cesarean section may be indicated.

While studies are limited, evidence appears to be against multiple attempts to deliver the baby vaginally with different instruments. A failed attempt at vacuum extractions followed by an attempt to deliver with forceps is often associated with an increase in maternal and newborn injury.[1] However, the sequential use of instruments is a provider decision, balancing the risks and benefits of neonatal and maternal morbidity. Each hospital should develop an interprofessional plan of care that addresses when attempts at an operative vaginal birth should be discontinued. Best practice recommendations include[2,12]:

- if the instrument does not apply easily
- The fetus does not descend easily with traction
- The fetus has not been delivered within 15 to 20 minutes of initiation of the operative birth

Nursing Management

The provider and the woman collaborate in decision making about the use of vacuum or forceps to assist in birth.[2,5,7,13] Although the RN is not responsible for obtaining informed consent for a nonemergent operative vaginal birth, verify that informed consent has been completed, and be certain that the woman understands the procedure, alternatives to the procedure, risks, and benefits. Refer to *Module 20* for further clarification for the nurse's role in informed consent. Nursing management includes maternal positioning to optimize alignment and traction, supporting the woman and pushing efforts, and assessment and document. Display 15.2 outlines specific nursing management responsibilities.

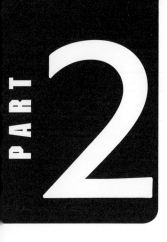

PART 2

Cesarean Birth

Cesarean birth is achieved through a surgical incision in the woman's abdomen. The purpose of the procedure is to preserve the health and well-being of the woman and/or the fetus. The rate of cesarean birth has risen over the last decade, and it is the most commonly performed surgical procedure in women.[14,15]

NOTE: In 2014, the overall cesarean birth rate was 32.2%. This represented greater than a 50% increase from a cesarean rate of 20.7% in 1996. This increase in the cesarean section rate has not demonstrated an improvement in maternal–newborn outcomes.[16]

• Why has the cesarean birth rate increased?

Reasons for the increase in cesarean birth rates are varied but are known to be associated with the following[13,17–19]:
1. Increased fear of litigation on the part of healthcare providers
2. Increased use of electronic fetal monitoring (EFM) with decreased tolerance of suspected fetal compromise in labor
3. Decreased tolerance of risks associated with breech, twin, operative vaginal birth, potential macrosomic infant, and TOLAC birth
4. Increased safety of anesthesia and operative care (use of antibiotics and availability of blood products)
5. Increased numbers of high-risk pregnancies
6. Theory that pelvic floor damage is related to labor and birth resulting in future urinary and fecal incontinence
7. Attempts to increase the woman's autonomy in decision-making about the mode of birth
8. Increased number of labor inductions
9. Increased use of neuraxial anesthesia, increased number of repeat cesarean births
10. Increased maternal body mass

NOTE: Many factors contributing to the increase in the cesarean birth rate are interrelated.

In recent years, there have been a number of initiatives to promote physiologic birth and decrease the primary cesarean birth rate. Many initiatives involve education of women *and* healthcare providers. Selected considerations for women and the interprofessional healthcare team that may have an impact are summarized in Display 15.5.

Lowering the incidence of cesarean births is a complex issue. Professional organizations, regulatory agencies, and payers have recently focused on reducing primary cesarean births as a strategy to decrease the overall cesarean section rate, maternal morbidity and mortality. Reduction of primary cesarean birth will require a change in current provider knowledge, skill and management of multiple gestations, fetal malpresentation, labor dystocia, potential macrosomia, and indeterminant or abnormal fetal heart tracings. While some organizations have published an "ideal" cesarean section rate there is no evidence to support an "ideal cesarean section rate" at this time.[20]

DISPLAY 15.5 EFFORTS TO REDUCE THE CESAREAN BIRTH RATE

Women and family considerations for promotion of physiologic birth[13,15,20,21]:
- Home environment for latent or early labor
- Reasons for admission to the hospital or birth center
- Techniques for coping and managing pain during labor and birth
- Facts about trial of labor and VBAC
- Advantages of vaginal birth
- The importance of choosing a care provider
- Development of a personal birth plan and discussion and agreement of plan with provider and care team

Interprofessional considerations for promotion of physiologic birth:
- Development of admission criteria
- The importance of assessments in determining labor status
- Individualized rationale for labor interventions
- Avoidance of automatic interventions
- Support of "one-on-one" care during labor
- Support and encouragement of positioning and nonpharmacologic pain relief measures
- Establishment of criteria for elective cesarean birth and trial of labor

From Piotrowski, K. (2012). Labor and birth complications. In Lowdermilk, D. L., Perry, S. E., Cashion, K., et al. (Eds.), *Maternity and women's health care* (10th ed., pp. 806–814). St. Louis, MO: Elsevier Mosby; Edmonds, J. (2014). Clinical indications associated with primary cesarean birth. *Nursing for Women's Health, 18*(3), 243–249; Caughey, A. B., Cahill, A. G., Guise, J. M., et al. (2014). Safe prevention of the primary cesarean section. *American Journal of Obstetrics and Gynecology, 210*(3), 179–193; Gei, A. (2012). Prevention of the first cesarean delivery: The role of operative vaginal delivery. *Seminars in Perinatology, 36*(5), 365–373.

• **What are the different types of cesarean birth?**

There are two types of cesarean surgical techniques.

1. The **classic incision** is made on the upper part of the uterus in the vertical midline (Fig. 15.4A). The classic incision is rarely used, except in an emergency situations requiring extremely quick access to the fetus or if alternate access to the fetus is needed (placental location, fetal presentation).

2. **Low-segment cesarean** may be done with either a **low transverse or low vertical incision** (Fig. 15.4B,C).

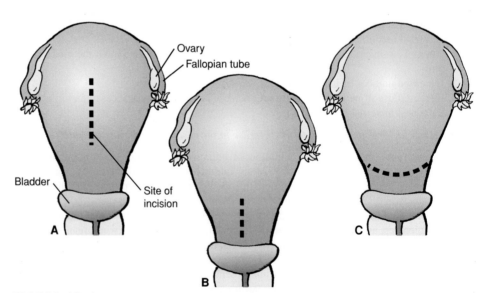

FIGURE 15.4 Cesarean birth uterine incisions. **A.** Classic. **B.** Low vertical. **C.** Low transverse. (From Orshan, S. A. (2008). *Maternity, newborn, & women's health nursing.* Philadelphia, PA: Lippincott Williams & Wilkins.)

NOTE: The incision that is visually apparent on the woman's skin may not be the incision on the uterus!

The low transverse incision is the most common incision for the following reasons.[13]
1. The incision is easier to perform and repair.
2. Less risk of uterine rupture in future pregnancies. (Lower uterine segment is less contractile.)
3. Less associated blood loss and postoperative infection.
4. The scar may be hidden in the pubic hair.

A *cesarean hysterectomy*, removal of the uterus after delivery of the fetus, may be performed in an obstetric emergency such as uterine hemorrhage, uterine rupture, placenta previa, or placenta accreta. Such conditions are rare.[22]

NOTE: Placenta accreta is an abnormal adherence of the placenta to the myometrium that may result in risks of prematurity for the fetus and severe hemorrhage for the woman. For additional information regarding abnormal placentation, refer to Module 16.

> **Important Terms**
> **Primary cesarean**—a woman's first cesarean birth.
> **Repeat elective cesarean**—a subsequent cesarean birth in the absence of any obstetric or maternal medical indications.

Cesarean Birth Upon Maternal Request

There is a growing rate of elective cesarean births for which there are no clear medical or obstetric indications.[14] These procedures, commonly referred to as "maternal choice" cesareans, are done primarily for convenience and pose ethical concerns for some care providers. Reasons offered for maternal choice cesarean section may include the ability to schedule the timing of the birth, decrease the risk of future maternal pelvic floor problems, fear of labor (pain, complications), and desire for control. Rationale for an elective cesarean section should be highly individualized. It is imperative that the woman and her provider discuss risks of a surgical procedure versus the natural process of birth, including the woman's desire for future pregnancies and potential for increased morbidity and mortality. The procedure should be performed after 39 weeks' gestation and the decision for an elective cesarean should not be based upon concern by the woman that pain medication will not be available.[20,25]

Indications/Risks for Cesarean Birth

Labor and birth complications are the most common reasons for cesarean birth. Relative contraindications include a nonviable fetus or a dead fetus. In these cases the maternal risks of surgery cannot be justified unless expedited removal of the fetus would improve maternal outcomes (e.g., maternal cardiopulmonary arrest, suspected amniotic fluid embolus) or if the woman was unable to deliver the newborn by vaginal birth (e.g., fetal malpresentation, provider diagnoses CPD).

• **What are the indications for a cesarean birth?[5,14]**

Cephalopelvic disproportion (CPD)—CPD is defined as an inadequate maternal pelvis in relation to the fetal head. CPD is a clinical diagnosis made by a physician and may be considered with a diagnosis of fetal macrosomia (estimated birth weight greater than 4,500 g in a woman with diabetes and at least 5,000 g in women without diabetes).

Fetal malpresentation—(see Module 2) Transverse and shoulder presentations make vaginal birth difficult and potentially dangerous. Vaginal breech delivery attempts are dependent on the skill and experience of the provider, fetal presentation, and estimated fetal weight.

Labor dystocia—Labor dystocia may be associated with CPD or fetal malpresentation, but can also include inadequate, ineffective uterine contractions and incomplete cervical dilatation without fetal descent (failure to progress, or failed induction). Soft tissue dystocia or obstructed labor due to excessive maternal adipose tissue or tumors may also necessitate a cesarean birth.

Changes in fetal status—May indicate that the fetus is not well oxygenated and thus requires careful evaluation and possible surgical intervention. See *Module 7* for EFM interpretation.

Congenital fetal anomalies—Some fetal anomalies such as conjoined twins and gastroschisis require controlled birth and immediate intervention by neonatal staff.

Obstetric indications—Umbilical cord prolapse, placenta previa, abruptio placentae, multiple gestation, uterine rupture, and hemorrhage are conditions which **may** contraindicate vaginal birth and require a rapid birth depending upon maternal and fetal status.

Maternal medical indications—Active herpes lesions, uterine or vaginal abnormalities, may require a surgical birth.

• What are the maternal and fetal risks of a cesarean birth?

Although cesarean birth seems to have been "normalized" as a viable birth option, it is a major surgical procedure and not without risks and complications. Display 15.6 outlines risks of cesarean birth. Cesarean birth may be of benefit to newborns and women and, in certain circumstances, has actually improved neonatal outcomes.[21]

DISPLAY 15.6 MATERNAL RISKS IN CESAREAN BIRTH

Anesthetic complications (aspiration, airway maintenance, and respiratory failure)
Laceration and injury to bowel, bladder
Hemorrhage
Wound complications (dehiscence)
Infection (uterine, bladder)
Thromboembolic complications
Increased risk for placenta previa, placenta accreta, and uterine rupture in subsequent pregnancies
Increased length of stay in the hospital
Increased costs
Increased chance of rehospitalization
Impaired maternal–newborn interaction (related to pain, fatigue, medication effects, difficulty breastfeeding)
Disruption of support network
Increased recuperation time
Negative emotional consequences of failure to achieve vaginal birth (anger, depression, grief, lowered self-esteem, altered body image, psychosomatic symptoms)

From Menon, J. R. (2000). Soft versus rigid vacuum cups for assisted vaginal delivery. *Cochrane Database of Systematic Reviews,* *2000*(2):CD000446; Piotrowski, K. (2012). Labor and birth complications. In Lowdermilk, D. L., Perry, S. E., Cashion, K., et al. (Eds.), *Maternity and women's health care* (10th ed., pp. 806–814). St. Louis, MO: Elsevier Mosby.

Neonatal risks include respiratory problems such as delays in neonatal transition, transient tachypnea, mild respiratory distress syndrome (RDS), iatrogenic prematurity (if gestational age is not certain), and lacerations occurring during surgery.[13]

Anesthesia for Cesarean Birth

• What type of anesthesia is used for a cesarean birth?[13]

Anesthesia selection for cesarean birth depends on the woman's current status, medical history, fetal status, and urgency of the procedure. The majority of women who undergo cesarean birth are administered neuraxial anesthesia (spinal, epidural, or combined spinal epidural block).

Neuraxial Anesthesia

- Has a lower risk of airway problems.
- Allows the woman to be awake and aware during the birth experience.
- Allows the woman to communicate with her support person and interact with her newborn immediately after birth, including initiation of skin-to-skin.

General endotracheal anesthesia is usually reserved for emergent problems requiring immediate delivery or in cases of maternal conditions that contraindicate neuraxial anesthesia.

NOTE: Fetal cord blood gases collected at a cesarean birth can demonstrate a lower pH in women administered with neuraxial anesthesia, but infants born to women under general endotracheal anesthesia may have lower Apgar scores.[13]

Nursing Considerations for Care of the Woman Undergoing Cesarean Birth

The nurse involved in the care of the woman experiencing a cesarean birth may assume varied roles. Most often, it is the labor nurse who prepares the woman, is in the operating room with the woman, and cares for her in the immediate postoperative period. In the operating room, this nurse is referred to as the *circulating nurse*. A nurse may also function as the *surgical nurse*. The surgical nurse is "scrubbed in," prepares the instruments and supplies, and assists the surgeon during the procedure with sterile instruments, sutures, and supplies. In addition, some obstetric nurses have expanded their practice to include first assisting skills with cesarean birth.[26] The first assistant:

- is knowledgeable about the procedure and the sequence of events
- is skilled at instrument handling and sterile technique
- communicates clearly and effectively with the surgical team
- provides adequate exposure and visualization of the surgical site while handling tissues safely
- assists with birth of the fetus and placenta
- assists with the repair of the surgical incision

Education and certification for first assistants varies according to state law, certifying agency, and institutional requirements.

Planned, Unanticipated, and Emergent Cesarean Births

Nursing care may need to be modified depending on whether the cesarean is planned, unanticipated, or emergent. If the procedure is planned (elective or scheduled), then the woman and family can be prepared with teaching. If the procedure is unanticipated or emergent, every attempt should be made to keep the woman and family informed, and allow her the opportunity to express concerns, ask questions, and make decisions as applicable.

In the event of an emergent cesarean birth, efforts are made to deliver the baby as quickly and safely as possible. During this time, many essential nursing tasks must be accomplished, yet communication with the woman and her family (or support person), the surgeon, anesthesiology, OR, and neonatal teams is of the utmost importance. The woman may have overwhelming stress and anxiety about the emergency procedure and for the safety of her baby. Expect to spend time after the procedure talking with the woman and her family about the events that led to the emergency situation.[5,13,15]

NOTE: The physician determines how quickly a cesarean section needs to be completed and jointly determines the plan of care with the woman, nursing, anesthesiology, and operative teams.

Phases of Nursing Care

- **What are the nursing responsibilities during a cesarean birth?**

To provide care to the woman undergoing a cesarean birth, principles of obstetric and surgical nursing care must be combined. Nursing care responsibilities during cesarean birth can be divided into three parts—preoperative, intraoperative, and postoperative.[5] These responsibilities are outlined in Display 15.7.

NOTE: The standards of care for the surgical and recovery areas in the birth setting are the same as those of the operating suites and PACU in a hospital! [5,13,24]

Family-Centered Care

- **How can the woman's family be involved in a cesarean birth?**

The woman and her family should be offered the same opportunities for participation in the birth and bonding with the newborn if the cesarean section is scheduled or unplanned without

---

DISPLAY 15.7 NURSING CONSIDERATIONS DURING
CESAREAN BIRTH

Preoperative Care
- Complete initial assessment per unit guidelines.
- Determine the last time the woman ate or drank.
- Verify that physician has obtained informed consent and the woman has signed the form.
- Initiate 20- to 30-minute baseline fetal heart rate tracing per EFM. If in active labor or tracing is not reassuring then continue monitoring until abdomen is scrubbed and prepped or provide fetal heart monitoring per unit policy.
- Initiate preoperative teaching for the woman, support person, and family about expected care, procedures, and noises before, during, and after the operative birth.
- Insert an intravenous line, at least 18 gauge, or ensure patency of existing line and initiate fluids.
- Draw and send ordered preoperative labs; view results prior to OR and notify obstetric physician and anesthesiology team of abnormal values.
- Clip abdominal and pubic hair as needed and indicated.
- Insert an indwelling Foley catheter; delay until after placement and dosing of neuraxial anesthesia, if possible.
- Administer ordered antibiotic 1 hr prior to incision (as determined by urgency of ordered cesarean birth). If cesarean birth follows labor or is ordered emergent, antibiotics may given by the anesthesiology team during the procedure.
- Gather appropriate maternal/newborn identification bracelets.
- Administer ordered preoperative medications including antithrombotic agents as indicated by risk factors.
- Complete preoperative briefing.
- Safely transport the woman to the OR suite.
- Document according to unit guidelines.

Intraoperative Care
- Assist with transfer to the OR table.
- Place the woman in a lateral position with uterine displacement utilizing a hip wedge.
- Remove intrauterine fetal and uterine monitoring devices prior to abdominal prep.
- Continue EFM until abdomen is prepped.
- Apply sequential compression stockings and turn on the device.
- Ensure appropriate placement and securing of the woman's arms on arm boards.
- Align the woman's legs and secure with appropriate restraint.
- Apply appropriate grounding device according to manufacturer's recommendations (NOTE: some ORs use a grounding pad under the patient).
- Scrub and prepare abdomen according to unit guidelines.
- Connect the suction and electrocautery units according to manufacturer's recommendations and set to the provider's preferred settings.
- Ensure that neonatal resuscitation equipment is in working order and all supplies are available.
- Notify other healthcare and surgical team members, neonatal staff as necessary to be present for birth.
- Position the woman's support person at the head of the OR table, behind the sterile screening drape.
- Assist with gowning and gloving of the surgical team as needed.
- Perform initial and subsequent sponge, needle, and instrument counts according to unit guidelines.
- Participate in OR "time out" to correctly identify woman, purpose, procedure, and participants.
- Document the events of surgery including: time the cesarean section was ordered, in room time; anesthesia start time; surgeon in room time; surgery start time incision, time of birth; time the surgery was completed; time the surgeon left the room; time the woman left the room.
- Encourage the woman and her support person.
- Support and assist surgical and anesthesia staff as needed.
- Support and assist neonatal staff as needed.
- Obtain umbilical cord blood samples and other pathology specimens such as the placenta, as ordered.
- Complete postoperative debriefing.
- Assist with placement of abdominal dressing.
- Note maternal and newborn status before transport to postanesthesia recovery unit (PACU).
- Safely transport the woman to the PACU.
- Document according to unit guidelines.

Postoperative Care
- Ensure that proper PACU equipment is available and functional.
- Perform and document postoperative assessments according to unit guidelines.
- Initial and ongoing assessments to include:
  - *Vital signs* and postpartum assessments per provider order and unit guidelines.
  - *Respiratory status:* airway patency, oxygen saturation, oxygen needs, rate, quality and depth of respirations, and auscultation of lungs.
  - *Circulatory status:* blood pressure, pulse, ECG, and skin color.

display continues on page 439

- *Level of consciousness:* orientation to person, place and time, response to stimulation.
- *Obstetric status:* position, height and tone of fundus, abdominal dressing, amount and color of lochia, maternal–newborn attachment, breastfeeding desires.
- *Motor status:* Level of sensation, movement and regression of anesthesia.
- *Intake and output:* intravenous fluids, urine output, and estimated blood loss.
- *Pain assessment:* report of pain; pharmacologic and nonpharmacologic interventions, and reassessment of pain.
- Encourage and facilitate interaction and closeness for the new family after birth including skin-to-skin care and early initiation of breastfeeding (within 1 hour) as per the woman's desires and condition.
- Discharge from PACU care after recovery period is complete, in collaboration with anesthesiology provider and obstetric physician, when the woman is stable and according to unit guidelines.
- Document according to unit guidelines.

NOTE: For additional information regarding postoperative care, refer to the *Module 17* on care of the woman during the immediate postpartum period.

From Simpson, K. R., & O'Brien-Abel, N. (2014). Labor and birth. In Simpson, K. A., & Creehan, P. A. (Eds.), *Perinatal nursing* (4th ed., pp. 403–425). Philadelphia, PA: Lippincott; Piotrowski, K. (2012). Labor and birth complications. In Lowdermilk, D. L., Perry, S. E., Cashion, K., et al. (Eds.), *Maternity and women's health care* (10th ed., pp. 806–814). St. Louis, MO: Elsevier Mosby; Association of Women's Health Obstetric and Neonatal Nurses. (2011). *Perioperative care of the pregnant woman: Evidenced based guidelines*. Washington, DC: Author.

anticipated maternal or fetal compromise.[5,12,13,25] Concepts of family-centered care during cesarean birth include:

- Have the support person present for education about the cesarean birth. Some units provide a video clip of a family-centered cesarean birth.
- Provide calming music in the OR for relaxation.
- Allow attendance of the support person at administration of neuraxial anesthesia and the cesarean birth. The support person is allowed to sit at the woman's head in the surgical suite behind the sterile screening drape.
- Place the blood pressure cuff on the woman's nondominant arm and ECG leads on the woman's back or laterally to allow for skin-to-skin contact without interference with maternal monitoring.
- Free the woman's dominant arm from arm board.
- If the woman desires, drop the surgical drape or have a clear plastic panel drape to allow the woman and support person to watch the birth.
- Immediately place the baby skin-to-skin on the woman's chest. If the woman is unable to provide skin-to-skin contact for any reason, consider initiation of skin-to-skin with the support person.
- Delay cord clamping to facilitate autotransfusion and increase newborn iron stores.
- Assessment of the newborn on the woman's chest by a nurse dedicated to the newborn care.
- Early initiation of breastfeeding (within 1 hour).
- Maintain skin-to-skin with transfer to PACU and during postoperative recovery.

While a cesarean birth experience may not be what the woman expected or desired, it can still be a positive and meaningful experience with family-centered nursing care, support, and education.

Vaginal Birth After Cesarean

• What is a VBAC?

Vaginal birth after cesarean (VBAC) has been a topic of much discussion since the 1980s. It was once thought that "once a cesarean, always a cesarean" due to the risk of uterine rupture with subsequent labor and birth. However, with data that indicate increased maternal morbidity and mortality of cesarean compared to vaginal birth, along with complications of repeated surgeries and subsequent pregnancies, consideration of VBAC is on the rise. Studies demonstrate a VBAC success rate of 60% to 80%.[23] VBAC is considered an accepted part of obstetric practice, with careful maternal selection, monitoring, and management.[23] Appropriate selection for **a trial of labor after a previous cesarean birth (TOLAC)** is paramount. The woman should have no other contraindications to labor and birth **and the provider should consider the following general criteria**[23,24]:

Knowledge of Prior Uterine Incisions

- A low-segment transverse uterine incision has the lowest risk of uterine rupture.
- A woman with no more than two prior low transverse cesarean births may attempt a TOLAC.
- A previous classic fundal uterine incision is a contraindication for TOL.
- The maternal pelvis should be clinically adequate, with no history of prior uterine rupture.

Setting for Delivery with TOLAC

- There must be an ability to perform an immediate **emergency cesarean birth** if needed.
- Appropriate surgical and anesthesiology staff must be available.
- Due to potential uterine rupture and subsequent blood loss, blood products should be readily available.
- Due to potential neonatal compromise, neonatal resuscitation staff must be readily available.
- With multiple cesarean births, the risk for placental implantation abnormalities including placenta previa and placenta accreta increases dramatically.[23] Placental implantation should be determined prior to birth. If a placental implantation abnormality is suspected, the birth should occur in a facility that has defined systems and processes in place to care for the woman and newborn.

Future family planning should be discussed with the woman when the risks and benefits of VBAC are discussed. Factors associated with VBAC success include:

- history of a previous vaginal birth with spontaneous, augmented, or induced labor.

OR

- the woman presents in spontaneous labor with this pregnancy.

Frequently Asked Questions about TOLAC and VBAC

- **Can a woman attempting trial of labor and vaginal birth after cesarean have labor induced?**

Induction of labor for maternal or fetal indications remains an option in appropriately selected and counseled women who desire to achieve a VBAC section. However, a woman undergoing labor induction or augmentation is less apt to be successful with a VBAC when compared to a woman of the same gestational age who begins labor spontaneously and is not augmented.[23]

NOTE: EXTREME CAUTION SHOULD BE USED IN MANAGING THE WOMAN WHO IS ATTEMPTING A VBAC WITH INDUCTION OR AUGMENTATION OF LABOR. EXCESSIVE USE OF OXYTOCIN AND UTERINE TACHYSYSTOLE SHOULD BE AVOIDED. The nurse is the primary care giver at the bedside and must be knowledgeable of guidelines for oxytocin management: competent with oxytocin administration; and vigilant with monitoring of the woman attempting an induced or augmented TOL. Charge nurses should make assignments and adjust staffing based on patient volume and acuity.[5]

- **Is a woman who has had two or more prior cesarean births a candidate for a TOLAC?**

Appropriately selected and counseled women with two previous low transverse cesarean births may be considered candidates for TOLAC.[23]

- **Is a woman with twins a candidate for TOLAC?**

Women with a twin pregnancy who have had one previous cesarean with a low transverse incision and who are appropriate candidates may be allowed a trail of labor.[23]

Nursing Considerations for Care of the Woman Undergoing VBAC

- Current opinion, based on the available literature and evidence, is that women with a history of a previous cesarean birth should have continuous electronic fetal monitoring [EFM] since the earliest indication of uterine rupture is an abnormal fetal heart tracing.[5,13,20]

- If the woman is undergoing cervical ripening, this should be done in an inpatient as opposed to an outpatient setting.
- There is no need for an intrauterine pressure catheter (IUPC) to be placed simply because the woman is attempting a VBAC. *IUPCs should be used for obstetric indications and do not provide evidence of uterine rupture.*
- VBAC attempt is not a contraindication for neuraxial anesthesia. However, the nurse should be aware *that pain associated with a uterine rupture may be masked or atypical in presentation.* Signs of uterine rupture are discussed in *Module 16.*

PRACTICE/REVIEW QUESTIONS

After reviewing this module, answer the following questions.

1. What constitutes an operative birth?

_____

_____

_____

2. For a woman undergoing an operative birth, the intrapartum nurse provides education to the woman and her support person about the procedure and prepares them for birth.

   a. True

   b. False

3. The nurse's role in an operative vaginal birth is to obtain informed consent.

   a. True

   b. False

For questions 4 through 13, match the following terms with the correct answer.

a. forceps
b. vacuum
c. outlet forceps
d. low forceps
e. midforceps

f. Simpson of Elliot forceps
g. Kielland or Tucker-McLane forceps
h. Piper forceps
i. 20 minutes
j. 10 minutes

4. Used when the leading part of the fetal head is at +2 station

5. Metal blades designed to curve around the fetal head and help facilitate birth

6. Used for outlet vaginal birth

7. A cup with a suction device attached that is placed on the fetal head to form a seal which will provide gentle traction to facilitate birth of the fetal head

8. Used for breech birth

9. Used when fetal head is visible at the vaginal introitus without separating the labia to guide and control birth

10. Used when the fetal head is engaged but above +2 station

11. Used for rotational birth

12. The maximum total time of vacuum application should not exceed

13. The time of maximum pressure force from vacuum application should not exceed

14. List the indications for the use of vacuum extraction or forceps.

    a. _____

    b. _____

    c. _____

    d. _____

15. List the conditions for which vacuum or forceps can be used.

    a. _____

    b. _____

    c. _____

    d. _____

16. List five contraindications for vacuum use.

    a. _____

    b. _____

    c. _____

    d. _____

    e. _____

17. List the more common risks to the fetus from a vacuum-assisted birth.

    a. _____

    b. _____

    c. _____

18. List five of the more serious risks to the fetus using a vacuum to assist with birth.

    a. _____

    b. _____

    c. _____

    d. _____

    e. _____

19. During a vacuum-assisted delivery if EFM is NOT being used the nurse should auscultate and document the FHR every 10 minutes.

    a. True

    b. False

20. The advantages of using a vacuum as opposed to forceps include _____ and _____.

21. List three things that the nurse should include in the documentation during an operative vaginal birth.

    a. _____

    b. _____

    c. _____

22. List nursing actions during a vacuum-assisted birth.

    a. _____

    b. _____

    c. _____

    d. _____

    e. _____

23. List possible maternal complications from a vacuum-assisted birth.

    a. _____

    b. _____

    c. _____

    d. _____

    e. _____

24. List three indications for when a forceps delivery is considered safer than vacuum-assisted birth.

    a. _____

    b. _____

    c. _____

25. After a delivery using forceps, the neonate should be assessed for:

    a. _____

    b. _____

    c. _____

26. After forceps-assisted birth, the woman should be assessed for:

    a. _____

    b. _____

    c. _____

    d. _____

    e. _____

27. State the purpose of a cesarean birth.

    _____

28. List five possible reasons for the increase in cesarean birth rate.

    a. _____

    b. _____

    c. _____

d. _____

e. _____

29. List three indications for a cesarean birth.

    a. _____

    b. _____

    c. _____

30. List five maternal risks of cesarean birth.

    a. _____

    b. _____

    c. _____

    d. _____

    e. _____

31. List three neonatal risks of cesarean birth.

    a. _____

    b. _____

    c. _____

32. List four of the advantages of using neuraxial anesthesia for a cesarean birth.

    a. _____

    b. _____

    c. _____

    d. _____

33. A low-segment transverse uterine incision has the highest risk of uterine rupture.

    a. True

    b. False

34. Factors associated with VBAC success include _____ and _____.

PRACTICE/REVIEW ANSWER KEY

1. Operative birth includes cesarean birth and vaginal birth assisted by vacuum or forceps.
2. a. True
3. b. False
4. d. Low forceps
5. a. Forceps
6. f. Simpson or Elliot forceps
7. b. Vacuum
8. h. Piper forceps
9. c. Outlet forceps
10. e. Midforceps
11. g. Kielland or Tucker-McLane forceps
12. i. 20 minutes
13. j. 10 minutes
14. a. Prolonged second stage of labor
    b. Change in fetal status
    c. Poor pushing effort (secondary to exhaustion or analgesia/anesthesia)

d. Maternal conditions (cardiac, pulmonary, cerebrovascular, or neurologic disease)

15. a. Vertex presentation
    b. Engaged with the fetal head position known
    c. Membranes must be ruptured
    d. Woman's cervix should be completely dilated
    e. Woman's bladder should be empty

16. a. Face or breech presentation
    b. Several maternal or fetal compromise requiring rapid delivery
    c. Evidence of CPD
    d. Fetal osteogenesis imperfecta
    e. Gestational age less than 34 weeks
    f. Bleeding disorders

17. a. Cup marks
    b. Bruising
    c. Minor lacerations

18. a. Cephalohematoma
    b. Subgaleal hematoma
    c. Retinal hemorrhage
    d. Intracranial hemorrhage
    e. Skull fractures

19. b. False

20. a. Easier to apply
    b. Less associated maternal trauma

21. a. FHR throughout the procedure
    b. The time of the first application of the vacuum or forceps
    c. A report to neonatal care staff that a vacuum or forceps was used during delivery

22. a. Providing education to woman and support person about the procedure and prepare her for vaginal birth.
    b. Prepare the room for the procedure, assemble the necessary equipment, and support the birth attendant as needed.
    c. Assess the fetal heart rate throughout the procedure.
    d. Be prepared for emergent operative birth, if necessary.
    e. Note and document the time of the first application of the vacuum.

23. a. Pain
    b. Extension of episiotomy
    c. Bladder trauma
    d. Perineal lacerations
    e. Soft tissue injuries to the vulva, vagina, cervix, and anal sphincter

24. Any three of the following:
    a. Assisted birth of the head in breech birth
    b. Preterm fetus
    c. Face presentation
    d. Suspected coagulopathy or thrombocytopenia of the fetus
    e. Maternal conditions that prohibit pushing
    f. Instrumented delivery with the woman under general anesthesia
    g. Cord prolapse in the second stage of labor
    h. Controlled delivery of the head during cesarean section

25. a. Bruising or abrasions at the site of application
    b. Cerebral or ocular trauma or skull fracture
    c. Nerve damage (facial palsy)

26. a. Vaginal and cervical lacerations
    b. Bruising
    c. Hematoma
    d. Increased bleeding
    e. Urinary retention from bladder trauma

27. To preserve the health and well-being of the woman or the fetus

28. Any five of the following:
    a. Increased use of EFM with decreased tolerance of fetal compromise in labor
    b. Decreased tolerance of fetal risks associated with potentially hazardous birth
    c. Increased safety of anesthesia and operative care
    d. Increased numbers of high-risk pregnancies
    e. Potential pelvic floor damage related to labor and birth
    f. Urinary and fecal incontinence
    g. Increased respect for the woman's autonomy in decision making about the mode of birth
    h. Increased numbers of labor inductions
    i. Increased use of regional anesthesia
    j. Increased number of repeat cesarean births
    k. Increased fear of litigation

29. Any three of the following:
    a. Cephalopelvic disproportion
    b. Fetal malpresentation
    c. Labor dystocia
    d. Abnormal fetal tracing
    e. Congenital fetal anomalies
    f. Obstetric indications
    g. Maternal medical indications

30. Any five of the following:
    1. Anesthetic complications
    2. Laceration and injury to bowel or bladder
    3. Hemorrhage
    4. Wound complications
    5. Infection
    6. Thromboembolic complications
    7. Increased risk for placenta previa, placenta accreta, and uterine rupture in subsequent pregnancies
    8. Increased length of hospital stay
    9. Increased costs
    10. Increased chance of rehospitalization
    11. Impaired maternal–newborn interaction
    12. Disruption of support network
    13. Increased recuperation time
    14. Negative emotional consequences of failure to achieve vaginal birth

31. a. Respiratory problems
    b. Iatrogenic prematurity
    c. Lacerations occurring during surgery

32. a. Lower risk of airway problems
    b. Allows the woman to be awake and aware of the birth experience
    c. The woman is able to communicate with her support person
    d. The woman is able to interact with her newborn after birth

33. b. False

34. History of previous vaginal birth with spontaneous, augmented, or induced labor; current pregnancy presenting in spontaneous labor

REFERENCES

1. Wegner, K. A., & Bernstein, I. M. (2014). *Operative vaginal delivery.* Retrieved from: www.uptodate.com
2. American College of Obstetrics and Gynecologists. (2002; reaffirmed 2012). Practice Bulletin No. 17. Operative vaginal delivery. *Obstetrics & Gynecology, 95*(6), 1–8.
3. Ali, U. A., & Norwitz, E. R. (2009). Vacuum-assisted vaginal delivery. *Reviews in Obstetrics and Gynecology, 2*(1), 5–17.
4. Menon, J. R. (2000). Soft versus rigid vacuum cups for assisted vaginal delivery. *Cochrane Database of Systematic Reviews, 2000*(2):CD000446.
5. Simpson, K. R., & O'Brien-Abel, N. (2014). Labor and birth. In Simpson, K. A., & Creehan, P. A. (Eds.), *Perinatal nursing* (4th ed., pp. 403–425). Philadelphia, PA: Lippincott.
6. Vacca, A. (2006). Vacuum-assisted delivery: An analysis of traction force and maternal and neonatal outcomes. *Australian and New Zealand Journal of Obstetrics and Gynecology, 46*, 124–127.
7. Incerpi, M. (2010). Operative vaginal delivery. In Goodwin, T. A., Montoro, M. N., Muderspach, L., et al. (Eds.), *Management of common problems in obstetric and gynecology* (pp. 41–44). Oxford, UK: Blackwell Publishing.
8. Nichols, C. M., Pendlebury, L. C., & Jennell, J. (2006). Chart documentation of informed consent for operative vaginal delivery: Is it adequate? *Southern Medical Journal, 99*(12), 1337–1339.
9. Yoemans, E. R. (2010). Operative vaginal delivery. *Obstetrics & Gynecology, 115*(3), 645–653.
10. Patel, R. R., & Murphy, D. J. (2004). Forceps delivery in modern clinical practice. *British Medical Journal, 328*, 1302–1305.
11. Simms, R., & Hayman, R. (2013). Instrumented vaginal delivery. *Obstetrics, Gynaecology, and Reproductive Medicine, 23*(9), 270–278.
12. American Academy of Pediatrics and American College of Obstetrics and Gynecologists. (2012). *Guidelines for perinatal care* (7th ed.). Elk Grove Village, IL: Author.
13. Piotrowski, K. (2012). Labor and birth complications. In Lowdermilk, D. L., Perry, S. E., Cashion, K., et al. (Eds.), *Maternity and women's health care* (10th ed., pp. 806–814). St. Louis, MO: Elsevier Mosby.
14. Clark, S. L., Belfort, M. A., Hankins, G. V., et al. (2007). Variation in the rates of operative delivery in the United States. *American Journal of Obstetrics & Gynecology, 196*(526), e1–e5.
15. Edmonds, J. (2014). Clinical indications associated with primary cesarean birth. *Nursing for Women's Health, 18*(3), 243–249.
16. Hamilton, B. A., Martin, J. A., Osterman, M. J., et al. (2015). *Births: Preliminary data for 2014* [National vital statistics reports; vol 64. No. 6]. Hyattsville, MD: National Center for Health Statistics.
17. Zhang, J., Troendle, J., Reddy, U. M., et al. (2010). Contemporary cesarean delivery practice in the United States. *American Journal of Obstetrics and Gynecology, 203*(326), e1–e10.
18. Marshall, N. E., Fu, R., & Guise, J. M. (2011). Impact of multiple cesarean deliveries on maternal morbidity: A systematic review. *American Journal of Obstetrics & Gynecology, 205*(262), e1–e8.
19. Walker, S. P., McCarthy, E. A., Ugoni, A., et al. (2007). Cesarean delivery or vaginal birth: A survey of patient and clinician thresholds. *Obstetrics and Gynecology, 109*(1), 67–72.
20. Gei, A. (2012). Prevention of the first cesarean delivery: The role of operative vaginal delivery. *Seminars in Perinatology, 36*(5), 365–373.
21. Caughey, A. B., Cahill, A. G., Guise, J. M., et al. (2014). Safe prevention of the primary cesarean section. *American Journal of Obstetrics and Gynecology, 210*(3), 179–193.
22. Cunningham, F. G., Leveno, K. J., Bloom, S. L., et al. (Eds.). (2010). Forceps delivery and vacuum extraction. *Williams obstetrics* (23rd ed., pp. 511–526). New York, NY: McGraw Hill.
23. American College of Obstetrics and Gynecologists. (2010). *Vaginal birth after previous cesarean section.* [Practice bulletin No. 115]. Washington, DC: Author.
24. Cunningham, F. G., Bangdiwala, S., Brown, S. S., et al. (2010). National institutes of health consensus development conference statement: Vaginal birth after cesarean: New insights. *Obstetrics & Gynecology, 115*(6), 1279–1295.
25. Association of Women's Health Obstetric and Neonatal Nurses. (2011). *Perioperative care of the pregnant woman: Evidenced based guidelines.* Washington, DC: Author.
26. Tharpe, N. (2007). First assisting in obstetrics: A primer for women's healthcare professionals. *Journal of Perinatal and Neonatal Nursing, 21*(1), 30–38.

Obstetric Emergencies

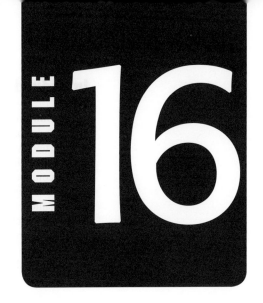

MODULE 16

SUZANNE McMURTRY BAIRD AND
BETSY BABB KENNEDY

Objectives

As you complete this module, you will learn:

1. The importance of rapid nursing responses and collaborative care during intrapartum emergencies
2. Risk factors for umbilical cord prolapse
3. Steps to take when a prolapse of the umbilical cord is suspected or has occurred
4. Factors that indicate a possible shoulder dystocia
5. Primary collaborative measures to relieve a shoulder dystocia
6. Techniques for McRoberts maneuver and suprapubic pressure
7. Guidelines for documenting an occurrence of shoulder dystocia
8. Current theoretical knowledge and pathophysiologic alterations that occur with an amniotic fluid embolism
9. Symptoms of amniotic fluid embolism
10. Supportive therapies for the women experiencing a possible amniotic fluid embolism
11. Priorities for treatment of obstetric hemorrhage
12. The "classic" symptoms of placental abruption
13. Etiologies of placental abruption
14. Criteria for classification of placental abruption
15. Treatment issues for placental abruption based on severity of symptoms
16. Incidence and risk factors for uterine rupture
17. Possible signs that a uterine rupture has occurred
18. Diagnostic criteria for postpartum hemorrhage
19. Predisposing factors for postpartum hemorrhage
20. Manipulative and pharmacologic measures to treat postpartum hemorrhage
21. The importance of maintaining family-centered care even during unexpected and emergency situations
22. The usefulness of team drills to improve outcomes in intrapartum emergencies

Key Terms

When you have completed this module, you should be able to recall the meaning of the following terms. You should be able to use the terms when consulting with other health professionals. Terms are defined in this module or in the glossary at the end of this book.

abruptio placentae (placental abruption)
accreta
amniotic fluid embolism (AFE)
increta
McRoberts maneuver
obstetric hemorrhage
percreta
prolapsed cord
shoulder dystocia
suprapubic pressure
uterine rupture
vasa previa

445

Introduction

Intrapartum emergencies are rare, but can be associated with significant maternal and fetal morbidity and mortality. It is important to know how to respond rapidly and appropriately. This module reviews selected issues and nursing care associated with emergencies in the intrapartum period, including cord prolapse, shoulder dystocia, amniotic fluid embolism (AFE), and hemorrhagic complications such as placental abruption, uterine rupture, vasa previa, and immediate postpartum hemorrhage (PPH). Other intrapartum emergencies such as a category III electronic fetal monitor strip (see Module 7), and eclamptic seizure (see Module 11) are presented in other modules. Simulation of potential obstetric emergencies is helpful to proactively assess systems, processes, communication, collaboration, and team member roles. If an obstetric emergency occurs, a debrief session is helpful to organize timing of event, management, and personnel involved. In addition, this discussion allows for all team members to discuss what went well and improvement opportunities.

Prolapsed Cord

Umbilical cord prolapse (UCP) may occur any time the maternal pelvis is not completely filled by the presenting fetal part. It occurs most often in fetal malpresentation, breech or transverse lie, or when the presenting part is not engaged. The most common cause of UCP is rupture of membranes, either spontaneously or artificially.[1] The umbilical cord can also prolapse as a result of obstetrical manipulation such as attempted rotation of the fetal head, external cephalic version, amnioinfusion, or placement of a cervical ripening balloon catheter, intrauterine pressure catheter, or fetal scalp electrode.[1] Other described risk factors for UCP include malpresentation, fetal anomalies, intrauterine growth restriction (IUGR), cord abnormalities, preterm labor/delivery, preterm premature rupture of membranes, multiple gestation, polyhydramnios, and grand multiparity.[1]

NOTE: A prolapsed cord means that the umbilical cord lies beside or below the presenting part of the fetus. The estimated occurrence rate is between 1.4% and 6.2% per 1,000 pregnancies.[2]

A prolapsed cord can:
- Pass through the cervix either before or alongside of the presenting part (overt; Fig. 16.1)
- Be palpable at the cervix (funic presentation; Fig. 16.2)
- Be hidden and not palpable (occult; Fig. 16.3)

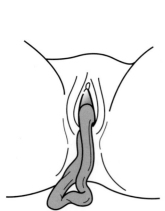

FIGURE 16.1 Prolapse of cord through the vaginal opening.

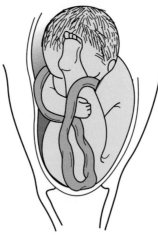

FIGURE 16.2 Prolapsed cord can be felt at the cervical opening.

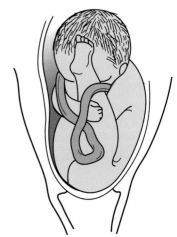

FIGURE 16.3 Hidden prolapsed cord.

NOTE: In fetal malpresentation, a cervical examination may be performed to evaluate for the presence of a prolapsed cord if membranes rupture spontaneously and a change in the fetal heart rate pattern occurs.

NOTE: Prompt recognition and management of UCP can minimize the effects of fetal hypoxia due to cord compression.

If a UCP occurs, the fetal heart rate monitor may demonstrate abnormal findings such as bradycardia or persistent variable decelerations.

• **What should the nurse do after detecting or suspecting a prolapsed cord?**

---

1. Notify a provider who has surgical privileges.
2. Call for help.
3. Place the woman in a position that uses gravity to reduce compression of the cord by the presenting part (Fig. 16.4A,B).

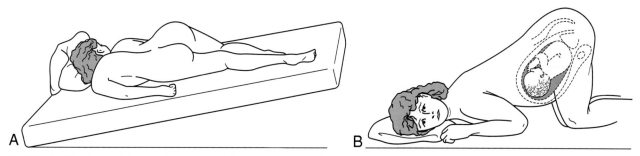

FIGURE 16.4 **A.** Sims position in Trendelenburg. **B.** Knee–chest position.

4. If a cord is felt, prepare the woman for an emergent cesarean birth. In rare circumstances, the physician may determine that vaginal birth may be more expeditious than cesarean if the woman is fully dilated and the presenting part has descended.
5. Perform a sterile-gloved vaginal examination. Place two fingers on either side of the cord or both fingers on one side of the cord to avoid compressing the cord and exert upward pressure against the presenting part to relieve pressure on the cord. Maintain elevation of the presenting part off the cord.
6. Try not to handle the cord because it can cause the cord to spasm, further impairing fetal blood supply.[3] If the cord protrudes outside of the vagina, replace cord into the vaginal vault with wet gauze if waiting for team arrival for emergent cesarean birth.[1]
7. Transport the woman to the operating room (OR) for an emergent cesarean birth.
8. Verify fetal heart rate in the OR.
9. Intrauterine fetal resuscitation measures may include oxygen delivered at 10 L by face mask and increased (or initiation of) intravenous fluid administration, but these measures should not delay transport of the woman to the operating room.
10. Educate and support the mother and family about the emergency and interventions.
11. Document events, interventions, and responses as soon as possible.

NOTE: Perinatal mortality rates with UCP have decreased to less than 10% due to the availability of operative and anesthesia teams as well as improved neonatal resuscitation techniques.[1,2]

Shoulder Dystocia

Management of shoulder dystocia in the absence of a primary care provider is discussed in Module 9. This module focuses on the responsibilities of the nurse when the birth attendant is present.

NOTE: Shoulder dystocia occurs when the fetal head is delivered, but the anterior shoulder is impacted or "stuck" on the pubic arch. Shoulder dystocia complicates up to 3% of vaginal births.[4]

Shoulder dystocia **cannot be reliably predicted or prevented**. In addition, there are no reliable risk identifiers or tools that have been proven effective to prevent most cases of newborn brachial plexus palsy, a condition associated with shoulder dystocia.[4] However, there are three clinical scenarios in which a provider may consider a varied birth plan[4]:

- Suspected fetal macrosomia defined as an estimated fetal weight of 5,000 g in a nondiabetic woman or 4,500 g in a woman with diabetes
- Prior shoulder dystocia
- Mid pelvic operative birth with an estimated fetal weight of 4,000 g

If one of these conditions exists and vaginal birth is anticipated, be prepared to act rapidly to reposition the woman and provide suprapubic pressure. Also, have an extra nurse at delivery, Anesthesiology to management maternal pain needs, and the newborn resuscitation team in case the baby is depressed at birth. Associated maternal and newborn risks of shoulder dystocia include the following.

Risks to the Mother

- Postpartum hemorrhage
- Third- or fourth-degree episiotomy and/or laceration

Risks to the Baby

- Brachial plexus injury
- Fracture of clavicle and/or humerus
- Cerebral hypoxia
- Death

A team approach and effective, calm communication during shoulder dystocia is essential. All staff should be prepared to respond emergently should a shoulder dystocia occur.

• What should the nurse do if shoulder dystocia occurs?

Primary nursing measures to relieve shoulder dystocia includes maternal positioning (McRoberts and Gaskin maneuvers) and suprapubic pressure. These maneuvers are considered to have the lowest risk with the highest rate of effectiveness. The *McRoberts maneuver* is accomplished by positioning the woman's legs back with the thighs on her abdomen. This straightens the sacrum and decreases the angle of incline of the symphysis pubis, making it easier to deliver the anterior shoulder (Fig. 16.5A to C). An alternative position is the "all fours" Gaskin maneuver, which has

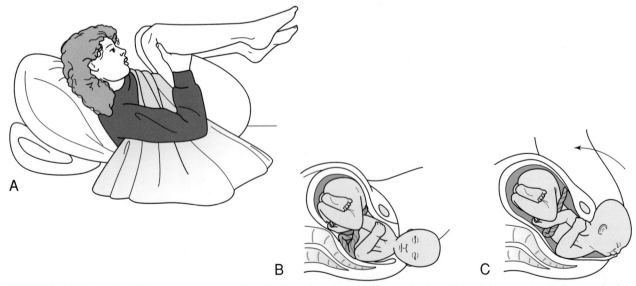

FIGURE 16.5 **A.** McRoberts maneuver position. **B.** Normal position of the symphysis pubis and the sacrum. **C.** The symphysis pubis rotates and the sacrum flattens.

a high success rate; however, it may be difficult to accomplish if the woman has a dense regional block.[5] The provider may also ask for suprapubic pressure over the anterior fetal shoulder. Downward and lateral pressure is applied in an attempt to dislodge the shoulder (Fig. 16.6). Lowering the bed and side rails may be helpful to accomplish these measures, but precautions should be taken to protect the mother and allow the delivering provider optimal alignment for additional maneuvers. A step stool may also be used to assist with elevation for suprapubic pressure.

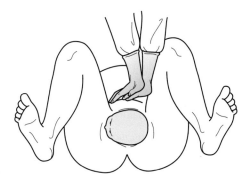

FIGURE 16.6   Suprapubic pressure.

NOTE: A combination of the McRoberts maneuver and suprapubic pressure may relieve more than 50% of shoulder dystocia cases.[4]

The provider determines the need and sequencing of additional measures if the shoulder dystocia is not relieved. These include the Rubin maneuver, delivery of the posterior arm (Jacquemier maneuver), Wood's screw maneuver, cephalic replacement (Zavanelli maneuver), symphysiotomy, and/or deliberate fracture of the clavicle.

NOTE: ACOG recommends antepartum screening for risk factors for shoulder dystocia and consideration of elective cesarean birth if the estimated fetal weight is above 5,000 g (4,500 g for diabetic women).[4]

• What should be documented about the occurrence of a shoulder dystocia?

Accurate documentation of the event is essential. Nursing documentation of the event should include the following:
- Specifics about nursing maneuvers performed, the order in which they were performed, who directed the maneuvers, and attempts to assess fetal status during the event
- Duration of the event (specifically the time from delivery of the fetal head to the delivery of the body)
- Team members involved and their role
- The anterior shoulder that was impacted (right or left)
- Fetal assessment prior to birth
- Umbilical cord gases
- Resuscitation measures for the newborn (newborn team documents care provided)
- Newborn assessment

IMPORTANT: NEVER USE FUNDAL PRESSURE DURING SHOULDER DYSTOCIA WHICH MAY FURTHER IMPACT THE ANTERIOR SHOULDER AND INCREASE THE RISK FOR BRACHIAL PLEXUS INJURY.

Be prepared to thoroughly assess the newborn at birth for signs of injury. (See Module 18 for additional information regarding newborn assessment.) Members of the team involved in the event should also take time to speak with the woman and family after the event to educate, explain, and support.

449

Amniotic Fluid Embolism

• What is an amniotic fluid embolism?

Amniotic Fluid Embolism (AFE) is a rare event with an estimated *incidence of 1 in 40,000 deliveries.*[6] Many aspects of AFE remain unknown, including risk factors for this devastating syndrome. Despite the name *amniotic fluid embolus,* this syndrome is not the result of amniotic fluid entrance into maternal circulation or embolism. Maternal pathophysiology is more likely related to an aggressive immunologic response to fetal tissue and massive release of endogenous and/or inflammatory mediators causing:

- Sudden maternal hypoxia
- Cardiovascular collapse
- Coagulopathy[7]

It has also been proposed that intrauterine infection may also be a signaling factor in the release of endogenous mediators resulting in a clinical picture similar to anaphylaxis or septic shock.[7]

NOTE: The maternal mortality rate with a diagnosis of AFE is between 20% and 60%, with only 15% of patients surviving neurologically intact in a national registry.[6]

• What are the most common symptoms of an AFE?[6]

The symptoms associated with AFE are listed in Table 16.1. These symptoms have an acute onset and lead to rapid maternal and fetal compromise.

TABLE 16.1 SYMPTOMS OF AFE AND RATE OF OCCURRENCE

SYMPTOMS OCCURRING FREQUENTLY (IN 80–100% OF CASES)	SYMPTOMS OCCURRING WITH MODERATE FREQUENCY (IN 20–80% OF CASES)	SYMPTOMS OCCURRING INFREQUENTLY (IN LESS THAN 20% OF CASES)
Hypotension	Dyspnea	Bronchospasm
Fetal compromise	Seizure, tonic–clonic	Transient hypertension
Pulmonary edema or acute respiratory distress syndrome	Atony	Cough
Cardiopulmonary arrest		Headache
Cyanosis		Chest pain
Coagulopathy		

From Clark, S. L. (2014). Amniotic fluid embolism. *Obstetrics & Gynecology, 123*(2), 337–348; Romero, R., Kadar, N., Vaisbuch, E., et al. (2010). Maternal death following cardiopulmonary collapse after delivery: Amniotic fluid embolism or septic shock due to intrauterine infection? *American Journal of Reproductive Immunology, 64,* 113–125.

• When does AFE usually occur?

In the national registry data, 70% of the women diagnosed with AFE were in labor, 19% of cases occurred during cesarean delivery, and 11% of cases occurred during the early postpartum period. AFE has also been reported to occur during amnioinfusion, termination of pregnancy, and abdominal trauma.

• What should the nurse do if the mother exhibits signs of AFE?[7]

Nursing care for the woman experiencing a possible AFE is focused on supportive therapy.

- Immediately call a rapid response or code as determined by the patient's status.
- Immediately notify the obstetric provider, anesthesia, and neonatal resuscitation staff (if patient is undelivered) and obtain a crash cart.
- Continuously monitor the fetus if the woman is undelivered and anticipate an emergency cesarean birth and neonatal resuscitation.
- Administer high-concentration oxygen by face mask to maintain normal saturation. Anticipate and prepare for intubation and ventilation.
- Initiate cardiopulmonary resuscitation (CPR) if the woman experiences cardiac arrest. If the mother does not respond to CPR, prepare for a perimortem cesarean section within

4 minutes following the maternal arrest since maternal and neonatal outcomes are linked to the time interval between maternal cardiopulmonary collapse and birth.

- Initiate peripheral intravenous access with a large-bore cannula. Anticipate central line placement and/or multiple peripheral lines.
- Treat hypotension with positioning and crystalloid boluses. Anticipate the need for massive blood product replacement, vasopressors, and inotropic agents.
- Anticipate arterial line placement for continuous blood pressure monitoring and access for blood gases and laboratory specimens.
- Prepare the woman and family for transfer to an intensive care environment or tertiary care center after initial stabilization.

Obstetric Hemorrhage

The following intrapartum emergencies are grouped together because they are all associated with complications from blood loss. Obstetric hemorrhage is the leading cause of maternal mortality **worldwide**, with one death occurring every 4 minutes. In the United States, the incidence of obstetric hemorrhage is 2.9% of all births and hemorrhage requiring blood transfusion has increased 114%.[8] Hemorrhage is responsible for approximately half of severe maternal morbidity such as acute respiratory distress syndrome (ARDS), acute kidney injury, and disseminated intravascular coagulation (DIC).[9] Although the maternal physiologic adaptations to pregnancy (Display 16.1) allows for compensation of blood loss at birth, if bleeding is excessive, previously effective compensatory mechanisms to maintain cardiac output (systemic vasoconstriction, tachycardia, and increased myocardial contractility) begin to fail and symptoms of shock and impaired organ perfusion become evident. Situational awareness and early recognition of maternal compromise is necessary to prevent maternal morbidity and mortality.

DISPLAY 16.1 HEMATOLOGIC ADAPTATIONS DURING PREGNANCY
Increased blood volume to 6–7 L
Increased plasma volume 40%
Increased red blood cell volume
Increased efficiency of clotting
Impaired fibrinolysis

From Sosa, M. E. (2014). Bleeding in pregnancy. In Simpson, K. R., & Creehan, P.A. (Eds.), *Perinatal nursing* (pp. 143–165). Philadelphia, PA: Wolters Kluwer; Francois, K. E., & Foley, M. R. (2012). Antepartum and postpartum hemorrhage. In Gabbe, S. G., Simpson, J. L., & Niebyl, J. R. (Eds.), *Obstetrics: Normal and problem pregnancies* (6th ed., pp. 415–444). New York: Churchill Livingstone.

Data have demonstrated that 54% to 93% of maternal deaths related to hemorrhage are preventable due to an under appreciation of blood loss and failure to provide adequate volume replacement in a timely manner.[8–10] Development and implementation of comprehensive, evidence-based hemorrhage protocols have been shown to improve recognition and management and decrease maternal blood transfusions and peripartum hysterectomy.[11] Therefore, The National Partnership for Maternal Safety recommends all the following[10]:

- U. S. Birthing Facilities have an obstetric hemorrhage protocol
- Hemorrhage kit or cart that contains appropriate medications and supplies
- Partnership with a local blood bank for blood products
- Active management of the third stage of labor

Assessing, recording, and reporting estimated blood loss (EBL) is one intervention in an obstetric hemorrhage protocol. Visual estimation can be extremely difficult to determine and may be underestimated by 30% to 50%.[12] Underestimation is especially prevalent in cases of hemorrhage and cesarean sections when there is mixing of blood with amniotic fluid and irrigation solutions. To improve accuracy and situational awareness, quantified blood loss (QBL) measurement is recommended with each birth or if obstetric hemorrhage occurs during the antepartum or postpartum periods. QBL is an objective tool that improves recognition and management of hemorrhage and may lead to a decrease in transfusions, surgical intervention, and length of stay.[13] QBL can be accomplished by weighing items soiled with blood, subtracting the dry weight of those items, and converting each gram to milliliter. Graduated under buttocks and operative drapes also assist with measurement.[13]

HELPFUL HINT: *Having a chart with the dry weights of commonly used linens and pads will assist in determining the QBL.*

NOTE: By the time a pregnant or postpartum woman exhibits signs of compromise such as dizziness, hypotension, and oliguria, the amount of blood loss is significant!

General nursing considerations for obstetric hemorrhage are as follows:

- Call a Rapid Response as indicated by maternal status and availability of team members.
- Place a Foley catheter and monitor intake and output every hour until stable. If urine output falls below 30 mL/hr, assess the woman for other signs and symptoms of volume depletion (tachycardia, tachypnea, weak peripheral pulses, dry mucus membranes).
- Quantitative, cumulative blood loss totals are helpful to anticipate maternal decompensation prior to laboratory analysis.
- Obtain intravenous access; multiple large-bore intravenous catheters or central line placement is necessary for class III or IV hemorrhage. Note: some hospitals use classes of hemorrhage to relate the amount of blood lost to maternal signs and symptoms. These classes are outlined in Table 16.2.

TABLE 16.2	CLASSIFICATION OF HEMORRHAGE	
CLASS	**BLOOD LOSS**	**PATIENT SYMPTOMS**
I	1,000 mL (15%)	Dizziness Palpitations Minimal blood pressure changes
II	1,500 mL (20–25%)	Tachycardia Tachypnea Weakness Narrowing pulse pressure ≤30 mm Hg Delayed capillary refill after blanching palm at base of fingers at ulnar margin Orthostatic hypotension
III	2,000 mL (30–35%)	Hypotension Marked tachycardia (120–160 beats/minute) Tachypnea (30–50 breaths/minute) Skin—cold, clammy, pale Restlessness
IV	≥2,500 mL blood loss (40%)	Symptoms of profound cardiogenic shock BP may be absent Peripheral pulses may be difficult to palpate Air hunger Oliguria or anuria

From Francois, K. E., & Foley, M. R. (2012). Antepartum and postpartum hemorrhage. In Gabbe, S. G., Simpson, J. L., & Niebyl, J. R. (Eds.), *Obstetrics: Normal and problem pregnancies* (6th ed., pp. 415–444). New York: Churchill Livingstone.

- Infuse crystalloid solutions to support cardiac output. Warm all fluids and blood products if massive volume replacement is anticipated.
- Use positioning to optimize cardiac output (left or right side; elevation of lower extremities).
- Obtain order for typing and cross-matching of blood and notify the blood bank of potential massive transfusion needs.
- Prepare for blood component therapy. Activate defined protocol for massive transfusion if transfusion of more than 4 units of blood products is anticipated. Commonly used blood products are described in Table 16.3.
- Monitor laboratory coagulation and electrolyte findings. During or immediately after hemorrhage, the hematocrit and hemoglobin values will be inaccurate due to the loss of plasma and red blood cells. It will take approximately 2 hours for the plasma volume to equilibrate to reflect the true values.[14] Therefore, it is recommended that blood product replacement be determined by maternal vital signs and QBL instead of laboratory evidence of anemia. Waiting for laboratory changes delays treatment.[13,15]

TABLE 16.3 COMMONLY USED BLOOD PRODUCTS

BLOOD PRODUCT	APPROXIMATE VOLUME PER UNIT (mL)	EFFECT
Packed red blood cells	240	Increases hematocrit 3% per unit
Platelets	50	Increases platelets 5,000–10,000 per unit
FFP (factor V, VIII, fibrinogen)	250	Increases fibrinogen 10 mg/dL per unit
Cryoprecipitate (factor VIII)	40	Increases fibrinogen 10 mg/dL per unit

From Martin, S. R. (2011). Transfusion of blood components and derivatives in the obstetric care patient. In Foley, M. R., Strong, T. H., & Garite, T. J. (Eds.), *Obstetric intensive care manual* (3rd ed.). New York: McGraw-Hill.

- Monitor maternal vital signs frequently until normalized and bleeding has decreased to an expected amount. Tachycardia and hypotension are signs of hypovolemia.
- Use warming devices to keep the patient warm and optimize oxygen transport. Monitor respiratory rate and SpO_2 trends assessing for potential respiratory compromise from pulmonary edema.
- Furosemide (Lasix) is not recommended to treat oliguria if a woman is hemorrhaging or has recently stopped. Oliguria with hemorrhage is best treated with additional fluids and/or blood.[15]
- Continuously monitor fetal status and employ intrauterine resuscitation techniques as indicated.
- Monitor arterial oxygenation saturation of hemoglobin (SpO_2) and maintain >95%.
- Monitor and manage maternal pain. Notify anesthesiology team for assistance with resuscitation and/or pain management needs as indicated.
- Prepare for emergent delivery and/or surgical intervention.
- Anticipate and prepare for possible invasive monitoring (e.g., arterial line, central line placement, and central venous pressure monitoring).
- Notify neonatal team of potential delivery if applicable.

NOTE: It is important to know and monitor for the desired effects of blood product administration including normalization of vital signs, urine output, pulse strength, and laboratory values.

If the woman refuses blood products due to cultural or religious beliefs, it is important to ensure the woman's wish is not confused with a lack of desire for all other interventions. Options to maintain cardiac output and oxygen transport such as auto transfusion and/or cell saving may be viewed as acceptable.

NOTE: Obstetric hemorrhage is not a diagnosis. It is a clinical sign that requires determination of the cause.[10]

Abruptio Placentae (Placental Abruption)

Placental abruption is a premature separation of a normally implanted placenta from the uterus (Fig. 16.7A to C). Depending on the degree of detachment, the loss of maternal–fetal surface

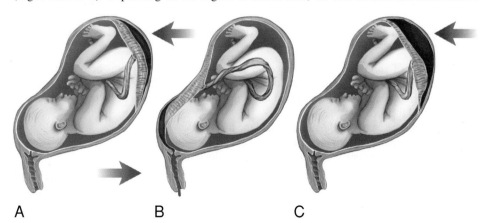

A   B   C

FIGURE 16.7 Placental abruption. **A.** Partial with concealed hemorrhage. **B.** Partial with apparent hemorrhage. **C.** Complete with concealed hemorrhage.

area for gas and nutrient exchange may deprive the fetus of essential blood and oxygen and lead to hypoxia, asphyxia, or death.[16] Placental abruption may be:
- **Revealed**—blood collects between the decidua and the membranes and passes out the cervix and vagina.
- **OR**
- **Concealed**—blood collects behind the placenta and there is no vaginal bleeding noted.

NOTE: The incidence of placental abruption varies but is approximately 1 in 100 pregnancies and is increasing in the United States due to gestational diabetes, preterm labor, and umbilical cord abnormalities.[17]

• What are the risk factors for abruption?

The primary etiology of placental abruption is unknown. Common factors that have been linked with abruption are outlined in Table 16.4.[17–21]

TABLE 16.4 RISK FACTORS FOR PLACENTAL ABRUPTION

RISK FACTOR	NOTES
Previous placental abruption	Recurrence risk 5–17%; if two consecutive abruptions the risk increases to 25%
Cocaine abuse	If used in the third trimester, abruption rate is 10%
Cigarette smoking	May be related to the number of cigarettes smoked each day
Maternal parity	The incidence in primigravid women is less than 1%; however, the percentage increases to 2.5% in grand multiparas
Chronic hypertension OR preeclampsia	Five fold increase as compared to normotensive women
Trauma	Sudden uterine decompression; falls, motor vehicle crash, violence
Preterm premature rupture of membranes (PPROM) <34 weeks EGA	2–5% incidence; intrauterine infection and oligohydramnios increase risk of abruption
Rapid uterine decompression	Rupture of membranes with polyhydramnios; delivery of first twin
Maternal thrombophilia	Inherited or acquired; increased risk with combination of thrombophilia types
Uterine malformation or fibroids	Placenta implants over malformation or fibroid

From Martin, S. R. (2011). Transfusion of blood components and derivatives in the obstetric care patient. In Foley, M. R., Strong, T. H., & Garite, T. J. (Eds.), *Obstetric intensive care manual* (3rd ed.). New York: McGraw-Hill; Kramer, M. S., Usher, R. H., Pollack, R., et al. (1997). Etiologic determinants of abruptio placentae. *Obstetrics & Gynecology, 89,* 221; Hulse, G. K., Milne, E., English, D. R., et al. (1997). Assessing the relationship between maternal cocaine use and abruptio placentae. *Addiction, 92,* 1547; Vintzileos, A. M., Campbell, W. A., Nochimson, D. J., et al. (1987). Preterm premature rupture of membranes: A risk factor for the development of abruptio placentae. *American Journal of Obstetrics & Gynecology, 156,* 1235–1238.

NOTE: If a woman presents with preterm labor, abdominal pain, vaginal bleeding, or trauma assess for signs and symptoms of abruption.

Suspicion of abruption may be based on clinical signs and symptoms before birth, but a definitive diagnosis comes with inspection of the placenta after delivery. Ultrasound detection rates have increased with improvements of imaging technology and may be helpful in diagnosing the location of the abruption[17]:
- Subchorionic: between the placenta and the membranes
- Retroplacental: between the placenta and the myometrium
- Preplacental: between the placenta and the amniotic fluid

Location and size of the abruption are linked to fetal survival, with retroplacental abruption associated with poorer outcomes. If suspected by the delivering provider, it is recommended that the placenta be sent to pathology for evaluation.[17]

NOTE: Abruption is a clinical diagnosis supported by risk factors, signs/symptoms, radiologic, laboratory, and pathology studies.

> • **What are the signs and symptoms of abruption?**

Presentation of placental abruption varies widely and depends on the location, gestational age, degree of separation, and blood loss. Signs and symptoms may progress if the placenta separation continues or with "chronic" decreased oxygenation of the fetus. Possible maternal and fetal signs and symptoms of abruption include the following[22]:

Maternal

- Uterine tenderness, backache, or shoulder pain
- Abdominal pain: sometimes described as sharp with sudden onset
- Vaginal bleeding: usually associated with uterine contractions
- Dark, blood ("port-wine")-stained amniotic fluid
- Increased uterine tone—described as "board-like"
- Low amplitude, high-frequency uterine contractions (sometimes called uterine irritability)
- Tachycardia
- Anemia and/or consumptive coagulopathy
- Shock and death

Fetal

- EFM changes associated with hypoxia: late decelerations, tachycardia, decreasing variability, bradycardia, sinusoidal (Fig. 16.8)
- Intrauterine growth restriction (IUGR)
- Oligohydramnios
- Death

Laboratory values may be evaluated to assist in the diagnosis and determine the extent of separation. Maternal serum values that may be monitored include fibrinogen, hematocrit, hemoglobin, and platelets. A Kleihauer–Betke test on maternal serum or vaginal blood to determine the presence of fetal red blood cells.

Placental abruption can be classified according to clinical assessments and laboratory findings and is defined in Table 16.5.

TABLE 16.5 GRADING OF PLACENTAL ABRUPTION

GRADE	MATERNAL EFFECTS	FETAL EFFECTS
1	Slight vaginal bleeding Uterine irritability Blood pressure unaffected Fibrinogen level normal	Heart rate pattern normal
2	Vaginal bleeding mild to moderate Uterine irritability, tetanic or frequent uterine contractions Elevated heart rate Blood pressure maintained Fibrinogen level may be decreased	Heart rate pattern with signs of fetal compromise
3	Vaginal bleeding moderate to severe; may be concealed Uterus firm to palpation and painful Maternal hypotension Fibrinogen levels often <150 mg/dL Other coagulation deficits present such as thrombocytopenia, clotting factor depletion	Category II or III EFM and/or fetal death has occurred

From Francois, K. E., & Foley, M. R. (2012). Antepartum and postpartum hemorrhage. In Gabbe, S. G., Simpson, J. L., & Niebyl, J. R. (Eds.), *Obstetrics: Normal and problem pregnancies* (6th ed., pp. 415–444). New York: Churchill Livingstone.

NOTE: *When there is more than a 50% separation of the placenta (Grade 3), the risk for fetal death is high.*

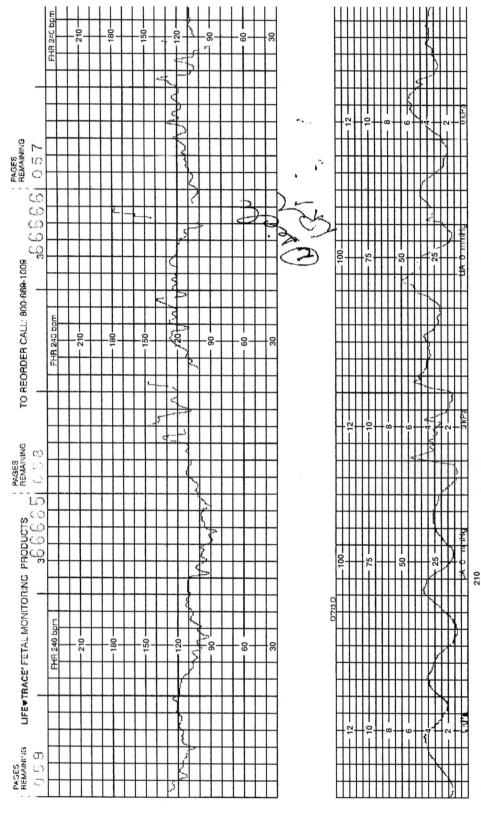

FIGURE 16.8 Electronic fetal monitoring tracing with evidence of placental abruption.

• **What should the nurse do if a placental abruption is suspected?**

Obstetric management of placental abruption is individualized based on the gestational age and the severity of maternal and fetal symptoms. For example, severe placental abruption will likely result in maternal and fetal compromise at any viable gestational age and is aggressively managed to achieve birth as soon as possible. If symptoms are mild and gestational age is preterm (20 to 34 weeks), a stable woman and fetus are managed conservatively to optimize neonatal outcome. If the woman is at term or near term and stable, and fetal status is reassuring, vaginal birth may be achieved.

Mild Symptoms

- Prepare to administer corticosteroids to promote fetal lung maturity if pregnancy is at less than 32 weeks of estimated gestational age (EGA).
- Closely monitor both maternal and fetal status.
- Measure and record all blood loss.
- Obtain an order to keep a current type and cross-match in the blood bank.
- Be prepared for a high-risk newborn.

Moderate/Severe Symptoms

- Ensure IV access with a large-bore catheter. Anticipate central line placement.
- Administer oxygen via nonrebreather face mask at 10 L/min.
- Assess vital signs frequently and initiate continuous pulse oximetry.
- Continuously monitor fetal status.
- Prepare for blood product replacement and notify the blood bank. Consider activation of the massive transfusion protocol.
- Anticipate cesarean birth.
- Manage the woman's pain.

In cases of severe placental abruption that results in fetal death, the woman may be allowed to deliver vaginally as long as she remains hemodynamically stable.

NOTE: There is a significant risk for maternal coagulopathy such as DIC if the fetus is an intrauterine demise. Be vigilant in monitoring the mother's vital signs, blood loss, and symptoms of DIC.

Uterine Rupture

• **What is a uterine rupture?**

Uterine rupture (Fig. 16.9) is defined as the symptomatic disruption and separation of the layers of the uterus or previous scar. Rupture may result in extrusion of the fetus or fetal parts into the

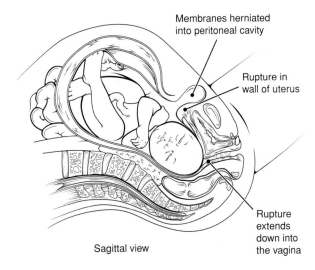

Membranes herniated into peritoneal cavity

Rupture in wall of uterus

Rupture extends down into the vagina

Sagittal view

FIGURE 16.9 Uterine rupture.

peritoneal cavity. Uterine dehiscence is the separation of a previous scar but the serosa layer of the myometrium remains intact, holding the fetus within the uterus.[23]

• How often does uterine rupture occur?

The overall incidence of uterine rupture is approximately 1%. Conditions associated with uterine rupture include the following[24]:
- Uterine scars—prior uterine surgery (e.g., cesarean birth, myomectomy)
- Prior uterine rupture, trauma, abortion, instrumentation injury or uterine perforation
- Grand multiparity
- Uterine over distention (macrosomic fetus, multiple gestation, polyhydramnios, fetal malpresentation)

NOTE: Induction of labor in women attempting a trial of labor after previous cesarean birth (TOLAC) is associated with higher rates of uterine rupture (0.4% spontaneous labor vs. 1% with induction).[25] The highest rates of uterine rupture during an TOLAC induction occurs with the combination use of prostaglandins and oxytocin.

For a discussion of vaginal birth after cesarean delivery (VBAC) and trial of labor (TOL), refer to Module 8.

• What is first sign/symptom of uterine rupture?

A category II or III fetal heart rate tracing is the first manifestation of uterine rupture in a laboring woman. It may be described as an abrupt decrease in FHR, late and/or variable decelerations, absent baseline variability, tachycardia or bradycardia, or an erratic fetal heart rate pattern. Any time an electronic fetal monitor strip exhibits these signs in a woman who is attempting a TOLAC, uterine rupture should be suspected. Timely notification and assessment by a physician with surgical privileges is necessary (Fig. 16.10).

• What other signs and symptoms might indicate a uterine rupture has occurred?

Other signs of uterine rupture may include the following:
- Loss of fetal station or no fetal descent
- Palpable fetal parts with maternal abdominal examination
- Vaginal bleeding—bright red
- Symptoms of maternal shock—hypotension, tachycardia
- Maternal pain—described as ripping or tearing sensation that is independent of uterine contractions, sudden sharp abdominal pain

NOTE: If the mother has neuraxial anesthesia for labor, she may not be able to report a sensation of pain, but may have other intense feelings such as anxiety and restlessness.

• What should the nurse do if a uterine rupture is suspected?

- Call a rapid response
- Notify the attending physician (a physician credentialed for cesarean birth) immediately
- Discontinue oxytocin
- Notify the anesthesia, operating room, and neonatal team to prepare for immediate birth
- Prepare the woman for an emergent cesarean section if vaginal birth is not imminent
- Administer oxygen by nonrebreather face mask at 10 L per minute
- Position the woman in left or right lateral recumbent position
- Administer crystalloid IV fluid bolus
- Anticipate blood product replacement
- Continuously monitor fetal status
- Prepare for a high-risk newborn

Postpartum Hemorrhage

• What is a postpartum hemorrhage (PPH)?

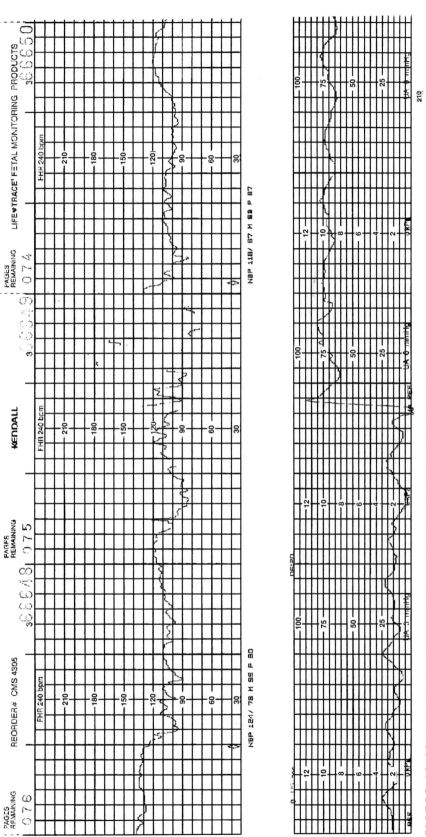

FIGURE 16.10 External electronic fetal monitor tracing prior to diagnosis of uterine rupture.

DISPLAY 16.2 UTERINE ATONY ETIOLOGY

Grand multiparity
Over distention of the uterus (large fetus, multiple gestation, polyhydramnios)
Precipitous labor or birth
Prolonged labor
Oxytocin induction or augmentation
Previous history of uterine atony
Full bladder after the birth

From Oylese, Y., & Ananth, C. V. (2010). Postpartum hemorrhage: Epidemiology, risk factors, and causes. *Clinical Obstetrics and Gynecology, 53*(1), 147–156.

Postpartum hemorrhage (PPH) is defined as blood loss of more than 500 mL after a vaginal birth or 1,000 mL with cesarean birth. PPH occurs in 2.9% of births and has increased 27.5% despite no changes in risk factors of women.[26,27] The most common cause of PPH is uterine atony. Uterine atony has many different etiologies. These etiologies are discussed in Display 16.2.

After delivery of the placenta, uterine contraction causes the myometrial fibers to constrict the spiral arterioles and control blood loss. If the uterus is unable to contract, increased blood loss will occur. PPH can occur *early* in the first 24 hours after delivery, or *late,* between 24 hours and 6 weeks postpartum. Causes of early and late PPH may include the following.

Early Causes

- Lacerations
  - Lower genital tract (perineal, vaginal, cervical, periclitoral, labial, periurethral, rectal)
  - Upper genital tract (broad ligament)
  - Upper urinary tract (bladder, urethra)
- Retained placental fragments
- Invasive placentation (placenta accreta, placenta increta, placenta percreta)
- Uterine rupture
- Uterine inversion
- Coagulation disorders (hereditary, acquired)

Late Causes

- Infection
- Retained placental fragments
- Placental site subinvolution
- Coagulation disorders

*NOTE: On admission, **BE AWARE** of any predisposing factors for PPH and **BE PREPARED** for a rapid response.*

• What should the nurse do in the event of a PPH?

As previously discussed in Module 5, active management of the third stage of labor decreases the risk of PPH. Oxytocin should be given prophylactically after birth of the baby or placenta to contract the uterus. Dosing for oxytocin and other uterotonic medications, along with nursing considerations, are presented in Table 16.6. If the woman is having continued, excessive vaginal bleeding after administration of oxytocin, empty the bladder and perform uterine massage. Uterine massage compresses and contracts the uterine muscle to lessen the bleeding and express clots. If the uterus remains "boggy"—soft and not contracted—notify the provider and activate the PPH protocol. If more than 1 dose of an additional uterotonic medication is needed and the mother continues to have excessive bleeding, call the provider and require them to emergently come to the bedside for assessment.[15] Thorough and frequent assessments should continue until bleeding has subsided. Review care of the postpartum woman in Module 17.

The provider may perform a bimanual pelvic and/or speculum examination to rule out lacerations (perineal, cervical, vaginal) or retained placental fragments. If manipulative and medication measures fail to control the bleeding, additional treatments are necessary. Intrauterine and/or vaginal tamponade balloon placement can be successful in temporarily treating acute refractory bleeding while initiating other measures (blood products, OR team availability).

TABLE 16.6 UTEROTONIC MEDICATIONS					
MEDICATION	**DOSE**	**ROUTES**	**FREQUENCY**	**SIDE EFFECTS**	**CONTRAINDICATIONS**
Oxytocin (Pitocin)	10–40 U	IV, IM	Continuous IV solution	Nausea and vomiting, water intoxication (high doses)	None
Misoprostol (Cytotec)	400–1,000 μg	Oral or rectal	Varies	Nausea, vomiting, diarrhea, fever, chills	None
Methylergonovine (Methergine)	0.2 mg	IM Do not give IV	Q 2–4 h for up to 5 doses	Hypertension, nausea and vomiting, myocardial ischemia	Hypertension (chronic or preeclampsia), coronary artery disease
15-methyl PGF2alpha (Carboprost, Hemabate)	0.25 mg	IM	15–90 mins (maximum of 8 doses)	Nausea, vomiting, diarrhea, flushing, fever, vasospasm, bronchospasm	Asthma, cardiac, pulmonary, renal, or hepatic disease

From Sosa, M. E. (2014). Bleeding in pregnancy. In Simpson, K. R., & Creehan, P. A. (Eds.), *Perinatal nursing* (pp. 143–165). Philadelphia, PA: Wolters Kluwer; Francois, K. E., & Foley, M. R. (2012). Antepartum and postpartum hemorrhage. In Gabbe, S. G., Simpson, J. L., & Niebyl, J. R. (Eds.), *Obstetrics: Normal and problem pregnancies* (6th ed., pp. 415–444). New York: Churchill Livingstone.

There are several manufacturers of uterine balloons and type is usually dependent on provider preference and rationale for use. These devices and supplies needed for insertion should be readily available on the unit (hemorrhage kit). Nurses working in obstetrics should be knowledgeable in assisting with placement, monitoring of continued blood loss, and troubleshooting. Most uterine balloons are left in for a 24-hour maximum time period and the mother monitored in a unit where staffing allows for frequent assessments.

NOTE: *In late pregnancy blood flow to the placenta is 750 to 1,000 mL/min, so there is great potential for significant blood loss in a short period of time.*[16]

Be prepared for rapid transfer to the OR for surgical management or an intensive care setting for hemodynamic stabilization if necessary. In addition, an OR setting may be utilized to provide for improved positioning, lighting, or examination with anesthesia. Angiographic arterial embolization may be considered to occlude the bleeding vessel and prevent surgical intervention. However, additional medical or surgical management should not wait in order for the interventional radiology team to assemble.[15]

Placenta Accreta

Placenta Accreta is a general term used to describe the abnormal, invasive placental chorionic villi growth that causes the placenta to adhere to the uterine lining. Accreta varies in degree of invasion (Fig. 16.11).
- **Accreta:** adherent placenta
- **Increta:** chorionic villi invade the myometrium

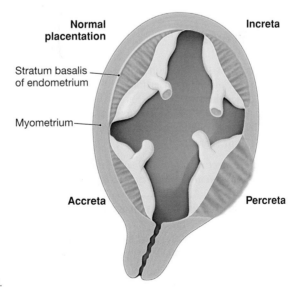

FIGURE 16.11 Placenta accreta.

- **Percreta:** chorionic villi grow through the myometrium and serosa; may attach to other organs and tissues

NOTE: Due to the rising cesarean birth rate, there is an alarming increase in the risk and diagnosis of placenta accreta.

- **What is the relationship between placenta accreta, previa, and previous cesarean birth?**[28]

If a woman has a diagnosis of placenta previa and a previous cesarean birth, placenta accreta should be considered and planned prior to scheduling her repeat cesarean section (Table 16.7). In the past, placenta accreta was diagnosed at birth, often resulting in maternal morbidity and mortality. However, with known risk factors and advances in radiologic technology, diagnosis is recommended in the antepartum period.[29] In addition, because of the potential for massive maternal hemorrhage at birth, a multidisciplinary approach for the care of these women has shown to improve outcomes such as massive transfusion, coagulopathy, postoperative admission, and length of stay in an intensive care unit, ureteral injury, or return to the OR.[30] Cesarean hysterectomy is usually required and should be planned in a hospital with full blood banking and laboratory capabilities and availability of dedicated Anesthesiology and surgical specialists such as Gynecology, Oncology, Urology, and Interventional Radiology.[15]

TABLE 16.7 RISK FOR PLACENTA ACCRETA WITH PLACENTA PREVIA AND A PRIOR CESAREAN BIRTH	
RISK FOR PLACENTA ACCRETA WITH PLACENTA PREVIA AND A PRIOR CESAREAN BIRTH	
NUMBER OF PRIOR CESAREAN BIRTHS	**PLACENTA ACCRETA RISK (%)**
0	3
1	11
2	40
3	61
4 or more	67

From Hull, A. D., & Resnick, R. (2010). Placenta accreta and postpartum hemorrhage. *Clinical Obstetrics and Gynecology, 53*(1), 228–236; Silver, R. M., Landon, M. B., Rouse, D. J., et al. (2006). Maternal morbidity associated with multiple repeat cesarean deliveries. *Obstetrics & Gynecology, 107*(6), 1226–1232; Warshak, C. R., Ramos, G. A., Eskander, R., et al. (2010). Effect of predelivery diagnosis in 99 consecutive cases of placenta accrete. *Obstetrics & Gynecology, 115*, 65.

NOTE: Obstetric teams in all hospitals need a process for care of an unexpected placenta accreta. It is also recommended that hospitals have a massive transfusion protocol. Display 16.3 is an example of an MTP.[15]

Vasa Previa

Vasa previa is the insertion of the umbilical vessels into the fetal membranes instead of the placenta (velamentous insertion) with the vessels crossing the cervical os below the presenting part.[16] Since the vessels are abnormally contained in the fetal membranes and not surrounded by the protective Wharton's jelly of the umbilical cord, sudden rupture of the vessels may occur (Fig. 16.12). If rupture and acute hemorrhage occur, it is usually with spontaneous or artificial rupture of membranes.[31]

*NOTE: Suspect vasa previa if rupture of membranes occurs, followed by the sudden onset of bright, red vaginal bleeding **and** indeterminate or abnormal EFM pattern.[16]*

- **What are the risk factors for vasa previa?**[16]

- Velamentous insertion of the cord
- Accessory placental lobes
- Placenta previa
- In vitro fertilization

Activate MTP

Determine Team Roles
- Team Leader
- Documentation
- Runner
- Blood Administration

Documentation
- RN - stands by Team Leader
- Notifies Blood Bank, Lab, RRT

Runner
Obtains MTP coolers from blood bank (can be nonlicensed personnel)

Team Leader
- Anesthesiologist or CRNA
- Obstetrician
- Intensivist

Blood Administration
NOTE: Labs prior and in between each cooler; do not wait for results to administer blood or continue MTP

Initial Labs
- Hg, Hct, platelets
- DIC panel: Fibrinogen, D-dimer, PT/INR, PTT
- ABG with metabolites (iCa, K, Glucose)

Initial MTP Blood Cooler
- 4 units RBC
- 4 units FFP
NOTE: If not previously typed and crossed, use O negative blood

Use Rapid Infuser Keep Patient Warm

Anticipate ongoing bleeding?

NO → **Team Leader Deactivates MTP**
Criteria: normalization of lab values and/or no evidence of ongoing bleeding

YES →

Repeat Labs
- Hg, Hct, platelets
- DIC panel: Fibrinogen, D-dimer, PT/INR, PTT
- ABG with metabolites (iCa, K, Glucose)

YES →

Subsequent MTP Blood Cooler(s)
- 4 units RBC
- 4 units FFP
- 1 apheresis platelet unit
- 1 dose cryoprecipitate

- Multiple gestation
- Fetal anomaly

• How do you manage a woman with vasa previa?

If diagnosed with color flow Doppler and ultrasound in the antepartum period, management is similar to a woman diagnosed with placenta previa. However, if undiagnosed and hemorrhage occurs during labor, an emergent cesarean birth is indicated since fetal hemorrhage and exsanguination is rapid.

***NOTE:** The overall perinatal mortality with vasa previa is 36%. Neonatal survival is 44% if diagnosed in labor. However, if antepartum diagnosis is made, neonatal survival is improved to 97%.*[32]

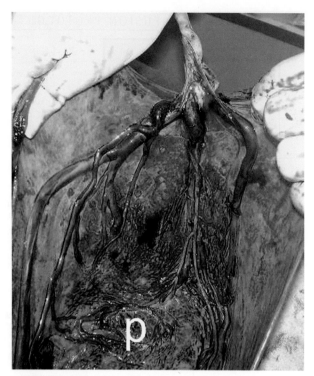

FIGURE 16.12   Velamentous insertion of the cord.

The Importance of Maintaining Family-Centered Care in an Intrapartum Emergency

Although any number of complications can place the woman in a dangerous emergency situation, remember that this is still a birth experience. Every effort should be made to keep the woman and her family/support person informed and educated. This requires skills that keep the woman and family always in focus. If a complication is anticipated based on risk factors, the woman can be adequately educated ahead of time. If this is not possible, then a collaborative debriefing should be done to inform the woman and family what has happened, what was done, and rational. When possible, the woman should be allowed contact with her newborn to facilitate attachment.

Strategies for Success in Intrapartum Emergencies

An intrapartum emergency not only causes fear and anxiety for the woman and family, it is also stressful for the healthcare team and increases the risk of errors. Therefore, hospitals need to have effective, efficient, and tested systems and processes in place to decrease delays in care and improve safety. The first strategy is to assess for risk factors of an obstetric emergency, communicate, and develop an interprofessional plan of care prior to the event. Second, early recognition of maternal compromise, communication of abnormal assessment parameters, and provider assessment has been shown to improve outcomes.[33]

A rapid, multifaceted response from the team is essential to success during intrapartum emergencies. The potential importance and effectiveness of periodic team drills to improve healthcare provider responses in emergencies has been established. The Joint Commission has recommended the use of drills since 2004 for common obstetric emergencies such as those presented in this module.

- **How can mock drills help the response to intrapartum emergencies?**

Drills for obstetric emergencies can potentially
- Increase the preparedness of the team
- Increase the confidence of the team

- Increase the effectiveness of the team
- Increase patient safety
- Reduce healthcare provider anxiety
- Promote collaborative care

AND

- Improve outcomes for mothers and babies
- Choose the most commonly experienced intrapartum emergencies
- Develop a list of roles and responsibilities of team members
- Develop algorithms or protocols for the sequencing of interventions
- Record the drill (scribe or video) for feedback
- Set reasonable goals for implementation
- Document and share successful programs for all to reap the benefits

For additional information on simulation, refer to Module 22.

PRACTICE/REVIEW QUESTIONS

After reviewing this module, answer the following questions.

1. Explain the first step that you would take when a prolapsed cord is detected.

    _____

2. If you suspect a prolapsed cord and the membranes rupture spontaneously, what should you do?

    _____

3. If the cord extends through the vagina and you are awaiting the OR team to arrive, what should you do?

    _____

4. Why is it not advisable to handle a prolapsed cord?

    _____

5. State five situations in which the danger of a prolapsed cord exists, necessitating a vaginal examination.

    a. _____

    b. _____

    c. _____

    d. _____

    e. _____

6. Shoulder dystocia occurs when

    _____

    _____

7. Shoulder dystocia can be predicted and prevented.

    a. True

    b. False

8. Even though shoulder dystocia cannot be reliably predicted or prevented, there are three clinical scenarios in which the provider may consider a varied birth plan. These include:

    a. _____

    b. _____

    c. _____

9. List the risks of shoulder dystocia to both the woman and baby.

    Woman   **Baby**

    _____   _____

    _____   _____

    _____   _____

    _____   _____

10. List actions to take if you anticipate a shoulder dystocia may occur.

    a. _____

    b. _____

    c. _____

11. Match the interventions for shoulder dystocia (Column A) with the provider (Column B).

    Column A   **Column B**

    _____ 1. Call for help.   a. nurse
                                      b. birth attendant
    _____ 2. Evaluate for   (midwife or
             episiotomy   physician)

    _____ 3. McRoberts maneuver

    _____ 4. Suprapubic pressure

    _____ 5. Manipulative maneuvers

    _____ 6. Remove posterior arm

    _____ 7. Roll mother to "all fours"

12. McRoberts maneuver is accomplished by positioning the woman's _____ on her _____.

    This makes it easier to deliver the anterior shoulder by

    _____ and _____ _____.

465

13. Documentation of the occurrence of a shoulder dystocia should include all of the following:

    a. _____

    b. _____

    c. _____

    d. _____

    e. _____

    f. _____

14. Fundal pressure should never be used in a shoulder dystocia due to risks to the woman and the baby.

    a. True

    b. False

15. Amniotic fluid embolism is likely related to an aggressive immunologic response to fetal tissue and massive release of endogenous and/or inflammatory mediators causing:

    a. _____

    b. _____

    c. _____

16. Maternal mortality with a diagnosis of AFE is:

    _____

17. Most AFEs occur during the immediate postpartum period?

    a. True

    b. False

18. The most common symptoms of AFE are:

    _____

    _____

    _____

19. If the intrapartum woman is not responding to CPR after a cardiac arrest caused by an AFE, a _____ may be performed to improve neonatal outcome.

20. List the maternal signs and symptoms of a class II hemorrhage (1,200 to 1,500 mL blood loss):

    a. _____

    b. _____

    c. _____

    d. _____

21. Maternal hypovolemic shock symptoms do not appear until approximately 40% of the circulating blood volume is lost.

    a. True

    b. False

22. The classic signs of a placental abruption are:

    a. _____

    b. _____

    c. _____

    d. _____

    e. _____

    f. _____

23. If the woman is experiencing mild to moderate vaginal bleeding, frequent uterine contractions, and an elevated heart rate, and the fetus demonstrates a change in heart rate baseline (tachycardia or bradycardia) and late decelerations, the placental abruption would likely be classified as:

    a. Grade 1

    b. Grade 2

    c. Grade 3

24. List five factors associated with placental abruption:

    a. _____

    b. _____

    c. _____

    d. _____

    e. _____

25. For the woman at 31 weeks' gestation with mild symptoms of placental abruption the nurse would anticipate administration of _____ to enhance fetal lung maturity.

26. A 28-year-old woman at 30 weeks' gestation has severe abdominal pain and palpable fetal parts outside the uterus. By definition, a disruption of the layers of the uterus allowing any portion of the fetal–placental unit outside is known as _____

    _____

27. Rank the following according to the highest incidence of uterine rupture with a history of a previous cesarean birth.

    a. no labor

    b. induction with prostaglandin

    c. induction without prostaglandin

    d. spontaneous labor

28. Changes in the electronic fetal monitor tracing which may indicate a uterine rupture include:

    _____

    _____

    _____

29. Postpartum hemorrhage (PPH) is defined as blood loss greater than _____ mL after birth, or a _____% change in admission and postpartum maternal hematocrit.

30. Explain how uterine atony may cause postpartum hemorrhage.

_____

_____

_____

31. A 20-year-old gravida 3 is having continued, excessive bleeding 45 minutes after a spontaneous vaginal birth of a baby girl. The first two nursing actions should be

a. _____

b. _____

32. Oxytocin may be given after delivery at a dose of _____ U to prevent postpartum hemorrhage.

33. Methergine should not be used in women with _____ or _____.

34. Administration routes for misoprostol include:

_____

PRACTICE/REVIEW QUESTION ANSWER KEY

1. Place the woman in a position that reduces compression of the cord by the presenting part. Use the extreme Trendelenburg or modified Sims position.
2. Perform a vaginal examination. If you encounter a prolapsed cord, leave your hand in the vagina, holding up the presenting part to alleviate compression on the cord.
3. Do not touch it. Cover the cord with a sterile gauze pad moistened with saline solution. Place the mother in the knee–chest or Sims position and call the provider.
4. Handling the cord can cause it to go into spasms, shutting off the fetal blood supply.
5. a. When there is unexplained fetal distress (especially when the presenting part is high)
   b. When membranes rupture with a high presenting part
   c. When membranes rupture in a woman with a malpresentation
   d. When the fetus is very premature
   e. In a twin gestation
6. The fetal head is delivered, but the anterior shoulder is impacted on the pubic arch.
7. b. False
8. a. Suspected fetal macrosomia defined as an estimated fetal weight of 5,000 g in a nondiabetic woman or 4,500 g in a woman with diabetes
   b. Prior shoulder dystocia
   c. Mid pelvic operative birth with an estimated fetal weight of 4,000 g
9. Woman—postpartum hemorrhage, third- or fourth-degree episiotomy/laceration

Baby—brachial plexus injury, clavicular fracture, cerebral hypoxia, death

10. a. Alert anesthesia staff to be present for the woman's pain management needs.
    b. Alert neonatal staff to be present to help with resuscitation of the newborn as needed.
    c. Empty the woman's bladder by catheterization to prevent possible obstruction or trauma.
11. 1. a
    2. b
    3. a
    4. a
    5. b
    6. b
    7. a
12. Thighs, abdomen, straightening the sacrum, decreasing the angle of incline of the symphysis pubis.
13. a. Specific maneuvers employed, order and number of attempts
    b. Duration of the event, time from delivery of the fetal head to the delivery of the body
    c. Team members involved
    d. Fetal arm impacted, left or right
    e. Umbilical cord pH
    f. Resuscitation measures for the newborn
14. a. True
15. Sudden maternal hypoxia and hypotension
    Cardiovascular collapse
    Coagulopathy
16. 60% to 80%
17. b. False
18. Hypertension, fetal distress, pulmonary edema or ARDS, cardiopulmonary arrest, cyanosis, and coagulopathy.
19. Perimortem cesarean section
20. a. Tachycardia
    b. Tachypnea
    c. Narrowing pulse pressure
    d. Delayed capillary refill
21. a. True
22. a. Uterine tenderness or abdominal pain
    b. Vaginal bleeding
    c. Increased uterine contractions
    d. Rigid, board-like abdomen
    e. Category II or II EFM pattern
    f. Maternal tachycardia
23. b. Grade 2
24. Any five of the following:
    a. Trauma
    b. Uterine or umbilical cord anomaly
    c. Maternal hypertension
    d. Cigarette smoking
    e. Maternal age and parity
    f. Cocaine use
    g. Premature rupture of membranes
    h. Placement of an intrauterine pressure catheter
    i. Previous cesarean birth
    j. Maternal thrombophilia
25. Corticosteroids

26. Uterine rupture
27. b, c, d, a
28. Abrupt decrease in FHR, late or variable decelerations, or an erratic FHR
29. 500 mL, 10%
30. Uterine atony can cause postpartum hemorrhage since the uterine vessels are not compressed when the uterine muscle is in a relaxed state.
31. Empty the woman's bladder and perform uterine massage
32. 10 to 40 U
33. Hypertension or coronary insufficiency
34. Oral, vaginal, or rectal

REFERENCES

1. Phelan, S. T., & Holbrook, B. D. (2013). Umbilical cord prolapse: A plan for an OB emergency. Contemporary OB/GYN. Retrieved from: http://contemporaryobgyn.modernmedicine.com/contemporary-obgyn/content/tags/bradley-holbrook-md/umbilical-cord-prolapse?page=full
2. Kahana, B., Sheiner, E., Levy, A., et al. (2004). Umbilical cord prolapse and perinatal outcomes. *International Journal of Gynaecology and Obstetrics, 84*, 127–132.
3. Lin, M. G. (2006). Umbilical cord prolapse. *Obstetrics and Gynecologic Survey, 61*, 269–277.
4. American College of Obstetrics and Gynecologists. (2014). Executive Summary: Neonatal brachial plexus palsy. *Obstetrics and Gynecology, 123*(4), 902–904.
5. Bruner, J. P., Drummond, S. B., Meenan, A. L., et al. (1998). All-fours maneuver for reducing shoulder dystocia during labor. *Journal of Reproductive Medicine, 43*, 439–443.
6. Clark, S. L. (2014). Amniotic fluid embolism. *Obstetrics & Gynecology, 123*(2), 337–348.
7. Romero, R., Kadar, N., Vaisbuch, E., et al. (2010). Maternal death following cardiopulmonary collapse after delivery: Amniotic fluid embolism or septic shock due to intrauterine infection? *American Journal of Reproductive Immunology, 64*, 113–125.
8. Callaghan, W. M., Creanga, A. A., & Kuklina, E. V. (2012). Severe maternal morbidity among delivery and postpartum hospitalizations in the United States. *Obstetrics & Gynecology, 120*, 1029–1036.
9. Grobman, W. A., Bailit, J. L., Rice, M. M., et al. (2014). Frequency of and factors associated with severe maternal morbidity. *Obstetrics and Gynecology, 123*(4), 804–810.
10. Kuklina, E., Meikle, S., Jamieson, D., et al. (2009). Severe obstetric morbidity in the U. S., 1998–2005. *Obstetrics and Gynecology, 113*, 283–299.
11. Shields, L. E., Wiesner, S., Fulton, J., et al. (2015). Comprehensive maternal hemorrhage protocols reduce utilization of blood products and improve patient safety. *American Journal of Obstetrics & Gynecology, 212*(3), 272–280.
12. Al Kadri, H., Anazi, B., & Tamim, H. (2011). Visual estimation versus gravimetric measurement of postpartum blood loss: A prospective cohort study. *Archives of Gynecology and Obstetrics, 283*, 1207–1213.
13. Grabel, K. T., & Weeber, T. A. (2012). Measuring and communicating blood loss during obstetric hemorrhage. *Journal of Obstetric, Gynecologic & Neonatal Nursing, 41*(4), 551–558.
14. Martin, S. R. (2011). Transfusion of blood components and derivatives in the obstetric care patient. In Foley, M. R., Strong, T. H., & Garite, T. J. (Eds.), *Obstetric intensive care manual* (3rd ed.). New York: McGraw-Hill.
15. Clark, S. L., & Hankins, G. D. (2012). Preventing maternal mortality: 10 clinical diamonds. *Obstetrics & Gynecology, 119*(2), 360–364.
16. Sosa, M. E. (2014). Bleeding in pregnancy. In Simpson, K. R., & Creehan, P. A. (Eds.), *Perinatal nursing* (pp. 143–165). Philadelphia, PA: Wolters Kluwer.
17. Francois, K. E., & Foley, M. R. (2012). Antepartum and postpartum hemorrhage. In Gabbe, S. G., Simpson, J. L., & Niebyl, J. R. (Eds.), *Obstetrics: Normal and problem pregnancies* (6th ed., pp. 415–444). New York: Churchill Livingstone.
18. Hull, A. D., & Resnick, R. (2010). Placenta accreta and postpartum hemorrhage. *Clinical Obstetrics and Gynecology, 53*(1), 228–236.
19. Kramer, M. S., Usher, R. H., Pollack, R., et al. (1997). Etiologic determinants of abruptio placentae. *Obstetrics & Gynecology, 89*, 221.
20. Hulse, G. K., Milne, E., English, D. R., et al. (1997). Assessing the relationship between maternal cocaine use and abruptio placentae. *Addiction, 92*, 1547.
21. Vintzileos, A. M., Campbell, W. A., Nochimson, D. J., et al. (1987). Preterm premature rupture of membranes: A risk factor for the development of abruptio placentae. *American Journal of Obstetrics & Gynecology, 156*, 1235–1238.
22. Oylese, Y., & Ananth, C. V. (2010). Postpartum hemorrhage: Epidemiology, risk factors, and causes. *Clinical Obstetrics and Gynecology, 53*(1), 147–156.
23. Lang, C. T., & Landon, M. B. (2010). Uterine rupture as a source of obstetrical hemorrhage. *Clinical Obstetrics & Gynecology, 53*, 237–251.
24. ACOG Practice bulletin no. 115. (2010). Vaginal birth after previous cesarean delivery. *Obstetrics & Gynecology, 116*(2 pt 1), 450–463.
25. Landon, M. B., Hauth, J. C., Leveno, K. J., et al. (2004). Maternal and perinatal outcomes associated with a trial of labor after prior cesarean delivery. For the NICHD Maternal Fetal Medicine Unit Network. *New England Journal of Medicine, 351*, 2581.
26. Callahan, W. M., Kuklina, E. V., & Berg, C. J. (2010). Trends in postpartum hemorrhage: United States, 1994–2006. *American Journal of Obstetrics and Gynecology, 202*(4), 353.e1–e6.
27. Bateman, B. T., Berman, M. F., Riley, L. E., et al. (2010). The epidemiology of postpartum hemorrhage in a large, nationwide sample of deliveries. *Anesthesia and Analgesia, 110*, 1368–1373.
28. Silver, R. M., Landon, M. B., Rouse, D. J., et al. (2006). Maternal morbidity associated with multiple repeat cesarean deliveries. *Obstetrics & Gynecology, 107*(6), 1226–1232.
29. Warshak, C. R., Ramos, G. A., Eskander, R., et al. (2010). Effect of predelivery diagnosis in 99 consecutive cases of placenta accrete. *Obstetrics & Gynecology, 115*, 65.
30. Eller, A. G. (2011). Maternal morbidity in cases of placenta accreta managed by a multidisciplinary care team compared with standard obstetric care. *Obstetrics & Gynecology, 117*(2), 331–337.
31. Comstack, C. H., & Bronsteen, R. A. (2014). The antenatal diagnosis of placental accreta. *British Journal of Obstetrics and Gynaecology, 121*(2), 171–181.
32. Oyelese, Y., Catanzarite, V., Perfumo, F., et al. (2004). Vasa previa: The impact of prenatal diagnosis on outcomes. *Obstetrics & Gynecology, 103*(5), 937–942.
33. Baird, S. M., & Graves, C. (2015). REACT: An interprofessional education and safety program to recognize and manage the compromise obstetric patient. *Journal of Perinatal and Neonatal Nursing, 28*(2), 138–148.

Assessment of the Newly Delivered Mother

JENNIFER DALTON

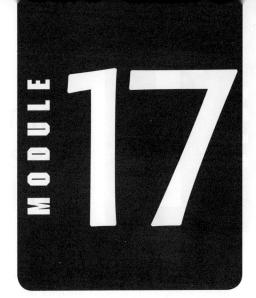

Objectives

As you complete Part 2 of this module, you will learn:

1. Components and expected findings of the physical assessment of a newly delivered mother
2. Variations from normal findings during the early postpartum period and familiarity with common interventions
3. Nursing interventions that promote parent–infant attachment
4. Techniques to assist the mother with the initiation of breastfeeding in the immediate postpartum period
5. Necessary interventions for women with recovery complicated by surgery, anesthesia, infection, or pregnancy-related hypertension
6. Ongoing needs of the newly delivered mother during postpartum hospitalization
7. General guidelines for discharge of mother and infant

Key Terms

When you have completed this module, you should be able to recall the meaning of the following terms. You should also be able to use the terms when consulting with other health professionals. The terms are defined in this module or in the glossary at the end of this book.

atony	involution
dermatome	lochia
preeclampsia	rubra
hematoma	tubal ligation

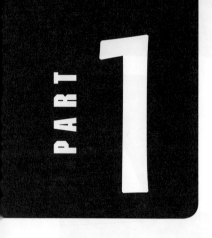

PART 1

Immediate Postpartum Assessment of the Mother

Immediately following the delivery of the placenta until maternal stabilization is a time of complex physiologic and psychosocial changes for the new mother. It is imperative that the nurse caring for the newly delivered woman has knowledge of the prenatal history as well as the intrapartum course.

• What are the components of the physical assessment of a newly delivered mother?

The nurse must be well versed in postpartum assessment and be able to identify subtle changes that could indicate a woman's deteriorating condition. Components of care should be standardized regardless of whether the recovery is done in a post-anesthesia care unit (PACU), a labor and delivery room or a postpartum room. According to the 2010 recommendations from the Association of Women's Health, Obstetric, and Neonatal Nurses (AWHONN), the nurse caring for the woman should not have any other patient or infant care responsibilities until an initial assessment is completed and documented, the repair of the episiotomy or perineal lacerations is complete and the woman is hemodynamically stable.[1]

The care provided should be family centered, which incorporates the needs of the woman and newborn as well as the family. The family consists of the woman and whoever she identifies as her family—this group of people is encouraged to take part in the care of both the woman and the newborn. Healthcare providers should listen to and honor the choices and perspectives of the family as a whole. The family's beliefs, values, and cultural backgrounds are then incorporated into the woman's plan of care. Findings of assessments and explanations of interventions should continue to be explained to the woman and family throughout the postpartum period.[2-5]

Assessments during the immediate postpartum period start from the delivery of the placenta and continue for at least 2 hours or until stable. Assessments should be orderly and ongoing so that timely identification can be made of any abnormal changes in the woman's clinical condition. Note the overall appearance of the woman, including skin color, motor activity, facial expression, speech, mood, state of awareness, and interactions with others. Any variation from normal assessment parameters requires reassessment, communication, and early intervention as indicated to prevent potentially serious consequences.[2-5]

NOTE: Assessments are done every 15 minutes in the first 2 hours.[4]

Vital Signs

Women undergo significant cardiovascular changes during the immediate postpartum period. Average blood loss for a vaginal birth is 400 to 500 mL. If the mother has additional blood loss, vital signs may change to reflect the mother's compensation to maintain cardiac output and tissue perfusion. In addition, blood flow that had been circulating in the uteroplacental vasculature is shunted back into the maternal system, increasing cardiac output.[2,3,5]

Normal Findings

- Systolic blood pressure between 90 and 140 mm Hg.
- Diastolic blood pressure between 60 and 90 mm Hg.
- Heart rate between 60 and 100 beats per minute.
- Respirations between 16 and 24 breaths per minute.
- Temperature between 97°F and 100.4°F.

NOTE: Tracking trends in vital signs are helpful when determining the cause of abnormal values.

Abnormal Findings

Blood Pressure

If blood pressure is elevated, assess the woman for pain and provide pain relief as indicated. Excessive pain may cause a temporary elevation in blood pressure. If blood pressure remains elevated after reassessment, notify the provider as elevated blood pressure in the postpartum period can be a sign of gestational hypertension or preeclampsia.

If a decrease in blood pressure (hypotension) is noted, immediately assess the amount of lochia and watch for signs of shock such as rapid pulse (tachycardia), confusion, clammy skin, rapid breathing (tachypnea), decreased pulse pressure (30 mm Hg or less), weak peripheral pulses, anxiety, or lightheadedness. If hypotension is reassessed, notify the provider to come to the bedside and call for additional assistance if blood pressure does not stabilize rapidly and is accompanied by excessive flow of lochia or signs of shock. The risk of **orthostatic hypotension** is increased in the postpartum period due to decreased vascular resistance in the pelvis. To prevent falls, assist the woman to the side of the bed in a sitting position prior to ambulation, and support her with the first ambulation.[2,3,5]

Heart Rate

Changes in intravascular volume may lead to tachycardia.
- **Hypovolemia signs and symptoms:** initial blood pressure increases followed by dropping blood pressure values, increased respiratory rate, narrowed pulse pressure (less than 30 mm Hg), weak peripheral pulses, dry mucous membranes, and decreased urine output.
- **Hypervolemia signs and symptoms:** increased blood pressure, increased respiratory rate, decreased pulse oximetry values, wide pulse pressure (greater than 70 mm Hg), bounding peripheral pulses, jugular venous distention, adventitious breath sounds, S3 heart sounds.

Respiratory Rate

Following birth, chest wall compliance improves with a decrease in upward pressure on the diaphragm. An elevated respiratory rate may indicate changes in intravascular volume. Other signs of respiratory compromise should be assessed. A decrease in respiratory rate may be caused by anesthetic and/or analgesic medication administration.

NOTE: If BP, HR, or RR is abnormal, reassess every 5 to 15 minutes until normal and notify the provider. With continued abnormal vital sign parameters, the provider should come to the bedside and evaluate the woman to determine the cause and develop an interprofessional plan of care.

Temperature

Take a temperature upon initiation of recovery and repeat in 1 hour, if normal, repeat at the end of recovery, if abnormal retake in 30 minutes. Remember that epidural anesthesia, hormone changes, muscle exertion, and some medications can cause an increase in temperature, but should remain below 100.4°F.

Abnormal Findings

Abnormal values must be evaluated to determine cause. Dehydration after a lengthy labor with inadequate fluid intake is a common cause of early postpartum fever. Women who have had epidural anesthesia may have fever unrelated to infection. Notify the provider and the newborn's pediatric provider if maternal temperature is higher than 100.4°F.

Breasts

During pregnancy, the breasts undergo changes to prepare for lactation. Assessment should include the following[2,3,5,6]:

- Inspection of the breasts for redness and the nipples for cracks, fissures, or blisters. Nipples may be erect, flat, or inverted. Flat nipples that cannot be made to protrude when gently squeezed just behind the nipple can cause difficulty with the infant latching onto the breast. An inverted nipple inverts further when this pinch test is attempted. A manual or electric breast pump can be used immediately before nursing to attempt to make the nipples easier for the infant to grasp.
- Palpation of the breasts for engorgement.
  - Breasts should palpate soft and nontender in the first 24 hours.
  - Postpartum day 2, the breasts are slightly firm and nontender as primary engorgement begins.
  - Postpartum day 3, the breasts are firm and tender. If breastfeeding, the breasts may be warm to touch.

See Figure 17.1.

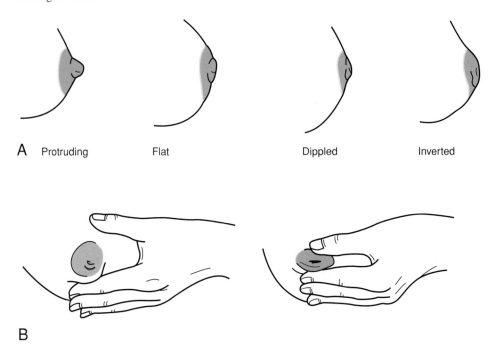

A   Protruding   Flat   Dippled   Inverted

B

FIGURE 17.1   **A.** Nipple shapes. **B.** *Left:* The mother can help the baby to latch on to an inverted nipple if she places her thumb above the areola and her fingers below and pushes the breast against her chest wall. *Right:* The mother should avoid squeezing her thumb and fingers together. The nipple might invert further. (Adapted from Huggins, K. [1990]. *The nursing mother's companion* [Rev. ed., pp. 29, 65]. Boston, MA: Harvard Common Press.)

The woman's decision on whether to breast or bottle feed determines breast care during the postpartum period. If the woman chooses to bottle feed, instruct on the following[2,3,5,6]:
- Wear a supportive bra 24 hours a day until the breasts become soft again.
- Ice packs can be applied to the breasts to reduce breast milk formation and discomfort.
- Do not manually express milk because this can stimulate milk production.
- Avoid heat to the breasts.
- Mild analgesic medications may be taken to ease discomfort.
- Breast engorgement usually decreases within 48 hours.

Uterus

Involution is the process of the uterus returning to its prepregnant state. Uterine tone should be assessed at least as frequently as vital signs, every 15 minutes in the first 2 hours.[4] Amount of blood loss should be assessed on an ongoing basis during this time. Uterine atony is the most common cause of postpartum hemorrhage, which remains a major cause of maternal morbidity and mortality.[7–9]

Evaluate the uterus by noting the fundal height, position, and tone. In order to do this, place one hand just above the symphysis pubis to "cup" the lower portion of the uterus. With the other hand palpate the abdomen starting above the umbilicus to locate the fundus. The fundal height is measured in relation to the umbilicus and is calculated in centimeters above or below the umbilicus. The tone should be firm. If the uterus is boggy (soft), massage until firm.[2,3,5,6]

Normal Findings

In the immediate postpartum period, the fundus should be:
- directly midline, not deviated to either side of the umbilicus;
- firm to the touch; and
- approximately 2 cm below the umbilicus.

Over the next 12 hours, the fundus will rise to approximately 1 cm above the umbilicus before it starts to descend at a rate of approximately 1 to 2 cm every 24 hours. Figure 17.2 indicates expected fundal height measurements during the postpartum period.[2,3,5,6]

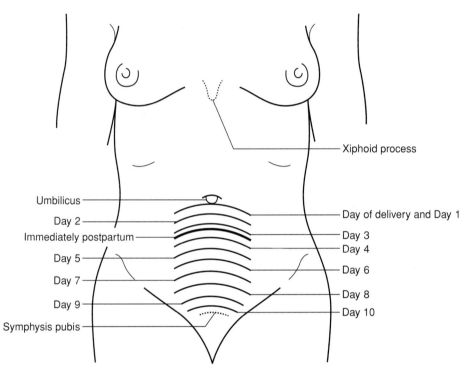

FIGURE 17.2 Fundal height and uterine involution. (Adapted with permission from Varney, H. [1997]. *Varney's midwifery* [3rd ed., p. 624]. Boston, MA: Jones & Bartlett.)

Abnormal Findings

A fundus that is higher than 2 cm above the umbilicus may indicate a distended bladder or a uterus that is filled with blood. After delivery of a large infant, the fundal height can be slightly elevated, and this may be a normal finding. Assist the woman to empty her bladder. Catheterize only if the woman is unable to void and the bladder is distended. Once the bladder is empty, reevaluate the fundal height. Massage the fundus in an attempt to expel any retained blood clots. Report increased fundal height that does not respond to intervention. A boggy uterus may indicate uterine atony, retained placental fragments, or clots. Boggy means the uterus feels spongy as it is not adequately contracted. The boggy uterus should firm up with massage by cupping one hand just above the symphysis pubis to stabilize the uterus and the other hand midline on the abdomen near the umbilicus and begin massaging the area. Moderate massage usually stimulates the relaxed uterus to contract. Massage only until firm. While massaging the uterus, continue to observe the perineum for the amount of bleeding and/or size of expelled clots. If uterine massage does not result in a firm uterus, notify the provider.[2,3,5,6]

Often, a uterotonic agent will be ordered to maintain a firmly contracted uterus. Some clinical situations that can predispose a newly delivered woman to uterine atony are prolonged labor, oxytocin induction of labor, magnesium sulfate therapy, large infant or multiple gestation, chorioamnionitis, or cesarean birth under general anesthesia.[6] For further discussion of postpartum hemorrhage, refer to Module 16 on Obstetric Emergencies.

NOTE: In most cases, postpartum hemorrhage related to uterine atony cannot be predicted before birth. Every newly delivery woman needs careful monitoring.[7–9]

Bowel

During the postpartum period, there is a decrease in gastrointestinal muscle tone and motility. Normal bowel function should return by the end of the second postpartum week. In addition to these changes, decreased activity, hydration, diet, perineal pain, and narcotic medications increase the risk of constipation. Note the date of her last bowel movement. This will be helpful information for continued postpartum care. Auscultate the woman's bowel sounds in all four quadrants. The postpartum woman should be able to pass flatus. Notify the provider if bowel sounds are absent.[2,3,5,6]

Bladder

Bladder distention, incomplete emptying, urine retention, and/or the inability to void may occur during the first few days postpartum. Within 12 hours of birth, changes in hormone levels (decreased estrogen and oxytocin) occur resulting in diuresis. Measure and record urine output in the first 24 hours post birth. A bladder scan can also be used at this time to assess for post void residual.[2,3,5,6]

Normal Findings

Gently palpate the lower abdominal area just above the symphysis pubis for bladder fullness or tenderness. The bladder should not be palpable or tender. The sensation of needing to void may be decreased as a result of pressure on the bladder during labor and birth or because of continued effects of neuraxial anesthesia.[2,3,5,6]

Abnormal Findings

The bladder may become distended from intravenous fluids administered during labor or from the diuresis that normally occurs postpartum. A distended bladder can interfere with uterine contractility and lead to uterine atony and excessive vaginal bleeding. Attempt to have the woman void either into a bed pan or assist with ambulation to the bathroom. Many women are able to void without the sensation of a full bladder. If the woman is unable to void or the bladder scan shows more than 150 mL remains in the bladder, a sterile in-and-out catheterization may be indicated. Avoid allowing the bladder to become over distended, which can lead to loss of muscle tone and continued difficulty with voiding. Burning with urination should be reported to the provider.[2,3,5,6]

Perineum

With adequate lighting and exposure, evaluate for edema and signs of *hematoma* (a discolored or bruised and edematous area). Provide privacy, and placing the woman in a side-lying position to separate the buttocks to expose the perineum for assessment.[2,3,5,6]

Normal Findings

Provide thorough perineal care to assist with visualization. The perineum should be pink, without signs of excessive bruising or findings of considerable edema. Inspection of an episiotomy or laceration repair should reveal approximated tissues with mild edema. An ice pack to the perineum during the first 24 hours may be used to improve comfort and decrease/prevent edema. Sitz baths may be ordered after 24 hours to promote circulation, healing, and comfort. Nonsteroidal anti-inflammatory medications may be ordered by the provider to reduce the inflammatory response and promote healing. Analgesics may be required to meet the woman's pain goals.[2,3,5,6]

To cleanse the perineum, instruct the woman to use a peribottle with warm water to rinse after voiding or bowel movements. The water should rinse in a "front to back" direction toward the rectum. Evaluate the peripad for lochia and instruct the woman to change the pad frequently.[2,3,5,6]

Abnormal Findings

Notify the provider of excessive perineal edema or symptoms of possible hematoma formation. A postpartum hematoma occurs when a blood vessel continues to bleed into the connective tissue of the vagina or perineal area. Risk factors for hematoma formation include the following[2,3,5,6]:

- Episiotomy
- Forceps birth
- Prolonged second stage of labor

A hematoma may be suspected if an area of the perineum becomes hardened, red, swollen, and the woman is complaining of excessive pain. Vaginal hematomas may not be visualized externally. Maternal cardiovascular compromise may occur with significant bleeding into the hematoma or if the hematoma displaces the uterus. Document the size and location of affected area for comparison during resolution. Large hematomas may have to be surgically drained and the bleeding vessel ligated. Observe for signs of distended bladder that may occur if edema is extensive and the woman is unable to void.[5]

Hemorrhoids may form during pregnancy and are often evident after vaginal birth. Note the presence, size, and pain associated with hemorrhoids.[2,3,5,6]

Lochia

Lochia, a Greek word that means "relating to childbirth," is blood, mucus, and sloughed-off tissue from the lining of the uterus that is expelled after birth. Identify the amount and color of the lochia and whether or not there are clots present.[2,3,5,6]

Traditionally, the amount of lochia has been determined by the quantity of saturation on the peripad:

- Scant (less than 2.5 cm)
- Light (less than 10 cm)
- Moderate (greater than 10 cm)
- Heavy (1 pad saturated within 2 hours)
- Excessive blood loss is one pad saturated in less than 15 minutes or pooling of blood under buttocks.

However, with the continued rise in maternal mortality and morbidity in the United States, it is now recommended that a quantified estimation of blood loss (QBL) be assessed for all women immediately postpartum and continuing into the extended postpartum period.[8]

NOTE: *Failure to recognize excessive blood loss during childbirth is a leading cause of maternal morbidity and mortality. Visual estimations of blood loss most often result in under-estimation of blood loss. Quantifying blood loss by weighing or using calibrated drapes reduces the chances of underestimating the amount of blood lost and facilitates early recognition and treatment of excessive blood loss.*[8]

Refer to Module 16 for additional information.

Normal Findings

Lochia should be red (*rubra*) and moderate in flow during the first hour not exceeding the saturation of two peripads in the first hour (Table 17.1).

Abnormal Findings

The most common cause of increased vaginal bleeding in the immediate postpartum period is uterine atony. Other causes that must be considered are retained placental fragments and bleeding from lacerations. If excessive lochia flow is identified, massage the fundus until firm. See Figure 17.3. Notify the provider if bleeding becomes heavy, if a pad is saturated within 15 minutes, or if large or persistent clots are expressed. Anticipate the need for an IV line, if not already available, or additional access. Monitor vital signs frequently and notify the provider if abnormal. Remember that in the postpartum period, significant blood loss can occur without a

TABLE 17.1	LOCHIA CHANGES		
TIMEFRAME	**LOCHIA STAGE**	**EXPECTED FINDINGS**	**ABNORMAL FINDINGS**
Days 1–3	Rubra	Dark red Moderate to scant flow Small clots Increased flow with position changes or breastfeeding Fleshy odor	Large/heavy amount Large clots Foul odor Tissue or possible placental fragments
Days 4–10	Serosa	Pink or brown color Scant amount Increased flow with physical activity Fleshy odor	Continued rubra color after fourth day Heavy amount: saturating peripad every hour Foul odor
After day 10	Alba	Yellow to white color Scant amount Fleshy odor	Bright red bleeding Heavy amount Foul odor

From Leifer, G. (2011). *Maternity nursing: An introductory text* (10th ed.). St. Louis, MO: Elsevier Science; Lowdermilk, D., & Perry, S. (2013). *Maternity nursing* (8th ed.). St. Louis, MO: Elsevier Health Sciences; Durham, R., & Chapman, L. (Eds.). (2014). *Maternal–newborn nursing: The critical components of nursing care* (2nd ed.). Philadelphia, PA: F.A. Davis; James, D. C. (2014). Postpartum care. In Simpson, K. R., & Creehan, P. A. (Eds.), *AWHONN's perinatal nursing* (4th ed., pp. 530–580). Philadelphia, PA: Lippincott.

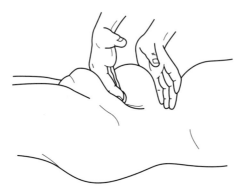

FIGURE 17.3 Placement of the hands for uterine massage.

decrease in blood pressure. Medications, as discussed in the section on decreased uterine tone, may be ordered. If bleeding continues despite a firm uterus, notify the provider and request them at the bedside for assessment. Further assessment of the perineum, vagina, and cervix for lacerations or evaluation of the woman for retained placental fragments may be necessary.[2,3,5–8] Anticipate the need to transfer to the operating room for further care as indicated. See Module 16 for more detailed information regarding postpartum hemorrhage.

Extremities

Women are at increased risk of thrombus formation during the postpartum period due to an increase in clotting factors during pregnancy. Assess for pain, swelling, tenderness, or warmth in lower extremities, which may indicate thrombus formation. Homan's sign, an assessment that requires dorsiflexion of the foot, is considered positive if pain occurs with the movement. To decrease the risk of thrombus formation, apply sequential compression devices if extended bed rest is anticipated and encourage early ambulation. Assess the legs for edema and varicosities.[2,3,5,6]

Pain

The woman may experience pain from perineal trauma (episiotomy, lacerations), incisions (cesarean birth or tubal ligation), hemorrhoids, intestinal gas (especially after cesarean birth), breast engorgement, or nipple irritation. In addition, after birth pains (moderate uterine contractions) occur as part of involution and increase in with frequency and intensity with breastfeeding due to oxytocin release with infant sucking. Adequately assess the report of pain, including perception of severity and location.[2,3,5,6]

NOTE: If there is an abnormal amount of pain reported after pain measures are implemented, notify the provider to determine the cause and to develop an interprofessional plan of care.

• Are there additional components of assessment after cesarean birth?

After a cesarean birth, the woman should be cared for in the PACU or an appropriately equipped labor and delivery room. Standards of care for these women are no different from the standards for any patient recovering from major surgery and anesthesia. Previously outlined reproductive and hemodynamic assessments and interventions for the postpartum mother also apply after a cesarean birth. Since postoperative hypothermia is common, assess the mother's temperature every 15 minutes until normothermic. Hypothermia interventions include the placement of warm blankets or forced-air warming devices, changing linen or the woman's gown if wet, and warming the room temperature. The woman will continue to receive IV fluids and have an indwelling urinary catheter. Intake and output totals should be assessed.

If the woman had general anesthesia, fundal massage will be painful. Give ordered pain medications as indicated, instruct the woman on breathing/relaxation, and explain the importance of assessment. If the uterus is contracted and lochia is small, massage should not be excessive or vigorous. The abdominal dressing condition should be assessed frequently noting any presence of blood. After the immediate postpartum period, the abdominal wound site should be inspected with other systems' assessments. Skin sutures or clips are usually removed on the fourth postoperative day unless there is concern for wound separation. Pneumatic compression devices should remain in place until ambulation. Early ambulation is encouraged to reduce the risk of thrombus formation and embolism, which is increased with cesarean birth. Laboratory evaluation of hematocrit is routinely done on postoperative day 1 or sooner if there is concern regarding blood loss.[2,3,5,6]

Routine separation of woman and infant is not necessary unless warranted by the condition of either the woman or the newborn. If the woman is planning on breastfeeding, the newborn should be placed to breast for feeding within the first hour. Provide support and encouragement with infant care.[6]

As anesthesia wears off during the early postpartum period, the woman will report pain or request pain medication. It is important for the nurse to know medications and dosing the woman received during surgery and which medications the anesthesiology provider has ordered for the immediate postpartum period. Some women might have received spinal or epidural narcotics that will decrease pain during the postpartum period, but may require anti-inflammatory agents to augment relief. Pain and/or discomfort are normal findings after surgery; a goal of care is to reduce the severity of the pain. Medicate the postpartum cesarean-delivered woman as needed to achieve comfort. An adequately medicated person experiences fewer complications related to immobility than a person in pain and recovers more quickly from surgery. Comfort measures, such as positioning and massage techniques, may be utilized as means of decreasing discomfort.

For a full discussion of intrapartum and operative care for the woman experiencing a cesarean birth, see Module 15.

• What are the components of assessment for a woman recovering from neuraxial anesthesia?

The plan for postpartum intermittent or continuous regional anesthesia for pain management is determined at birth by the anesthesiology provider and in conjunction with the woman's pain goals. If the woman has an uncomplicated vaginal birth, medication administration by an epidural pump is usually discontinued. The following outlines the nurse's responsibility for assessment of regional anesthesia recovery during the immediate postpartum period[10]:

- Assessment of vital signs as previously outlined
- Assessment of current pain level and notification of appropriate provider if pain needs are not met
- Monitor the level of mobility
- Removal of epidural catheter according to hospital/agency policy
- Communication of abnormal assessment parameters to appropriate provider and according to provider orders

As a component of the recovery assessment from neuraxial anesthesia, it is important for the nurse to know the type of anesthetic used since length of action for different anesthetics and the time of last dose affects the length of the recovery period. Most neuraxial anesthetic medications will wear off within 2 hours after discontinuation/last dose. If the woman's sensory and mobility do not return within 2 hours, the anesthesiology provider should be notified.

For post cesarean birth, women who have received neuraxial (spinal or epidural) anesthesia, the sensory level of the block should be evaluated by the anesthesiology provider upon admission to the PACU. Often, the anesthesiology provider will use dermatome levels to document the current sensory level (see Fig. 17.4). The chart is used to identify areas of the skin that correspond to the area of innervation in the spine. Assessment of the spinal level of the anesthetic may be performed by using an alcohol pad to touch the abdomen until sensation is identified by the woman. The level at which sensation is felt corresponds to the spinal level. As anesthesia wears off, the spinal level decreases. Sensation and the ability to move the legs indicate that the level of anesthesia is diminishing.

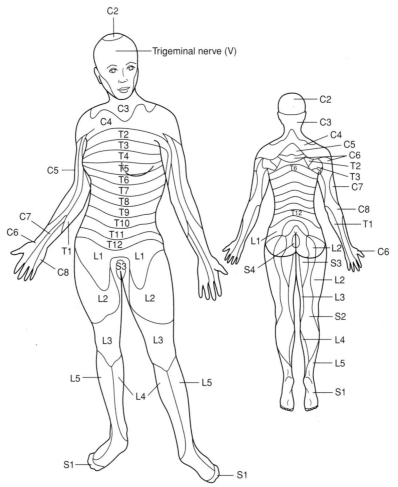

FIGURE 17.4   Segmental dermatome distribution of spinal nerves. C, cervical segments; L, lumbar segments; S, sacral segments; T, thoracic segments. (Adapted with permission from Thibodeau, G. [1987]. *Anatomy and physiology* [p. 71]. St. Louis, MO: Mosby.)

Careful attention to positioning of the lower extremities to prevent injury is also important until full sensation has returned. Ambulation should not be attempted until full control of the legs returns. Even after motor control has returned, sensation in the lower body can be diminished increasing the risk of the woman falling.

An epidural hematoma is a rare complication of neuraxial anesthesia, with an increased risk in women with coagulation deficits or after receiving anticoagulation therapy. Bleeding and hematoma formation in the epidural space can lead to irreversible neurologic damage due to compression on the spinal nerves, ischemia, and infarction. If sensory regression is not evident during the postpartum period, the nurse should notify the anesthesiology provider and have them come to the bedside to assess the woman since early diagnosis and resolution improve outcomes.

NOTE: Due to the fall risk and increased nurse to patient ratios after the initial recovery period, it is recommended that discharge from anesthesiology care does not occur until the woman has recovered from the effects of anesthesia.[1]

• What are the components of assessment for a woman recovering from general anesthesia?

Recovery from general anesthesia occurs in a specially equipped and appropriately staffed PACU area. Emergency resuscitation supplies and equipment should be readily available and include the following[4,11]:

- Artificial airways
- Oxygen
- Suction
- Blood pressure, pulse, temperature, and pulse oximetry monitoring
- Glucometer

One-to-one nurse-to-patient ratio should be assigned until the mother is stable and all critical elements of maternal care have been met. In addition, one nurse should be assigned to care for each newborn until the newborn critical elements are met. Once the critical elements are met, one nurse can take care of the mother/baby duo with a second nurse available as needed (Table 17.2).[1,6]

TABLE 17.2 CRITICAL ELEMENTS DURING THE IMMEDIATE POSTPARTUM PERIOD	
MATERNAL CRITICAL ELEMENTS	**NEWBORN CRITICAL ELEMENTS**
Report from the anesthesiology provider has been completed, questions answered, and the transfer of care has occurred	Report from the newborn nurse has been received, questions have been answered, and the transfer of care has occurred
The woman is conscious and her respiratory status is within defined parameters	The initial newborn exam has been completed and documented
The initial assessment is completed and documented	Identification bracelets have been placed
The woman is hemodynamically stable	The newborn's condition is stable

From Association of Perioperative Registered Nurses. (2012). *Perioperative standards and recommended practices for inpatient and ambulatory settings.* Denver, CO: Author.

Any nurse working in PACU should have specialized training in the monitoring of postoperative women and emergency resuscitation.[6]

Most hospitals require a systematic assessment to determine the readiness for post-anesthesia discharge. The Aldrete Scoring System is a common tool used with score of greater than or equal to 8 as the usual score required for discharge (Table 17.3).[12]

• What are the components of postpartum care for women with obstetric, medical, or surgical complications in the postpartum period?

Puerperal Infection

Puerperal infection is a term used to describe any bacterial infection of the genital tract in the postpartum period. Infection during the birth process is most commonly chorioamnionitis, an infection of the fetal membranes that can occur after prolonged rupture of membranes or multiple vaginal examinations. The infection usually begins to resolve after birth but may necessitate administration of antibiotics and progressive infection in the mother. The pediatric care provider should be notified of infections in the mother.[5,6] See Module 12 for additional information regarding infections.

An oral temperature of greater than 100.4°F (38°C) is considered fever and should be reported to the provider. Other signs of infection can include tachycardia, tachypnea, unusual pain, or a tender uterus. Risks of endometritis include the following[5,6]:

- Previous diagnosis of chorioamnionitis
- Prolonged labor and/or rupture of membranes
- Frequent cervical exams

TABLE 17.3	MODIFIED ALDRETE SCORE	
	CRITERIA	**SCORE**
Respiration	Able to breathe deeply and cough freely	2
	Dyspnea, shallow, or limited breathing	1
	Apnea	0
Oxygen saturation	Able to maintain oxygen saturation greater than 92% on room air	2
	Needs oxygen inhalation to maintain oxygen saturation greater than 90%	1
	Oxygen saturation less than 90% even with oxygen supplementation	0
Consciousness	Fully awake	2
	Arousable on calling	1
	Not responding	0
Circulation	Blood pressure ±20 mm Hg preanesthetic level	2
	Blood pressure ±20–49 mm Hg preanesthetic level	1
	Blood pressure ±50 mm Hg preanesthetic level	0
Activity	Able to move four extremities	2
	Able to move two extremities	1
	Able to move zero extremities	0
		TOTAL

- Lacerations during birth
- Internal monitoring or procedure (fetal scalp electrode, intrauterine pressure monitoring, amnioinfusion)
- Hemorrhage
- Underlying medical problems that may compromise healing or host defense (e.g., diabetes)
- Anemia

Other causes of postpartum infection include the following[5,6]:
- Urinary tract infection (UTI) (cystitis or pyelonephritis)
- Pneumonia
- Wound (episiotomy/laceration, cesarean section)
- Mastitis
- Pelvic thrombophlebitis
- Necrotizing fasciitis

NOTE: *Indwelling urinary catheter should be removed as soon as possible in the postpartum period to decrease the risk of UTI.*

The provider will consider the cause of the fever and, if infection is suspected, may order broad-spectrum antibiotics. Fluids may also be ordered, either intravenously or by mouth. In addition, antipyretic medication may be ordered to reduce fever. Monitoring of the course of the infection by evaluation of vital sign and laboratory trends is important to determine the effectiveness of treatment.

Preeclampsia

The cure for preeclampsia is birth. Usually, a woman rapidly improves after the birth; however, the risk for seizures continues, especially in the first 24 hours. Women with preeclampsia need careful assessment and monitoring of vital signs, especially blood pressure, in the early postpartum period. Assessment of trends in blood pressure values is important for these women. The provider will define parameters of blood pressure readings that are acceptable and parameters that require notification. Reports of headache and visual changes by the mother are also important to consider in the overall assessment of recovery. Intake and output should be strictly monitored every hour. Urine output should be greater or equal to 30 mL per hour. Breath sounds should be monitored and pulse oximetry values checked with the increased risk of pulmonary edema associated with preeclampsia.[2,3,5]

NOTE: *Refer to Module 11 on hypertensive disorders of pregnancy for a more complete description of preeclampsia and the necessary assessments, interventions, and magnesium sulfate administration.*

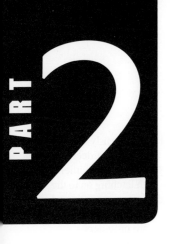

PART 2

Role of the Nurse in Postpartum Care

- ### What can the nurse do to promote infant attachment?

The bond between parents and their infant begins from conception and continues to develop during infancy. Sometimes referred to as the "sacred hour," the first hour after birth is a special time for an infant and the new family. For healthy newborns, the best place for them is skin to skin with the mother. Place the baby supine on the woman's chest. All assessments on the stable newborn can be done in this location.[9,13]

Skin-to-skin contact provides the best environment for the stabilization of the newborn after birth. Being skin-to-skin[9,13]:
- helps stabilize respiration and oxygenation,
- reduces incidence of hypoglycemia,
- helps maintain normal temperature,
- reduces stress hormone, and
- decreases crying.

The nurse can promote this attachment to the newborn in simple ways. Parents and family need access to their infant. Well newborns should remain in the woman's room. Many hospitals encourage this practice with AWHONN-recommended nurse-to-patient ratios and by organizing care for both in the woman's room.[1] If an infant must be cared for in the nursery, it is important that policy allows either parent to visit at any time and to call as needed.

Parents need opportunities to get to know their newborn and to learn to feel confident in caring for the infant's needs. The nurse can arrange these opportunities and give positive reinforcement. For example, the father gains confidence and learns much more about his new infant if he is assisted in changing the baby's diaper than if the expert nurse does the job. It is important for the nurse to observe the interactions between parents and newborn during the postpartum stay and to notify pediatric and obstetric care providers of observed difficulties with attachment.

- ### How can the nurse assist the woman in initiating breastfeeding in the immediate postpartum period?

The decision to breast or formula feed is often made in the prenatal period. A discussion of the value of breastfeeding with the obstetric and/or pediatric provider is an important part of prenatal education. AWHONN and the American Academy of Pediatrics recommend exclusive breastfeeding for at least 6 months.[14,15] There are many short- and long-term newborn benefits to breastfeeding.[14,15]

Short-Term: decreased risk of gastrointestinal infections (gastroenteritis, necrotizing enterocolitis), ear infections, pain with minor procedures, hospital readmission, respiratory infections, sudden infant death syndrome (SIDS), and urinary tract infections.

Long-Term: decreased risk of asthma, atopic dermatitis, cardiovascular disease, celiac disease, diabetes, obesity, and sleep disordered breathing; also associated with increased cognition and neurodevelopment.

The only true contraindications to breastfeeding are rare and include[14]:
- infants with galactosemia,
- mothers who are seropositive for human immunodeficiency virus (HIV),
- mothers with human T-cell lymphotropic virus type I or II,

- mothers who require chemotherapy or radiation cancer treatments,
- mothers with untreated tuberculosis,
- illicit substance abuse by the mother, and
- presence of herpes simplex lesions on the breast(s).

Initiation of breastfeeding during the first hour of the infant's life and frequent early nursing are associated with fewer problems with lactation. Early breastfeeding also helps to decrease postpartum bleeding and more rapid uterine involution. Artificial nipples (e.g., bottles, pacifiers) should be avoided during the early postpartum period to prevent problems with latching on to the breast. Supplementation with formula or water in the early postpartum period is unnecessary and can interfere with successful lactation. Breastfeeding is a learned activity for both the woman and newborn. This process takes time and assistance from knowledgeable care providers.

Determine the readiness of the woman and infant to breastfeed and as soon as possible after birth and encourage initiation of breastfeeding. During this first hour, the newborn is typically in the quiet/alert state and is receptive to breastfeeding. Assist the woman to a comfortable position. Sitting in an almost upright position is often a position that is good for early nursing. The mother can see her infant, and the nurse can easily observe the nursing couple. Use pillows to position the mother and infant comfortably. The newborn should be positioned so that the infant's body faces the woman's body and the infant's head is in a straight line with his or her own body (Fig. 17.5). The cradle hold, the cross-cradle hold, and the football hold are all good positions for early nursing. Have the woman gently stroke the infant's lower lip until the infant opens the mouth wide. While the infant's mouth is wide open, instruct the woman to quickly move the infant toward the breast. The woman can cup her breast with her hand to guide the breast, grasping the breast with four fingers below and the thumb above the areola (see Fig. 17.5). Fingers need to be kept well back from the areola (the pigmented area of the breast that surrounds the nipple).

The newborn should draw 0.5 to 1 inch of the areola into the mouth. At this first feeding, allow the newborn to nurse on one breast for as long as the baby continues to actively nurse,

Assist the mother to position the infant's body to face the mother's body.

Show the mother how to grasp the breast with four fingers below and the thumb above.

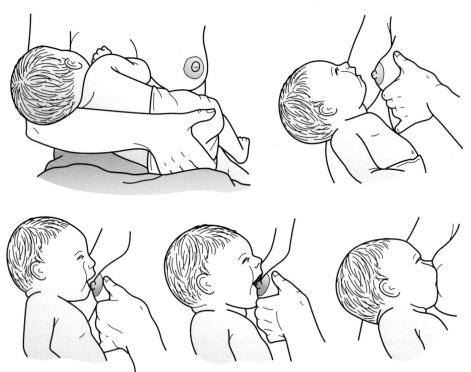

Instruct the mother to touch the nipple to the infant's lower lip.

When the infant's mouth opens wide, instruct the mother to pull the baby in to latch on.

FIGURE 17.5 Positioning for breastfeeding. (Adapted from Huggins, K. [1990]. *The nursing mother's companion* [Rev. ed., p. 43]. Boston, MA: Harvard Common Press.)

then assist the woman to position the newborn at the opposite breast. The newborn may or may not vigorously nurse both breasts at this first feeding. Remind the woman to begin nursing with this second breast at the next feeding. Allow the newborn to learn to nurse during this early feeding. Duration of the feeding is not as important as is the stimulation of the breasts and the learning process. Teach the woman to break the newborn's suction by inserting the tip of her finger into the corner of the infant's mouth when feeding is complete.

Encourage the woman to breastfeed frequently during the hospital stay. Have her offer the breast every 2 to 3 hours and teach her cues that the newborn is waking and getting ready to feed. It is easier to learn to nurse a calm infant who is not crying with hunger. Some newborns do not readily nurse for several feedings. Explain to the woman that this is normal behavior and that her baby is also tired from birth. Most infants nurse vigorously by 12 to 24 hours after birth. Continued difficulties should be referred to a lactation consultant or care provider experienced in lactation assistance. It is important that newborns are feeding well before discharge from the hospital and that the woman knows how to get assistance if needed. A woman should also be taught that the use of any medications while breastfeeding be discussed with the baby's provider.

• What is the role of the nurse in postpartum sterilization?

The decision for postpartum sterilization is most appropriately made during the antepartum period and includes the process of informed consent. Informed consent is obtained by the physician and includes information that the woman can understand about the risks and benefits of a procedure and any alternatives to the procedure. The woman is allowed the opportunity to ask questions and then make her decision. A permit for the procedure is the documentation of this process of education, decision, and consent.

Tubal ligation (the interruption of the course of the fallopian tube) may be performed in the immediate postpartum period if a regional anesthetic has been used for the delivery and if the condition of the mother and infant is satisfactory. If an anesthetic must be initiated for the surgery, the anesthesia care provider will consider the risks and benefits of the timing of this procedure.

Preoperative assessments include a review of the permit and evaluation of the woman and newborn's status in the immediate postpartum period. Vital signs, fundal height, and lochia flow are evaluated. The woman's bladder should be assessed for distention. The woman should be encouraged to empty her bladder immediately before being transferred to the operating room. Allow the woman the opportunity to ask questions about the procedure.

The anesthesia care provider or obstetrician may order preoperative medications. It is important to notify the care provider of any variations from the normal postpartum assessments of the woman or any problems of the newborn before tubal ligation is performed. Postoperative interventions are also similar to care after a cesarean birth. Pain can usually be managed with oral medications.

Refer to the assessments of a woman recovering from cesarean birth for postoperative assessments following tubal ligation. The incision is smaller, and pain is typically less severe. Often, women report pain localized to the right side of the abdomen after tubal ligation. A catheter in the bladder is not always used during the procedure. Therefore, the woman's bladder should be assessed to prevent distention and increased uterine bleeding.

• What are the woman's ongoing needs during postpartum hospitalization?

The period of postpartum hospitalization is commonly at least a 24-hour stay. Women remain in the hospital during that time when intensive postpartum care is required and return to their home environments to recover completely. During the hospital stay, the newly delivered woman recovers physically and should also demonstrate the capability to care for herself and her newborn. Rubin's identified periods of the postpartum, *taking in* and *taking on,* identify maternal readiness for self-care and newborn care. During *taking in,* the woman is more passive and focuses primarily on her physical needs. In the *taking-on* period, the woman begins to assume the care of herself and her infant. The woman is commonly discharged during the taking-in period or the early taking-on period and is not ready for assuming total care of herself or her infant. The family needs to understand the new mother's need for help with her care and the newborn's care during this early phase of the postpartum period.[2,3,5]

Education

The educational needs of the new family have always been a concern and the responsibility of the postpartum and newborn nurse. As length of the postpartum stay has decreased, so have the opportunities for education. New research supports the need for thorough prenatal education in postpartum and newborn care. In the early postpartum period, the newly delivered woman is only able to assimilate information that is reinforcement or review of that previously learned. Topics of education that are important for reinforcement of previous teaching include physical care of the woman, physical care of the newborn, warning signs of problems of both newborn and woman, infant nutrition, family adjustments, birth control, and needs for continued care. A simple technique that is effective for education of the new family is for the nurse to explain the care given as it is being provided. The woman has an immediate opportunity to ask questions.[2,3,5]

Rest and Comfort

The physical needs of woman and newborn during the hospital stay include the needs of the woman for rest and nourishment. The nurse evaluates the continued recovery from birth and monitoring the return to the prepregnant state. Variations from normal assessments should be discussed with the provider before discharge. Newborn needs are similar and include the need for the establishment of nourishment. Whether the newborn is breastfed or bottle fed, patterns of feeding need to be observed by the nurse and assistance provided to the parents.

Immunizations

Rubella

During the prenatal period, the woman will be tested for rubella immunity. If she is rubella "Non immune," she should receive a rubella immunization prior to discharge for protection in future pregnancies. Women who contact rubella in the first trimester in pregnancy risk transmitting the infection to the fetus which may result in birth defects such as[5]:
- Deafness
- Blindness
- Heart defects
- Mental retardation

Following immunization, women should avoid becoming pregnant for 3 months.

Varicella

It is also recommended by the Centers for Disease Control and Prevention (CDC) for women to be assessed for immunity to the varicella virus.[16] If the woman is not immune, she should receive the first of 2 doses of the live virus prior to discharge. The second dose is then given at the woman's postpartum visit.[16]

Influenza

Lastly, if the woman has not received an influenza vaccination and it is during "flu" season, it is recommended for her to receive the immunization prior to discharge.[16]

Prevention of Rh Isoimmunization

If the postpartum woman is Rh-negative and has given birth to an Rh-positive baby, Rho (D) immune globulin (RhoGAM®) should be administered within 72 hours of birth to prevent Rh isoimmunization and hemolytic anemia in a future pregnancy. Administration prevents the woman from producing anti-Rh (D) antibodies. Rho (D) immune globulin may be dispensed by the blood bank or pharmacy.[5]

NOTE: *If the woman requires Rho (D) immune globulin and immunization for rubella or varicella, titers for immunity should be checked after 6 to 8 weeks since seroconversion may be impaired. This is due to potential interference of the Rho (D) immune globulin since both are live viruses.*[17]

> • **How can the postpartum nurse begin to prepare the woman for the transition to care at home?**

A well-organized and coordinated system of maternity care is needed to ensure that mothers and infants receive the follow-up care necessary to meet the needs of the early postpartum period. Healthcare systems are responding to these needs for follow-up care in a variety of ways. Home visits by specially trained home health nurses, sometimes called "perinatal community nurses," are available for some women. Follow-up phone interviews to identify problems are another method used by care systems.

Every woman, before discharge, needs to know how she can obtain further care for herself and her newborn. Schedules for needed follow-up visits for woman and infant are important. Written lists of community resources and emergency phone numbers are also helpful. This information needs to be discussed with the new family and should also be provided in writing (Table 17.4).[2,3,5]

TABLE 17.4 EXAMPLE DISCHARGE TEACHING CATEGORIES

EXAMPLE DISCHARGE TEACHING CATEGORIES

Woman	Discharge process and preparations
	Lochia changes
	Self-care: breasts, perineum, bladder, wound
	Fundal massage
	Afterbirth pain
	Diet and nutrition
	Physical activity and exercise
	Changes in mood and emotions including signs/symptoms of postpartum mood disorders
	Signs/symptoms of complications
	• Fever: temperature ≥100.4 degrees
	• Swelling and pain in lower extremities
	• Wound drainage
	• Increased vaginal bleeding
	Sexual activity including plans for contraception
	Pain management
	Medications
	Need for follow-up care with provider
Newborn	Infant safety and security
	Proper hand hygiene
	Feeding method and techniques
	Changes in stool
	Urination
	Bathing
	Skin care
	Diapering
	Warmth
	Proper car seat use: car seat challenge test as applicable
	Soothing techniques
	Sleep patterns and positioning
	Signs/symptoms of complications
	• Fever: include how to take temperature
	• Inability to eat
	• Jaundice
	• Decreased urination
	• Lethargy
	Exposure to second hand smoke
	Immunizations
	Medications and/or lab testing
	Need for follow-up care with provider

From Leifer, G. (2011). *Maternity nursing: An introductory text* (10th ed.). St. Louis, MO: Elsevier Science; Lowdermilk, D., & Perry, S. (2013). *Maternity nursing* (8th ed.). St. Louis, MO: Elsevier Health Sciences; Durham, R., & Chapman, L. (Eds.). (2014). *Maternal–newborn nursing: The critical components of nursing care* (2nd ed.). Philadelphia, PA: F.A. Davis.

PRACTICE/REVIEW QUESTIONS

After reviewing Part 2, answer the following questions.

1. It is not unusual to be unable to palpate the uterus immediately after birth. During this time, the uterus is often boggy and difficult to locate.

   a. True

   b. False

2. A distended bladder is suspected if the fundal height is above the umbilicus and deviated to the right of the midline.

   a. True

   b. False

3. During the first postpartum hour, the vital signs should be evaluated at least every 15 minutes.

   a. True

   b. False

4. Excessive edema of the perineum should be reported to the physician or midwife.

   a. True

   b. False

5. It is not uncommon for the newly delivered woman to have heavy vaginal bleeding during the first postpartum hour.

   a. True

   b. False

6. A newly delivered woman must be separated from her ill infant. The nurse can facilitate attachment by:

   a. arranging a visit to the nursery as soon as the woman is physically able

   b. reassuring the woman that her infant is being well cared for by the newborn nurses

   c. explaining to the woman that bonding with the newborn can wait until the infant is well

7. A woman is concerned that her newborn did not vigorously nurse at the first feeding and may be hungry. You tell the woman:

   a. she might have to supplement breastfeeding with formula until the newborn begins to nurse more effectively

   b. newborns are learning to nurse at the first feeding and will learn with time; colostrum will meet the newborn's nutritional needs

   c. you will let the pediatric provider know about the problem

8. A mother who is breastfeeding should be taught to check with her physician, midwife, or primary care provider before taking any medications.

   a. True

   b. False

9. Breast shells should be worn if the woman who is breastfeeding has inverted nipples.

   a. True

   b. False

10. Fewer problems with breastfeeding occur if the newborn nurses during the first hour of life.

    a. True

    b. False

11. Informed consent for sterilization includes:

    a. information on the risks of the procedure

    b. reasons to have the surgery done

    c. alternatives to the surgery

    d. a decision by the woman to have the surgery done

    e. all of these

12. Immediately after a cesarean birth, the newly delivered woman:

    a. can return to her postpartum room

    b. should be cared for in a recovery room (PACU) or an appropriately equipped LDRP room depending on anesthesia provided during the cesarean birth

13. A family experiencing a perinatal loss will:

    a. experience the grief process

    b. have no special needs during the postpartum

    c. request early discharge

14. Postpartum education for the new family should include:

    a. infant care

    b. care of the new mother

    c. infant feeding

    d. contraception

    e. A, B, and C

    f. all of these

PRACTICE/REVIEW ANSWER KEY

1. b. False. Immediately after birth, the uterus should be firm and easily palpable in the midline.
2. a. True
3. a. True
4. a. True
5. b. False
6. a
7. b
8. a. True
9. a. True
10. a. True
11. e
12. b
13. a
14. f

R E F E R E N C E S

1. Association of Women's Health, Obstetric and Neonatal Nurses. (2010). *AWHONN's guide for professional registered nurse staffing for perinatal units.* Washington, DC: Author.

2. Leifer, G. (2011). *Maternity nursing: An introductory text* (10th ed.). St. Louis, MO: Elsevier Science.

3. Lowdermilk, D., & Perry, S. (2013). *Maternity nursing* (8th ed.). St. Louis, MO: Elsevier Health Sciences.

4. American Academy of Pediatrics, American College of Obstetricians and Gynecologists. (2012). *Guidelines for perinatal care* (7th ed.). Elk Grove, IL, Washington, DC: Authors.

5. Durham, R., & Chapman, L. (Eds.). (2014). *Maternal–newborn nursing: The critical components of nursing care* (2nd ed.). Philadelphia, PA: F.A. Davis.

6. James, D. C. (2014). Postpartum care. In Simpson, K. R., & Creehan, P. A. (Eds.), *AWHONN's perinatal nursing* (4th ed., pp. 530–580). Philadelphia, PA: Lippincott.

7. Department of Health and Human Services. (2014). Evidence-based practice center systematic review protocol. Project title: Management of postpartum hemorrhage. www.effectivehealthcare.ahrq.gov. Accessed August 5, 2014.

8. Association of Women's Health Obstetrics and Neonatal Nursing. (2015). Quantification of blood loss: Practice Brief Number 1. *Journal of Obstetric, Gynecologic, and Neonatal Nursing, 44*(1), 1–3.

9. The American Congress of Obstetricians and Gynecologists. (2012). Optimizing protocols in obstetrics: Management of obstetric hemorrhage. ACOG. www.acog.org. Accessed August 5, 2014.

10. Association of Women's Health Obstetrics and Neonatal Nursing Position Statement. (2015). Role of the registered nurse in the care of the pregnant woman receiving analgesia and anesthesia by catheter techniques. *Journal of Obstetrics and Gynecology, 44*(1), 151–154.

11. American Society of Anesthesiologists. (2007). Practice guidelines for obstetrical anesthesia: An updated report by the American Society of Anesthesiologists Task Force on Obstetrical Anesthesia. *Anesthesiology, 106*, 843–863.

12. Association of Perioperative Registered Nurses. (2012). *Perioperative standards and recommended practices for inpatient and ambulatory settings.* Denver, CO: Author.

13. Phillips, R. (2013). The sacred hour: Uninterrupted skin-to-skin contact immediately after birth. *Newborn and Infant Nursing Reviews, 13*(2), 67–72.

14. American Academy of Pediatrics. (2012). Breastfeeding and the use of human milk. *Official Journal of the American Academy of Pediatrics, 129*(3), e827–e841.

15. Association of Women's Health Obstetrics and Neonatal Nursing Position Statement. (2015). Breast feeding. *Journal of Obstetrics and Gynecology, 44*(1), 145–150.

16. Centers for Disease Control and Prevention (CDC). (2012). In Atkinson, W., Jamborsky, J., & Wolfe, S. (Eds.), *Epidemiology and prevention of vaccine-preventable disease* (12th ed.). Washington, DC: Public Health Foundation. Retrieved from: www.cdc.gov/vaccines/pubs/pinkbook/index.html

17. Kroger, A. T., Sumaya, C. V., Pickering, L. K., et al. (2011). General recommendations on immunization: Recommendations of the advisory committee on immunization practices (ACIP). *Morbidity and Mortality Weekly Report, 2*(11), 1–60.

Assessment and Care of the Term Newborn Transitioning to Extrauterine Life

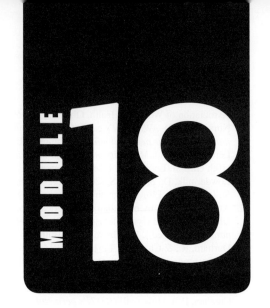

MODULE 18

LUCINDA STEEN STEWART AND
ERIN RODGERS

Objectives   *As you complete this module, you will be able to:*

1. Discuss newborn physiologic adaptations to extrauterine life
2. Understand assessment of the transitioning newborn and how to intervene when indicated
3. Identify common newborn procedures and medications performed during the transition period; why and how they are performed or administered
4. Recognize which newborns require umbilical cord blood gases, be exposed to the procedure of obtaining blood gases, and begin basic interpretation of blood gas values
5. Identify the importance of when and who to notify when a newborn does not transition as expected

Introduction[1-3]

The birth of a baby is a life-changing event for a family, a life event that may have been anticipated for months or even years or may have been completely unplanned. Families transition to their new roles of mother, father, grandparent, or sibling in many different ways depending on cultural conventions, family traditions, personal decisions, and life circumstances. During this transition period, the nurse provides care to the newborn and family unit to optimize adaptations to extrauterine life. Not only does the nurse provide essential physical newborn care but also incorporates sensitive social, emotional, cultural, and spiritual care to the mother and family unit. This chapter contains information to guide the nurse in safe, client-centered care of the term newborn and family.

• Who provides nursing care for the newborn?[1-3]

As early as 1991, the World Health Organization (WHO) and United Nations Children's Emergency Fund (UNICEF) began to promote the global "Baby-Friendly Hospital Initiative." The main purpose of this initiative is to promote practices that support breastfeeding in hopes of mothers exclusively breastfeeding and breastfeeding for a longer duration. Since that time, many hospitals have changed long-standing philosophies, policies, and practices of newborns being whisked off to the nursery for the first several hours of life, to having the newborn stay with the mother continuously throughout the hospital stay. In addition, extensive literature supports the importance of early contact between the newborn and the mother. Through such measures as early skin-to-skin contact and breastfeeding, maternal–infant bonding is enhanced.

These changes in practice oftentimes left the labor and delivery nurse to simultaneously care for the immediate postpartum woman as well as the transitioning newborn. In response to promoting patient care safety during this highly crucial transitioning time for mother and newborn, AWHONN's *Guidelines for Professional Registered Nurse Staffing for Perinatal Units* (2010) recommends that one RN provide care for the immediate postpartum woman and a second RN be assigned to care for the newborn.[3] Many institutions use either an additional labor and delivery nurse or a newborn nursery nurse to provide care for the transitioning newborn. Which nurse provides care for the newly born infant will depend upon philosophy of the facility, physical layout of the unit and staffing patterns. Each facility needs clearly outlined guidelines to define who is responsible for providing this care for each patient.

NOTE: Regardless of the nurse's role, the criteria for care of the transitional newborn care remains the same.

Transition to Extrauterine Life

• What are the expected responses of the newborn to extrauterine life?

As the newborn takes its first breaths and the umbilical cord is clamped, a separate human life is begun.[4-6] The newborn is expected to breathe spontaneously, cry, maintain a heart rate range of 100 to 180 bpm, demonstrate flexion of the extremities and have reflexes present, all within the first few minutes of life. With adequate respirations and circulation, color gradually changes from dusky blue/pink immediately after birth to the overall color normal for the newborn's ethnicity. Lips and tongue should be pink for all ethnicities with transitional acrocyanosis expected.

Multiple physiological adaptations occur simultaneously due to mechanical, chemical, thermal, and sensorial stimuli. As the fetus is delivered vaginally or by cesarean birth, pressure on the newborn thorax is released and passive recoil of the chest allows intake of air. The very low fetal pO_2, high pCO_2, stimulate chemoreceptors in the respiratory center of the brain to also initiate inspiration at birth (in the absence of acidosis). Continued respirations provide positive pressure to sustain alveolar inflation.

At the same time as these respiratory changes are occurring, fetal circulation also begins adapting to newborn circulation patterns. With cord clamping the umbilical artery, vein and ductus venosus close and will become ligaments over the next several weeks. Initial inspiration decreases intrathoracic pressure allowing decreased pulmonary resistance and increased pulmonary capillary filling. These adaptations lead to decreased right-sided heart pressures, thus permitting functional closure of the foramen ovale. When the newborn pO_2 increases to approximately 50 mm Hg, the ductus arteriosus closes which allows for increased pulmonary circulation and increased circulation of oxygenated blood systemically, thus resulting in the newborn becoming pink in the first few minutes of life.

The newborn must also accomplish the essential adaptations of clearing the airway, regulating temperature, maintaining blood glucose control, and learning how to coordinate the suck and swallow reflex for successful breast- or bottle feeding. The nurse continuously assesses for the expected newborn adaptations and intervenes to promote optimal transitioning to extrauterine life.

Initial Assessment and Care of the Newborn[4,6–18]

• **How can the nurse support the newborn in expected transition to extrauterine life?**

During the initial newborn period, if an infant is transitioning well, the following sequence of events can be expected. Throughout this period, it is crucial that a nurse experienced in newborn care be vigilant in assisting this transition.

Initial drying and skin-to-skin contact: Newborns demonstrating an expected transition to extrauterine life are encouraged to remain with the woman for routine newborn care. Upon delivery, the infant is immediately placed prone, skin-to-skin, on woman's bare abdomen. During this time the newborn is dried with blankets and a cap is placed on the newborn's head. Removal of wet blankets and placing a warm dry blanket over the newborn and woman will help to prevent heat loss. The drying of the newborn also provides appropriate stimulation for spontaneous respirations. During this time, the nurse is continuously assessing the newborn. If the newborn is able to clear his/her own secretions without difficulty, then routine bulb suctioning is not warranted.

Cord clamping: There is much debate and controversy regarding the ideal time for cord clamping. When the umbilical cord is clamped too soon after birth, there is the potential for the newborn to not receive a sufficient amount of blood from the placental circulation and subsequently develop anemia and decreased iron stores. Other studies conclude that delaying the cord clamping allows too much blood to be delivered from the placenta to the newborn, resulting in polycythemia, and potential significant hyperbilirubinemia. The nurse caring for a newborn can expect either immediate cord clamping, within 15 to 20 seconds of birth, or delayed cord clamping, up to several minutes after birth depending on provider preferences and the newborn's condition. (See *Module 5* for additional information regarding delayed cord clamping.)

Initial assessment—Apgar scoring: At 1 minute of age, the initial Apgar score is assigned. The Apgar score is a quick assessment of five criteria, used to evaluate the newborn's transition to extrauterine life. Introduced in 1952 by Dr. Virginia Apgar, the five criteria are outlined in Table 18.1: heart rate, respiratory rate, muscle tone, reflex irritability, and color, with each criteria scored from 0 to 2. The highest possible Apgar score is 10. The blanket covering the newborn is removed for this assessment. The Apgar score will be repeated at 5 minutes of age. If newborn condition warrants intervention, do not wait until 1-minute Apgar to begin resuscitation. The Apgar score is helpful in evaluating the newborn's adjustment to extrauterine life. It is an indicator for neither implementation of neonatal resuscitation nor of future neurological outcome.[18] As the Apgar score does require some subjective evaluation of the newborn's physiological condition, the assessment should be done by a nurse experienced in newborn care or a neonatal team member.
  • Total score of 7 to 10: Adjusting well to extrauterine life
  • Total score of 4 to 6: Moderate difficulty adjusting to extrauterine life
  • Total score of 0 to 3: Severe distress

TABLE 18.1 CRITERIA FOR APGAR SCORING			
SIGN	**SCORE 0**	**SCORE 1**	**SCORE 2**
Heart rate	Not detectable	<100	>100
Respiratory rate	Absent	Slow, irregular	Good, crying
Muscle tone	Flaccid	Some extremity flexion	Active motion
Reflex irritability			
Response to tap on sole of foot	No response	Grimace	Grimace
Response to catheter in nostril (after oropharynx is cleared)	No response	Cry	Cough or sneeze
Color	Blue, pale	Body pink, blue extremities	Completely pink

Reprinted with permission from Apgar, V. (1953). A proposal for a new method of evaluation of the newborn infant. *Current Researches in Anesthesia and Analgesia, 32*(4), 260–267.

Newborn identification: In order to protect the safety of the newborn, early and accurate identification is imperative. This will include applying matching identification bracelets on the newborn, mother, and support person. This is done in the delivery area, prior to any separation from mother or transport to another unit. Often, the newborn has a bracelet applied to each ankle, or to an ankle and wrist, and should be secured tight enough to remain on the infant with anticipated weight loss but should not impair blood flow to the extremity. In addition, some hospitals have electronic infant security systems that require bands that remain in constant contact with the newborn's skin to prevent alarming. It is important to be knowledgeable of hospital policies and provide consistent infant identification and security measures.

Early breastfeeding: Breastfeeding during the immediate postpartum period should be encouraged and supported by nurses. AWHONN supports breastfeeding as the optimal method of infant nutrition. If the women wishes to breastfeed and the newborn is transitioning well to extrauterine life, breastfeeding can begin within a few minutes of birth. Breastfeeding in the first hour of life can improve success rate and duration of breastfeeding.

Apgar at 5 minutes of age: As the nurse continues to closely monitor the newborn, a second Apgar score is assessed at 5 minutes of age. This score can be obtained as the newborn and mother continue skin-to-skin contact. If the 5-minute Apgar is less than 7, it is recommended by the American Academy of Pediatrics (AAP) to repeat the Apgar score every 5 minutes up to 20 minutes. In addition, other supportive measures per Neonatal Resuscitation Program (NRP) guidelines are continued to facilitate transition. Factors that may influence the Apgar score are outlined in Table 18.2.

First set of vital signs: Though protocol can vary for different institutions, it can be expected that the first set of vital signs will be obtained at 30 minutes of age. This will include heart rate, respiratory rate, and temperature. Axillary temperature is an accurate and safe method to measure body temperature in the newborn. Many institutions require initial temperature to be measured at 15 minutes of age. If the newborn continues to transition well, vital signs are obtained every

TABLE 18.2 FACTORS INFLUENCING APGAR SCORES	
Factors that can cause variations in Apgar scores	
Several factors can cause variations in Apgar scores and may not indicate a need for resuscitation. An overall clinical evaluation is important in these situations when considering the care of the infant. Some of these factors include the following:	
Gestational age	The standard Apgar goal of 10 points might not be an appropriate gauge of fetal well-being for babies of less than 31–34 wks' gestation. These infants often lack the tone of a term infant and the ability to respond appropriately when reflex irritability is tested.
Intubation and cord visualization	Meconium-stained amniotic fluid may indicate the need for immediate intubation and suctioning of the hypopharynx and trachea. Intubation often produces stimulation of the vagus nerve and subsequent temporary lowering of the heart rate. Newborns usually recover from this intervention spontaneously, but this temporary slowing of the heart rate can affect Apgar scoring.
Congenital defects	Newborns with congenital defects of the heart or neuromuscular or cerebral malformations may have Apgar scores that do not reflect a need for resuscitation. These infants need further evaluation.
Infection	Infection in the newborn may affect tone, color, and reflexes.

TABLE 18.3	NEWBORN VITAL SIGNS	
NEWBORN VITAL SIGNS	**AVERAGE FINDINGS**	**ACCEPTABLE VARIATIONS**
Heart rate: count for a full minute	Apical heart rate: 120–160 bpm, when awake	*Variations*: Heart rate can increase to 180 bpm with crying and decrease to 100 bpm with sleeping.
Respiratory rate: count for a full minute	30–60 breaths/min	*Variations*: Periodic breathing (irregular rate and rhythm) can occur. RR can increase with crying, and decrease with sleeping. Sometimes rate is elevated just after birth, but decreases to a normal range by 1–2 hrs old. *Triggers*: Respiratory distress or apnea greater than 15 sec is not an expected variation.
Temperature:	Axillary: 36.5–37.2°C or 97.7–99°F	*Triggers*: Hypothermia, hyperthermia, or temperature instability can be related to infection or uncontrolled environmental temperature.

RR, respiratory rate.

30 minutes until the newborn has remained stable for 2 hours. In addition to vital signs, the nurse will continue to assess skin color, respiratory effort, muscle tone, and level of activity every 30 minutes as well. Vital signs can be measured while the newborn remains skin-to-skin (Table 18.3).

• **What parameters should be assessed in the transitioning newborn?**

Physical assessment: After the initial transition period and family bonding has occurred, the nurse should complete a head to toe physical assessment within the first 1 to 2 hours of life. Physical assessment of the newborn is conducted in a quiet, warm environment that is well lit. It is important to proceed in an orderly progression to ensure that a complete and thorough examination occurs. The parents or key support people can remain in the room for the examination, allowing the nurse the opportunity to share the examination findings with the family. All findings, including expected variations of normal, are accurately recorded. In order to have an accurate and complete assessment, the newborn must be fully undressed. It is imperative that the nurse keep the newborn warm and prevent cold stress by keeping him/her covered with blankets and a cap as much as possible.

The examination begins with the overall general appearance of the newborn. Before touching the newborn, the nurse inspects noting the color, respiratory effort, position, level of alertness, activity level, and muscle tone. This inspection is done with the newborn both prone and then supine. The nurse next auscultates both the cardiac and respiratory systems. Though this is out of the typical order of assessment of a body system/organ of inspect, palpate, and then auscultate, this is done to hear accurate cardiac and respiratory sounds ideally while the newborn is resting quietly. At this point the nurse can begin a head to toe assessment going from least to most invasive in the following order: inspect, palpate, auscultate. Throughout the examination, the nurse continues to assess skin with each system/body part inspected. Table 18.4 provides further information regarding newborn assessment.

Newborn Medications

• **When, what, why, and how are newborn medications administered?**

Eye Prophylaxis[4,6,17–20]

Due to the risk of a neonate potentially developing a vision-threatening eye infection, routine administration of antimicrobial eye ointment is mandated by most, if not all, states in the United States. Erythromycin 0.5% ophthalmic ointment is the drug of choice, and is a safe and effective method to reduce gonococcal or chlamydial eye infections. Other treatment options may include silver nitrate 1% solution or tetracycline 1% ophthalmic ointment; however, chemical conjunctivitis is more common with these medications. Application of prophylactic medication should occur

TABLE 18.4	NEWBORN ASSESSMENT
Measurements	Accurate measurement of weight, length, and head circumference (HC) contributes to an accurate picture of the overall well-being of a newborn
Weight	Zero scale immediately before weighing infant. Consideration of safety when weighing (fall risk and infection risk from scale)
Length	Measure from top of the head to the bottom of the feet with the newborn's legs fully extended
Head circumference	Frontal–occipital measurement is taken at the widest part of the head
Head	Inspect size, shape, and symmetry, noting any variations such as cephalohematoma or caput succedaneum
	Palpate anterior and posterior fontanel, suture lines
Face	
Eyes:	Inspect for symmetry, placement on face, movement
	Sclera noting color/hemorrhages
Ears:	Inspect for position, malformations, patency
	Palpate entire pinna
Nose:	Inspect for symmetry
	Palpate for patency of both nares
Mouth:	Inspect lips for color and symmetry noting rooting/sucking; inspect mucous membrane, frenulum of tongue
	Palpate soft and hard palate with gloved finger, noting strength and coordination of the suck
Neck	Inspect for symmetry and range of motion, turning newborn's head to face each shoulder
	Palpate neck
Clavicles	Palpate along both clavicles noting crepitus, pain, or possible fractures
Chest	Inspect chest wall for symmetry, nipple placement
Respiratory:	Inspect for respiratory effort
	Count respiratory rate for full minute due to expected irregular rate of newborn respirations
	Auscultate all lung fields
Cardiac:	Inspect precordium
	Palpate for apical pulse
	Auscultate with both bell and diaphragm of a neonatal stethoscope, noting heart sounds including S1, S2, extra heart sounds, murmurs
Abdomen	Inspect for size and symmetry
	Inspect umbilical cord for number of vessels, size, and condition of cord
	Auscultate bowel sounds prior to palpation
	Palpate four quadrants
Genitalia	
Male:	Inspect penis, noting foreskin and urethral opening/meatus; scrotum noting color, rugae
	Palpate for descended testicles
Female:	Inspect external genitalia and separating labia to further inspect
Anus	Inspect for patency of anus
Extremities upper and lower	Inspect for limb position, symmetry of movement
	Inspect hands and feet noting number of digits and palmar and plantar creases
	Inspect feet noting position
Hips	Inspect: Symmetry of leg length. While supine with knees bent up and feet flat on bed, compare knee height
	Inspect: Compare for symmetry of gluteal folds. Roll newborn to prone position with legs extended
Trunk and spine	While baby in prone position, note any hair/nevus/lesion/pigmentation along lower spine
	Palpate length of spine
Neurological	Note level of alertness
	Tone and pitch of the cry
	Assess for pain using neonatal pain scale
	Assess reflexes: Rooting, suck, swallow, Babinski, plantar grasp, palmar grasp, and Moro

REMEMBER: Be familiar with the policies, procedures, equipment and medications at your institution to safely perform these skills.

shortly after birth, up to 1 hour of life for all infants, regardless of the route of birth. In order to promote maternal and infant bonding and promote breastfeeding, this can occur up to 1 hour after birth.

SKILL UNIT 1 | EYE PROPHYLAXIS WITH ERYTHROMYCIN OINTMENT

ACTIONS	REMARKS
1. Don clean gloves.	Always follow universal precautions.
2. Cleanse eyes with gauze pad.	Cleanse from inner to outer canthus.
3. Open eye and place an inch ribbon of medication in the lower conjunctival sac.	Place from inner to outer canthus. Hold tip of medication tube at least 1 in to avoid injury to eye.
4. After 1 min excess medication may be wiped off.	Gently wipe off with gauze pad.

Vitamin K Injection[6,20–24]

Vitamin K (phytonadione) is an essential component in the clotting cascade to prevent hemorrhage. Production of vitamin K begins with the presence of bacteria in the intestines. Since the gut of the newborn is sterile until bacteria is introduced, the newborn is unable to make sufficient amounts of vitamin K until about 8 days old. Because of this naturally occurring low level of newborn vitamin K, exogenous vitamin K administration is recommended. When vitamin K is not routinely administered to all newborns, they are at risk for vitamin K deficiency bleeding (VKDB). Potential complications of this deficiency include intracranial hemorrhage, intra-abdominal hemorrhage, overt bleeding, bruising, lethargy, vomiting, poor feeding, and pallor. Because of these factors, vitamin K administration has been recommended by the AAP since 1961.

Vitamin K 1 mg is recommended via intramuscular (IM) injection soon after birth for all newborns weighing more than 1.5 kg. This injection may be delayed until after the initial skin-to-skin contact and breastfeeding have occurred. The vastus lateralis is the preferred site for injection due to larger muscle mass and less risk of hitting a nerve or major vessel. Both the gluteus medius and deltoid muscles are poorly developed in newborns and thus are not recommended for use in newborns.

SKILL UNIT 2 | PROCEDURE FOR VITAMIN K (PHYTONADIONE) INJECTION

ACTIONS	REMARKS
1. Gather supplies: Vitamin K Alcohol pad Syringe with 25–27-gauge, ½- to 5/8-in needle Bandage	Vitamin K comes prepared in prefilled syringes at some hospitals. Read package instructions to administer it correctly
2. Don clean gloves and locate injection site in vastus lateralis	Always practice universal precautions
3. Draw up vitamin K if not in a prefilled syringe	If medication comes in an ampule, be sure to use a filtered needle to draw up the medication and change to the correct size needle for injection
4. Clean site with alcohol pad and let dry	Drying of the alcohol kills bacteria
5. While stabilizing leg, inject vitamin K into the vastus lateralis slowly.	Current evidence-based practice supports no aspiration prior to IM injections
6. Withdraw needle and apply gentle pressure to site	Gentle pressure helps decrease medication seeping out and may increase absorption
7. If site continues to bleed after gentle pressure, apply bandage	Bandages can cause trauma to skin, so only use if needed
8. Observe site for edema and erythema	Rare adverse effects include hemolysis, hyperbilirubinemia, and jaundice

REMEMBER: All healthcare providers need to wear gloves while handling the infant until the bath is completed. Only infants with an infectious disease such as hepatitis B, HIV, or herpes simplex need to have a bath during this initial transition period.

Care for the Newborn Who Does Not Follow Expected Transition

• When can problems be anticipated?[3,4,6,7,25–27]

Although it is impossible to completely predict all infants who will require resuscitation, many times, a difficult transition can be anticipated. Knowledge of gestational age, maternal health history, prenatal course, and intrapartum events can prepare you to anticipate many of these difficulties with transition. Below is a list of some situations that are likely to require extra interventions for the newborn at birth.

- Preterm
- Congenital anomalies
- Intrauterine growth restriction (IUGR)
- Category III fetal heart rate (FHR) tracing (See *Module 7* on External Fetal Monitoring)
- Operative delivery (forceps or vacuum)
- Emergency cesarean delivery
- Maternal chorioamnionitis
- Maternal hypertensive disorders
- Maternal diabetes

• What is needed for preparation for birth?

In order to provide immediate newborn care, each birthing room and operating room should be stocked with emergency equipment, supplies, medications, and the personnel to perform newborn assessment and resuscitation as indicated. AWHONN recommends one RN to be assigned to provide immediate care for the woman and another to provide care for the newborn until stabilization. At least one staff member should be present who is capable of initiating resuscitation of the newborn. This includes being able to perform chest compressions and competency using a continuing positive airway pressure (CPAP) bag. An additional staff member needs to be readily available to perform full neonatal resuscitation measures including endotracheal intubation, ventilation, and emergency medications as needed. When the need for resuscitation is anticipated, the trained resuscitation person or team should be present just prior to birth to set up equipment and supplies. Some institutions require all nurses who provide care for newborns to be certified in neonatal resuscitation. See *Module 5* for additional information regarding anticipation of and preparation for potential newborn compromise. During labor, the obstetric and newborn nurses assigned for birth should communicate regarding anticipation of birth.

• What nursing interventions are essential when a newborn does not transition as expected?

The purpose of this section is to provide education and review of basic assessment and interventions for the newborn. NRP guidelines are not discussed here. The nurse's duty is to constantly balance the need for mother–infant bonding and skin-to-skin contact with safety for the infant. If a newborn does not respond effectively to being dried, stimulated, and placed skin-to-skin with the woman, then further assessment is required. Below are basic steps to assist in this process.

- Place infant in an open bed warmer for better visualization of color, respiratory effort, and heart rate. This space will also provide easier access if more invasive interventions are required.
- Continue drying infant and remove all wet blankets and caps.
- Initiate interventions in which you are trained and call for another healthcare provider trained in neonatal resuscitation who has been trained to start IV lines, intubate, and/or administer medications as needed.
- Keep family informed of newborn's condition, what is being done to assist infant, and which other staff members have been notified. Timely communication with the family in emergency events can assist them in understanding and coping with the situation. When the newborn stabilizes, he/she may be returned skin-to-skin with the woman with continued observation by the nurse caring for the newborn.
- Document time, assessment, interventions, newborn responses to interventions, and staff notified.

- **What is an umbilical cord blood gas and which newborns need to have one?**

Umbilical cord blood sampling is a laboratory test performed on blood from the umbilical cord that is a beneficial addition to Apgar scoring in the evaluation of the fetal condition at the time of birth. Results provide objective assessment of the metabolic condition of a newborn as well as a reflection of placental functioning. ACOG[25] recommends that umbilical cord blood gases be obtained anytime the newborn is not transitioning in the expected manner or has known complications. If unsure, a cord blood gas will need to be sent, the delivering healthcare provider can go ahead and double clamp and cut a 10- to 20-cm (8- to 10-in) section of umbilical cord to have, if needed. The cord segment may be discarded if the 5-minute Apgar is >7 and the newborn is vigorous.

- **Do you need both arterial and venous cord blood samples?**

A complete cord blood gas panel includes: pH, pO_2, pCO_2 and base deficit or base excess. A sample is taken from both an umbilical artery and the umbilical vein. Remember the two umbilical arteries carry the **deoxygenated** blood from the fetus back to the placenta while the umbilical vein carries the **oxygenated** blood from the placenta to the fetus. Thus, arterial values reflect fetal condition while venous values reflect placental function. If a sample is obtained from only one vessel there can be confusion in values as to whether it is an arterial or venous sample. When both arterial and venous samples are obtained, a comparison of values can better determine the source of the blood gas; however, even this method has a measure of error. Since the arterial sample reflects fetal status it is the most essential blood gas sample to obtain (Fig. 18.1).

SKILL UNIT 3 | UMBILICAL CORD BLOOD GAS SAMPLING

ACTIONS	REMARKS

1. Gather supplies:
    Obtain either:
    A prepackaged blood gas kit with two
        heparinized syringes
    OR
    Two 3-mL syringes with 22–23-gauge
        needles AND a vial of heparin
        1,000 units/mL
    Two patient labels and laboratory
        requisitions
    Personal protective equipment (PPE)
	If available at your institution, the prepackaged kit allows for less
	    handling of needles.
	Know your institution's policy if cord blood should be labeled
	    with maternal or newborn name and medical record number.
	Fill out labels and lab requisitions prior to delivery when possible
	Identifying each sample as either "venous" OR "arterial."
	Always use universal precautions when drawing cord blood
	    gases. Gloves are always indicated. Mask and eye protection
	    may also be indicated.

2. Prepare syringes (as indicated):
    Flush both syringes with heparin solu-
        tion. Eject heparin and air from
        syringe so that only a small coating is
        left in syringe
	No preparation is required for prepackaged heparinized syringes.
	Too much heparin left in syringes can alter blood gas results.
	    With no heparin the blood sample will usually clot before
	    getting to the lab.

3. Receive specimen:
    A 10–20-cm clamped segment of cord is
        passed off the delivery table
    Place cord on a well-lit, solid, flat surface
	This segment of cord is double clamped and cut per birth attendant.
	The blood gas in a clamp cord will stay stable up to 60 min.
	Obtain blood sample as soon as you receive it whenever pos-
	    sible.

4. Obtain blood sample:
    With the bevel up insert needle into
        one of the two arteries
    Withdraw 1–2 mL of blood (at least
        0.5 mL)
    Carefully eject any air and cap
    Repeat these steps for the venous
        sample
	Remember, there are two arteries which are smaller and darker
	    than the vein.
	Do not hold cord in your hand or with your fingers for risk of
	    needle stick.
	Do not recap specimen with a needle or send it to the lab with a
	    needle still attached.
	Uncapped specimens quickly mix with air, and blood gas results
	    will be altered.

5. Send labeled cord blood gas to lab with
    corresponding requisition
	Know your hospital policy if cord gases are allowed to be sent
	    via pneumatic tube system or need to be hand carried to the
	    lab.
	Send to lab as soon as possible.

• **How do you interpret umbilical cord gas values?**

A complex physiological relationship exists in maintaining acid–base balance in the fetus as it experiences the stresses of labor. Each value is assessed in relationship to the others in order to determine how the newborn has tolerated the intrauterine environment and labor. Module 7 previously discusses aerobic and anaerobic metabolism, physiologic mechanisms in the development of respiratory, metabolic, and mixed academia, and interpretation of values. To review, steps for interpretation include:

- Step 1 pH: To evaluate the blood gas, ask yourself if the pH is low, high, or normal. If the pH is low, then the subsequent values are assessed to determine if the source of the acidemia is from respiratory, metabolic, or mixed causes. A pH within the usual range would be considered normal, high would be alkalotic, and low would be acidotic.
- Step 2 pO_2: It is not unusual for many healthy newborns to be have some level of hypoxemia at birth until respirations have been established; thus, some experts consider this value unnecessary for evaluating arterial cord blood gases.
- Step 3 pCO_2: If pCO_2 is elevated then a respiratory source for acidosis is suspected. Since the placenta functions as the lungs for the fetus, high pCO_2 accompanied with acidemia correlates with respiratory acidosis. These findings are most commonly associated with inadequate gas exchange of CO_2 at the placenta. The FHR tracing may exhibit repetitive variable decelerations, indicative of umbilical cord compression. Newborns that have respiratory acidosis may or may not have a low 1-minute Apgar. They exhale the extra CO_2 when respirations are established and usually recover quickly.
- Step 4 Base: Base excess or base deficit calculates the amount of base that is present in the blood with bicarbonate accounting for a large portion of base. The significance of the base excess or base deficit value is to determine the source of the acidosis as respiratory or metabolic. Whether the acidosis is from purely metabolic causes or mixed respiratory and metabolic acidosis, these newborns frequently will have low 1- and 5-minute Apgar scores, will require resuscitative measures, and require ongoing care in the NICU for stabilization. Clinical significance of acidosis is discussed in Table 18.5.

TABLE 18.5 CLINICAL SIGNIFICANCE OF UMBILICAL CORD BLOOD GAS VALUES

TYPE OF ACIDOSIS	LAB VALUES	NEWBORN CLINICAL ASSESSMENT	SIGNIFICANCE
Respiratory acidosis	pH–low pCO_2–high Base excess–normal	May have low 1-min Apgar but quickly equilibrate pH with strong respiratory effort. 5-min Apgar usually ≥7.	Not associated with significant newborn complications or long-term injury.[5]
Metabolic acidosis	pH–low pCO_2–normal Base excess–high	Frequently have low 1- and 5-min Apgars, and require some resuscitative assistance.	The lower the pH and higher the base deficit the slower the recovery. pH of <7 with base excess of −12 mol/L have increased risk of newborn complications.
Mixed acidosis	pH–low pCO_2–high Base excess–high	Usually have low 1- and 5-min Apgars and require significant resuscitative assistance.	The lower the pH and higher the base deficit the slower the recovery. pH of <7 with base excess of −12 mol/L have increased risk of newborn complications.

Blood Glucose Screening

• Which newborns need a blood glucose check?

In the past, all newborns were screened for hypoglycemia, a complication that if left untreated for a prolonged period of time, can result in long-term neurologic damage.[4–7,28–30] According to the AAP[29] universal blood glucose screening of the newborn is no longer recommended. Only infants that fall into a high-risk group or are symptomatic (jitteriness, tachypnea, lethargy, hypotonia, poor feeding, eye-rolling, cyanosis, seizures, and/or apneic spells) need to have a blood glucose test performed.

Neonatal hypoglycemia occurs when glucose is used faster than it can be maintained. Infants of diabetic mothers (particularly those who have had poor glycemic control) are at greatest risk because maternal elevated blood glucose crosses the placenta and, in response, the fetal pancreas produces more insulin to keep up with the high glucose level. When the umbilical cord is clamped and cut at delivery, the maternal glucose supply is cut off, but the fetal pancreas is still producing high levels of insulin and thus blood glucose begins to drop.

Newborns recommended for a blood glucose testing:
- Preterm/late preterm
- Intrauterine growth-restricted (IUGR)
- Infants of diabetic mothers (IDM)
- Large for gestational age (LGA)—above 90th percentile
- Small for gestational age (SGA)—below 10th percentile
- Perinatal stress (hypoxia, respiratory distress syndrome [RDS])
- Symptomatic newborn (jitteriness, lethargy, poor feeder, hypothermia, hypotonia, etc.)

• When should a blood glucose check be performed?

Most experts recommend that capillary blood glucose be checked within 1 hour of birth for those newborns that have an indication. If within normal limits and infant is asymptomatic then frequent repeated checks until neonate is stable for several hours is usually recommended. Point-of-care newborn blood glucose sampling is performed via heelstick with a lancet and utilizing a capillary blood glucose monitor.

SKILL UNIT 4 | PROCEDURE FOR OBTAINING BLOOD GLUCOSE FOR INITIAL SCREENING

ACTIONS	REMARKS
1. Gather supplies: Bedside blood glucose monitor Alcohol pad, lancet, cotton ball or gauze pad, bandage Reagent strip Heel warmer	Perform quality control test per institution policy and manufacturer's instructions Some states require annual point-of-care testing certification for nurses to perform blood glucose
2. Place heel warmer securely around heel Leave in place for 5 or more minutes	Warming heel promotes vasodilation, thus improves blood flow for obtaining sample Read manufacturer's directions for use
3. Choose puncture site on heel Use lateral aspect of either heel	Avoid using the middle of the heel as the puncture site due to potential for artery and/or nerve trauma, and potential necrotizing osteochondritis
4. Don clean gloves	Always practice universal precautions
5. Clean heel site with alcohol pad AND let dry completely	Drying of the alcohol kills bacteria
6. Puncture with lancet	Puncture needs to be deep enough to draw blood but not so deep as to cause trauma Automatic spring-loaded devices may offer a more accurate puncture and less pain

skill unit continues on page 499

ACTIONS	REMARKS
7. Let first drop of blood form and wipe it off with cotton ball or gauze pad	Not all manufacturers require this step
8. Apply the second drop of blood to the reagent strip	As directed by manufacturer
9. Insert into blood glucose monitor	As directed by manufacturer
10. Wait for value to display on monitor	Know your institution's policies for when to notify the health care provider and what interventions should be performed
11. Apply bandage to heel	Applying pressure assists puncture to stop bleeding

Evaluation of Newborn Blood Glucose

Several issues make neonatal hypoglycemia difficult to define. One of the innate problems with blood glucose monitoring in neonates is that point-of-care testing of capillary blood in neonates can be unreliable, especially at very low concentrations. Values may vary as much as 10 to 20 mg/dL, so a blood glucose of 30 mg/dL with a bedside blood glucose could be 15 mg/dL when verified by laboratory enzymatic testing. Secondly, it is also noted that clinical symptoms of hypoglycemia and blood glucose values frequently do not correlate with long-term neurological outcomes. Thirdly, healthy newborns will frequently have blood glucose levels as low as 30 mg/dL in the first hour or two after birth and with normal feeding will subsequently rise to 45 mg/dL by 12 hours of age.

NOTE: It is essential to note that any point-of-care values that are outside of normal range need to be followed up with blood or plasma glucose laboratory studies; however, treatment for these low bedside values should not be delayed while waiting on laboratory verification.

Interventions for Hypoglycemia

Clinical practice for management of neonatal hypoglycemia continues to have limited empirical data to define precise timing of screenings, absolute values for long-term neurologic damage, and glucose concentrations requiring therapeutic intervention. The AAP has developed some general guidelines for prevention and management of neonatal hypoglycemia based on the research that is available. Three main categories intervention are outlined: early feeding, screening, and intervention for low blood glucose values or symptomatic high-risk newborns.

It is important to note that newborns of diabetic mothers may develop hypoglycemia within the first hour after birth. As we discussed earlier, healthy, stable newborns are encouraged to breastfeed within the first hour of life. If the newborn has risk factors for hypoglycemia, it then becomes essential that they either consume breast milk or formula within the first hour of age, followed by a blood glucose evaluation 30 minutes later. If initial blood glucose is less than 25 mg/dL, then IV glucose is indicated. For a blood glucose between 25 and 40 mg/dL, it is appropriate to refeed the newborn or start IV glucose and then recheck the blood glucose in 1 hour. Asymptomatic high-risk newborns should continue to be fed every 2 to 3 hours with a blood glucose check prior to each feed.

REFERENCES

1. World Health Organization, UNICEF. (2009). Baby-friendly hospital initiative: Revised, updated and expanded for integrated care. Retrieved from: http://www.who.int/nutrition/publications/infantfeeding/bfhi_trainingcourse/en/
2. Kinsey, C., & Hupcey, J. (2013). State of the science of maternal–infant bonding: A principle-based concept analysis. *Midwifery, 29*(12), 1314–1320.
3. *AWHONN's Guidelines for Professional Registered Nurse Staffing for Perinatal Units.* (2010). Washington, DC.
4. Lowdermilk, D., Perry, S., Cashion, K., et al. (2012). *Maternity and women's health care* (10th ed.). Mosby: Inc., an affiliate of Elsevier Inc., printed in USA.
5. Gabbe, S. G., Niebyl, J. R., Simpson, J. L., et al. (2012). *Obstetrics: Normal and problem pregnancies* (6th ed.). Saunders, an Imprint of Elsevier Inc.: printed in Canada.
6. Simpson, K., & Creehan, P. (2014). *Perinatal nursing* (4th ed.). Philadelphia, PA: Wolters Kluwer.
7. American Academy of Pediatrics (APA), American College of Obstetrics and Gynecology (ACOG). (2012). Guidelines for Perinatal Care (7th ed.).
8. Moore, E. R., Anderson, G. C., Bergman, N., et al. (2012). Early skin-to-skin contact for mothers and their healthy newborn infants. *The Cochrane Database of Systematic Reviews, 5,* CD003519.
9. Newman, J., & Kernerman, E. (2009). The importance of skin to skin contact. International Breastfeeding Centre. Retrieved

from: http://www.nbci.ca/index.php?option=com_content&id=82:the-importance-of-skin-to-skin-contact-&Itemid=17

10. Kattwinkel, J. (2008). Neonatal resuscitation guidelines for ILCOR and NRP: Evaluating the evidence and developing a consensus. *Journal of Perinatology, 28*(suppl 3), S27–S29.

11. Mercer, J. S., Erickson-Owens, D. A., Graves, B., et al. (2007). Evidence-based practices for the fetal to newborn transition. *Journal of Midwifery & Women's Health, 52*(3), 262–272.

12. Committee on Obstetric practice, The American College of Obstetricians and Gynecologists. (2012). Committee Opinion No. 543. Timing of umbilical cord clamping after birth. *Obstetrics & Gynecology, 120*, 1522–1526.

13. Apgar, V. (1953). A proposal for a new method of evaluation of the newborn infant. *Current Researches in Anesthesia & Analgesia, 32*(4), 260–267.

14. American Academy of Pediatrics, Committee on Fetus and Newborn, American College of Obstetricians and Gynecologists and Committee on Obstetric Practice. (2006). The Apgar score. *Pediatrics, 117*(4), 1444–1447.

15. World Health Organization. (2014). Early initiation of breastfeeding. Retrieved from: http://www.who.int/elena/titles/early_breastfeeding/en/

16. Durham, R., & Chapman, L. (2014). *Maternal-newborn nursing* (2nd ed.). Philadelphia, PA: F.A. Davis Company.

17. Hockenberry, M., & Wilson, D. (2011). *Wong's nursing care of infants and children* (9th ed.). St. Louis, MO: Elsevier.

18. American Academy of Pediatrics (AAP). (2012). Prevention of neonatal ophthalmia. In Pickering, L. K. (Ed.), *Red Book: Report of the Committee on Infectious Diseases* (29th ed., p. 880). Elk Grove Village, IL: American Academy of Pediatrics…

19. Workowski, K. A., & Berman, S., Centers for Disease Control and Prevention (CDC). (2010). Sexually transmitted diseases treatment guidelines, 2010. Retrieved from: http://www-ncbi-nlm-nih-gov.proxy.library.vanderbilt.edu/pubmed?term = 21160459

20. Echegaray, C. (2014). Vanderbilt pediatricians call for a tracking system for babies not getting vitamin K shot. VUMC Reporter. Retrieved from: http://news.vanderbilt.edu/2014/05/vanderbilt-pediatricians-call-for-a-tracking-system-for-babies-not-getting-vitamin-k-shot/

21. American Academy of Pediatrics (AAP), American College of Obstetricians and Gynecologists (ACOG). (2012). *Guidelines for perinatal care* (7th ed.). Elk Grove Village, IL: AAP.

22. Rishovd, A. (2014). Pediatric intramuscular injections: Guidelines for best practice. *The American Journal of Maternal/Child Nursing, 39*(2), 107–112.

23. Centers for Disease Control and Prevention. (2009). Pink book vaccine guidelines: Appendix D. Retrieved from: http://www.cdc.gov/vaccines/pubs/pinkbook/downloads/appendices/appdx-full-d.pdf

24. American Academy of Pediatrics. (2014). Immunization training guide and practice procedure manual. Retrieved from; http://www2.aap.org/immunization/pediatricians/pdf/immunizationtrainingguide.pdf

25. American College of Obstetricians and Gynecologists (ACOG). (2006). (reaffirmed 2012). Committee Opinion, Number 348. *Umbilical blood gas and acid-base analysis.* Retrieved from: http://www.acog.org/~/media/Committee%20Opinions/Committee%20on%20Obstetric%20Practice/co348.pdf?dmc=1&ts=20140918T1408094108

26. Freeman, R. K., Garite, T. J., Nageotte, M. P., et al. (Eds.). (2012). Umbilical cord blood gases to assess fetal condition at birth. In *Fetal heart rate monitoring* (4th ed.). Princeton, NJ: Lippincott Williams & Wilkins.

27. Armstrong, L., & Stenson, B. J. (2007). Use of umbilical cord blood gas analysis in the assessment of the newborn. Retrieved from: http://www.ncbi.nlm.nih.gov/pmc/articles/PMC2675384/

28. McKee-Garrett, T. M. (2014). UpToDate. Overview of the routine management of the healthy newborn infant. Retrieved from: http://www.uptodate.com/contents/overview-of-the-routine-management-of-the-healthy-newborn-infant?source=search_result&search=healthy+newborn+infant&selectedTitle=1~150

29. American Academy of Pediatrics (AAP). (2011). Postnatal glucose homeostasis in late-preterm and term infants. *Pediatrics, 127*(3), 575–579.

30. Woo, H., Tolosa, L., El-Metwally, D., et al. (2014). Glucose monitoring in neonates: Need for accurate and non-invasive methods. *Archives of Disease Childhood Fetal and Neonatal, 99*(2), F153–F157.

Maternal Transport

SUSAN DRUMMOND

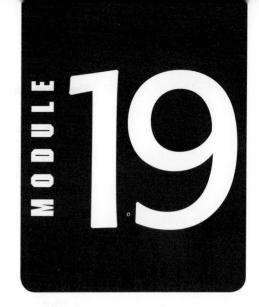

MODULE 19

Key Terms

When you have completed this module, you should be able to recall the meaning of the following terms. You should also be able to use the terms when consulting with other health professionals. The terms are defined in this module or in the glossary at the end of this book.

inborn neonate	mortality
morbidity	outborn neonate

Determining the Need for Maternal Transport

• What is maternal transport?

An essential component of any perinatal care system is the capability of providing interhospital transport of pregnant women and neonates.[1] *Maternal transport* refers to the process of transferring the pregnant woman under the supervision of skilled medical personnel from a level I or level II institution (referring hospitals) to a level III institution (receiving hospital). Each situation is considered individually. The transfer can be accomplished by private vehicle, ambulance, rotary-wing aircraft (RWA) (helicopter), or fixed-wing aircraft (FWA). The decision regarding the type of vehicle depends on the condition of the pregnant woman and fetus as well as distance and travel time. It is a decision that should be shared jointly by the referring care provider and flight personnel or receiving physician.

• What are the advantages of maternal transport?

Over the last few decades, the transport of the premature or sick newborns to intensive care units of regional centers after birth has become widely accepted. These babies are often referred to as **outborn neonates**, in distinction to those born within the referral hospital (i.e., **inborn neonates**). The survival rates and quality of life for the high-risk neonate have improved significantly. However, neonates born to women transported prior to birth have better survival rates and decreased risks of long-term complications than those transferred following birth.[1] A recent meta-analysis shows that very low–birth-weight (VLBW) infants born at non level III hospitals have higher odds of death during the neonatal period or prior to hospital discharge compared to infants born at level III hospitals.[2] Morbidity and/or mortality are decreased by delivering an infant in a facility that has the equipment, staffing, and resources appropriate for optimal care.[3–5]

Transport of the neonate involves not only the availability of a local neonatal intensive care unit (NICU), but also the complication risk during transport, the need for highly skilled personnel and specialized equipment, and the expense of the transport. In utero transport of selected risk pregnancies is strongly recommended. Therefore, when possible, the primary emphasis should always be on prenatal diagnosis and subsequent maternal transfer. Even with advanced training and technologies, women usually make the best transport incubator.[6] Transport within regionalized perinatal care networks allows for benefits of high-technology maternity and fetal/neonatal care and services, while presumably reducing costs and decreasing duplication of services within a region. Perinatal outreach education has been shown to be an effective strategy to promote transfer of pregnant mothers so that VLBW infants are born at level III centers.[7]

Interfacility transport also benefits the woman. An increase in the prevalence of high-risk conditions such as hypertension, diabetes, obesity, and abnormal placentation has contributed to a recent rise in maternal morbidity and mortality.[8] Over the past 20 years, the U. S. pregnancy-associated mortality ratio has doubled to 14.3 per 100,000.[9] In one study, transport of women with pregnancy complications to an appropriate facility has resulted in a reduction of maternal mortality.[10]

Advantages include several considerations:
- If the baby is transferred in utero, the need for sophisticated equipment and the risk of neonatal problems during transport are reduced. Advanced testing and treatment at the center enable a more accurate assessment of when and how to deliver the baby.
- Advanced therapeutic techniques can be provided for the high-risk woman.
- If an ill or severely preterm baby is delivered, immediate steps can be taken to stabilize and treat the newborn without losing precious time during transport.
- The hospital stay of the woman and her newborn tends to be shorter, resulting in a reduction of hospital costs.
- Finally, maternal transport ensures that the woman and newborn are together during the first few days after birth. This provides the opportunity for the woman and newborn to become acquainted and attached to each other in the unique process of bonding.

• Are there disadvantages of maternal transport?

Probably the greatest concern in transferring the undelivered woman to a regional center is the physical separation from family and friends. If possible, a family member should accompany the woman or follow in a car at the time of transport. The woman and/or her newborn, after receiving specialized care at a referral center, may be back transported (returned) to the original referring hospital for continuing care after the complications that required the transfer have been resolved. This may result in a decreased amount of time that the woman and newborn are separated from family and community.

NOTE: The referring nursing staff and transport personnel must help to reduce the disruption and stress for the pregnant woman and her family during transfer. Create a quiet private place to explain to the expectant woman and her family why the transfer is necessary and exactly how it is going to take place. Stress any positive aspect of the clinical situation (e.g., the baby is doing well presently).

The rate of admissions to NICUs increases with a maternal transport system. A great percentage of these newborns have extremely low birth weights. In the past, these babies did not survive. They require special care, which is met in tertiary care centers that have established maternal–fetal medicine programs. Resource management to maximize efficiency, effectiveness, and safety is essential.[1]

Timing of Maternal Transport

• When is the best time to transport the woman?

Transport of the undelivered woman to a regional center should be considered in the following situations:
- It is anticipated that the newborn might require intensive care not available at the referring hospital.
- The obstetric, medical, or surgical needs of the woman require diagnosis, treatment, and care using highly specialized equipment, skills, and staff not available at the referring hospital.

When possible, referral should be made while the woman and fetus are in a stable condition and birth is not expected to occur within a reasonable time frame that transport could occur. This presents a low risk for transferring the woman and fetus. It is optimum, of course, to refer early enough to allow beginning assessment and treatment at the receiving hospital, thus preventing a crisis situation for either woman or fetus when they reach the receiving hospital. Transport team members should be selected from appropriately trained, licensed healthcare providers.[1]

High-reliability perinatal units promote clinical practices based on nationally recognized guidelines and espouse a team philosophy of "safety first." One feature of such perinatal units is that "patients are transferred in a timely and reliable way" to facilities that can care for all potential problems rather than operating on the hope "that the disaster will not occur."[11] (Behavioral scientists define *high-reliability organizations* as those with "the ability to operate technologically complex systems essentially without error over long periods."[11]) "Hope" is never a "plan."

Transfer of patients in early labor is recommended in the following circumstances:
- Time for transport will take less than 2 hours.
- The woman's condition is stable.
- Birth is not anticipated for 4 to 6 hours.
- A professional attendant, such as a nurse, physician, or trained emergency medical technician, can accompany the woman.

High-risk transport situations include the following:
- The woman's condition is unstable.
- Time of birth is unpredictable.

In high-risk transport situations, the decision as to whether the woman is stable enough for transport and who should accompany the woman should be made by the perinatal specialist and transport team experienced in such decision-making.

In either of these high-risk situations, it is highly recommended that the woman be accompanied by the following:
- Referring physician or designate
- Nurse, nurse practitioner, or neonatologist with the skill and experience to manage resuscitation and care of the newborn

NOTE: Maternal transport might be contraindicated in women who are too unstable at the time of the transport request. For example, a woman in premature labor who is dilated beyond 5 cm should be evaluated carefully. Decisions depend on the makeup of the transport team, distance, and time. Safety of the woman and the fetus is the primary consideration. It may be advisable to have the newborn transport team dispatched prior to an anticipated high-risk birth so that this highly skilled team can provide immediate resuscitation and stabilization to the newborn.

Other contraindications may include women with the following:
- Actively bleeding placenta previa
- Abruptio placentae
- Unstable fetal condition

Many times, the transport team will need to make critical decisions before leaving the referring hospital.

REMEMBER: Critical factors in successful maternal transport are appropriate treatment of the mother before transport and attendance by skilled personnel.

Conditions Requiring Transport to a Regional Center

• What conditions in the mother require referral to a regional center?

The majority of maternal transports will be carried out because of concern for a potentially compromised fetus. Prematurity remains the predominant cause of neonatal morbidity and mortality. In 2010, preterm births represented 12% of all births in the United States. Although the rate of preterm births increased approximately 30% from 1981 to 2006, in 2007 this trend began to reverse. The U. S. preterm birth rate decreased for the fourth consecutive year in 2010.[12] The downward trend is continuing. In 2013, preterm births represented 11.4% of births, although the range among the states was 8.1% to 16.6%.[13] Preterm infants also constitute approximately 75% of neonatal mortalities. Statistics from selected regional centers indicate uniformly better outcomes for in utero fetal transport (i.e., the mortality risk for fetuses transported in utero is approximately half that of newborns transported after birth).

Other conditions that may require the woman to be transported to a regional center for high-risk care are outlined as follows.[14–16]

Obstetric Complications

- Preterm premature rupture of membranes occurring before 34 weeks' gestation or with a fetus estimated to weigh less than 2,000 g. (For additional information on management and complications of preterm premature rupture of membranes, refer to Module 10.)

NOTE: Management varies with gestational age. At 34 weeks' gestation or greater, birth is recommended for all women with ruptured membranes.[16] A vaginal/rectal culture for group B streptococcus (GBS) should be obtained using a sterile cotton-tipped applicator on women when presenting with preterm premature rupture of membranes. Infection with GBS is responsible for serious neonatal morbidity and mortality.[17] See Module 12 for GBS discussion.

- Any condition in which the probability exists for the birth of an infant less than 34 weeks' gestation or weighing less than 2,000 g, such as the following:
  - Preeclampsia with severe features or other hypertensive complications
  - Certain anticipated multiple births (e.g., discordancy, higher-order multiples)
  - Poorly controlled or severe diabetes mellitus
  - Intrauterine growth restriction
  - Some women with third trimester bleeding
  - Rh isoimmunization
  - Severe oligohydramnios

- A woman at high risk for hemorrhage (e.g., placenta accreta or >3 previous C/S) as many community hospitals do not have a blood bank supply to respond to such an emergency

Maternal Medical Complications

- Infection or sepsis
- Severe organic heart disease
- Acute or chronic renal failure
- Drug overdose
- Some women with carcinoma
- Morbid obesity
- Uncontrolled diabetes mellitus or diabetic ketoacidosis

Maternal Surgical Complications

- Trauma requiring intensive care or surgery beyond the capabilities of local facilities or where the procedure can result in the onset of premature labor
- Acute abdominal emergencies at less than 34 weeks' gestation or with a fetus estimated to weigh less than 2,000 g
- Thoracic emergencies requiring intensive care or surgical correction

Fetal Complications

- Fetal congenital anomalies diagnosed by ultrasound can dictate the need for maternal transport so that the newborn can be cared for immediately following birth by the appropriate neonatal services specific for the condition (e.g., gastroschisis, cardiac defects).

NOTE: Transfer from a level II institution should be considered for the following:
- *Any fetus anticipated to require long-term ventilation support after birth.*
- *Any fetus anticipated to require neonatal care at less than 28 to 34 weeks' gestation. (This will depend on the skilled personnel and advanced technology of the institution.[18])*
- *Suspected genetic or congenital disorder requiring further evaluation.[18]*

The need to transfer to a higher level of care may not be anticipated before birth.

After birth, many babies are cyanotic, often peripherally. Typically, cyanotic babies have the following characteristics[19]:
- Premature, have experienced a difficult birth or ingested meconium, or had premature rupture of membranes
- Marked respiratory distress
- Radiographic evidence of lung disease
- Elevated PCO_2 levels
- PO_2 increases with 100% oxygen

On the other hand, a newborn with an unknown cardiac abnormality usually has the following characteristics[19]:
- Term
- Uncomplicated birth
- Little respiratory distress
- Cyanosis, which is central and disproportionate to distress; tongue and mucous membranes are blue
- No radiologic evidence of lung disease

When born with cyanotic congenital heart disease in a level I or level II hospital, the newborn should be transported by a neonatal transport team to a higher level of care appropriate to the condition of the newborn. Most babies should be referred to a major pediatric cardiac unit with surgical capabilities.[19] **IT IS FAR BETTER TO ANTICIPATE THIS NEED WHEN POSSIBLE AND TRANSPORT THE MOTHER BEFORE BIRTH.**

Recently, the U. S. Health and Human Services Secretary approved the recommendation that all newborns be screened for critical congenital heart disease (CCHD) using pulse oximetry.[20] Many states are utilizing perinatal regionalization programs to educate community hospitals regarding this recommendation.

Glucocorticoid Therapy for Fetal Maturation

Administration of glucocorticoids (corticosteroids), such as betamethasone or dexamethasone, to a pregnant woman 24 to 48 hours prior to birth has been shown to stimulate surfactant production and decrease respiratory distress syndrome (RDS) in the premature newborn. Clinical recommendations are as follows[21,22]:

- All pregnant women between 24 and 34 weeks' gestation who are at risk for preterm birth within 7 days should be considered for antenatal treatment with a single course of corticosteroids. Optimal benefit from such therapy lasts 7 days.
- Treatment consists of 2 doses of 12 mg of **betamethasone** given intramuscularly 24 hours apart **OR** 4 doses of 6 mg of **dexamethasone** given intramuscularly 12 hours apart.

For additional information regarding corticosteroid administration, refer to Module 10.

> If preterm birth is anticipated, the first dose of corticosteroids should be administered prior to maternal transport if possible. In addition, communication to the receiving facility with documentation of administration should be provided.

Fetal Echocardiography

The use of fetal echocardiography is currently evolving and requires extensive experience by the diagnostician to accurately diagnose some congenital cardiac abnormalities. A diagnosis by an inexperienced individual can be wrong or incomplete. When a cardiac abnormality is suspected in utero in a facility other than a tertiary care center, maternal transport is indicated.[19]

Responsibilities of the Referring and Receiving Centers

> • **What steps should be taken by the referring physician and hospital in initiating the transport?**

The decision to transport the pregnant or laboring woman should be made jointly by her provider and the physician to whom the referral is being made. The situation should be discussed with the woman and/or her family.

In 1986, Congress enacted the Emergency Medical Treatment & Labor Act (EMTALA) to ensure public access to emergency services regardless of ability to pay. Section 1867 of the Social Security Administration (SSA) imposes specific obligations on Medicare-participating hospitals that offer emergency services to provide a medical screening examination (MSE) when a request is made for examination or treatment for an emergency medical condition (EMC), *including active labor,* regardless of an individual's ability to pay. Hospitals are then required to provide stabilizing treatment for patients with EMC/s. If a hospital is unable to stabilize a patient within its capability, or if a patient requests, an appropriate transfer should be implemented (www.cms.hhs.gov). If an unstable patient is to be transferred, the treating provider is expected to document the reasons and that the risk/benefit ratio favors patient transfer to a facility with the capacity to provide the care the patient needs.

The following guidelines for the organization of the transport are divided into **referring center** responsibilities and **receiving center** responsibilities.[18,23]

Referring Center Responsibilities

- The referring provider confers with the receiving physician by phone. This should assist the receiving physician in developing a treatment plan to maintain stabilization of the patient before and during transport. It is the referring center's responsibility to follow COBRA/EMTALA guidelines.
- An ambulance is the most appropriate vehicle for the majority of maternal transports. Helicopter and fixed-wing aircrafts are also used for the safe transfer of obstetric patients.[24,25] The mode of transport/type of vehicle used should be chosen based on safety and efficiency taking into account the weather, terrain, etc.[26]

- The composition of the transport team should be a joint decision between the referring and receiving care providers based on the condition of the woman and/or fetus and may include physicians, nurse practitioners, registered nurses, respiratory therapists, and/or emergency medical technicians.[1]
- If the transport is done by the referring hospital, the referring physician and hospital retain responsibility until the transport team arrives with the patient at the receiving hospital. If the transport team is sent by the receiving hospital, the receiving physician or designee assumes responsibility for patient care from the time the patient leaves the referring hospital.[1]
- The woman is transported from the obstetric unit of the referring center or provider's office to the obstetric unit of the receiving hospital. This reduces the risk of unnecessary delays in the emergency department or admitting office.

REMEMBER: *Adequate documentation of the woman's health status is essential for developing a treatment plan at the receiving center. Send all available medical records and complete prenatal records, including any ultrasonography reports and laboratory test results.*

NOTE: *A member of the woman's family should be encouraged to accompany her. If the mother requires care by the ambulance attendants, the family member may sit with the ambulance driver or follow in a car.*

Receiving Center Responsibilities

- **What steps should be taken by the receiving physician and hospital in accepting the transport?**

- The receiving center is responsible for updating the referring provider with access by telephone on a 24-hour basis to communicate with receiving obstetric and neonatal units.[1]
- The receiving physician is responsible for accepting the referring care provider's request for transport and for making preparations to receive the transport.
- Shared responsibility for the patient by the receiving provider (usually a physician) and the referring provider begins on initial consultation and acceptance for the transfer. Full responsibility begins with admission to the receiving center.
- Every woman accepted by transport from a referring hospital should be seen by a provider within 30 minutes of arrival.
- Communication by telephone, letter, or fax with the referring care provider should occur after admission.
- If the woman is discharged undelivered, communication should occur before the discharge.
- A discharge summary including diagnosis, an outline of the hospital course, and recommendations for ongoing care of both woman and newborn should be sent to the referring provider.
- The woman should return to the care of the referring provider as soon as possible. Separation of the woman and newborn should be avoided when possible.
- If the woman needs to be referred to the receiving center or provider again, the referral process begins again with a provider-to-provider phone call.

Nursing Care in Maternal Transport

- **How can the nurse assist the woman and her family through the transfer process?**

The process of being transferred from one hospital to another increases the woman's and family's awareness of the medical problems accompanying the pregnancy. At the same time, geographically distancing women and members of her family reduce the opportunity for mutual support. Coping abilities of both parties can suffer. It is important that communication between woman and father or other family members be facilitated throughout the stay at the high-risk center. Many transport teams have printed information for the woman and family that can be helpful.

Nursing Interventions Throughout the Stay at the Referring Hospital[27]

These interventions are aimed at preparing the family for the transport.
- Ensure that the woman and her family understand the reasons for the transfer. **Ask the woman to say why she is being transported.** *This is important.*

- Inform the family about the regional hospital to which the transfer is being made. Information should include the following:
  - The name of the physician and a primary nurse at the receiving hospital (sometimes this is unknown)
  - The type of care given at the receiving hospital (teaching facility or private hospital)
  - How the woman will be transported (e.g., ambulance, helicopter)
  - How long the trip will take
  - When the trip is to occur
  - Who will accompany her (check with the transport team to see if someone is allowed)
  - Hospital unit policies, including visiting hours and telephone numbers
  - How family members can travel to the receiving hospital by car or mass transportation
  - Cost of transport and whether covered by insurance
  - Encourage the woman to discuss her fears and concerns with you. Be able to answer questions regarding her diagnosis and proposed plan of care

Nursing Interventions at the Receiving Hospital

Patients/families under great stress have difficulty dealing with more than a few people. Ideally, one nurse should be assigned initially to assist the woman and her family.

- Welcome the woman and her family while orienting them to the unit.[27]
- Review unit policies and encourage the mother's support person to visit as often as is appropriate.
- Facilitate telephone communication with family members as appropriate.
- Promote prebirth bonding of the woman and family to the fetus by discussing the fetus' unique characteristics, such as activity levels and times of quiet.

Have the neonatal nurse practitioner or neonatologist speak to the woman and family members regarding their concerns for the premature newborn. Arrange a tour of the NICU if the condition of the mother permits. Parents need to be assisted to identify the fetus as a developing individual—a part of the family—even with a fetus that is greatly compromised during the pregnancy.

- After the birth, promote parent–infant interaction at whatever level is appropriate. If the newborn is in an NICU, do the following:
  - Encourage parental visits.
  - Take a picture of the newborn for family members to see.
  - Have the NICU nurse report to or write down information about the newborn's progress.
  - Involve parents, when possible, with decisions about their newborn's care.
  - Provide opportunities for parents to care for their newborn at whatever level appropriate.
  - Allow the woman and family to discuss their fears, concerns, and anxieties.
  - Provide the family with some privacy during visits.
  - Assist the woman with the initiation of breastfeeding including the pumping and storage of breast milk if this is the woman's choice.
  - Assist the family to contact the appropriate support services (e.g., social service, clergy, psychologists, parent groups).
  - Facilitate continuity of care for the newborn and parents if the infant is transferred back to the referring hospital for final recovery closer to the parent's home.

Optimizing Safe Transport

Transport team members should have the collective expertise sufficient to provide the following, if necessary: (1) monitoring of blood pressure, uterine contractions, deep tendon reflexes, and fetal heart rate; (2) monitoring the administration of intravenous infusions and usage of tocolytic, antihypertensive, and anticonvulsant medications; and (3) care for a wide variety of emergency conditions, including birth and neonatal resuscitation.[18]

• What basic equipment is needed for maternal transport?

Most ambulances have basic life support (BLS) equipment adequate for the majority of maternal transports. The referring physician should be familiar with the availability of BLS and advanced life support (ALS) ambulances in the area. Equipment should also be available for anticipated complications such as birth, seizure, and hemorrhage. Organization and maintenance of additional transport equipment is the responsibility of the transport team. The Tennessee Perinatal Care System *Guidelines for Transportation*[18] lists additional equipment that may be necessary for maternal transport in Table 19.1.

TABLE 19.1 MATERNAL TRANSPORT SUPPLIES AND EQUIPMENT	
ITEM	**NOTES**
Precipitous birth kit	If the woman is in labor during transport, a birth kit from the referring hospital should include: cord clamps scissors to cut the cord suction bulbs blankets and hat for the newborn[18]
Newborn resuscitation supplies and equipment	• Neonatal-dosed medications for resuscitation • Pressure gauge • Flowmeter • Oxygen analyzer • Oxygen blender • Oxygen tubing • Oxygen masks (preterm and term neonatal) • Infant positive-pressure bag and mask • Suction catheter (#6, #8, and #10 F)
Newborn transport incubator	In transporting a high-risk laboring woman who has the possibility of birth before reaching the referral hospital, a *transport incubator* should be part of the equipment. The incubator must be capable of the following: • Providing a stable, adjustable heat source • Providing constant and adjustable oxygen • Providing good visibility of the newborn • Being easily transported • Providing easy access to the newborn for care and treatment • Operating on DC sources of electric power while in transport and AC sources for hospital use ***NOTE:** If used in RWA and/or FWA, the incubator should meet FAA requirements for crashworthiness and should be tested by an FAA certified mechanic to assure equipment does not interfere with navigational instruments.*[18]
Doppler or fetal monitor	Fetal assessment should continue during transport
Reflex hammer	If the woman is on magnesium sulfate, continue to assess DTRs every 1 hr
Infusion pump Latex-free supplies	Keep all infusions on a pump unless a bolus line is needed
Medications Uterotonic agents	• Oxytocin (Pitocin) • Methergine • Misoprostol • Hemabate
Magnesium sulfate	Premixed bag (20 g in 500 mL for a concentration of 1 g in 25 mL)
Calcium gluconate	Include dosing to be given if magnesium toxicity is suspected.

table continues on page 510

ITEM	NOTES
Tocolytic agents	In addition to magnesium sulfate, include the following tocolytic medications: • Nifedipine • Brethine (for SQ administration) • Indocin
Antihypertensive agents	• Apresoline • Labetalol
Antibiotics	Continue previous dosing regime

NOTE: In all transport situations, the mother should be encouraged to avoid positions that compromise maternal blood flow. Keep the mother in a semi-Fowler's or left side-lying position. This displaces the gravid uterus off the vena cava, promoting optimal maternal cardiac output.

An important step in the preparation for transfer is to carefully label any bag of intravenous fluid just before transport. In addition, the transport service must have a method of assuring that all medications and intravenous fluids are appropriately calculated.[28] Oxygen administration is advised in any clinical situation for which there is concern about potential fetal compromise.

Specific Liability Issues Related to Transport[1]

Every nurse and provider involved in transport should be keenly aware of liability issues. Such sensitivity may serve to sharpen all facets of clinical practice to the benefit of both the patient and healthcare personnel.

    Specific liability issues include the following:
• Use of treatment protocols or algorithms
• Lack of informed consent
• Failure to stabilize before transport
• Failure to diagnose or delay in diagnosing a problem more significant than what was relayed by the transferring hospital
• Equipment issues
• Delay in treatment or transfer
• Actual error (e.g., wrong medication or dose)
• Liability transfer from referring facility to receiving facility

The Commission of Accreditation of Medical Transport Systems (CAMTS) offers a program of voluntary evaluation of compliance with accreditation standards with measureable criteria for medical transport that are designed to address issues of patient care and safety. This provides medical professionals involved with air and ground transport systems to improve services and can serve as a marker of excellence for federal, state, and local agencies, as well as to the public.[28] See "Resources of Note" for further information.

Outreach Education

Indispensable to the appropriate use of a regional perinatal referral center is a program to educate the communities about its capabilities.[1] Outreach education should include information about the referral center's personnel and capabilities and also continuing education about current treatment modalities for high-risk situations. The S.T.A.B.L.E. program, taught by many outreach education programs, focuses exclusively on the post resuscitation/pre transport stabilization care of sick neonates which can improve outcomes for outborn neonates.[29]

Summary

Establishing national levels of maternity care has been successfully done in other specialties such as trauma, stroke, and neonatology should improve maternal care and therefore also improve neonatal outcomes.[8] Recently, the American College of Obstetricians and Gynecologists (ACOG) and the Society for Maternal–Fetal Medicine (SMFM) published an Obstetric

Care Consensus on levels of maternal care.[30] This document introduces uniform designations for levels of maternal care, describes standard definitions for facilities that provide each level of care, and provides consistent guidelines for service.[30] Descriptions exist for birth centers, level I (basic care), level II (specialty care), level III (subspecialty care), and level IV (regional perinatal centers). The goal of regionalized maternal care is for pregnant women with complications to receive care in facilities prepared to provide the level of care needed. Hospitals are encouraged to carefully evaluate the Consensus on maternal levels of care and be prepared to transfer those patients that they are not adequately prepared to care for so that safety for the mother is enhanced.

PRACTICE/REVIEW QUESTIONS

After reviewing this module, answer the following questions:

1. What is the primary advantage of transporting the high-risk woman to a regional center before the baby is born?

   _____

2. What is the primary disadvantage of transporting the high-risk woman to a regional center?

   _____

   _____

3. Describe a *low-risk* maternal transport situation.

   _____

   _____

   _____

4. Under what conditions should the *high-risk* woman in *early* labor be transported?

   a. _____

   b. _____

   c. _____

   d. _____

5. Describe a *high-risk* maternal transport situation.

   _____

   _____

   _____

6. The obstetric complications necessitating high-risk care involve conditions occurring before _____ weeks' gestation or an estimated birth weight below _____ g.

7. List several *obstetric complications* that require high-risk care and therefore maternal transport from community hospitals in some cases.

   a. _____

   b. _____

   c. _____

   d. _____

   e. _____

8. Briefly list *medical* and *surgical complications* necessitating high-risk care.

   Medical Complications

   a. _____

   b. _____

   c. _____

   d. _____

   e. _____

   Surgical Complications

   a. _____

   b. _____

   c. _____

9. What fetal situations necessitate the transfer of a mother from a level II to a level III institution?

   a. _____

   b. _____

10. Newborns often experience cyanosis after birth, often peripherally. List three characteristics of cyanotic babies, who are generally not experiencing a cardiac abnormality.

    a. _____

    b. _____

    c. _____

11. A newborn with a cyanotic congenital heart abnormality needs to be kept at the level I or level II hospital until he or she is stabilized. After stabilization, the baby may be transferred.

    a. True

    b. False

12. Cyanosis of mucous membranes and the tongue in a term baby who has no radiologic evidence of lung disease is suspicious for:

    a. cardiac abnormality

    b. peripheral cyanosis, common in many babies

13. Current recommendations from the NIH (2000) advise antenatal treatment for all pregnant women between

511

_____ weeks' gestation and _____ weeks' gestation who are at risk for preterm delivery within _____ days and that they be considered for treatment with a single course of corticosteroids.

14. Corticosteroid therapy (e.g., betamethasone, dexamethasone) brings about a significant decrease in RDS in infants born between 29 and 34 weeks' gestation.

    a. True

    b. False

15. A *single course* of treatment with *betamethasone* consists of _____ doses of _____ mg given intramuscularly _____ hours apart.

16. A single course of treatment with *dexamethasone* consists of _____ doses of _____ mg given intramuscularly _____ hours apart.

17. The referring physician must initiate the transport by contacting the receiving physician.

    a. True

    b. False

18. A health professional should always accompany the mother during transport.

    a. True

    b. False

19. The mother's record and laboratory data should be sent to the high-risk center by mail.

    a. True

    b. False

20. The woman should be taken to the emergency room of the receiving hospital.

    a. True

    b. False

21. A discharge summary sheet should be sent to the referring care provider.

    a. True

    b. False

22. A woman who is a gravida 3, para 2, is at a level I hospital in her 34th week of pregnancy. She is dilated 6 cm, and her preterm labor is complicated by severe preeclampsia. The receiving and referring physicians have agreed on maternal transport by helicopter to the high-risk regional center, which is 40 miles away. Who is the most appropriate member of the health team to accompany the woman?

    _____

    Why? _____

23. List eight nursing interventions that the nurse at the referring hospital can do to assist the woman and her family in the transfer to the high-risk regional center.

    a. _____

    b. _____

    c. _____

    d. _____

    e. _____

    f. _____

    g. _____

    h. _____

24. List eight nursing interventions designed to assist the woman in adjusting to the high-risk regional center after transfer.

    a. _____

    b. _____

    c. _____

    d. _____

    e. _____

    f. _____

    g. _____

    h. _____

25. List five specific liability issues related to transport.

    a. _____

    b. _____

    c. _____

    d. _____

    e. _____

PRACTICE/REVIEW ANSWER KEY

1. Survival rates and quality of life (long-term sequelae) for the high-risk neonate are improved.
2. The woman is separated from friends and family.
3. The low-risk transport situation is one in which the woman and fetus are in a stable condition and birth is not expected during the immediate 24-hour period.
4. a. Transport will take less than 2 hours.
   b. The woman's condition is stable.
   c. Delivery is not anticipated for 4 to 6 hours.
   d. An experienced health professional can accompany the woman.
5. The high-risk transport situation is one in which the woman's or fetus' condition is unstable (e.g., actively bleeding with a placenta previa or in active labor and dilated 5 cm or beyond) and the time of birth is unpredictable.
6. 34: 2,000

7. Answers should include:
   a. Premature rupture of membranes before 34 weeks' gestation or with a fetus thought to weigh less than 2,000 g
   b. Premature labor before 34 weeks' gestation
   c. Conditions in which the infant might deliver before 34 weeks' gestation or weigh less than 2,000 g (e.g., severe preeclampsia or hypertensive disorder, multiple gestation, poorly controlled or severe diabetes mellitus, intrauterine growth restriction with signs of fetal distress, bleeding in the third trimester, Rh isoimmunization, severe oligohydramnios)
8. **Medical Complications**
   a. Infections that can result in premature birth
   b. Severe heart disease
   c. Renal disease with deteriorating function or increasing hypertension
   d. Drug overdose
   e. Some patients with carcinoma
   Surgical Complications
   a. Trauma that requires care or surgery beyond what the local hospital can provide
   b. Acute abdominal problems at less than 34 weeks' gestation or a baby weighing less than 2,000 g
   c. Thoracic emergencies
9. a. Any fetus anticipated to require long-term ventilatory support after birth
   b. Any fetus anticipated to require neonatal care at less than 30 to 34 weeks' gestation (this depends on the skilled personnel and advanced technology of the institution).
10. Any three of the following:
    a. Are premature, had a difficult delivery, experienced meconium passages in utero, had premature rupture of membranes
    b. Are in marked respiratory distress
    c. Have radiologic evidence of lung disease
    d. Have an elevated PCO_2 level
    e. Have PO_2 increases with 100% oxygen
11. b. False—The infant is going to get worse with time.
12. a
13. 24; 34; 7
14. a. True
15. 2; 12; 24
16. 4; 6; 12
17. a. True
18. b. False—This depends on the circumstances under which the woman is being transported. Occasionally, a private car may be used, in which case the health professional would not accompany the woman.
19. b. False
20. b. False
21. a. True
22. A physician
    This represents a high-risk maternal transport.
23. Any eight of the following:
    a. Ensure that the woman and her family understand the reasons for the transfer.
    b. Inform the family about the regional hospital to which the woman is being transferred.

c. Give the names of the physician and a primary nurse at the regional center.
d. Discuss the type of care given.
e. Tell the woman how she will be transported and how long the trip will take.
f. Tell the woman when the trip is to occur and who will be accompanying her.
g. Familiarize the woman with the hospital unit policies, including visiting hours and telephone numbers.
h. Discuss how family members can get to the regional center and where they might be able to stay.
i. Allow the woman to discuss her fears and concerns with you.
24. Any eight of the following:
    a. Welcome the woman and her family while orienting them to the unit.
    b. Review unit policies and promote visiting of the woman's support person as appropriate to her level of illness.
    c. Facilitate telephone communication with family members as appropriate.
    d. Promote prebirth bonding of the woman and family to the fetus by discussing the fetus' unique characteristics, such as activity levels and times of quiet.
    e. Promote parent–infant interaction at whatever level is possible and appropriate.
    f. Encourage the woman and family to discuss their fears, concerns, and anxieties.
    g. Provide the family with some privacy during visits.
    h. Assist the family to contact appropriate support services (e.g., social service, clergy, psychologists, parent groups).
    i. Facilitate continuity of care for infant and parents if the newborn is transferred back to the referring hospital for final recovery.
25. Any five of the following:
    a. Use of treatment protocols or algorithms
    b. Lack of informed consent
    c. Failure to stabilize
    d. Failure to diagnose or delay in diagnosing a problem more significant than what was relayed by the transferring hospital
    e. Equipment issues
    f. Delay in treatment or transfer
    g. Actual error (e.g., wrong drug or dose)
    h. When does liability transfer from the referring facility to the receiving facility?

REFERENCES

1. American Academy of Pediatrics and the American College of Obstetricians and Gynecologists. (2012). Maternal and neonatal interhospital transfer. In *Guidelines for perinatal care* (7th ed., pp. 77–93). Washington, DC: Author.
2. March of Dimes. (2010). *Towards improving the outcome of pregnancy III. March of dimes foundation.* White Plains, NY: Author.
3. Clement, M. S. (2005). Perinatal care in Arizona 1950–2002: A study of the positive impact of technology, regionalization and the Arizona Perinatal Trust. *Journal of Perinatology, 25*, 503–508.

4. Clement, M. S. (2002). *Perinatal transport in Arizona.* Phoenix: Office of Women's and Children's Health, Arizona Department of Health Services.

5. Hohoagschwandter, M., Husslein, P., Klebermass, K., et al. (2001). Perinatal mortality and morbidity: Comparison between maternal transport, neonatal transport and inpatient antenatal treatment. *Archives of Gynecology and Obstetrics, 265*(3), 113–118.

6. Ohning, B. L., & Driggers, K. P. (2001). Transport of the critically ill newborn. *EMedicine Journal, 2*(5). Available from: www.emedicine.com/ped/topic2730.htm

7. Binder, S., Hill, K., Meinzen-Derr, J., et al. (2011). Increasing VLBW deliveries at subspecialty perinatal centers via perinatal outreach. *Pediatrics, 127*(3), 487–493.

8. Hankins, D. V., Clark, S., Pacheco, L. D., et al. (2012). Maternal mortality, near misses and severe morbidity. *Obstetrics and Gynecology, 120*(4), 929–934.

9. Berg, C. J., Callaghan, W. M., Syverson, C., et al. (2010). Pregnancy related mortality in the United States, 1998–2005. *Obstetrics and Gynecology, 116*(6), 1302–1309.

10. Schoon, M. G. (2013). Impact of inter-facility transport on maternal mortality in the Free State Province. *South African Medical Journal, 103*(8), 534–537.

11. Knox, G. E., Simpson, K. R., & Garite, T. J. (1999). Highly reliable perinatal units: An approach to the prevention of patient injury and medical malpractice claims. *Journal of Healthcare Risk Management, 19*(2), 24–27.

12. Morbidity and Mortality Weekly Trend. (2013). Preterm births—United States 2006 and 2010. Retrieved from: www.cdc.gov

13. National Vital Statistics Reports. (2014). Births: Preliminary data for 2013. Available from: www.cdc.gov

14. Rehm, N. E. (1987). Indications for maternal transport—the Utah experience. In Coulter, D. M. (Ed.), *Current concepts in transport: Neonatal, maternal, administrative* (3rd ed., pp. 297–298). Salt Lake City: Perinatal Transport Service, University of Utah Medical Center.

15. American College of Obstetricians and Gynecologists. (2002). Prevention of early-onset group B streptococcal disease in newborns. *Committee Opinion, 279*, 1–8.

16. American College of Obstetrians and Gynecologists. (2013). Premature rupture of membranes. *Practice Bulletin, 139*, 1–13.

17. Centers for Disease Control and Prevention. (2002). Prevention of perinatal group B streptococcal disease: A public health perspective. *Morbidity and Mortality Weekly Report, 51*(RR-11), 1–22.

18. Tennessee Perinatal Care System. (2014). *Guidelines for transportation* (6th ed.). Nashville: Tennessee Department of Health, Maternal and Child Health. Prepared by the Subcommittee on Perinatal Transportation of the Perinatal Advisory Committee.

19. Orsmond, G. S. (1995). Management of cyanotic heart disease. In Trautman, M. S. (Ed.), *Current concepts in transport. Neonatal syllabus* (7th ed., pp. 16–20). Salt Lake City: University of Utah.

20. Morbidity and Mortality Weekly Report. (2012). Newborn screening for critical congenital heart disease: Potential roles of Birth Defects Surveillance Programs—United States, 2010–2011. Available from: www.cdc.gov

21. National Institutes of Health. (2001). Antenatal corticosteroids revisited: Repeat courses. *NIH Consensus Statement Online 2000, 17*(2), 1–10.

22. American College of Obstetricians and Gynecolists. (2011). Antenatal corticosteroid therapy for fetal maturation. *Committee Opinion, 475*, 1–3.

23. Strobino, D. M., Frank, R., Oberdorf, M. A., et al. (1993). Development of an index of maternal transport. *Medical Decisions Making, 13*(1), 64–73.

24. O'Brien, D. J., Hooker, E. A., Hignite, J., et al. (2004). Long-distance fixed-wing transport of obstetrical patients. *Southern Medical Journal, 97*(9), 816–818.

25. Ohara, M., Shimizu, Y., Satoh, H., et al. (2008). Safety and usefulness of emergency maternal transport using helicopter. *The Journal Of Obstetrics and Gynaecology Research, 34*(2), 189–194.

26. Wilson, A., Hillman, S., Rosato, M., et al. (2013). A systematic review and thematic synthesis of qualitative studies on maternal emergency transport in low- and middle-income countries. *International Journal of Gynecology and Obstetrics, 122*, 192–201.

27. Davis, D. H., & Hawkins, J. W. (1985). High-risk maternal and neonatal transport: Psychosocial implications for practice. *Dimensions of Critical Care Nursing, 4*(6), 373–379.

28. Commission on Accreditation of Medical Transport Systems. (2006). *Accreditation standards of the commission on accreditation of medical transport systems* (7th ed.). Anderson, SC: Author.

29. Taylor, R. M., & Price-Douglas, W. (2008). The STABLE Program post resuscitation/pretransport stabilization care of sick infants. *The Journal of Perinatal & Neonatal Nursing, 22*(2), 159–165.

30. American College of Obstetricians and Gynecologists and Society for Maternal Fetal Medicine. (2015). Obstetric care consensus: Levels of maternal care. *American Journal of Obstetrics and Gynecology, 125*, 502–515.

RESOURCES OF NOTE

Commission on Accreditation of Medical Transport Systems. (2006). *Accreditation standards of the commission on accreditation of medical transport systems. mission statement.* Anderson, SC: Author.

Conference. (Annual). *Current concepts in transport (neonatal, pediatric).* Sponsored by the Pediatric Education by the Pediatric Education Services at Primary Children's Medical Center, University of Utah, School of Medicine, Salt Lake City, Education Department. Phone: 801–588–4060.

Tennessee Perinatal Care System. (2012). *Guidelines for transportation* (7th ed.). Subcommittee on Perinatal Transportation of the Perinatal Advisory Committee. Tennessee Department of Health, Maternal and Child Health. Address: 425 5th Avenue North, 5th Floor, Cordell Hull Building, Nashville, TN 37247–4701.

Liability Issues in Intrapartum Nursing

SUZANNE McMURTRY BAIRD,
BETSY BABB KENNEDY, AND
SUSAN L. BAUDHUIN, ESQ.

MODULE 20

Objectives

As you complete this module, you will learn:

1. Why malpractice suits are a nursing concern
2. Common areas of litigation for intrapartum nurses
3. Components of informed consent
4. Circumstances that require consent
5. When informed consent is not necessary
6. Issues related to informed consent
7. The functions of the medical record
8. The relationship that exists between standards of nursing practice and documentation of care
9. Information that must be documented in the medical record by nurses during care of the woman in the intrapartum period
10. The general guidelines for documentation in a medical record
11. Tips for countersigning documentation, documenting verbal orders, and telephone triage
12. Strategies for avoiding malpractice claims
13. What to do if you are named in a malpractice suit

Key Terms

When you have completed this module, you should be able to recall the meaning of the following terms. You should also be able to use the terms when consulting with other health professionals. The terms are defined in this module or in the glossary at the end of this book.

addendum	fraud
capacity	information
collusion	informed consent
competence	malpractice
confidentiality	negligence
conservator	standard of practice
documentation	therapeutic privilege
duress	voluntariness
emancipated	

Introduction

The intrapartum nurse faces high risk for involvement in a malpractice suit. The alarming number of cases alleging malpractice in obstetrics as a whole may be the result of a number of factors.

- Childbirth is an intense, emotional experience and parents have high expectations for a "perfect" birth and newborn. Poor outcomes are not usually anticipated.
- Parents may be well-informed consumers of health care.
- Obstetrics is a high-pressure, rapidly changing specialty. Accidents, errors in judgment, and negligence do occur.
- There is increasing accountability and autonomy in nursing practice.

This module is divided into four parts, reviewing the components of malpractice, general areas of nursing liability, issues unique to intrapartum nurses, and strategies to avoid malpractice claims. Display 20.1 describes the legal process of a malpractice claim. Note: this process may vary slightly for each state.

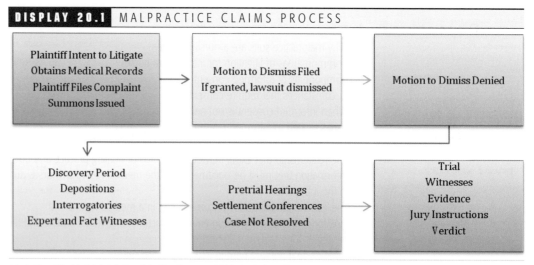

DISPLAY 20.1 MALPRACTICE CLAIMS PROCESS

| Plaintiff Intent to Litigate / Obtains Medical Records / Plaintiff Files Complaint / Summons Issued | Motion to Dismiss Filed / If granted, lawsuit dismissed | Motion to Dimiss Denied |
| Discovery Period / Depositions / Interrogatories / Expert and Fact Witnesses | Pretrial Hearings / Settlement Conferences / Case Not Resolved | Trial / Witnesses / Evidence / Jury Instructions / Verdict |

Adapted from Westrick, S. J. (2014). *Essentials of Nursing Law and Ethics* (2nd ed.). Burlington, MA: Jones & Barlett.

Components of Malpractice

• How are medical malpractice and negligence defined?[1]

Medical malpractice is any act or omission by a healthcare professional during treatment of a patient that (1) deviates from accepted norms of practice (or standards of care) in the medical community, *and* (2) causes an injury to the patient. Such deviations are known in the legal realm as "**negligence.**" Negligence in the nursing realm would be the failure to act as a reasonably prudent nurse would act under the same or similar circumstances. In simple terms, as a nurse you are held to certain professional standards that impose a legal duty to act or refrain from acting in any way that endangers the patients for whom you are providing care.

• What is standard of care?[1]

Nursing standards of care are qualitative guidelines for providing safe care and should reflect a desired and achievable level of performance against which actual performance can be compared. The purpose of a standard of care is to guide professional nursing practice. Nursing standards do not require outstanding or above average care—they are used to determine what is "reasonable" under the circumstances. Standard of care for nurses in the legal context is defined as the degree of skill, care, and judgment used by an "ordinary, prudent" nurse under same or similar circumstances. In every nursing malpractice lawsuit, there will be an allegation that the nurse breached a duty owed to the patient by failing to meet the applicable standard of care. Thus, these standards of care become the criteria used in medical negligence lawsuits to describe in what way(s) the nurse failed in his or her duty.

NOTE: Know and follow your state's nurse practice act and your facility's policies and procedures.

• Where are nursing standards found?

Nursing standards are found within state statutes (nurse practice acts), hospital policy, procedures, and protocols, national professional organizations (e.g., American Nurses Association), and specialty nursing organizations (e.g., Association of Women's Health, Obstetrics and Neonatal Nursing, Association of Critical Care Nurses). When no written policy addressing a particular situation exists, the standard of care is what a reasonably prudent nurse would do under the same or similar circumstances, and is established in court through the testimony of nursing experts.

• What are the key elements of professional negligence suits?[1]

In a malpractice lawsuit, the plaintiff (person filing the lawsuit) must establish *all* of the following elements:
- ***duty*** to the patient
- ***breach*** of that duty
- ***injury*** to the patient
- ***causal link*** between the breach and the patient's injury

General Areas of Nursing Management Cited in Legal Cases

Improper Medication Administration

Errors in medication administration are commonly occurring adverse events that result in patient harm. Many initiatives have been implemented in healthcare organizations to attempt to decrease the occurrence. However, errors in practice still exist at an alarming rate due to the complex and unpredictable environment in which nurses are working.[2,3]

In addition, intrapartum nurses administer several high-alert medications routinely in practice. Often, these medications are at the center of allegations in a medical malpractice case. These include:
- Magnesium sulfate
- Oxytocin
- Insulin
- Heparin

Registered nurses (RNs) are expected to adhere to professional standards and to advocate for and participate in activities to create safe medication systems within their practice setting. To safeguard against medication errors, here are some helpful tips:
- Always practice the seven rights of medication administration and defined protocols, even when you are busy or fatigued.
  - Right medication
  - Right dose
  - Right route
  - Right time
  - Right patient
  - Right reason
  - Right documentation
- Have policies and protocols and standardized administration in place for high-alert medications.
- Check the order and clarify with the provider if you have any questions.
- Check the label before administration.
- Look up the medication if not familiar with all seven rights. Know WHY you are administering a medication.
- If it seems wrong, double check with another nurse, provider, or the pharmacist.

- Complete double checks as indicated for high-alert medications and document.
- Omit or delay the medication administration as warranted by patient assessment and notify the provider.
  - Example: hold brethine if maternal heart rate greater than 120 beats per minute.
- Know the woman's allergy profile.
- Use checklists as indicated.
  - Example: Oxytocin Pre-Use and In-Use Checklists

Failure to Assess and Monitor for Side Effects of Medication or Interventions

Medication practice is much more than just the technical task of giving a pill or giving an injection. Assessment following medication administration or titration of a medication based on the woman's assessment is an important aspect of nursing care. Reassessment following administration of a medication allows for the continued formation of the plan of care and other needed communication or intervention. The titration of oxytocin based on maternal and fetal assessments is a high liability area for obstetric nurses.

NOTE: Nurses have the educational preparation to make patient-specific range-related medication decisions.

Improper Use of Equipment or Availability of Equipment

The use of any piece of equipment with patient care requires the following:
- Knowledge of the manufacturers' recommendations and facility policy for use
- Routine monitoring for proper working function (as indicated and outlined by the facility's policy)
- Recognition of equipment malfunction
- Training and competency of proper use
- Knowledge and competency of how to interpret data obtained from the equipment

NOTE: Be specific about your request and the time frame for response! Always clarify, confirm, and restate any orders given.

Poor or Inadequate Communication and/or Collaboration

There is a legal duty to notify the appropriate physician and/or midwife in a timely manner of any significant, abnormal assessment data that does not respond to routine nursing intervention. Failure to notify of abnormal assessment findings may lead to poor outcomes and increase the chances for malpractice litigation. The Joint Commission has identified miscommunication among caregivers as a primary cause of perinatal events, including infant death and injury.[4,5] In the intrapartum setting, communication among all caregivers is essential to optimize outcomes. Communication occurs in the medical record and verbally. Common breakdowns in RN to physician/midwife communication may involve the following situations:
- Nurse is busy providing urgent care to patient
- Nurse is convinced that physician/midwife will not act on assessment data
- Nurse fears that the physician/midwife will become angry regarding communication
- Nurse does not want to interrupt physician/midwife
- Nurse fails to see the relevance of assessment data
- Nurse fails to persist in communication
- Nurse fails to request the physician or midwife to come to the bedside for patient assessment

Effective communication techniques that nurses, nurse midwives, and physicians can use include the following[5-8]:
- In all communication, focus on the woman
- Speak clearly using a congenial tone
- Use professional behaviors
- Be aware of negative body language
- Present facts in an organized manner presenting all relevant facts, abnormal assessment findings, and specific concerns
- Agree upon the plan of care. If you disagree with the plan, state your rationale(s)
- Be an active listener
- Keep an open mind and consider alternatives
- Ask for clarification if communication is unclear

- If the woman, fetus, or both are at risk, tell the provider to report to the hospital to assess the patient immediately, and document the conversation
- Inform the provider if you plan to communicate up the chain of command

NOTE: Be specific about your request and the time frame for response! Always clarify, confirm, and restate any orders given.

Example Documentation of Assertive Communication:
"Dr. _____, I'm really uncomfortable with the fetal heart rate pattern. The variability is minimal and there are repetitive late decelerations. I have put on oxygen, repositioned the woman, and turned off the oxytocin. However, the decelerations have continued and the variability remains minimal. I think this woman needs your personal assessment regarding labor progress and the plan of care. I want you to come in now."

Ultimately, all care providers have the same goal: a healthy woman and baby. It is important to remember this goal in communicating and collaborating with members of the health care team. Using effective, standardized methods of communication such as SBAR (Situation, Background, Assessment, Recommendation) can enhance patient safety, improve outcomes, and reduce liability.[9]

The most common communication between nurses is report, hand-off, or hand-over, when care of the woman is transferred between providers, shifts, or units. The purpose of the hand-off is to pass along woman-specific information to ensure continuity of care and safety. *Hand-off reports should be standardized to minimize gaps in information that could contribute to inappropriate care of the patient.* The SBAR technique is one format that has been utilized for effective communication between nurses and between nurses and physicians or midwives. As an adjunct to the SBAR technique is bedside report. Participating in the hand-off at the woman's bedside allows her and/or her family members to ask questions, clarify assessment parameters, and understand the plan of care. Display 20.2 is an example of SBAR.

DISPLAY 20.2 SBAR EXAMPLE

SBAR TECHNIQUE FOR EFFECTIVE COMMUNICATION BETWEEN NURSES AND OTHER NURSES, PHYSICIANS, OR MIDWIVES

S—Situation	*Who are you?*
	What is your role in the care of the patient?
	Who is the patient?
	What is the reason for the call or transfer of care?
	(e.g., category III EFM pattern, bleeding, elevated blood pressure, transfer to another shift or unit)
B—Background	*What is the clinical context?*
	What is the woman's pertinent medical and obstetrical history?
	(e.g., gravida status, parity, gestational age, history of preeclampsia, previous cesarean birth, plan of care)
A—Assessment	*What is the current concern?*
	What is your assessment of the situation?
	(e.g., complete description of EFM parameters, vital signs, other symptoms, lab results, transferring care to the next shift)
R—Recommendation	*What needs to be done to correct it?*
	What are you requesting?
	(e.g., "I need you to come and assess the patient now"; "I need you to come and assess the EFM tracing now"; "I need this order changed"; "These labs need to be drawn in the next shift.")

NOTE: Being well prepared and organized to give a report during a hand-over or before making a call to the provider is important. If you are unsure of your assessment, discuss the situation with your charge nurse or preceptor. Avoid giving report on a woman for another nurse unless it is an emergent situation.

Failure to Act as a Patient Advocate and Initiate the Chain of Command

Every hospital should have a written chain of command policy/procedure for nurses to follow in order to properly escalate concerns. Nurses may become liable when a disagreement regarding clinical management occurs and they fail to initiate the defined chain of command. *Chain of command activation is indicated when there is potential for the maternal and/or fetal condition to rapidly deteriorate causing harm, and discussions with the appropriate provider have failed to provoke a proper plan of care. Display 20.3 is an example chain of command.*

DISPLAY 20.3 EXAMPLE CHAIN OF COMMAND

Example Chain of Command

1. Conflict regarding nursing and medical management.
2. Conversation between primary nurse and physician/midwife.
3. Notification of charge RN.
4. Notification of nurse manager/supervisor.
5. Discussion by charge RN and/or nurse manager with physician/midwife.
6. Discussion by charge RN and/or nurse manager with Chief of Obstetrics.
7. Chief of Obstetrics discusses plan with physician/midwife.
8. Notification of Hospital Administrator by Nursing and/or Chief of Obstetrics.
9. Hospital Administrator assists with resolution of conflict.

NOTE: Prior to activating the chain of command, the nurse should discuss care concerns with the provider. If the concern is not addressed, then the nurse should inform the provider that she is activating the chain of command.

Failure to Follow Provider Orders

Provider orders should comply with hospital policy and be based on evidence or best practice recommendations. The nurse may be held liable if provider orders are not followed and injury occurs as a result of not following the orders. If there is concern regarding a specific provider order, the nurse should notify the provider and discuss the rationale for the order. Liability may also occur if the provider order is clearly contraindicated by normal practice and the nurse follows the order. Communication regarding the plan of care includes a clear understanding of provider orders.

Failure to Verify Informed Consent

Obtaining informed consent is required by law.[1,10] Providers are obligated, prior to delivering certain types of treatment, to inform the woman about the risks and benefits of the proposed treatment, along with the risks and benefits of forgoing treatment, and any alternatives. Only after the woman has voluntarily consented may the provider proceed. All states provide exceptions in the case of emergencies, or when the woman has been declared mentally incompetent by a court of law, or if the woman lacks physical capacity. Providers who fail to properly obtain informed consent are subject to legal actions for malpractice and/or criminal battery (unlawful contact). It is crucial to understand the necessary content, applicability, and the nurse's role and responsibility in this area.

• **What are the components of informed consent?[1,10]**

For valid informed consent, the woman must be legally and physically capable of making the decision, the proper information must be conveyed, and the consent must be given voluntarily. The question of whether a woman is legally able to make a treatment decision involves a number of factors. First, the woman must be of legal age. Eighteen is recognized as the legal age for decision making in most states, but a woman under 18 may be considered "emancipated" and thus legally able to make her own treatment decisions if she meets certain criteria set by state law. In many cases, emancipation requires a court order. Do not *ever* assume a woman under 18 years is emancipated based on your assessment of her situation without knowing the laws regarding emancipated minors in your state.

The next part of the assessment involves whether the woman is capable of comprehending the information presented such that she can meaningfully consent. You will hear this referred to as "capacity" or "competence." While the terms are used interchangeably, they are different. To distinguish, "capacity" is a medical term referring to the determination made by *providers* as to whether an individual is capable of making medical decisions. "Competence" is a legal term referring to judicial determination. Even though questions of competency are legal in nature, usually a provider makes the assessment in the process of deciding whether the woman is mentally able to assess and make choices about her own care. The inquiry is whether the individual understands the treatment choices, risks, and alternatives; and whether she understands the significance and consequences of her decision. If you have concerns about the woman's ability to process information and make decisions, you should notify the treating provider.

The issue of meaningful consent does not present only with women who are underage, mentally ill, or mentally or physically challenged. Courts have invalidated a woman's consent where certain conditions rendered the patient unable to meaningfully process the information; thus, the consent given was not legally binding. Some examples of situations where courts invalidated a patient's informed consent are: being under great amounts of stress or in extreme pain (e.g., labor); being medicated/sedated; being intoxicated or under the influence of drugs; or being in a semiconscious state.

NOTE: States vary in the requirements for informed consent. It is the responsibility of the physician and nurse to know the laws regarding informed consent in their own state of practice.

Information refers to the content of the explanation given to the woman. Failure to provide reasonable and relevant information *in language the woman can understand* exposes providers to possible legal action. While states vary in their approaches to informed consent, the information given during an informed consent discussion should include the following:

- The nature of the individual's condition, the diagnosis, or suspected diagnosis
- The nature and purpose of the proposed treatment, including who will perform the treatment
- Expected outcomes and benefits
- Major risks, complications, and side effects of the proposed treatment
- Reasonable alternatives
- The right to refuse treatment
- Possible consequences of refusing treatment

Voluntariness refers to the circumstances under which the woman gives consent. All patients have the right to weigh decisions about their medical care after full disclosure of all relevant information, freely, and without being pressured or deceived. If fraud (deception), duress (forcing the woman to agree through the use of pressure, threats, coercion, violence, and restraints), or collusion (usually arises when family members work with providers in secret to direct treatment) is present, the consent is invalid. Remember that an individual can refuse further treatment or withdraw consent for a particular procedure at any time. Withdrawal can be given verbally, in writing, or by gesture (e.g., shaking head "no," withdrawing arm from nurse's hand). If the woman indicates a withdrawal of consent, the procedure should be discontinued as soon as safely possible. Extenuating circumstances in a life-threatening situation can negate the woman's refusal of treatment.

NOTE: The patient may prevail in a malpractice lawsuit if the patient did not consent to a procedure or was poorly informed by the provider.

REMEMBER: A positive outcome of a procedure does not protect you from a lawsuit.

IMPORTANT CONCERNS: Barriers of language, hearing, and vision must be addressed through interpreters, use of available technology, and services in order to assist the woman in understanding and consenting to treatment.

• Are there exceptions to informed consent?[1,10]

It is not absolutely necessary to obtain consent when delay will cause death or seriously jeopardize the patient's health. Another exception of sorts is *"therapeutic privilege,"* which occurs when a healthcare provider does not fully inform a patient about a treatment or procedure because the provider believes that complete disclosure would be harmful or extremely emotionally upsetting. Because in the United States all patients have the right to be informed about and make treatment decisions (including refusal of treatment), today's courts almost never recognize this exception.

- **Under what circumstances may another individual give informed consent for treatment of an adult?**[1,10]

When an adult is mentally incompetent or physically unable to give consent (i.e., comatose), a legal guardian, conservator, a legally designated power of attorney for health care, or judge may provide consent. These are the *only* sources for such consent. Family members do not automatically have the right to give consent. The court can overrule a competent adult's decision about a treatment, but such a judicial determination is made only when the state's interest of preservation of life is counter to the woman's wishes.

*NOTE: The preservation of life concept is the basis for many court decisions involving the fetus and/or newborn after the age of viability has been achieved. **EXAMPLE:** A woman who refuses a cesarean birth when the fetus is at term and a placenta previa is evident.*

- **Who should obtain informed consent for treatment or a procedure?**[1,10]

Providers (physician, certified nurse midwife, or nurse practitioner) are responsible for obtaining informed consent for medical procedures or treatments because only a treating provider has the required training, expertise, and knowledge regarding the woman's condition. In most instances, all treatment and care provided by a nurse is covered by a general consent to treatment. Nurses are often involved in the informed consent process, however.

Nurses are frequently requested to witness informed consent. In addition, in some settings, the provider might delegate the task of obtaining a woman's signature on a consent form to nursing personnel. If this is the policy and procedure of the institution, prior informed consent must have been obtained by the provider during prenatal care. **THE GUIDELINES FOR OBTAINING CONSENT IN THESE CASES MUST BE SPECIFICALLY WRITTEN FOR THE PROCEDURE, APPROVED, AND SIGNED BY MEDICAL AND NURSING ADMINISTRATION. If the woman questions the information provided, or she is unclear in her understanding, or refuses to sign the consent, you must not only refrain from trying to educate or persuade the woman, but are OBLIGATED, BOTH LEGALLY AND ETHICALLY, TO INFORM THE ATTENDING PROVIDER OF THE WOMAN'S INQUIRIES AND/OR REFUSAL TO SIGN. The provider is the only person legally responsible for giving additional information or answering the woman's questions about treatment.**

NOTE: Remember that a nurse simply obtaining a woman's signature on a consent form does not transfer the legal liability for informed consent from the provider to the nurse.

- **Under what circumstances should informed consent be obtained?**[1,10]

Many professionals believe that consent must be obtained only for major interventions (e.g., surgery, chemotherapy). This is incorrect. A written format is not necessary for every contact, but you should get consent before any patient contact. Prior to initiating any invasive treatment (like administering an injection or starting an IV), explain in simple terms what you are about to do and make sure the woman does not object. The woman may give consent verbally or by actions that imply consent (e.g., extending an arm for you to draw blood). Documenting that you explained your treatment with no objections should protect you from any allegation of failing to obtain consent for your nursing care.

NOTE: Informed consent is not a one-time event—the process should be ongoing throughout the woman's treatment.

Verbal and Telephone Orders

Although technology has decreased the need for telephone or verbal orders, in many settings this type of order may still be used.[11] However, there are many opportunities for misinterpretation of orders. If a telephone or verbal order is unavoidable, most institutions have policies governing time frames for the provider cosigning the order (e.g., verbal orders for medications must be cosigned within 24 hours). When taking a verbal order, write down the order, restate the order verbatim, including the patient's name, ask for confirmation, and clarify any questions. In charting the order, indicate "repeated and confirmed."

Timely or Inaccurate Assessment

The frequency of assessment should be determined by the woman's risk status and based on best practice recommendations. Risk status determined on admission may change during the course of labor and may require increased frequency of assessments. Nurses may also be liable for inaccurate assessment. A common complaint against the nurse is inaccurate fetal heart rate (FHR) monitoring interpretation. Inaccuracy of assessment may lead to a failure to intervene to improve maternal/fetal status or delay communication to the provider.

Lack of Knowledge and Clinical Competency

When a malpractice case proceeds, knowledge or competency of nurses is a common issue if inaccurate assessments have been performed. It is imperative that you maintain knowledge and skills involved in the care of your patient population. Documentation of orientation completion and continuing education is important. These documents may be requested if you are involved in the patient's care.

Whereas responsibility is shared among all team members to improve any system or process that impacts patient safety and outcomes, leadership should facilitate rapid changes in complex systems that interfere with safe care. In addition, leadership needs to be aware of clinical care issues and staffing patterns in order to optimize performance and outcomes.

Legal Issues Unique to Intrapartum Care

Triage of Pregnant Women

Women may present to an obstetric triage or labor and delivery unit not only for obstetric issues, but also for medical or surgical complications. Hospitals should have a defined and a consistent process in which to triage pregnant women. Following a basic initial assessment of the pregnant woman, priority and appropriate environment for care should be determined based on acuity and gestational age. The basic initial assessment should include maternal vital signs, FHR, and if the woman is having uterine contractions.[12,13]

There are several common allegations with obstetrical triage.

Failure to Advise the Woman to Seek Medical Treatment
Because diagnosing conditions by telephone cannot be done accurately or reliably, it has been recommended that when calls come in to an intrapartum setting, the woman should be instructed to come in for evaluation or to contact their provider. If a telephone discussion with a woman occurs, documentation in the medical record should include:
- Date and time
- Name of the caller
- Reason for the call in the caller's words
- Pertinent information about the problem (e.g., signs/symptoms, onset, duration, frequency; actions that alleviate or increase symptoms)
- Instructions given to the individual, including when and where to seek additional evaluation and care
- The person's response to instructions

NOTE: It is critical to document the person's response to the instructions. A documented refusal to comply when there is an adverse outcome demonstrates the individual's contributory negligence to the situation. Also, a woman who requests a visit should be directed to the most expedient source of evaluation.

Failure to timely and accurately assess maternal–fetal status in the triage area
Without defined processes, women may not be assessed in a timely manner and may be evaluated on a "first come, first serve" basis. This type of process does not allow for acuity

assignment, and prioritization of women who have more urgent needs and outcomes may be compromised.[13]

Failure to require a provider to assess maternal–fetal status if assessment data falls outside defined normal parameters or if the woman is high risk.
Under the Emergency Medical Treatment and Active Labor Act (EMTALA), RNs may serve as a **Qualified Medical Provider** and complete the medical screening examination if the following criteria are met[14,15]:
- Hospital and nursing policy specifically outline the scope of practice and requirements
- Education and competency to complete the medical screening examination
- A discussion occurs between the nurse and provider regarding the assessment data
- Discharge orders from the provider are obtained and documented in the medical record

If assessment parameters fall outside of defined norms, a provider must assess the woman.[12] Nurses and hospitals may become involved in a malpractice suit if abnormal assessment parameters or risk factors are present, the nurse is the only person to perform an assessment, the woman is discharged home, and there is a poor outcome. Table 20.1 is an example of nursing competency criteria as a qualified medical provider.

Failure to provide timely and effective communication to the obstetric provider
Following the initial assessment, the obstetric provider should be promptly notified if any of the following are assessed[12]:
- Vaginal bleeding
- Acute, abdominal pain
- Temperature of 100.4°F or higher
- Preterm labor
- Hypertension (BP greater than or equal to 140/90)
- Category II or category III EFM pattern
- Imminent birth

Following notification, you should expect the provider to come into the hospital and assess the woman. Hospitals should have a policy in place that defines how quickly a provider should arrive at the hospital after notification and/or coverage by another, if unavailable.

Failure to comply with EMTALA *requirements*, which include[14,15]:
- provision of an adequate medical screening examination by a qualified medical provider
- stabilization treatment within the capabilities of the institution with an emergency medical condition
- transfer/discharge according to outlined EMTALA guidelines

Transfer and/or discharge of a woman in active labor based on her inability to pay for medical expenses.[14,15]
The medical screening exam should not be delayed in order to obtain information regarding the woman's ability to pay medical expenses. Transfer may be requested by the provider if the woman's condition requires care outside of the hospital's capabilities, the provider's best clinical judgment determines that transfer is safe, and a receiving hospital has accepted the transfer. However, the purpose of the EMTALA law was to prevent transfer based solely on the woman's ability to pay. For further information about transport of the woman, refer to *Module 19 Maternal Transport*.

Change in Maternal Status

Birth is an evolving process with changes in maternal physiologic status occurring throughout. Frequent, regular assessments are recommended during the intrapartum period to determine if and when changes in maternal/fetal status occur and whether the assessment data fall outside the realm of normal. Nurses are often brought into a malpractice suit due to their failure to perform assessments or appreciate abnormal maternal/fetal assessment parameters and communicate these changes to the primary provider.

CRITICAL THINKING CASE EXAMPLE: A laboring woman has been ruptured for 8 hours. Her heart rate has been trending up and is now 118 beats per minute. The nurse attempts to determine why her heart rate is elevated and takes the woman's temperature. Her temperature is now 101°F and the nurse notifies the provider. The provider orders antibiotics and acetaminophen for presumed chorioamnionitis. To follow up, the nurse will continue to reassess the woman's vital signs at frequent intervals until normalized.

TABLE 20.1	MEDICAL SCREENING EXAM FOR LABOR BY QUALIFIED MEDICAL PERSONNEL

Registered Nurse: _____

COMPETENCY	SECOND VERIFY	DATE	SECOND VERIFY	DATE	SECOND VERIFY	DATE
Prenatal record review						
Identifies significant medical/surgical history						
Estimation of gestational age						
Head to toe physical assessment						

Assessment of uterine contractions
    Frequency
    Intensity
    Duration
    Resting tone						

Assessment of FHR tracing
    Baseline rate
    Baseline variability
    Accelerations
    Decelerations						

Assessment of vaginal discharge and/or bleeding						

Cervical exam
    Dilation
    Effacement
    Position
    Consistency						

Presenting part						
Fetal position						
Fetal station						

Point of care testing
    Nitrazine
    Urine
    Glucose						

Identification of risk factors						
Identification of abnormal assessment parameters						
SBAR communication with physician/certified nurse midwife (CNM)						
Appropriate disposition of the woman						

Labor: defined as spontaneous uterine contractions resulting in cervical change

I deem that _____, RN meets the qualifications and competencies of a

Qualified Medical Provider and can provide a Medical Screening Exam for labor.

Director of Obstetrics: _____

Date: _____

Administration of Uterine Stimulants

One of the most common allegations against obstetric nurses is the misuse of a uterine stimulant medication when less-than-optimal pregnancy outcomes have occurred. Some *common allegations with uterine stimulants are:*

- *Failure to accurately assess maternal/fetal status and appreciate signs of fetal hypoxia and possible metabolic acidosis*
- *Fetal injury related to prolonged hypoxia (as evidenced by changes in the FHR pattern) due to prolonged uterine tachysystole*

- *Fetal injury related to the continued use of a uterine stimulant with evidence of a category III EFM tracing*
- *Maternal and/or fetal injury related to the use of a uterine stimulant when it was contraindicated*

*NOTE: Use caution when administering uterine stimulants and avoid prolonged uterine tachysystole. **The safest method for administration of any uterine stimulant is the lowest possible dose that effects cervical change and labor progress.** The nurse should titrate the dose based on uterine activity, fetal response, and cervical change. For additional information regarding management of a uterine stimulant such as oxytocin or misoprostol, refer to Module 8.*

Shoulder Dystocia

When shoulder dystocia is diagnosed by the physician or midwife, prompt interventions are recommended to decrease the risk of maternal–fetal injury and liability. Even though shoulder dystocia is **unpredictable**, the nurse may be named in a malpractice case due to actions taken at delivery, and/or documentation of events. Refer to *Module 16 Intrapartum Emergencies* for a complete discussion of shoulder dystocia. Nursing actions that may decrease liability for the nurse when shoulder dystocia occurs include the following:

- Remain calm
- Call for additional nursing (RN) and physician assistance (determined by availability)
- Call for the neonatal team and prepare for newborn resuscitation

NOTE: Consider having one emergency response for all notifications to get the appropriate team members at the bedside.

- Place the woman in McRoberts position
- Provide correct suprapubic pressure; avoid fundal pressure
- Assist physician/midwife with patient positioning for additional maneuvers such as the all-fours Gaskin maneuver
- State out loud the maneuvers you are assisting with. For example, "I am applying suprapubic pressure."
- Reassure the woman and family
- Debrief with the team as soon as possible after the birth

Documentation should occur as soon as possible after debriefing of events. Once the timing and sequence of events are agreed upon by all team members, the following parameters of the document should be completed:

- Fetal assessment and/or attempts to obtain fetal assessment data during maneuvers
- Time when calls for help were sent out and when help arrived
- Timing and sequence of nursing maneuvers. **The provider should document all internal maneuvers**
- Timing of birth—head to body time
- Health team members present during birth
- Family members present during birth
- Newborn resuscitation measures utilized

NOTE: Avoid fundal pressure—which may further impact the shoulder.

Management of the Second Stage of Labor

During the second stage of labor, rapid changes in maternal and fetal condition may occur.[16] Continuous nursing presence at the bedside not only provides the woman and family reassurance during this time, but also allows for frequent assessments and interventions as indicated. Common allegations during the second stage of labor include the following:

- *Failure to appreciate a deteriorating fetal status*
- *Failure to notify the appropriate physician/midwife in a timely manner* (maternal or fetal assessments that fall outside of normal values)
- *Failure to anticipate neonatal resuscitation needs*

To decrease liability related to nursing management during the second stage of labor:

- Accurately assess uterine activity and fetal status. Adjust oxytocin dose based on assessments.
- Report any fetal and/or maternal concerns to the provider in a timely manner and have them come to the bedside.
- Consider using delayed pushing method ("laboring down") with concerns regarding maternal and/or fetal status.

- Anticipate the need for neonatal resuscitation and request neonatal resuscitation team to be present at delivery, if indicated.
- Avoid the supine lithotomy position.
- Continuously support the woman's efforts.
- Know where the delivering physician/midwife is located.

NOTE: If the provider orders "continuous fetal monitoring," the order should be carried out to the best of your ability, even if the woman is moved to another environment for birth, such as an operative suite.

Change in Fetal Status and Intrauterine Fetal Resuscitation Measures

Failure by the nursing staff to recognize and appreciate fetal compromise may increase liability exposure, especially if an adverse perinatal outcome occurs. Common allegations related to recognition and treatment of abnormal FHR patterns include, but are not limited to the following:

- Failure to accurately assess fetal status
- Failure to appreciate a deteriorating fetal status
- Failure to provide appropriate intrauterine resuscitation measures for the EFM pattern
- Failure to timely notify the provider regarding a change in fetal status
- Failure to require the provider to come to the bedside to assess fetal status

Appropriate intrauterine resuscitation measures, as indicated by the EFM pattern, are discussed in detail in *Module 7*. Interventions may include, but are not limited to[17]:

- Repositioning the mother
- Administration of an intravenous fluid bolus
- Initiation of oxygen at 10 L per minute via nonrebreather face mask
- Evaluation of uterine activity and decrease or discontinuation of oxytocin infusion or other uterine stimulants as indicated
- Administration of brethine in the presence of prolonged uterine tachysystole and as indicated by provider order and maternal condition
- Assessment of cervical status for prolapsed cord, rapid change, and/or fetal descent
- Assessment of maternal blood pressure; comparison with baseline; notification of anesthesia team if hypotension occurs with regional anesthesia
- Notification of the provider

If there is a change in FHR pattern, analysis to determine the cause assists in development of a plan of care, guide interventions, and decreases liability. The following illustrates suggested progressive steps for EFM assessment:

1. What is the baseline FHR?
2. Is the baseline rate within normal limits?
3. If not, what clinical factors (maternal or fetal) could be contributing to this baseline rate?
4. What is the baseline variability?
5. If the baseline variability is minimal or absent, does fetal scalp stimulation elicit an acceleration of the FHR appropriate for gestational age?
6. What clinical factors could be contributing to the baseline variability?
7. Are accelerations or decelerations present?
8. If decelerations are present, what type?
9. What are the appropriate interventions for this type of deceleration?
10. Is uterine activity normal in frequency, duration, intensity, and resting tone?
11. What is the FHR response to uterine activity?
12. If the FHR pattern is abnormal, what are the appropriate interventions to resolve the situation? Will the interventions resolve the situation?
13. Is the FHR pattern such that notification of the physician/midwife or ancillary services (NICU, OR team) is warranted?

NOTE: Ongoing fetal assessments should be made at the woman's bedside instead of the surveillance computer screen at the nurse's station.

NOTE: If "continuous fetal monitoring" is ordered and there is difficulty in tracing the FHR continuously, documentation should reflect these difficulties and actions taken to attempt a continuous tracing. For example: "Pt. repositioned on right side. Difficult to maintain continuous EFM tracing due to fetal movement. Plan to continue adjustment of US to attempt continuous tracing. When tracing, EFM Category I."

Signal Ambiguity

Signal ambiguity may become a legal issue with an unexpected newborn outcome and a seeming normal electronic FHR strip. With advanced sensitivity technology of electronic fetal monitors, maternal heart rate instead of FHR may begin to trace. Often, this occurs with maternal or fetal repositioning during the second stage of labor (Fig. 20.1). If a nurse becomes suspicious that maternal heart rate is tracing instead of fetal, the nurse may (1) palpate the woman's pulse and compare to the FHR, (2) utilize maternal pulse oximetry or electrocardiographic monitoring, or (3) place a fetal scalp electrode depending on the maternal and fetal status.[18] In addition, if a nurse is monitoring multiple fetuses, the electronic signal may become difficult to discriminate. In this situation, ultrasound assessment may be utilized to determine fetal positioning and the likelihood of monitoring separate heart beats.[18]

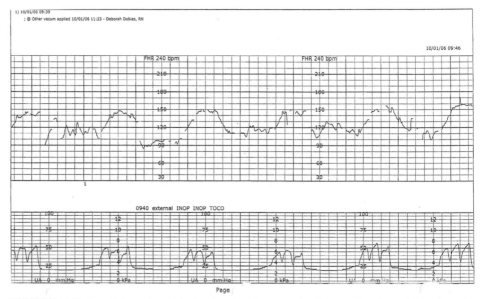

FIGURE 20.1 FHR tracing with signal ambiguity. Note the FHR accelerations with each pushing effort of the woman.

Operative Vaginal Birth

Operative vaginal birth refers to use of a vacuum extractor or forceps to facilitate birth. Nursing responsibilities during an operative vaginal birth include:
- Verification of the woman's informed consent obtained by the provider
- Verification of fetal station (exam may be done by the provider)
- Requesting appropriate personnel to attend the birth as indicated by risk factors and plan of care
- Maternal positioning

For additional information regarding operative vaginal birth, refer to *Module 15.*

NOTE: The physician performing the operative vaginal birth should document events such as the number of pulls, forceps placement, vacuum pressures, and progress with attempts. Conflicting documentation of events may increase liability for the nurse, hospital, and physician. The nurse should document positioning and labor support provided. Family members and other healthcare team members present should also be documented.

Anticipation of Neonatal Compromise

It is estimated that approximately 10% of newborns will require some assistance to begin breathing at birth.[12,19] For high-risk births, a team of neonatal providers or specially trained personal should be present prior to birth for optimal neonatal resuscitation and outcomes. A set of predefined criteria to notify the neonatal team decreases variation, improves performance, and optimizes outcomes. By receiving notification prior to birth, neonatal response team members can proceed immediately to the birth location, receive critical information about either the maternal or fetal status, and prepare for resuscitation. Refer to *Module 5* regarding maternal and/or fetal conditions that may indicate the need for additional resuscitation needs at birth.

Timing of Cesarean Birth

Timing of when to do a cesarean birth is determined by a physician. However, language that describes the urgency in which a cesarean birth occurs drives the coordination of care and should be consistent among care providers.[20] Table 20.2 is an example.

TABLE 20.2	URGENCY OF CESAREAN BIRTH TERMINOLOGY	
URGENCY	**DEFINITION**	**CATEGORY**
Emergent	Immediate threat to life of mother or fetus	1
Indicated	Indicated, but no immediate threat to life of mother or fetus	2
Scheduled	Scheduled	3

Guidelines for Documentation of Care

• What are the functions of the medical record?

The medical record may be written or computerized and serves the following purposes[21,22]:
- Provides an ongoing record of the patient's status, care provided, and outcomes of interventions
- Documents that appropriate standards of care were implemented by a qualified professional
- Provides a permanent legal record of care while in the healthcare system
- Serves as a means of communication from one care provider to another
- Can be used for reimbursement purposes
- Can be a source for research data
- Can be used for quality assurance monitoring

DISCUSSION: Everyone has heard the saying "If it wasn't charted, it wasn't done." In practice, this may not always be the case, but omissions in documentation can be used to allege a breach of the standard of care. You may provide perfect care for the mother and baby, but if it was not charted, you may not be able to "prove" it in court. Care providers may testify that something was done, but the omission in documentation will be criticized in the courtroom. In addition, a legal proceeding may not take place until years after the care was provided and your recollection of events and timing of care provided may be diminished.

• What are the Components of Nursing Documentation?

From the time of admission until discharge from the unit, documentation should cite information on the woman and fetus(es), which includes but is not limited to:
- The nurse's assessment (subjective and objective)
- Interprofessional plan of care
- Interventions (actions)
- Outcomes of care (responses)

Your *evaluation* should include assessment of both maternal and fetal status. Much of the woman's history may be reviewed in the prenatal records. Specifically, you should review or take a history and perform a physical examination that meets the standards of practice as outlined by hospital policies and unit guidelines.

1. **Presenting complaint** in the woman's words
2. **History**
   - **Family history:** genetic and congenital abnormalities, neurologic or cognitive disorders, metabolic problems

- **Medical history:** allergies, diabetes, hypertension, cardiac disease/lesions, herpes simplex virus, HIV, exposure to infectious diseases, deep vein thrombosis, asthma, stroke
- **Surgical history**
- **Sensory and motor:** notation of any loss of function; presence of prosthesis, dentures, glasses, contact lenses, ambulatory needs
- **Social history:** smoking, alcohol or nonprescribed/illicit drug intake, support, person for labor, labor preparation, abuse profile
- **Laboratory Studies:** blood type, Rh status, antibody status, serology titer, rubella titer, hemoglobin/hematocrit, genetic or congenital anomaly screening, HIV testing, and culture results for chlamydia, gonorrhea, and group B streptococcus)
- **Obstetric History:**

Gravida _____

Term _____

Preterm _____

Abortion _____ (spontaneous or elective)

Living _____ (current living children)

In addition, type of delivery, newborn weight, complications during pregnancy or childbirth should also be determined.

Current pregnancy: last menstrual period, expected date of delivery, weight gain, infections, gestational diabetes, hypertension, vaginal bleeding, results of ultrasound examinations, and results of most recent antenatal testing (e.g., nonstress test, contraction stress test, amniocentesis, biophysical profile)

Current history: onset of uterine contractions, frequency, duration, quality, vaginal discharge or bleeding consistency and amount, status of membranes rupture time, color of fluid, fetal activity, oral intake of liquid and/or solids, any concurrent symptoms of visual disturbance, headache, or dysuria

Current medications including over-the-counter preparations, herbs with dosage, and time last taken

Obstetric care provider: name, title, date and time of notification, and by whom
Birth Plans
Infant care plans: feeding, breast/bottle, circumcision, pediatric care provider; adoption plans
3. **Physical Examination**
   - Height and current weight
   - Vital signs
   - Deep tendon reflexes
   - Urine dipstick results
   - Systems assessment (NOTE: In some settings, head, eyes, ears, nose, throat, breast, heart and lungs, abdomen (general), and extremities may be examined by other care providers according to unit policies. However, the nurse must be aware of the findings and their impact on the nursing assessment and plan.)
   - **Fetal assessment:** EFM (heart rate, baseline rate, variability, accelerations, decelerations), position, and presentation.
   - **Uterine assessment:** contractions, frequency, intensity, duration, and resting tone; tenderness
   - **Cervical examination:** effacement, dilatation, fetal station and presentation, membra**nes** status (**i**f ruptured, amniotic fluid amount, color, odor, results of Nitrazine or fern tests), and the collection of cultures when appropriate.

When the provider is notified of a deviation from normal assessment, his or her response should be noted in the record. *It is essential to provide evidence of your critical thinking and clinical decision making in your documentation.* For example, if the nurse observes a change in the fetal status, a phone call may be made to the provider. Examples of ineffective nurse documentation are "Physician aware, no orders received"; "Midwife notified"; or "Dr. Smith called." In these notations, there is no documentation of the conversation, the nurse's clinical reasoning, actions taken, plan of care, or responses in the notation. Although no one advocates "over charting" or "double charting," a narrative note may be the best way to provide evidence of your sound clinical judgment. Therefore, adequate space to accomplish this should be provided for in the documentation system.

Effective and efficient documentation systems for emergency situations should be planned and practiced prior to an event (e.g., shoulder dystocia, hemorrhage, maternal cardiopulmonary arrest). Summary notes are acceptable if contemporaneous charting is not possible, but the chronology of events should be correct.

• What are the General Guidelines for Medical Record Documentation?

- Record only factual information.
- Never make entries for another person.
- Avoid biased language against the patient and other healthcare providers.
- Document discussions that affect the plan of care. Use quotation marks for patient statements if needed.
- An addendum made after the record is requested for legal action is suspect.
- Use documentation to demonstrate your sound clinical reasoning and critical thinking.
- Document often enough to show the whole picture.
- Identify by name any individuals referenced—don't just say "Provider notified" or "nursing supervisor aware."
- Always be mindful that your documentation paints a picture of the care you give and makes a lasting impression of your professional competence.
- If using a paper medical record:
  - Make entries legible.
  - Avoid gaps in documentation that can be filled in later or used for speculation about what happened.
  - Use only standard abbreviations. Be aware of the official "Do not use" list.
  - Include the accurate date, time, and your (the recorder's) name and title.
  - To correct an error, draw a line through the incorrect information, write "error" above it, write the date and time, and initial the entry. *The accurate information is entered as an* **addendum**.
  - Enter an addendum at the next available space on the chart form. Use the current date and time for the new entry. The content can be referenced to the previous material.
  - *When there is a delay in entering chart information, write the phrase "late entry" at the beginning of the note.* Enter the note at the next available space on the chart form. *Use the current date and time for the entry.* Explain the delay in recording the information and cross-reference it to the area of the record where it should have appeared in chronologic order.

• What are Some Common Issues Related to Electronic Documentation?

- Never share your access code or password for the system.
- Access information ONLY as part of your job function.
- Do not ignore computer alerts about data entry, missing data, or best practice recommendations.
- Use correct procedures for adding late entry information to a record. All electronic systems will have a timed, tracking process that will record when you entered a chart and what you charted. This record is sometimes produced in a medical malpractice case.
- Maintain competencies in system use.

Remember, the record you create today is the one you may go into court with in the future. Make sure it reflects your critical thinking and the plan of care.

• What are Some Considerations Regarding Countersigning Notes?

When policies of an institution require the nurse to countersign or sign off for other personnel, consider the following:
- Countersigning means that you have reviewed the entry and consider it accurate.
- It also means that you have approved the care provided by the other person.
- Make sure the note indicates who provided the care.

Strategies to Avoid Malpractice Claims

1. **Review your institutional policies, guidelines, and protocols.** Make sure they are current and reflect evidence and/or best practice recommendations. Be certain they are aligned with recommendations from national professional organizations and regulatory boards such as AWHONN, ACOG, ACNM, AORN, and The Joint Commission. Know and use them.
2. **Perform only those skills you know to be within your scope of practice.** Know the scope of practice for your role in providing care. Know your strengths and weaknesses. Work with your preceptors and charge nurse to gain experience and confidence in areas where you feel weak.
3. **Stay current in obstetrics and with technological advances by attending continuing education conferences, seminars, and in-services.** Continuous learning demonstrates a commitment to providing excellent, safe patient care, and to the practice of professional nursing.
4. **Be clear about who is managing the patient.** Everyone on the healthcare team should know at all times who is responsible for the patient. Communication is automatically improved if you know you are talking to the right person.
5. Follow-up on any tasks you have delegated to others. Many malpractice claims can be traced back to instances where someone "dropped the ball."
6. **Be a patient advocate and know how to use the chain of command.** To use the chain of command effectively, you must be confident in your assessments and clinical reasoning. Overcoming fear of conflict and being assertive is easier if you know the "HOW" and "WHY." Don't be afraid to advocate for the patient when you feel the outcome is dependent upon your actions.
7. **Learn and use good communication skills.** Technical expertise is expected, but communication skills can make the difference in whether or not you get sued. Whether communicating a plan of care to an oncoming shift during report, communicating with the patient and family, or communicating with a provider about a concerning maternal/fetal status, say what you mean.
8. **Document.** Your charting should be accurate and complete. Never chart ahead of time. Review your charting and imagine you were defending it in front of a jury. Does it reflect your critical thinking and plan of care?
9. **Get to know your patients.** Use clear and respectful communication skills with patients and families. Be mindful of both verbal and nonverbal communication. Patients who feel as if their needs are not being met, whether or not it is an accurate perception, become angry. Your interactions with the patient and family frame their perception of the quality of care they are receiving. Always treat patients with dignity, respect, and compassion. A little compassion goes a long way.
10. **Don't make excuses.** Understaffing should never be an excuse for delivering poor quality care.
11. **Report near-miss situations and be proactive to search for solutions to fix the issue before injury occurs.**
12. **The Golden Rule.** Remember the golden rule we learn early in life: Treat others as you would like to be treated.

NOTE: PROVIDE SAFE, INDIVIDUALIZED, QUALITY CARE to every woman and family. Of all the strategies to avoid a malpractice claim, this is the most basic and important.

What to Do if You are Called to Testify

In-depth information about depositions or testifying in a malpractice suit is beyond the scope of this module. However, some broad guidelines are as follows:

Notify your professional insurance carrier (if applicable).
- Notify your employer's Risk Manager/Department.
- Do not discuss the case with anyone except your insurance carrier, claims representative, attorney, or risk manager.
- Review the patient's medical record when instructed by Risk Management.
- Review the institution's policy and procedure manual for the year in which the incident occurred.
- Have a current curriculum vitae including your continuing education.

PRACTICE/REVIEW QUESTIONS

After reviewing this module, answer the following questions.

1. List three components of informed consent.

   a. _____

   b. _____

   c. _____

2. List the type of information that should be included when obtaining informed consent.

   a. _____

   b. _____

   c. _____

   d. _____

   e. _____

   f. _____

   g. _____

3. Describe the exceptions to informed consent?

   _____

   _____

4. Who may give consent for treatment when an adult is mentally incompetent?

   _____

5. Who is responsible for obtaining consents for medical procedures or treatments?

   _____

6. State at least three important functions of the medical record from a legal standpoint.

   a. _____

   b. _____

   c. _____

7. In general, what are the nurse's responsibilities for documentation in the medical record?

   _____

   _____

8. When medications or procedures are withheld, what action should the nurse take?

   _____

   _____

9. How should an error in charting be corrected?

   _____

   _____

10. What three circumstances should be present when a nurse countersigns another person's notes?

    a. _____

    b. _____

    c. _____

11. State the precautions to be taken when accepting a verbal order.

    a. _____

    b. _____

    c. _____

12. In handling a telephone triage, what information is needed about the current problem?

    a. _____

    b. _____

13. List items to review in preparation for giving a deposition or testimony.

    a. _____

    b. _____

14. What criteria will be used to judge a nurse's practice?

    _____

    _____

15. List four of the areas of nursing management that are most often cited in legal actions.

    a. _____

    b. _____

    c. _____

    d. _____

16. List three reasons why intrapartum nurses face high risk for involvement in a malpractice suit.

    a. _____

    b. _____

    c. _____

17. Define *negligence.*

    _____

    _____

18. List the four key elements in a *malpractice suit.*

    1. _____

    2. _____

    3. _____

    4. _____

19. List five sources of nursing standards.

    a. _____

    b. _____

    c. _____

    d. _____

    e. _____

20. List eight common allegations faced by intrapartum nurses.

    a. _____

    b. _____

    c. _____

    e. _____

    f. _____

    g. _____

    h. _____

21. Describe the safest method for administration of uterine stimulants.

    _____

    _____

22. List five nursing actions to decrease liability in the event of a shoulder dystocia.

    a. _____

    b. _____

    c. _____

    d. _____

    e. _____

23. When is activation of chain of command recommended?

    _____

    _____

    _____

    _____

24. List six effective communication techniques.

    a. _____

    b. _____

    c. _____

    d. _____

    e. _____

    f. _____

PRACTICE/REVIEW ANSWER KEY

1. a. Capacity
   b. Information
   c. Voluntariness

2. a. The nature of the individual's condition
   b. The purpose of the treatment
   c. Expected outcomes
   d. Major risks
   e. Reasonable alternatives
   f. Right to refuse treatment
   g. Possible outcomes of refusing treatment
3. When delay will cause death or serious jeopardy to the patient's health.
4. Only a legal guardian, conservator, the patient's power of attorney, or a judge
5. The physician
6. Any three of the following:
   a. Provides an ongoing written record of the patient's status, care provided, and the outcomes of the interventions.
   b. Documents that appropriate standards of care were implemented by a qualified professional.
   c. Provides a permanent legal record of the patient's course while in the healthcare system.
   d. Serves as a means of communication from one care provider to another.
7. Nurse's assessments, interventions, and the outcomes of care for the woman and the fetus
8. Document in the chart the reasons that the medication or procedure was not administered.
9. Draw a line through the incorrect information, write "error" above it, write the date and time, and initial the entry. The accurate information is entered as an addendum.
10. a. It is a requirement of the institution's policies and procedures.
    b. The nurse has reviewed the content of the note.
    c. The nurse approves the care provided to the patient.
11. a. Restate the order, including the patient's name.
    b. Ask for confirmation.
    c. Chart "repeated and confirmed."
12. a. Signs/symptoms, onset, duration, and frequency
    b. Actions that alleviate or increase the signs and symptoms
13. a. The patient's chart
    b. Policy and procedure manual enforced at the time of the incident
14. Current national standards as developed by national professional organizations such as AWHONN
15. Any four of the following:
    a. Incomplete documentation
    b. Medication errors
    c. Violation of national standards of practice
    d. Improper use of equipment
    e. Failure to notify the appropriate professionals when maternal or fetal status falls outside normal parameters
    f. Failure to follow physician orders, hospital policies, and hospital procedures
    g. Failure to recognize and respond to cases of fetal distress
    h. Failure to intervene appropriately in the presence of negligence on the part of the providers

16. Any three of the following:
    Childbirth is an intense, emotional experience and parents have high expectations for a "perfect" birth and newborn.
    Poor outcomes are not tolerated well.
    Parents may be well-informed consumers of health care.
    Obstetrics is a high-pressure, rapidly changing specialty; accidents, errors in judgment, and negligence do occur.
17. Negligence is the failure to act as a reasonably prudent nurse under the same or similar circumstances
18. a. Duty to the patient
    b. Breach of duty
    c. Injury to the patient
    d. Causal link between the breach and the patient's injury
19. Any five of the following:
    a. State statutes (nurse practice acts)
    b. American Nurses Association (ANA)
    c. National professional and specialty nursing organizations
    d. Joint Commission for Accreditation of Healthcare Organizations
    e. Hospital policy and procedures
    f. Testimony from expert witnesses
20. a. Failure to appreciate a change in maternal status
    b. Failure to appropriately administer uterine stimulants
    c. Failure to initiate appropriate shoulder dystocia maneuvers
    d. Failure to provide adequate screening for obstetric maternal triage (telephone or inpatient)
    e. Failure to initiate chain of command
    f. Failure to notify physician/midwife
    g. Failure to appropriately manage the second stage of labor
    h. Failure to recognize a category III EFM tracing and provide appropriate intrauterine fetal resuscitation
21. Use the lowest possible dose that effects cervical change and labor progress.
22. Any five of the following:
    a. Remain calm
    b. Call for RN/physician assistance
    c. Call for neonatal team and prepare for newborn resuscitation
    d. Avoid fundal pressure
    e. Provide firm suprapubic pressure
    f. Position patient for McRoberts maneuver
    g. Assist physician/midwife with patient positioning for additional maneuvers such as the all-fours Gaskin maneuver
    h. State out loud the maneuvers you are assisting with. For example, "I am applying suprapubic pressure."
    i. Reassure patient
    j. Debrief with all team members following the event
23. Chain of command activation is recommended when there is potential for the maternal and/or fetal condition to rapidly deteriorate causing harm, and discussions with the appropriate physician or midwife have failed to provoke an agreeable action plan.
24. Any six of the following:
    a. Speak clearly

b. Speak using a congenial tone
c. Be courteous and professional
d. Present facts in a methodical or chronological style—organization
e. Ask for clarification if communication is unclear
f. Communicate all relevant facts, abnormal findings, and specific concerns
g. State your reasons if you disagree with a treatment plan
h. If the mother or fetus (or both) is at risk, tell physician to report to the hospital to assess the patient immediately and document your discussion.
i. Inform the provider if you plan to communicate up the chain of command

REFERENCES

1. Westrick, S. J. (2014). *Essentials of nursing law and ethics* (2nd ed.). Burlington, MA: Jones & Barlett.
2. Jones, J. H., & Treiber, L. (2010). When the 5 rights go wrong: Medication errors from the nursing perspective. *Journal of Nursing Care Quality, 25*(3), 240–247.
3. Committee on Patient Safety and Quality Improvement. (2012). Committee opinion No. 531: Improving medication safety. *Obstetrics and Gynecology, 120*(2 pt 1), 406–410.
4. The Joint Commission. (2013). *Sentinel event statistics data root causes by event type 2004–2013.* Oakbrook Terrace, IL: Author. Retrieved from: http://www.jointcommission.org/assets/1/18/Root_Causes_by_Event_Type_2004–2Q2013.pdf
5. Joint Commission on Accreditation of Healthcare Organizations. (2005). *Preventing infant death and injury during delivery, sentinel event alert no. 30.* Oakbrook Terrace, IL: Author.
6. Lyndon, A., Zlatnik, M. G., & Wachter, R. M. (2011). Effective physician nurse communication: A patient safety essential for labor and delivery. *The American Journal of Obstetrics and Gynecology, 205*(2), 91–96.
7. Institute for Healthcare Improvement. Develop a culture of safety. Retrieved from: http://www.ihi.org/IHI/Topics/PatientSafety/SafetyGeneral/Changes/Develop+a+Culture+of+Safety.htm
8. Lyndon, A., Johnson, M. C., Bingham, D., et al. (2015). Transforming communication and safety culture in intrapartum care: A multi-organization blueprint. *Journal of obstetric, gynecologic, and neonatal nursing, 44*(3), 341–349.
9. Joint Commission on Accreditation of Healthcare Organizations. (2005). The SBAR technique: Improves communication, enhances patient safety. *Joint Commission Perspectives on Patient Safety, 5*(2), 1–8.
10. Menendez, J. B. (2013). Informed consent: Essential legal and ethical principles for nurses. *JONAS Healthcare Law, Ethics, and Regulation, 15*(4), 140–144.
11. Joint Commission on Accreditation of Healthcare Organizations. (2006). Guidelines for accepting and transcribing verbal or telephone orders. *The Source, 4*, 6–10.
12. American Academy of Pediatrics and the American College of Obstetricians and Gynecologists. (2012). *Guidelines for perinatal care* (7th ed.). Washington, DC: Author.
13. Paisley, K. S., Wallace, R., & DuRant, P. G. (2011). The development of an obstetric triage acuity tool. *The American Journal of Maternal/Child Nursing, 36*(5), 290–296.
14. Compilation of the Social Security Laws: Examination and Treatment for Emergency Medical Conditions and Women in Labor. (1986). Sec. 1867.[42 U.S.Code 1395dd]. Retrieved from: https://www.ssa.gov/OP_Home/ssact/title18/1867.htm

15. Angelini, D., & Howard, E. (2014). Obstetric triage: A system-actic review of the past fifteen years: 1998-2013. *MCN, 39*(5), 284–297.

16. Association of Women's Health, Obstetric and Neonatal Nurses. (2008). *Nursing management of the second stage of labor (evidence-based clinical practice guidelines)* (2nd ed.). Washington, DC: Author.

17. Lyndon, A., & Ali, L. U. (2015). *AWHONN fetal monitoring principles and practice* (5th ed.). Kendall Hunt.

18. Chez, B. F., & Baird, S. M. (2011). Electronic fetal heart rate monitoring: Where are we now? *Journal of Perinatal and Neonatal Nursing, 25*(2), 180–192.

19. Wyckoff, M. H., Aziz, K., Escobedo M. B., et al. (2015). 2015 American Heart Association Guidelines for cardiopulmonary resuscitation and emergency cardiovascular care science; Part 13: neonatal resuscitation. *Circulation, 132*(2), S543–S560.

20. Royal College of Obstetricians and Gynaecologists. (2010). *Classification of urgency of caesarean section—a continuum of risk. Good Practice No. 11.* 1-4. Retrieved from: https://www.rcog.org.uk/globalassets/documents/guidelines/goodpractice-11classificationofurgency.pdf

21. Patient safety and health information technology. (2015). Committee Opinion No. 621. American College of Obstetricians and Gynecologists. *Obstet Gynecol, 125*, 282–283.

22. Association of Women's Health, Obstetric and Neonatal Nurses. (2011). Health information technology for the perinatal setting. Position Statement. *Nursing for women's health, 15*(4), 346–348.

A D D I T I O N A L   R E S O U R C E S

Association of Women's Health, Obstetric and Neonatal Nurses. (2011). Nursing support of laboring women. An official position statement of the Association of Women's Health, Obstetric & Neonatal Nursing. Position Statement. *Journal of obstetric, gynecologic, and neonatal nursing, 40*(5), 665–666.

Association of Women's Health Obstetric and Neonatal Nurses. (2012). Quality patient care in labor and delivery: A call to action. *Journal of obstetric, gynecologic, and neonatal nursing, 41*, 151–153.

American Nurses Association. (2010). *Nursing: Scope and standards of practice* (2nd ed.). Silver Spring, Maryland, MD.

Association of Women's Health, Obstetric and Neonatal Nurses. (2009). *Standards and guidelines for professional nursing practice in the care of women and newborns* (7th ed., pp. 1–43). Washington, DC: Author.

Association of Women's Health, Obstetric and Neonatal Nurses. (2010). *Guidelines for professional nurse staffing.* Washington, DC: Author.

Berkowitz, R. L. (2011). Of parachutes and patient care: A call to action. *American Journal of Obstetrics & Gynecology, 205*(1), 7–9.

Institute for Safe Medication Practices. www.ismp.org

National Council of State Boards of Nursing (NCSBN): http://www.ncsbn.org

The American Association of Nurse Attorneys (TAANA): http://www.taana.org

Perinatal Grief and Loss

SUZANNE McMURTRY BAIRD,
MEGHAN BERTANI-YANG, AND
BETSY BABB KENNEDY

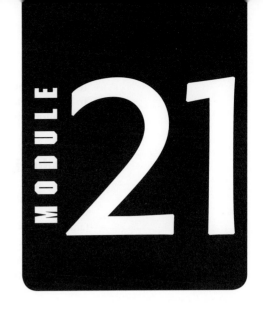

MODULE 21

Part 1
Caring for the Dying Newborn

Part 2
Caring for the Dying Mother

Part 3
Caring for the Care Provider

Objectives

As you complete this module, you will learn:

1. Spiritual and cultural considerations for loss and grief
2. Types of perinatal loss
3. Communication techniques with families experiencing perinatal loss
4. Essential elements of palliative care for newborns including symptom management
5. The significance of bereavement care
6. End-of-life care in the event of maternal death
7. Support mechanisms for care providers

Key Terms

When you have completed this module, you should be able to recall the meaning of the following terms. You should also be able to use the terms when consulting with other health professionals. The terms are defined in this module or in the glossary at the end of this book.

advanced directives
durable power of attorney
end of life

Living Will
palliative care
postmortem care

To Cure Sometimes
To Relieve Often
To Comfort Always
                    —Hippocrates

Introduction

Pregnancy and birth are usually a time of happiness and celebration. The death of a pregnant woman or her newborn is an unexpected, tragic event that profoundly affects the lives of her family, friends, healthcare providers, and the community.

It is important to develop and implement a comprehensive, individualized plan of care incor porating the physical, emotional, cultural, and spiritual aspects of care in collaboration with other healthcare team members. Figure 21.1 is a conceptual model for grief care.

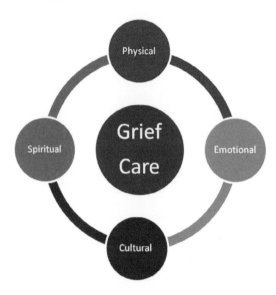

FIGURE 21.1   Grief care conceptual model.

Spiritual and Religious Needs

While a woman's spiritual and religious beliefs and preferences may provide comfort and hope for both her and her family, they inform care provided by the healthcare team. Hospital chaplains or the family's private spiritual leader provide invaluable guidance to the healthcare team by exploring the family's beliefs, values, and religious practices, while offering spiritual support. It is important for all care team members to evaluate their own personal attitudes and beliefs, and how they may influence the spiritual care provided to a grieving family.

Cultural Differences in Grief

Women and their families possess diverse cultural attitudes and beliefs. Understanding their attitudes, beliefs, and traditions is necessary for the healthcare team to provide comprehensive care during times of grief and end of life (EOL). While anticipating common grief practices and reactions among various cultures can be helpful, it is important to remember individual differences prohibit generalizations to every member of each culture. Therefore, the most effective way to provide the most supportive care for the woman and her family is to not make assumptions, but to ask what would be most helpful for them. The use of qualified, on-site, medical translators, and/or electronic language assistant systems is helpful for effective communication if required during this distressing time. Most hospitals/agencies advise against noncertified members of the healthcare team and/or family members serving as an interpreter. In addition, some cultures do not fully disclose disease or care information and the care provider should understand the wishes of the woman/family. Care providers should respect cultural and personal values, beliefs, and family preferences. All care, treatment, and services should be in a manner that meets both oral and written communication needs.

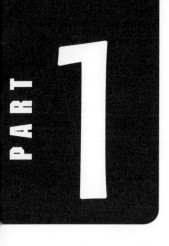

PART 1

Caring for the Dying Newborn

SELF-ASSESSMENT QUIZ	TRUE	FALSE
1. Chronically ill newborns become tolerant of painful procedures.	☐	☐
2. A fetus can feel pain as early as 20 weeks' gestation.	☐	☐
3. Newborns experience less pain than adults because of immature neurologic systems.	☐	☐
4. Morphine is never the drug of choice to treat pain because of the side effect of respiratory depression.	☐	☐
5. Newborns in intensive care units (ICUs) are subjected to up to 130 procedures every 24 hours many of which are painful.	☐	☐
6. Dying newborns need 130 cal/kg/day for maintenance nutrition.	☐	☐
7. All families should be at the bedside of a dying newborn.	☐	☐

Answers may be found at the end of this module. If you answered all statements correctly, you are well on your way to providing excellent comfort care for the dying newborn

> **"Those we have held in our arms for a little while, we hold in our hearts forever."**
>
> **—Author Unknown**

> **"Each new life, no matter how brief, forever changes the world."**
>
> **—Author Unknown**

> **"How very quietly you tiptoed into our world, silently, only a moment you stayed. But what an imprint your footprints have left upon our hearts."**
>
> **—Author Unknown**

Perinatal Loss

Perinatal losses are not an uncommon event. According to Callister,[1] around 7 million perinatal losses occur throughout the world. In the United States, the perinatal mortality rate in 2011 was 6.26 per 1,000 births.[2] It is difficult to obtain an accurate rate for perinatal losses due to various definitions of what constitutes a perinatal loss. The American Academy of Pediatrics (AAP) states three recognized definitions[3]:

- Perinatal death, definition I, includes infant deaths that occur at less than 7 days of age and fetal deaths with a stated or presumed period of gestation of 28 weeks or more.
- Perinatal death, definition II, includes infant deaths that occur at less than 28 days of age and fetal deaths with a stated or presumed period of gestation of 20 weeks or more.
- Perinatal death, definition III, includes infant deaths that occur at less than 7 days of age and fetal deaths with a stated or presumed gestation of 20 weeks or more.

It should be noted that these definitions do not include early losses (less than 20 weeks' gestation), so it can be presumed that the perinatal mortality rate is much higher than what is reported. These data highlight the importance for medical staff to be educated and trained on how to care for a woman and her family experiencing a loss; there is a high likelihood that medical staff will encounter these situations many times throughout their careers.

AWHONN uses the classification system in Table 21.1 to describe perinatal losses and includes early losses.[4]

TABLE 21.1 PERINATAL LOSS	
TYPE OF LOSS	**DEFINITION**
Ectopic pregnancy	Implantation occurs outside of the uterus
Miscarriage (i.e., spontaneous abortion)	Loss occurs at ≤20 wks' gestation
Stillbirth	Loss occurs at >20 wks' gestation
Neonatal death	Loss occurs after birth through the first 28 d of life

From Association of Women's Health, Obstetric and Neonatal Nurses. (2006). *Perinatal loss: A continuum of loss.* www.awhonn.org/Resources_Documents_pdf_2_DOD_POEP10_PerinatalLoss.pdf. Accessed January 18, 2015.

Miscarriages and stillbirths precipitate bereavement, as they are often unexpected and sudden. The cause may never be known, but the loss is typically never forgotten by the woman or her family.[5] Most families that choose the palliative care option for their fetus or infant with a known life-limiting condition usually experience either a stillbirth or neonatal death.

Another type of perinatal loss is a medical interruption of a pregnancy (sometimes referred to as elective abortion). There may be many reasons why a woman chooses to end a pregnancy, one of which is because the fetus has a congenital abnormality that may be incompatible with life or result in a poor quality of life (i.e., a life-limiting condition). When the diagnosis is made in utero, many women cannot imagine continuing the pregnancy. They are afraid of becoming so attached to the baby only to have the newborn not survive for very long after birth. It is just as important to support these women and their families as research has found that those who terminated their pregnancies experienced higher levels of trauma. However, almost 88% of those women stated they would make the same decision again as they felt that it was easier than delivering a malformed baby.[6] Many times it is assumed that because a woman is choosing to terminate her pregnancy, she must not love or want her baby. For the majority of women this is untrue. Unfortunately, because of this assumption, these women do not receive the same type of support from the medical staff and/or family and friends. They are not offered keepsakes or educational materials about grief. This can be devastating for these women who are already at high risk for depression and other negative effects. Recommendations for the healthcare providers involved in the care of women during and after termination of pregnancy for fetal anomaly (TOPFA) include the following[6–8]:

1. Develop protocols for care of the woman, family, and disposition of remains.
2. Ensure a supportive care provider.
3. Provide continuity of care.
4. Supply appropriate educational materials before and after the procedure.
5. Offer anticipatory guidance about what to expect.
6. Create/collect and deliver meaningful keepsakes.
7. Conduct follow-up calls.
8. Provide compassionate care, demonstrated through listening, therapeutic touch, and presence.

• How can the nurse assist parents who experience a perinatal loss?

The delivery of a miscarriage, stillborn, or a terminally ill infant is an event that produces enormous stress for the new mother and family. Women may remember details of their loss as well as the care they received during the loss throughout their lives.[9] The intrapartum and perinatal nurses must function as a care provider, support person during the grief process, patient advocate, and coordinator of care.[7] The nurse should assess the woman's needs and proceed with developing a patient-centered plan of care as soon as it is known that the demise has occurred.[10] Genuine listening and presence of the nurse with the woman, her partner, and family cannot be underestimated. Many hospitals have developed bereavement programs to assist parents with the grief process through coordination of services and ongoing sensitive care. Bereavement checklists can help in provision of consistent, comprehensive, and complete care.

Immediately after the birth of a demised infant, both parents are in the shock phase of grief. Additionally, the woman is concerned with her own personal health and safety, as after any birth. Questions relating to the reason for the death arise and are often difficult or impossible to answer. The nurse's role during this initial phase is both to provide physical care for the woman and to assist with the process of grief. There are many manifestations of grief that may present in the woman, partner, and family, but it is important to remember there is no "usual" or "normal" way to express grief. Each woman, partner, and family may demonstrate different feelings and behaviors. Examples of manifestations across psychosocial, physical, cognitive, and behavioral domains include:

- Feelings of sadness, anxiety, hopelessness, detachment
- Tightness in the throat or chest, fatigue, weakness, shortness of breath
- Confusion, distractedness
- Sleep disturbance, appetite disturbance, withdrawal, avoidance, crying

To begin to grieve for the infant lost, it is necessary for the parents to create memories of the child. Parents should be offered adequate time to hold and touch the newborn in a *private setting*. The family may wish to view the infant multiple times. The nurse can wrap the infant in a blanket and remain with the family, if needed or requested, to answer questions. It is common for parents to remark on the gender of the child, the perfection of hands or feet, and family resemblance—in effect, to claim the child as their own. Naming the child is another activity that assists parents with this process of claiming the child who has died.

The nurse has ongoing responsibilities in coordinating care for the woman and her family. Decisions about location of the postpartum stay, notification of hospital staff who will be in contact with the woman, and notification of support services (e.g., social services, clergy, grief counselors) are tasks for the nurse. The woman may not wish to stay in the obstetric setting and prefer to recover during her postpartum stay in another area, away from the newborn nursery. It is important for all care providers to be aware of the family's loss. The hospital should devise a system for alerting other healthcare providers and staff that a loss has occurred, hopefully prevent awkward and painful encounters. The nurse must also facilitate and allow ample time for decisions to be made about disposition of the infant's remains.

Finally, perinatal nurses must consider their own feelings related to the loss. Just as parents search for the answers to why the loss occurred, so do care providers. It is also common for nurses to avoid the family because of the uncertainty of how to help or feelings that medical care has failed this family. The belief that every pregnancy should or will have the outcome of a healthy infant is common, but not realistic. Nurses need to examine their role in good outcomes, while accepting the fact that poor outcomes cannot always be prevented. A hospital with a carefully considered plan for assisting families with perinatal loss also considers these needs of the care providers. Strategies for supporting care providers are presented later in this module.

- ### How should the nurse communicate with parents who experience a perinatal loss?

Perhaps, one of the most difficult aspects of caring for a family experiencing a perinatal loss is not knowing what to say. Many times people are afraid of saying the wrong thing; therefore, it leads to silence. Silence can be detrimental to the family, as they may perceive that silence means their nurse either does not recognize their loss or does not care about it.[11] While silence is harmful, so is saying something wrong. The attitude of the nursing staff can directly affect how a family copes with the loss, which has long-term implications. Therefore, it is important for nurses to receive education and training in communication during bereavement situations, which lead to more confidence and increased levels of comfort in these situations. What women and their family need the most is for the nurse to have a positive perspective and to reassurance the patient that she is not at fault.[5]

- ### What should a nurse say to grieving parents and what should be avoided?[11]

Table 21.2 provides guidance for talking to women and families experiencing a perinatal loss.

NOTE: Families often ask nurses for advice and help in decision-making. It is important for the nurse to refrain from giving personal advice, but appropriate to speak about what other families have found helpful.

Palliative Care of the Fetus or Newborn

Despite recent advances in medical technology, many lethal conditions that a baby can develop in utero have no cure. These medical advances have led to an increase in the ability to make these diagnoses prenatally, therefore, allowing parents to have the time to prepare for the birth and to

TABLE 21.2 COMMUNICATION DO'S AND DON'TS	
DO'S	**DON'TS**
Do listen more than you talk	Don't dominate the conversation
Do allow for silence	Don't ask one question after another without a break
Do answer their questions and refer them to the most appropriate people	Don't use clichés such as: "I know just how you feel" "At least you have other children" "You can always have another baby" "At least you didn't really know your baby" "This will bring your family closer"
Do refer to the baby by name (if they have named the baby) and talk about special features of the baby	Don't avoid them because you are uncomfortable (avoidance adds pain; acknowledgment of their loss is what they need)
Do be genuine and caring	Don't change the subject when they talk about their dead baby
Do allow them to express their feelings and tell their story without passing judgment	Don't answer a question you don't have the answer to
Do encourage them to be patient with themselves and not expect too much	Don't give advice or relay personal experiences.
Do ask about the funeral or memorial service	Don't make comments that suggest they or their baby received inadequate care
Do ask about other family members (siblings, spouses, grandparents)	Don't make comments that they should have received care sooner (they already have doubt and guilt)
Do ask if they have any special requests of you	Don't talk only with mothers (include fathers, children)

From Wilke, J., & Limbo, R. (2012). *Resolve through sharing (RTS): Bereavement training in perinatal death* (8th ed.). La Crosse, WI: Bereavement and Advance Care Planning Services, Gunderson Lutheran Medical Foundation, Inc.

make a decision as to the best plan of care for their child. In order to help parents through this difficult time, they should be referred to a palliative care team. A palliative care team is an inter-disciplinary team that often comprised a palliative care physician, nurse practitioner/advanced practice nurse, bedside nurse, social worker, chaplain, and other members to help provide psychosocial care for the family (e.g., a child life specialist to support any siblings of the newborn).

• What is perinatal palliative care?

Perinatal palliative care is a compassionate model of care that begins with diagnosis in the womb and continues through the birth and death of the baby. One major objective of perinatal palliative care is to help the family to celebrate their baby for whatever length of time they have together. The overall purpose is alleviate suffering of the infant, emotionally support the family, and make sure the family is given honest information in a timely manner.[12]

When the parents first meet with the palliative care team, they are often in shock and perhaps even in denial, so it is important for the team to make sure the parents have a clear understanding of the diagnosis. This is a crucial aspect of the process as the only way the parents can make the most appropriate decision for them is if they have a full understanding, which also helps to ensure the most informed decision. It is also vital for the team to be aware that when the parents received the diagnosis, the grief process began. Therefore, the team should respond with empathy and to understand how difficult it may be for the parents to comprehend the entire situation. When the option of comfort-only, or palliative care, is presented to parents, it can cause some angst as it goes against what parents instinctually want to do for their baby—protect them and save them from anything that will cause harm.

NOTE: *It is difficult at first for parents to understand how doing "nothing" for their baby is actually doing "something."*

Palliative care involves providing interventions that limit the amount of pain and suffering a baby may experience during the dying process and ensures the best quality of life. This is done by providing pain medication, nutrition, and other measures to make the baby comfortable. The main objective of comfort care is to limit and preferably to prevent any medical procedures that may cause discomfort or pain, such as placing IVs.

Ideally, the palliative care team meets with the parents several times before developing the care plan for the baby. Once the family has chosen the option of comfort care, the plan is discussed with the entire team to help the family decide on all the various details. A comprehensive plan of care when providing comfort care only at birth should include the following components:

- Information about the diagnosis
- Woman's preferences during labor and birth (e.g., monitoring or no monitoring of the fetal heart rate)
- Method of birth (vaginal birth is preferred in these situations in order to minimize complications for the woman)
- Care of the baby after birth (e.g., how to provide nutrition, pain medication)
- Family members and others who will be present during and/or after birth
- Spiritual care needs (e.g., baptism or other religious rituals/ceremonies)
- Keepsakes/mementos desired
- Postmortem care (e.g., autopsy, funeral arrangements)
- Plans for hospice care if baby survives until discharge

Once the plan has been developed, it can be helpful and beneficial for the family to continue to meet with the palliative care team or to at least stay in contact with some of the members and continue to receive ongoing support. Anticipatory grief can be as difficult to deal with as grief that is experienced after the death. Many families report that the time spent waiting between diagnosis and the birth is the most difficult.[12] Families oftentimes feel a sense of relief after the baby has been born and has died because they no longer have to experience the anticipatory grief and can move forward along the grief recovery continuum.

The overall goal of palliative care in the obstetric setting is to give parents some control in a very difficult situation and to provide some normalcy in an otherwise abnormal situation. The birth of a baby is usually a joyous time for a family and that joy is taken away when that baby has been diagnosed with a life-limiting condition. However, with a well-developed care plan, the family can have a positive experience and be able to celebrate the life of their child, no matter how long or short it is. A review of the literature has found that the families' response to the palliative care model is "overwhelming positive."[6] Figure 21.2 presents a flowchart for newborn palliative care.

Implications for Nursing Practice

A nurse caring for a family experiencing palliative care of a fetus/newborn or perinatal loss should be aware of the desired plan of care and advocate for that plan to be followed. These women and their families are under a tremendous amount of stress and can experience a lot of anxiety, making it difficult to answer questions or make decisions. The nurse may alleviate some stress and anxiety by promotion of care aligned with the birth plan and through patient education.

A nurse may also help the family experience birth as any other woman would. It can be challenging for a nurse to be in such an emotionally charged situation, and tempting to avoid the family as much as possible. However, the nurse is a critical source of support in providing a hand to hold, especially during the birth, as families are excited to meet their new baby. Also, at this time, the nurse may feel fear in the unknown regarding how long the baby will survive. By treating the newborn as any other baby, the nurse gives parents the strength and encouragement to interact with their baby.

Nurses report a major barrier to having confidence in working with families in a comfort care only birth situation is a lack of education and training.[6] Therefore, nurses can encourage their leaders to conduct training sessions and ongoing educational opportunities or seek out opportunities in other venues. With education, nurses are more equipped to provide that positive experience for the family in the midst of a difficult situation.

Relieve Often

For many years, it was thought that newborns did not experience discomfort or pain due to an immature central nervous system.[12] Procedures were performed without regard to the newborn's

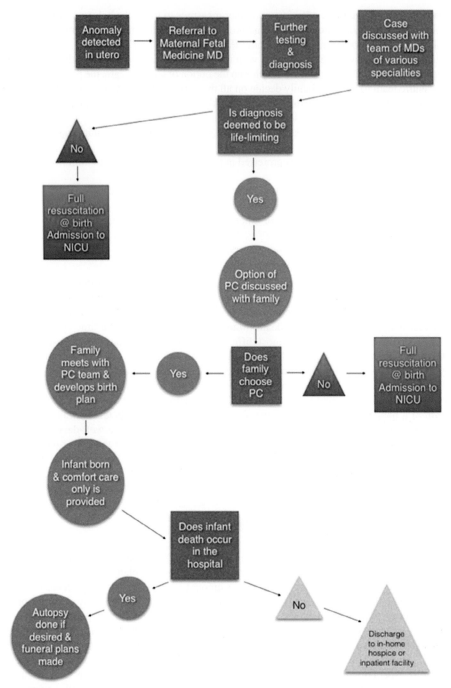

FIGURE 21.2 Process for implementing palliative care in the perinatal setting.

comfort or level of pain. Current evidence-based practice mandates vigilant nursing assessment and management to prevent and relieve unnecessary infant pain or discomfort.

Hunger

Some newborns with life-limiting conditions may still express signs of what we believe to be hunger. Allowing sucking or feeding (orally or by nasogastric tube) may bring about a sense of satiation or fullness to the infant and thus comfort to both infant and family. Although the goals of feeding an infant who is very near death are not the same as for those whose growth and development are considerations, feeding a baby is a fundamental act of nurturing in which many families need, and choose, to participate. Mothers should be given the opportunity to put the baby to breast to attempt feeding. Even if the newborn is unable to breastfeed, it can provide comfort and bonding for both the woman and the baby. Families need to be educated that feeding the newborn will not prolong life, but it is provided as a means of comfort. It will be important to teach family members to monitor signs of feeding intolerance, which will likely increase as the baby approaches the EOL, and can contribute to potentially severe discomfort for the infant. Frequent regurgitation of formula, choking, and lack of hunger cues may all be indications that the frequency, quantity, route, and/or viability of feedings needs to be reevaluated. In the face of feeding intolerance, but continued agitation/restlessness, comfort feedings via a syringe, eyedropper, or perhaps the sucking of a pacifier or finger may provide family with additional opportunities for memory making.[13] Conversely, the decision to withhold feedings in a newborn who will not survive is also to be acknowledged and respected, after appropriate communications between family and the care team.

Mouth Care

For those newborns not feeding, periodic moistening of the lips and tongue may be helpful. Use moist gauze wrapped around a finger or moistened small cotton swabs to gently wipe around the mouth area.

Skin Care

Although bathing is not necessary, it may be the parents' desire to either have this done or participate in grooming their newborn. Wiping with a warm, moist washcloth or applying nonperfumed lotion may be satisfactory. Provide routine care for diaper changes.

Eye Care

In the event of eyelid nonclosure, artificial tears may be helpful.

Symptom Management

As a newborn nears death, there may be physiologic clues that, when recognized, can provide valuable opportunities to assist families in caring for their baby and to attend to symptoms that may need to be treated, ameliorated, or palliated.[12]

Symptoms that may occur include the following:
- Bluish discoloration of skin, particularly around the mouth
- Breathing becomes irregular, may be labored, "gasping," or noisy
- Temperature instability
- Lethargy
- Agitation/restlessness/irritability

Symptom management:
- Swaddling, positioning
- Pharmacologic methods—After attempts to otherwise comfort, medication may be necessary to relieve restlessness or discomfort. Commonly ordered sedatives for neonates include (dosage based on weight). Preferred delivery method should not include any painful procedures. Therefore, PO medications are preferred.
  - Sedatives
    - midazolam (IV or nasal drops)
    - lorazepam (Ativan) (IV or PO)
    - phenobarbital (IV or PO)
  - Analgesics
    - morphine (IV or PO)
    - fentanyl (IV)
  - Seizures may be treated with diazepam, lorazepam, or phenobarbital as indicated.

Keepsakes

The loss of a child, especially an infant, does not fit into the construct of the normal life cycle. The loss of a baby invokes intense grief. Parents not only grieve for the loss of their child, they also grieve for the loss of what could have been, and the chance to create memories with their child. It is important and beneficial for parents to be able to have keepsakes of their baby. Keepsakes can be tangible items, such as photos, locks of hair, imprints of hand and feet, plaster moldings of hand and feet, and jewelry. These help to create an ongoing connection to the baby as well as facilitate making memories.[14] This is why it can be beneficial for the parents to actively participate in the creation of the keepsakes as it increases the connection felt to the keepsakes and increases their therapeutic value. Another way to increase the therapeutic value is to have the keepsakes touch the baby in some way. For example, the nurse might place a ring or bracelet on the baby when taking photos and then give it to the family. When families have an item that makes them feel connected to a loved one, it facilitates the grief process.[14]

Another contributing factor to this intense grief is that this type of loss is typically not recognized by society, especially when the loss occurs through a miscarriage or stillbirth. When grief goes unrecognized, it only intensifies it and can lead to disenfranchised grief, making it even more complicated and difficult to cope with. Having tangible items, such as photos, ink prints, and plaster moldings help to validate what the parents already feel—that it was a real baby and that it is a real loss. Dressing the baby in clothes, even small fetuses, helps the family to feel that their baby is being recognized as a real baby. Photos, prints, and moldings can be done with the smallest of fetuses, even early in the second trimester. Therefore, it is important to offer keepsakes to families experiencing a loss at any stage of pregnancy. It should never be assumed that they cannot be done and consequently not be offered to a family. Even if a loss occurs early on in the pregnancy (during the first trimester), keepsakes can still be given to families. They may not be those tangible items, but items such as love tokens, ceramic hearts, and baby rings can still serve as a connection to the baby.

What if the family refuses any keepsakes? It is helpful for the family to discuss the benefits of having keepsakes before they make any final decisions. When it is a sudden, unplanned loss, families are understandably in shock and are not able to think clearly, making decision making virtually impossible. Many times once a family learns of the benefits and has been given some time to think about it, they choose to have keepsakes. It is important not to pressure families into getting keepsakes, but it has been found that the biggest regret families have in the future is not having anything to help remember their baby, especially in regards to photographs. If families are unsure, keepsakes can still be done and either kept at the hospital or can be given to a member of the extended family to keep in case the family changes their mind. However, it is crucial to be aware of a family's religious or cultural beliefs. Some religions and cultures do not accept keepsakes for a variety of reasons, such as not touching the body after death. Some families may not feel it is a loss; therefore, they should not be made to feel that they should be mourning. Still others truly feel that having keepsakes would just make the loss that much more difficult for them as they want to cope by not even dwelling on the loss. Therefore, it is imperative to be able to fully assess the families' needs, situation surrounding the loss, beliefs, and coping style to be able to best support families in their decision.

Family Support

Most often during a perinatal loss, the focus of the support is understandably on the parents of the newborn. However, it is important to remember that other family members are grieving as well. Grandparents experience a tremendous amount of grief because they have dual pain; not only are they grieving the loss of their grandchild, they are also grieving for their own child's suffering.[13] They are unable to protect their own child from one of the most painful experiences one can have in life and that can lead to feelings of such helplessness. It can be beneficial for the nurse to provide specific tasks for grandparents to do to be able to support their child during and after the loss.

Other family members that are typically forgotten are the siblings of the baby. Siblings usually are not adequately supported during a perinatal loss because of the belief that they do not understand what is happening; therefore, they are not grieving. Even though siblings may not have a complete concept of death, it does not mean they are not grieving. Many times when parents are expecting a new baby, they include other siblings by taking them to doctor appointments, letting them help to choose a name for the baby, and feeling the baby kick mommy's tummy. Siblings often share in the excitement of the impending birth and feel much disappointment and sadness when they learn that their new baby will not be coming home. That is a loss in and of itself and any type of loss elicits feelings of grief.

Since children do not have the ability to think abstractly until adolescence, they do not have a full understanding of death. This leads to misconceptions about what has happened to the baby, which can lead to increased anxiety and fear. Therefore, it is vital for the parents to have an open and honest discussion with the siblings using developmentally appropriate terms about what happened to the baby. Parents and other adult family members should be careful to not use vague terms when discussing death with the siblings. It is very common in many cultures to not discuss death, so this leads to phrases being used such as "passed away" and "went to sleep." Adults use these terms to "soften" death, but these phrases can be very confusing for siblings. Children are concrete thinkers; therefore, they take words and phrases literally. Telling a child that the baby went to sleep will lead to a child who is afraid to go to sleep ever again. Or by saying "we lost the baby" invokes feelings of fear and anxiety because no one is looking for their lost baby. Parents need to be encouraged to use the actual words "dead" and "death" in order to facilitate the best understanding for the siblings.[15]

In order to help siblings cope with their grief, they should be involved in the bereavement process as much as possible. It can be beneficial for them to see the baby, even after it is deceased, as this helps them to understand that the baby was real. It can be difficult for them to conceptualize a baby being in their mommy's tummy, so seeing the baby eases the confusion. It also provides them with a memory of their brother or sister, which is a key component in positive long-term coping. This is why it is also important for siblings to have keepsakes of the baby. Photos, ink prints, and plaster hand and foot moldings are tangible items that not only help them understand the baby is real, they also provide a connection to the baby once they are old enough to have a full understanding of death. Just as it is beneficial for the parents to be involved in the making of the keepsakes, the same is true for the siblings. They should also be included in any rituals of the family, such as funerals and memorial services.

Siblings are often left out of the bereavement process and are prohibited from seeing the baby out of fear that it will be traumatizing for the siblings. However, with proper information and age-appropriate preparation for what they will see and experience, siblings often have a positive experience and one that will last them for a lifetime. This is also vital for their ability to cope with the loss in the long term. Child life specialists, who have backgrounds in child development and helping children understand the hospital experience, can be helpful in assisting families to facilitate positive coping for the siblings.

While parents should receive the main focus of support at the time of a perinatal loss, nurses should also remember to provide support to other members of the family. Utilization of the interdisciplinary team can assist the nurse with this. The positive coping of the parents is aided in the presence of other members of the family who are supported and coping well.

Answers to Self Assessment Quiz

F, T, F, F, T, F, F

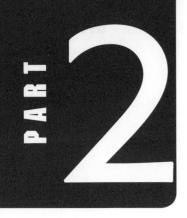

PART 2

Caring for the Dying Mother

Since pregnancy-related death remains an infrequent event, providers may lack the knowledge, skills, and awareness of palliative needs, end of life (EOL), and postmortem care. However, due to earlier diagnosis and advances in health care, more women now survive childhood and chronic medical disorders to reach childbearing age and often become pregnant. Pre-existing conditions, such as obesity, heart disease, thrombophilia, diabetes, and chronic hypertension, place the pregnant woman at increased risk for mortality. The physiologic changes associated with pregnancy and childbirth may exacerbate such conditions and increase risk. Other circumstances such as preeclampsia, infection, hemorrhage, embolism, and trauma may affect a previously healthy woman during pregnancy and often are associated with serious sequelae. In addition, the maternal mortality in the United States has steadily increased, such that the perinatal nurse should be familiar with grief issues related to the death of a woman in the intrapartum setting.

NOTE: There have been numerous case reports of the indefinite extension of life for a pregnant woman, who legally meets the criteria of death, usually to extend the gestational period and facilitate fetal growth and maturity.[16]

Decisions Related to End of Life

The Patient Self-Determination Act (PSDA), federal legislation enacted in December 1991, requires institutions to notify patients about the process for initiating advanced directives.[17] The purpose of the PSDA is to promote the opportunity for patients to discuss treatment options and plans with their healthcare providers, leading to the promotion and consummation of advanced directives prior to illness. Most states have enacted legislation that promotes living wills and/or a durable power of attorney. However, unless a woman has a major pre-existing medical condition, death is not anticipated during pregnancy and birth, and EOL decisions have never been formally determined. There are several types of advanced care planning documents. The term "patient" is used in generic discussion of these documents.

Living Will

A Living Will is a written, legal document that outlines medical treatments and healthcare wishes for the patient if they are unable to make those decisions. Living Wills usually outline wishes for resuscitation, extended ventilation, nutrition (tube feeding), antibiotics, palliative care, organ donation, and any other specifics that the patient preplans with her healthcare provider and family.

Durable Power of Attorney

A patient may have an identified medical power of attorney, which is a type of advanced directive that identifies a specific person to make healthcare decisions for that person if they are unable to do so.

Do Not Resuscitate Order

Do not resuscitate orders (DNR) may be derived from a patient's Living Will or based on the patient's physical condition. Each hospital should have a specific policy/procedure in place that addresses how DNR orders are written and carried out. A DNR policy should address specifics about physician orders, variations in resuscitation (e.g., do not intubate; no chest compressions) and how a DNR is communicated to all healthcare team members. The decision to forego resuscitative measures is ideally made jointly among the woman, family, and healthcare team. If a patient is incompetent, the decision may be made between a family member designated as a surrogate decision-maker and the physician.

Palliative and End-of-Life Care

Palliative care measures provide symptom and pain relief to improve quality of life for women and families during a life-threatening illness and at EOL. Interventions to save or prolong life often cause pain and suffering for the patient. Providers should be aware of assessment parameters that have been frequently described immediately prior to death. These include the following:
- Discolored skin: described as blue, particularly around the mouth
- Irregular breathing patterns: described as labored, gasping, and noisy
- Temperature instability
- Lethargy
- Agitation, restlessness, and/or irritability

Table 21.3 provides a sample EOL plan of care.

TABLE 21.3 END-OF-LIFE PLAN OF CARE

END-OF-LIFE PLAN OF CARE

Communicate with the woman/family regarding disease state, condition, and care choices.
- Ensure a quiet and private location for communication
- Speak while sitting down
- Use easy to understand terminology
- Provide risks, benefits, and alternatives of treatment
- Allow time for questions
- Express empathy
- Demonstrate active listening

If the woman doesn't have the capacity to make decisions and/or no previous wishes have been documented, appoint a surrogate decision maker regarding care issues. (State law dependent)

Ask about cultural and/or religious needs

Respect woman/family wishes for care and comfort

Encourage the presence of family and friends at the bedside unless otherwise specified

Follow agency policy/protocol

Obtain informed consent for postmortem exam and disposition of remains

Develop a plan of care based on EOL discussions

Suggest resources for woman/family such as Chaplain, Social Work

Protect the woman and family's privacy

From Hill, P. E. (2011). Support and counseling after maternal death. *Seminars in Perinatology, 36*(1), 84–88.

Comfort-Centered Care for the Dying Woman

EOL symptom management is an essential ethical obligation of the healthcare team in order to decrease stress and suffering in the dying, as well as the family.[18,19] Many EOL symptoms occur in clusters and present a challenge in management.

NOTE: *An important nursing function is to teach and reassure the family that medications given to manage EOL symptoms do not hasten death.*[18]

Pain

Since pregnancy-related death is often unanticipated in a previously healthy, young woman, prolonged resuscitation interventions to sustain life are often carried out. With this in mind, care providers need to be cognizant of symptoms that may indicate pain and suffering and promptly treat. Morphine is a common medication used to relieve EOL pain and should be titrated as needed.

Dyspnea

Dyspnea is a common symptom in dying women and may be frightening to them and their family. To treat respiratory symptoms in EOL settings, morphine is typically the drug of choice. Morphine is administered PO or IV 1 to 2 mg/hour and titrated as needed. Oxygen does not relieve dyspnea unless it is due to hypoxia. Congested breathing, sometimes called the "death rattle," is the result of pooled secretions in the throat. Suctioning is not recommended as it may cause pain, agitation, and increased secretion production. Treatment may also include the placement of a scopolamine patch behind the woman's ear or glycopyrrolate (Robinul) administration to reduce secretions.[18,19]

Agitation

Managing agitation in EOL is essential to keep the woman safe without using restraints. Haloperidol is the most effective medication, but benzodiazepines or sedating neuroleptics may be used.[18,19]

Palliative Sedation

Palliative sedation is utilized when other interventions to reduce EOL symptoms have failed. It is important to know that palliative sedation does not hasten death. Palliative sedation medications include midazolam and barbiturates, alone or in combination. Since the death of a pregnant woman is usually unanticipated, most will have cardiopulmonary arrest, advanced cardiac life support measures, be intubated, and sedated at the time of death.[16] Therefore, the decision to initiate palliative sedation is usually not required.

Supporting Family-Centered Care

Often EOL care occurs in a busy ICU with monitoring of vital signs, noisy alarms, and restricted family visitation. In most adult ICUs, a dying mother would not be allowed to hold her newborn due to hospital policy or staff concerns of harm to the child. These concerns and practices are not supported with evidence. In fact, many families may find comfort in having the baby stay in the mother's room. Allowing the woman to hold the newborn and the family to take pictures is a lasting memory.

There have long been liberal family visitation policies in intrapartum settings recognizing the essential role of a supportive presence for the mother. In the event of an adverse occurrence necessitating cardiopulmonary resuscitation or other life-saving measures, family, and others providing support for the woman are usually escorted from the area to wait. Recent recommendations for the continued presence of family members during a resuscitative event, however, are based on growing evidence that their presence has many benefits.[20] The woman may be comforted, family members may experience decreased anxiety, fear, and suspicion regarding resuscitative efforts, while also decreasing unrealistic expectations, all without disruption of care activities.[20,21]

Communication, presence, and attentiveness to family needs are the hallmarks of providing EOL care.[22] Nurses must keep families informed and respond promptly to questions or facilitate the presence of other members of the healthcare team to provide information. Simply being present with families in their moments of grief may provide comfort.

Postmortem Care

Providing care after death is emotional for all nurses. Respectful and thoughtful personal care may include bathing and dressing the woman prior to the family spending time with her.[23] The family may wish to be involved in providing personal care if possible. Maternal death is an unusual occurrence in the perinatal setting, thus, if death occurs in an area not accessible to the family or in a busy section of the unit, clear the hallways of visitors and take the body to a private area of the unit, preserving dignity and privacy, so the family can spend time together.[23] Positioning the deceased's body in a manner that is visually comforting and aesthetically acceptable indicates sensitivity and respect.[22] It is important to offer the family any keepsakes they would like to have, such as plaster moldings of the hands, as these can be important mementos for any surviving children. This can be especially meaningful for a surviving baby to have a tangible item of remembrance from his/her mother. Transportation and final preparation of the body for the morgue are determined by hospital procedure, policy, or coroner involvement.

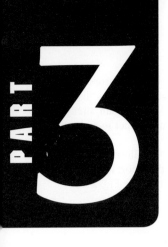

PART 3

Caring for the Care Provider

Nurses have always prioritized care for the woman and family. More recently, in the event of a maternal or perinatal death, there is emphasis on caring for the care provider as well. Typical steps included the first focus on the event itself. Debriefing after a critical event was added as a mechanism to explore both successes in provider actions and opportunities for improvement in care. Debriefing increased awareness of triggers that may cue providers to impending maternal compromise. Now, there is recognition of care provider needs for mechanisms of support in the event of a critical incident. Figure 21.3 represents a comprehensive view of these elements. This section provides an overview of mechanisms that contribute to a culture of support that benefits providers in the wake of perinatal or maternal death.

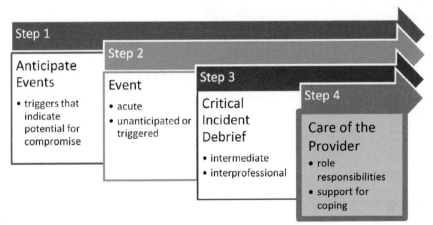

FIGURE 21.3   Critical event elements.

Pregnancy and birth are normal, natural processes. Even though obstetrical nurses are trained to attend to care needs during an emergency, the death of a mother or her newborn is not an expected outcome, stressing the members of the healthcare team as well as the system. Nurses involved in these often-unanticipated **acute events** may perceive stress related to the event itself; the need to identify, mobilize, and organize additional resources, while ensuring that safe care is still provided for other women; the performance of skills; the transfer to an intensive care environment; or death.[24]

Immediately post event, the nurse may remain focused on completing various tasks, many of which may be unfamiliar such as required documentation, forms, and postmortem care.[24] In addition to the stress evoked by the actual event, members of the healthcare team may perceive additional stress related to the often unpredictable, strong emotions exhibited by the woman and family.

It is important for each member of the healthcare team who participated in the emergency or its immediate aftermath, to be provided with an opportunity to **debrief** and discuss the event. During the debrief session, team members may express feelings, concerns, and identify opportunities for improvement.[25] In addition, the debrief session is a time when discussion of "what went well" may comfort providers involved in the event.

Coping with the outcome of the event, as well as the behavior and emotions of a stressed and possibly grieving woman and family, compounds the stress perceived by members of the healthcare team. Delaying or failing to identify and manage event-related stressors during this time may lead to burnout, turnover, complicated grief, and posttraumatic stress disorder (PTSD). During this phase, the nurse may need to take time off work and regain strength, energy, and confidence. Grief counseling services may also be a helpful adjunct to assist the nurse in returning to work.

Reintegration to the work environment can be difficult for a nurse following an unexpected death of a woman or newborn. It is at this time that unit leadership support is imperative to understand the emotions of the nurse and assist her/him to return to work (see Fig. 21.4).

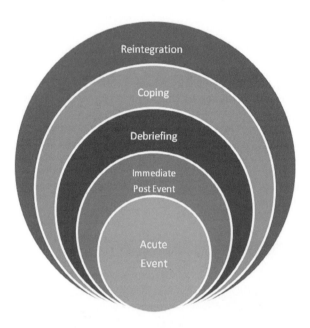

FIGURE 21.4 Critical incident phasing.

Following a critical incident, there is often role confusion for each team member. Clarifying anticipated roles of all team members can lead to more rapid and effective response, and recognition of grief in the care provider. Examples of role responsibilities are presented in Tables 21.4 and 21.5.

TABLE 21.4 CHARGE NURSE RESPONSIBILITIES

CHARGE NURSE RESPONSIBILITIES
"TEAM LEADER"[24]

- Confirm appropriate number and skill mix responding to the emergency. Notify other needed team members as indicated.
- Once appropriate team members are present, return to unit functions. There should be adequate providers involved in the emergent situation without having the Charge RN to assume a role in the emergency. This allows for continued unit functions.
- Inform all staff of emergency and rearrange assignments to cover patients for nurses involved in the emergency care.
- Evaluate the need to "hold" elective procedures and admissions until adequate staffing (this may include stopping oxytocin administration if unable to assess and titrate as recommended).
- Notify Chaplain and Social Work to assist with the family and visitors (if not previously notified in a code alert).
- Limit visitors in hallways, close doors, and ensure privacy.
- Reassure other women and families if they ask about the emergency.
- Designate a "safe room" for debrief.
- Assign support staff to assist those involved in care (e.g., runner, clean up).
- Evaluate the staff members' ability to return to work and assume care of another patient.
- Confirm that a risk management report has been completed prior to leaving work.
- Consider future assignments for staff involved in care. Example, don't assign another patient that is experiencing a perinatal loss in the near future.

TABLE 21.5	NURSE LEADER RESPONSIBILITIES

NURSE LEADER RESPONSIBILITIES
"TEAM SUPPORTER"[24]

• Determine the need for additional staffing to resume care needs on the unit. Coordinate with the Charge RN.
• Check in with the staff members involved after the emergency and make sure their needs are met.
• Be understanding and supportive of the staff members' grief.
• Communicate what went well during the event and compliment care providers involved.
• Anticipate schedule changes as needed for staff time off.
• Lead a debriefing session after the event. An additional meeting at a later date may include other leadership members, but it is important to discuss care needs during the shift they occur in order to gather details.

Other tools that may be helpful include the following[24]:
• Develop checklists for staff to organize responsibilities in a critical event.
• Develop a staff self-care checklist which may include the names of counselors in the area of perinatal grief, relaxation, nutrition, and exercise.

Summary

Although rare, perinatal and maternal deaths are significant events with profound and lasting impact on the women, families, and care providers involved. Knowledge of appropriate EOL care, comprehensive palliative care planning, critical incident management guidelines, and resources for staff coping provide a foundation for provision of comfort, care, and support for all.

Acknowledgement

*With acknowledgment of the contributions of Mary Jo Gilmer and Angel Carter.

PRACTICE/REVIEW QUESTIONS
After reviewing the module, complete the following questions:

1. Match the definition in Column B with the correct term in Column A.

Column A	**Column B**
1. _____ Ectopic pregnancy	a. Loss occurs at ≤20 weeks' gestation
2. _____ Stillbirth	b. Implantation occurs outside of the uterus
3. _____ Miscarriage	c. Loss occurs after birth through the first 28 days of life
4. _____ Neonatal death	d. Loss occurs at >20 weeks 'gestation

2. List recommendations for the healthcare providers involved in the care of women during and after termination of pregnancy for fetal anomaly (TOPFA):

1. _____
2. _____
3. _____
4. _____
5. _____

6. _____
7. _____
8. _____

3. Describe different ways the woman, partner, and/or their families may manifest grief.

_____
_____
_____

4. True or False. The best way for nurses to communicate with families experiencing loss is to offer advice in decision-making.

5. Describe the purpose of perinatal palliative care.

_____
_____
_____

6. List at least six components of a perinatal palliative plan of care.

1. _____
2. _____
3. _____

4. _____

5. _____

6. _____

7. True or False. Children in the family should be protected from the perinatal death of a sibling and protected from grief.

8. The term Living Will refers to which one of the following?

   A. A written, legal document that outlines medical treatments and healthcare wishes for the patient if they are unable to make those decisions.

   B. A type of advanced directive that identifies a specific person to make healthcare decisions for that person if they are unable to do so.

9. Describe beneficial reasons for maintaining family presence during the event of cardiopulmonary resuscitation.

   _____

   _____

10. Delaying or failing to identify and manage event-related stressors related to a maternal or perinatal loss may lead to:

   ._____

   _____

11. Differentiate the roles of a "team leader" and a "team supporter" with regard to nursing responsibilities in a critical incident.

   _____

   _____

PRACTICE/REVIEW ANSWER KEY

1. 1. b
   2. d
   3. a
   4. c
2. Develop protocols for care of the woman, family, and disposition of remains.
   Ensure a supportive care provider.
   Provide continuity of care.
   Supply appropriate educational materials before and after the procedure.
   Offer anticipatory guidance about what to expect.
   Create/collect and deliver meaningful keepsakes.
   Conduct follow-up calls.
   Provide compassionate care, demonstrated through listening, therapeutic touch, and presence
3. Feelings of sadness, anxiety, hopelessness, detachment, tightness in the throat or chest, fatigue, weakness, shortness of breath, confusion, distractedness, sleep disturbance, appetite disturbance, withdrawal, avoidance, crying

4. False
5. To alleviate suffering of the infant, emotionally support the family, and make sure the family is given honest information in a timely manner
6. Information about the diagnosis
   Mother's preferences during labor and birth
   Method of delivery
   Care of the newborn after birth
   Family members and others who will be present during and/or after delivery
   Spiritual care needs
   Keepsakes/mementos desired
   Postmortem care
   Plans for hospice care if baby survives until discharge
7. False
8. A. A written, legal document that outlines medical treatments and healthcare wishes for the patient if they are unable to make those decisions.
9. The woman may be comforted, family members may experience decreased anxiety, fear, and suspicion regarding resuscitative efforts, while also decreasing unrealistic expectations.
10. Burnout, turnover, complicated grief, and PTSD.
11. See tables in Module.

REFERENCES

1. Callister, L. C. (2014). Global perspectives on perinatal loss. *MCN, The American Journal of Maternal Child Nursing, 39*(3), 207.
2. Gregory, E., MacDormand, M., & Martin, J. (2014). *Trends in fetal and perinatal mortality in the United States, 2006–2012. NCHS Data Brief, no. 169.* Hyattsville, MD: National Center for Health Statistics.
3. Barfield, W. D. (2011). Clinical report: Standard terminology for fetal, infant, and perinatal deaths. *Pediatrics, 128*(1), 177–181. Reaffirmed January 2015.
4. Association of Women's Health, Obstetric and Neonatal Nurses. (2006). *Perinatal loss: A continuum of loss.* www.awhonn.org/Resources_Documents_pdf_2_DOD_POEP10_PerinatalLoss.pdf. Accessed January 18, 2015.
5. Evans, R. (2012). Emotional care for women who experience miscarriage. *Nursing Standard, 26*(42), 35–41.
6. Wool, C. (2011). Systematic review of the literature: Parental outcomes after diagnosis of fetal anomaly. *Advances in Neonatal Care, 11*(3), 182–192.
7. Limbo, R., & Kobler, K. (2010). The tie that binds: Relationships in perinatal bereavement. *The American Journal of Maternal Child Nursing, 35*(6), 316–321.
8. Cacciatore, J. (2010). Stillbirth: Patient-centered psychosocial care. *Clinical Obstetrics & Gynecology, 53*(3), 691–699.
9. Wool, C. (2015). Clinician perspectives of barriers in perinatal palliative care. *The American Journal of Maternal Child Nursing, 40*(1), 44–50.
10. Smart, C. J., & Smith, B. L. (2013). A transdisciplinary team approach to perinatal loss. *MCN, The American Journal of Maternal/Child Nursing, 38*(2), 110–114.
11. Wilke, J., & Limbo, R. (2012). *Resolve through sharing (RTS): Bereavement training in perinatal death* (8th ed.). La Crosse, WI: Bereavement and Advance Care Planning Services, Gunderson Lutheran Medical Foundation, Inc.

12. Sudia-Robinson, T. (2011). Ethical implications of newborn screening, life-limiting conditions, and palliative care. *The American Journal of Maternal/Child Nursing, 36*(3), 188–196.

13. Carter, B. S., Brown, J. B., Brown, S., et al. (2012). Four wishes for Aubrey. *Journal of Perinatology, 32*, 10–14.

14. Miller, L. H., Lindley, L. C., Mixer, S. J., et al. (2014). Developing a perinatal memory-making program at a children's hospital. *MCN, The American Journal of Maternal Child Nursing, 39*(2), 102–106.

15. Jones, B. L., Gilmer, M. J., Parker-Raley, J., et al. (2011). Parent and sibling relationships and the family experience. In Wolfe, J., Hinds, P., & Sourkes, B. (Eds.), *Textbook of interdisciplinary pediatric palliative care* (pp. 135–147). Philadelphia, PA: Elsevier.

16. Hill, P. E. (2011). Support and counseling after maternal death. *Seminars in Perinatology, 36*(1), 84–88.

17. Patient self-determination act, in the Omnibus Budget Reconciliation Act of 1990, P.L.I01–50S, sections 4206,4751, enacted November 5, 1990.

18. D'Arcy, Y. (2012). Managing end-of-life symptoms. *American Nurse Today, 7*(7), 22–26.

19. American Society of Pain Management Nursing position statement on pain assessment in patients who cannot self-report, Herr, K., Coyne, P. J., McCaffery, M., et al. (2011). Pain assessment in the patient unable to self-report: Position statement with clinical practice recommendations. *Pain Management Nursing, 12*(4), 230–250.

20. Jabre, P., Belpomme, V., Azoulay, E., et al. (2013). Family presence during cardiopulmonary resuscitation. *New England Journal of Medicine, 368*(11), 1008–1018.

21. AACN Practice Alert. (2010). *Family presence during resuscitation and invasive procedures.* http://www.aacn.org/wd/practice/docs/practicealerts/family-presence-during-resuscitation-invasive-procedures.pdf. Accessed July 15, 2015.

22. Williams, C. M. (2005). The identification of family members' contribution to patients' care in the Intensive Care Unit: A naturalistic inquiry. *Nursing in Critical Care, 10*(1), 6–14.

23. Henry, C., & Wilson, H. (2012). Personal care at the end of life and after death. *Nursing Times, 108.* Online issue. http://www.nursingtimes.net/Journals/2012/05/08/h/i/z/120805-Innov-endoflife.pdf.

24. Foreman, S. (2014). Developing a process to support perinatal nurses after a critical event. *Nursing for Women's Health, 18*(1), 61–65.

25. Blacklock, E. (2012). Interventions following a critical incident: Developing a critical incident stress management team. *Archives of Psychiatric Nursing, 26*, 2–8.

ADDITIONAL RESOURCES

Agency for Healthcare Research and Quality: www.ahrq.gov
Includes Evidence-Based Practice Centers (EBC), which review all relevant scientific literature on clinical, behavioral, and organization and financing topics to produce evidence reports and technology assessments.

American Academy of Hospice and Palliative Care: www. aahpm.org
Prevention and relief of patient and family suffering by providing education and clinical practice standards, fostering research, facilitating personal and professional development, and by public policy advocacy.

ELNEC: End-of-Life Nursing Education Consortium: www.aacn.nche.edu/elnec
The End-of-Life Nursing Education Consortium (ELNEC) project is a national education initiative to improve end-of-life care in the United States.

Children's Hospice International: www.chionline.org
Provides resources and referrals to children with life-threatening conditions and their families.

Bereavement services: www.bereavement.net
Offers support groups, private counseling, educational seminars, and workshops tailored to meet the needs of the bereaved and those wishing to learn more about the grief process.

Growth House, Inc.: www.growthhouse.org
Strives to improve the quality of compassionate care through public education and global professional collaboration from people who are dying.

International Journal and Online Forum of Leaders in End-of-Life Care: www.edc.org/lastacts
Features peer-reviewed articles striving to enhance comfort and dignity of dying persons and their families.

Medically Induced Trauma Support Services: http://www.mitsstools.org

National Hospice and Palliative Care Organization: www. nhpco.org

Perinatal Hospice and Palliative Care: www.perinatalhospice.org/FAQs.html#what_is_perinatal_hospice.

Implementing a Perinatal Education Program

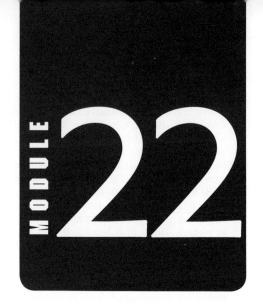

JULIE MARTIN ARAFEH AND
DINEZ SWANSON

Skill Unit 1

Scenario Template: Managing an Unexpected Birth

Skill Unit 2

High-Risk Scenario Template: Hemorrhage

Objectives

As you complete this module, you will:

1. Review characteristics of the adult learner
2. Define simulation-based training
3. Describe how to utilize various educational modalities to plan educational opportunity for various levels of intrapartum nurses

Key Terms

When you have completed this module, you should be able to recall the meaning of the following terms. You should also be able to use the terms when consulting with other health professionals. The terms are defined in this module or in the glossary at the end of this book.

adult learning theory   simulation
debriefing   nursing orientation

Overview

The learning needs of staff in intrapartum units are varied from students, to new graduates, to experienced nurses. Intrapartum units require different types of programs to meet the educational needs of the staff. This text has been designed to address different educational levels in a variety of formats.

- New graduate residency program
- Self-directed continuing education for the experienced nurse
- Continuing education program for intrapartum staff in a facility
- Perinatal outreach program

This module reviews the basic concepts of adult learning theory including characteristics of the adult learner, application of theories in practice, and how the text can be used to support the development of cognitive, technical, and behavioral skills in intrapartum staff or students of intrapartum nursing.

Adult Learning Theory

In the development of any educational program, the needs of adult learners should be considered and concepts of adult learning theory utilized in designing the program. The characteristics of the adult learner reflect a group that is internally motivated, is self-directed, and seeks new knowledge for immediate application.[1] It is important to be cognizant of the need to develop critical thinking skills through the use of this text. The cognitive domain can be broken into two levels: the primary and the most basic level consisting of knowledge, comprehension, and application, and the higher level consisting of analysis, synthesis, and evaluation.[2] Traditionally, the bulk of education has concentrated on the lower level despite the fact that practitioners operate at the higher level during patient care. It is important to challenge the learners with an opportunity to put the new knowledge gained from reading this text into practice either through case review or simulation. Much of the literature in adult education reflects the importance of hands-on experience as a means to acquire and refine new knowledge. Experiential learning also leads to longer retention of new skills for a longer period of time when compared with traditional didactic presentations.[3–8]

Simulation-Based Training

Simulation-based training (SBT) is an education methodology that incorporates experiential learning. During SBT, the learner is placed in a realistic setting that supports practice of concepts that have been studied. The objectives for the learner in SBT are often divided into three categories: cognitive, technical, and behavioral.

- Cognitive learning objectives are what the learner needs to know.
- Technical learning objectives are what skills the learner needs to be able to perform.
- Behavioral learning objectives cover nontechnical skills such as communication.[9]

Experts in human performance training have suggested that 10 behaviors are critical to effective, efficient, and safe team performance.[10] These skills can best be taught in SBT. Behavioral skills identified as important include the following:

1. Know your environment
2. Anticipate and plan
3. Assume the leadership role
4. Communicate effectively
5. Distribute work load optimally
6. Allocate attention wisely
7. Utilize all available information
8. Utilize all available resources
9. Call for help early
10. Maintain professional behavior

These three categories of learning objectives inform all aspects of SBT and are the most important part of the scenario, the working tool of SBT. The scenario contains the topic of the SBT (such as shoulder dystocia or eclampsia) in the form of the patient story or history and learning objectives written to cover critical aspects of that topic. For any given topic of SBT, learning objectives can be written to cover a wide range of learner experience from nursing student to expert.

Debriefing occurs immediately after the end of the scenario and is facilitated by one of the instructors. Debriefing allows the learners to review and reflect on the events that occurred during the scenario. The debriefing should occur in a location that provides confidentiality to encourage an honest and open discussion about the events in the scenario. In addition to a secure location, all attending the debriefing should sign a confidentiality agreement that states the performances in the scenario, and the conversation in the debriefing will not be discussed outside of SBT. Assurance that performance issues or discussion during SBT will be held confidential creates a safe learning environment for those involved.[11]

SBT is uniquely able to combine cognitive, technical, and behavioral skill practices. The addition of video recording of training scenarios allows all participants to constructively review the session and discuss actions of the team during debriefing. These sessions can advance individual performance and performance of the interdisciplinary team as a whole. All learners and instructors should sign a consent form before video recording giving permission for the recording and detailing if the recording will be destroyed after debriefing or retained. If retained, the learners need to be informed how the recording will be used. The learners have the right to deny any use of the recording outside of debriefing without their permission. Samples of confidentiality and consent to video forms can be found in Displays 22.1 and 22.2.

DISPLAY 22.1 CONFIDENTIALITY AGREEMENT FOR SIMULATION

Center for Advanced Pediatric & Perinatal Education

CONFIDENTIALITY AGREEMENT

During your participation in training in a simulated medical environment at the Center for Advanced Pediatric and Perinatal Education (CAPE) at Lucile Packard Children's Hospital at Stanford, you will be both an active participant in realistic scenarios and an observer of others immersed in similar situations (either in real time or on videotape). The objective of this training program is to train individuals to better assess and improve their performance in difficult clinical situations. It is to be understood that the scenarios to which you and your colleagues will be exposed are designed to exacerbate the likelihood of lapses and errors in performance. Because of these issues you are asked to maintain strict confidentiality regarding both your performance and the performance of others, whether witnessed in real time or on videotape. Failure to maintain confidentiality may result in unwarranted and unfair defamation of character of the participants. This could cause irreparable harm to you and your colleagues and would seriously impair the effectiveness of this simulation-based training program.

While you are free to discuss in general terms the technical and behavioral skills acquired and maintained during training at CAPE, you are required to maintain strict confidentiality regarding the specific scenarios to which you are both directly and indirectly exposed. The development of challenging scenarios is extremely labor intensive and any foreknowledge by participants of what is to be presented to them will defeat the purpose of this type of training.

The bottom line: All that takes place in the simulator stays in the simulator.

By signing below, you acknowledge having read and understood this statement and agree to maintain the strictest confidentiality about the performance of individuals and the details of scenarios to which you are exposed.

Signature: _____   **Date:** _____

Print name: _____

Email: _____

Please turn off all CELL PHONES and PAGERS unless they are immediately required for professional or personal circumstances.

Used with permission from CAPE: Center for Advanced Pediatric and Perinatal Education.

Topics for intrapartum scenarios can include shoulder dystocia, precipitous birth, hemorrhage, or any of the topics covered in the modules of this text. Sample scenarios can be found in the Skills Units at the end of this module. The sample scenarios can be used as a template to create other scenarios for the different modules in the text. Educators running an SBT program

---

DISPLAY 22.2 AUTHORIZATION AND CONSENT TO PHOTOGRAPH AND PUBLISH

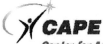

CAPE

Center for Advanced Pediatric & Perinatal Education

AUTHORIZATION AND CONSENT TO PHOTOGRAPH AND PUBLISH

The undersigned hereby authorizes the staff of the Center for Advanced Pediatric and Perinatal Education at Lucile Packard Children's Hospital at Stanford to photograph or permit other persons to photograph

_____

PRINT NAME

While participating in its training programs. The undersigned agrees that the staff of the Center may use and permit other persons to use the negatives, prints, videotape or films prepared from such photographs for the purposes and manner as either may deem appropriate. The undersigned agrees the photographs may be used for purposes including, but not limited to, dissemination to the hospital staff, physicians, health professionals and members of the public for educational, treatment, research, scientific, public relations, advertisement, promotional and/or fundraising purposes, and that such dissemination may be accomplished in any manner. Such use is subject only to the following limitations:

_____

The undersigned has entered into this agreement in order to assist scientific treatment, education, public relations, promotional and/or fund raising goals and hereby **waives any right to compensation** for these uses by reason of foregoing authorizations, and the undersigned and his or her successors hereby hold the staff of the Center and their successors, harmless from and against any claim for injury or compensation resulting from the activities authorized by this agreement.

The term "photograph" as used in this agreement shall mean still photography or video in any format, including any physical or digital means of recording and reproducing images.

Date: _____ Time: _____

Signature: _____

Street Address: _____

City, State, Zip:_____ Email:_____

Yes, you may use my video for educational purposes.

No, you may not use my video for educational purposes.

Please turn off all CELL PHONES and PAGERS unless they are immediately required for professional or personal circumstances.

Used with permission from CAPE: Center for Advanced Pediatric and Perinatal Education.

---

should have experience with SBT or attend a simulation instructor program. In addition, evaluation of the program is important to improve future simulations. An example evaluation tool is outlined in Table 22.1.

Nursing Education Programs

The goal of nursing education is to facilitate development of individual knowledge, attitude, and skills that allow a nurse to provide safe, effective, evidence-based care.[12,13] There continues to be a decrease in focus on specialty area education such as obstetrics or pediatrics in pre licensure nursing education; however, a generalist knowledge base may be assumed of the graduate nurse. Any graduate or experienced nurse entering an intrapartum unit should be teamed with a mentor/preceptor for support and guidance. Ongoing, continuing education provides nurses with the opportunity to further develop and refine nursing skills leading to expertise; a comprehensive knowledge base, experience with common and less common technical skills and well versed in team and leadership skills.

Student Nurse Education Program

Student nurses experience learning in both the classroom and clinical or simulated clinical setting. The student nurse is frequently assigned to the intrapartum setting in an observational role.

TABLE 22.1 SIMULATION EVALUATION TOOL

EVALUATION FOR SIMULATION-BASED TRAINING

Program Title: _____

Date: _____ Participant name: _____

KEY:

5 Strongly agree
4 Agree
3 Neither agree nor disagree
2 Disagree
1 Strongly disagree

1. The skills and content presented are relevant to my practice.
   1 2 3 4 5
   Comments:

2. This format was helpful with learning and retention of skills.
   1 2 3 4 5
   Comments:

3. The debriefing sessions were a valuable component of the simulation.
   1 2 3 4 5
   Comments:

4. Review of skills/use of video was helpful in incorporating new behaviors.
   1 2 3 4 5
   Comments:

5. This simulation will assist me in providing better care to intrapartum patients.
   1 2 3 4 5
   Comments:

6. Review of the module before simulation training was helpful.
   1 2 3 4 5
   Comments:

7. It is helpful to review skills with other intrapartum colleagues.
   1 2 3 4 5
   Comments:

8. The faculty facilitated the learning process and skill retention.
   1 2 3 4 5
   Comments:

With unpredictable census and acuity, the setting may provide limited learning opportunities. It is also considered a "high-risk" area where maternal and/or fetal status may rapidly change.[14] Accessibility of patient care experiences for nursing students is also influenced by factors such as workplace culture, patient satisfaction targets, patient refusal, limited practice settings, and liability issues. In women's health clinical rotations, the clinical group of nursing students is often divided into three or four areas of the hospital, including intrapartum, antepartum, and mother–baby (postpartum, newborn nursery). With the student dividing time between multiple units, some of which are observational experiences only, the amount of "hands-on" time the student has to learn in any one women's health area is limited. Partnership between academia, hospitals, and staff nurse preceptors may facilitate the clinical learning experiences for students.

New-Graduate Residency Program

New-graduate nurses are the largest pool of nurses available for recruitment across the nation. However, upon entry into practice, new-graduate nurses face many challenges including role transition, high-performance expectations in an increasingly high acuity environment, and an increased level of accountability as it relates to nursing quality indicators.[15] The Institute of Medicine strongly recommends the development and implementation of nurse residency programs (NRPs) to improve retention of nurses and expand existing competencies, leading to improved patient outcomes. Nursing staff turnover has significant financial implications for healthcare institutions. A stressful work environment and increased workload have resulted in high turnover of new graduate nurses at a rate of 35% to 65% per year within the first year of employment.[16]

A graduate nurse residency program should provide the new nurse with critical thinking, delegation, priority skill setting, and conflict resolution skills, while building confidence and providing a mentoring relationship. The NRP aims to help new graduates:

- Transition from advanced beginner nurse toward competent professional nurse in the clinical environment.
- Develop effective decision-making skills related to clinical judgments and performance.
- Provide clinical leadership at the point of patient care.
- Strengthen their commitment to nursing as a professional career choice.
- Formulate an individual development plan related to the nurse's new clinical role.
- Incorporate research-based evidence into their practice.

New graduates begin with a rather prescriptive and linear approach to both their thinking and their practice. While they adjust to changing roles, routines, responsibilities, and relationships, new graduate nurses require all their energy and focus for specific tasks such as administering medications, speaking with physicians, or performing a dressing change.[17,18] Goals for the new graduate nurse include enhancing their knowledge, and identifying new competencies specific to the role. Simulations may be used to enhance new graduate nurses' competencies.

Nurse Residency Curriculum

A graduate nurse residency program should include a logical progression of caring for laboring woman without complications to caring for laboring women experiencing complications. A sample curriculum plan might consist of online and face-to-face modules, skills competency assessment, pre/post content assessments, direct hands-on experience, and simulation. The new graduate works closely with a clinical coach on the unit, and is usually assigned an additional mentor, who may or may not be on the unit, to serve as a resource and guide during the process of socialization. The Association of Women's Health, Obstetrics and Neonatal Nursing's (AWHONN) Didactic and Clinical Competencies can serve as a resource for development of curriculum for new graduate nurses or modified for experienced nurses transferring to perinatal nursing.[19]

Ideally, the new graduate nurse will be exposed to all areas of nursing in women's services. Following these experiences, the graduate nurse and education coordinator can determine the best fit for the new nurse and develop detailed pathway for that particular area. One way to transition the new graduate nurse to increase job satisfaction and reduce turnover is to assign a consistent clinical coach once the specific area is determined.[20] The clinical coach is selected by input from the new graduate and education coordinator. NRPs are successful when an experienced and trained clinical coach guides the graduate nurse into practice. Having one consistent coach, rather being passed from nurse to nurse during orientation is shown to alleviate frustration and improve satisfaction of nurse graduates.[21] The selected coach should be aware of differences between experienced and novice nurses, and have an understanding of how to transition the new graduate through the stages of skill acquisition. Training programs for clinical coaches ensures appropriate coaching capabilities and improve outcomes for the new graduate nurse.[22] Elements of a training program for clinical coaches might include principles of teaching–learning, effective communication, role socialization, reflective practice guidance, delegation and accountability, quality and safety tenets, teamwork, and patient-centered care.[23] Development of these programs to support clinical coaches increases their confidence levels as well as understanding the critical nature of their role.[24] A mentor may also be assigned to the new graduate nurse in a residency program. Mentoring provides resources and a supportive environment for new graduate nurses. The role of the mentor differs from that of clinical coach in function. Mentors are nurses who provide a sounding board giving the new nurse someone to go to when they are experiencing distress and may be purposefully assigned such that they are not based in the same unit as the new graduate. Socializing the new nurse is one of the most important things that can be done to decrease feelings of distress and low self-esteem, increase job satisfaction, and reduce the turnover rate.[20,25]

One method that can be used to determine how new nurses are progressing in their role is the Casey–Fink tool, validated with new graduate nurses. The Casey–Fink tool consists of five sections, including new graduate demographic information, comfort with skills and procedures, job satisfaction, open-ended questions, and 25 questions with Likert-scale responses. Five factors are measured in the Casey–Fink tool:

- Support
- Patient safety
- Stress
- Communication/leadership
- Professional satisfaction[26]

Continuing Education for Intrapartum Staff: Self-directed, Team Training, and Outreach

The modules in the text are designed for either self-directed review or as an adjunct to other educational offerings to provide cognitive content and skills review with experiential learning that occurs with SBT. For example, prior to SBT the modules that will be included in the scenario can be assigned for study and review. Questions can be found in each module to provide self-assessment of the concepts presented in that module or the questions can be used by an educator to assess the learner's grasp of the cognitive content. Knowledge and cognitive skills are the basis for decision-making in training sessions and ultimately at the bedside.

The modules can also be used to augment the learner's existing knowledge base to support development and refinement of technical skills specific to intrapartum nursing. Review of the skill units in the text that are applicable to the scenario, in conjunction with a technical skills practice session, will engage both visual and auditory learners. Ideally, a skills practice session can be conducted immediately before the scenario where the skill will be used. This allows the learner to review the basics of the skill, then employ it in a similar manner to actual patient care.

Sample Agenda for SBT

8:00–8:15	Introductions, Review of Agenda
8:15–8:45	Review of assigned modules, Question and Answer
8:45–9:45	Review of skills
9:45–10:00	Briefing for SBT
10:00–11:00	Scenario#1 with video debriefing
11:00–11:45	Scenario #2 with video debriefing
11:45–12:00	Question and Answer, Evaluation

Selection of scenario topic used for interdisciplinary or outreach training is best based on the needs of the staff being trained. Determination of educational and SBT need can be accomplished several ways. A survey can be sent to the staff to determine what they perceive their needs are. Data can be examined from the departments of Risk Management, Infection Control, or Quality Improvement/Patient Safety. A review of sentinel events or poor patient outcomes can also be done. Regardless of the method used to select the scenario topic, it should be a topic that is seen as relevant and important to intrapartum staff. Once a topic is selected, the patient history and course of events used in the scenario can mimic actual patient cases. Then, if the topic of the scenario is questioned by the staff, the instructors can relay how and why the topic was selected and the scenario written.

Once a scenario topic is selected, it will need to be adapted to match the unique circumstances the staff practices in. For example, the scenario will be written differently if the unit has 24-hour in-house provider coverage or if providers are called when needed. Each unit functions with a minimum level of staff, so this will need to be taken into consideration. For example, if a postpartum hemorrhage scenario is being conducted for a staff where the minimum is two nurses and there are four roles to be filled, part of the scenario will require the two nurses to activate a plan to bring the correct number of nurses to the patient to meet the standard of care. Rehearsal of the scenario with experienced staff before using it for training will help to insure all unit circumstances have been taken into consideration.

During debriefing the staff may uncover issues with the unit system that interfere with patient care or that may inhibit the staff from meeting patient care standards. These issues need to be noted in detail and given to administrators that can address them. Prior to beginning SBT whether for the instructors' intrapartum unit or for a unit from an a different facility for outreach, a discussion should occur with the legal representatives for the facility to ensure that all components of SBT, particularly debriefing and any issues that are uncovered during debriefing, remain nondiscoverable in a court of law. Legal representatives will need to be made fully aware of the type of training that will be conducted, the content that will be covered, and the possibility that system issues may be uncovered. A discussion of this detail will allow the staff to participate in educational and quality improvement exercises without fear of reprisal.

SKILL UNIT 1 | SCENARIO TEMPLATE: MANAGING AN UNEXPECTED BIRTH

Scene
A 32-year-old G3 P2 presents to labor and delivery in labor at term gestation with intact bulging bag of waters. Vital signs are within normal limits and the fetal monitoring strip is a category I. The woman states an urge to push. During the cervical exam spontaneous rupture of membranes occurs and the infant is born precipitously.

Level of Difficulty
It is important to be aware of the experience level of the learner. Learning objectives for each category will be divided into those for student or new learners and those for experienced learners. For experienced learners, the intensity and complexity of the scenario can be increased by including one or more of the following options:
- Family member present
- Woman speaks a different language than the learners
- Equipment malfunction

LEARNING OBJECTIVES
Cognitive
For student/new learners:
- Signs of precipitous birth including vaginal exam and appearance of bulging perineum
- Cardinal movements of the fetus before and during birth

For experienced learners:
- Describe situations that can result in a precipitous birth, including differences in labor patterns between nulliparous and multiparous women
- List complications that can occur, for example shoulder dystocia or meconium-stained fluid

Technical
For students/new learners:
- Assembly of supplies at the bedside for a precipitous birth
- Describe actions to assist more experienced staff with birth

For experienced learners:
- Review the steps to assist the woman with the birth
- Describe how to create a safe environment for the woman and newborn during birth
- Discuss care of the woman and newborn immediately after birth

skill unit continues on page 564

Behavioral

For all learners:
- Call for help indicating what staff members are needed for birth
- Use of clear, concise communication among team during crisis

For experienced learners:
- Assumption of leadership role
- Ability to delegate tasks based on skill sets

Expected Critical Actions

- Call for help
- Woman positioned for birth in a manner that is safe and comfortable for her
- Perineum cleansed
- Gloves and necessary drapes placed for birth
- Determine position of fetus
- Support the perineum with nondominant hand
- Instruct the woman in clear, concise manner
- After birth of the head, check for nuchal cord
- Clamp and cut nuchal cord
- Support fetal head during restitution
- Support the fetal body during birth
- After birth, secures infant in an arm hold with head slightly down
- Cord clamped
- Warm, dry, and stimulate infant
- Control delivery of the placenta with steady downward traction with one hand and support of the fundus with the other hand
- Evaluate for perineal tears
- Evaluate bleeding

NOTE: Consider the use of video to record the scenario in order to review learners' performances. This provides the learners with the unique opportunity to see themselves in action and gain insight into their strengths and weaknesses. Reflection on performance followed by additional practice allows the learner to process new information leading to the ultimate goal of this manual: acquisition and retention of new skills and improved critical thinking.

SKILL UNIT 2 | HIGH-RISK SCENARIO TEMPLATE: HEMORRHAGE

Scene

A 40-year-old G3 now P3 delivered a viable, term infant 30 min ago. Her past history is unremarkable with the exception of uterine atony leading to hemorrhage after her last birth that resolved with uterotonic agents and required two units of packed red blood cells. Quantified blood loss after this birth has been 550 mL. Her most recent vital signs are blood pressure of 110/80, pulse of 110, and respiratory rate of 32. At her next assessment she has a bulging bladder with a boggy uterus at three fingerbreadths above the umbilicus. A large amount of bright red vaginal bleeding is noted and she is complaining of feeling weak and dizzy.

Level of Difficulty

Learning objectives for each category will be divided into those for student or new learners and those for experienced learners. For experienced learners, the intensity and complexity of the scenario can be increased by including one or more of the following options:
- Hemorrhage does not respond to uterotonic agents
- Family member is upset and interferes with patient care
- Newborn is in room and is hypothermic

LEARNING OBJECTIVES

Cognitive

For student/new learners:
- List common causes of postpartum hemorrhage and risk factors
- Describe changes in vital signs associated with hemorrhage

skill unit continues on page 565

For experienced learners:
- State the stages of hemorrhage and corresponding patient signs and symptoms
- List management strategies to manage hemorrhage including uterotonics, tamponade devices, and surgical interventions

Technical

For students/new learners:
- Demonstrate proper technique for uterine massage and detection of full bladder
- Correctly administer uterotonic medications

For experienced learners:
- Assist with assembly and placement of uterine tamponade devices
- Implement massive transfusion guidelines
- Locate, assemble, and utilize rapid infuser

Behavioral

For all learners:
- Call for help indicating what staff members are needed for hemorrhage
- Clear, concise communication among team during crisis

For experienced learners:
- Assumption of leadership role
- Ability to delegate tasks based on skill sets

Expected Critical Actions

- Recognize signs and symptoms of hemorrhage
- Begin uterine massage and palpate for full bladder
- Call for help (including provider of record), uterotonic medications, and hemorrhage supplies/cart
- Assign roles to nursing staff upon arrival including medication administration, intravenous fluids/blood administration, recorder, vital sign assessment, empty bladder, provider assistance
- Administer uterotonic agents per unit protocol
- Start second intravenous line with normal saline and blood tubing, send labs per order
- Continue to measure blood loss
- Start oxygen as needed
- Cover patient with warm blankets as much as possible to conserve heat
- Call for massive transfusion if ordered
- Assemble rapid transfuser and prime for fluid administration
- Assemble and assist with placement of uterine tamponade device
- Prepare for surgical therapy as needed

Evaluation of Training

The questions on the form in Table 22.1 will assist in evaluating the relevancy of the skills/simulation in enhancing clinical knowledge and skills. The learner's answers will provide a basis for evaluating the effectiveness of this format for intrapartum education. In addition, this survey offers regional centers or agencies a means of determining the degree of participant satisfaction. This form may be duplicated as needed.

CONCLUSION

The ultimate goal of this text is to improve patient safety through increased content knowledge, acquisition of new skills, and the eventual transfer to the clinical environment. The Joint Commission (TJC) conducted a root cause analysis of 71 cases of perinatal morbidity and mortality.[27] Causes topping the list included communication, staff competency, and training. This text directly addresses these issues through up-to-date information related to best practices as well as recommendations for interactive teaching methods within this module. Team training through multidisciplinary drills on scenarios such as the one listed in Appendices that follow will assist teams in meeting TJC's recommendations to improve perinatal outcomes.[28]

Acknowledgement

*The authors would like to acknowledge Kimberly Yaeger MEd, RN, for her contribution to the adult learning and simulation-based learning sections of this module.

REFERENCES

1. Knowles, M. S. (1984). *Andragogy in action.* San Francisco, CA: Jossey-Bass.
2. Bloom, B. S., & Krathwohl, D. R. (1956). *Taxonomy of educational objectives: The classification of educational goals, by a committee of college and university examiners. Handbook 1: Cognitive domain.* New York, NY: Longmans.
3. Draycott, T. J., Crofts, J. F., Ash, J. P., et al. (2008). Improving neonatal outcome through practical shoulder dystocia training. *Obstetrics & Gynecology, 112,* 14–20.
4. Wagner, B., Meirowitz, N., Shah, J., et al. (2011). Comprehensive perinatal safety initiative to reduce adverse obstetric events. *Journal for Healthcare Quality, 34*(1), 6–15.
5. Riley, W., Davis, S., Miller, K., et al. (2011). Didactic and simulation nontechnical skills team training to improve perinatal patient outcomes in a community hospital. *Joint Commission Journal on Quality and Patient Safety, 37*(8), 357–364.
6. Deering, S., & Rowland, J. (2013). Obstetric emergency simulation. *Seminars in Perinatology, 37,* 179–188.
7. Gardner, R., & Raemer, D. B. (2008). Simulation in obstetrics and gynecology. *Obstetrics and Gynecology Clinics of North America, 35,* 97–127.
8. Rosen, M. A., Hunt, E. A., Pronovost, P. J., et al. (2012). In situ simulation in continuing education for the health care professions: A systematic review. *The Journal of Continuing Education in the Health Professions, 32*(4), 243–254.
9. Halamek, L. P. (2007). Teaching versus learning and the role of simulation-based training in pediatrics. *The Journal of Pediatrics, 151,* 329–330.
10. Helmreich, R. L., & Foushee, H. C. (1993). Why crew resource management? Empirical and theoretical bases of human factors training in aviation. In Weiner, E. L., Kanki, B. G., & Helmreich, R. L. (Eds.), *Cockpit resource management* (pp. 3–45). San Diego, CA: Academic Press.
11. Fanning, R. M., & Gaba, D. M. (2007). The role of debriefing in simulation-based learning. *Simulation in Healthcare: Journal of the Society for Simulation in Healthcare, 2,* 115–125.
12. Strong, M., Kane, I., Petras, D., et al. (2014). Direct care registered nurses' and nursing leaders' review of the clinical competencies needed for the successful nurse of the future: A gap analysis. *Journal for Nurses in Professional Development, 30*(4), 196–203.
13. Yanhua, C., & Watson, R. (2011). A review of clinical competence assessment in nursing. *Nurse Education Today, 31,* 832–836.
14. Raines, D. A. (2010). Obstetrical nursing experience simulation. Filing the gap. *Nursing for Women's Health, 14*(2), 113–119.

15. Theisen, J. L., & Sandau, K. E. (2013). Competency of new graduate nurses: A review of their weaknesses and strategies for success. *Journal of Continuing Education in Nursing, 44*(9), 406–414.
16. Giallonardo, L. M., Wong, C. A., & Iwasiw, C. L. (2010). Authentic leadership of preceptors: Predictor of new graduate nurses' work engagement and job satisfaction. *Journal of Nursing Management, 18*(8), 993–1003.
17. Boychuk Duchscher, J. E., & Cowin, L. (2008). Multigenerational nurses in the workplace. *Journal of Nursing Administration, 34*(11), 493–501.
18. Duchscher, J. E. B. (2009). Transition shock: The initial stage of role adaptation for newly graduated registered nurses. *Journal of Advanced Nursing, 65*(5), 1103–1113.
19. Association of Women's Health, Obstetric and Neonatal Nurses. (2013). *Basic, high-risk and critical-care intrapartum nursing clinical competencies and education guide* (5th ed.). Washington, DC: Author.
20. Ferguson, L. M. (2011). From the perspective of new nurses: What do effective mentors look like in practice? *Nurse Education in Practice, 11*(2), 119–123.
21. Dyess, S. M., & Sherman, R. O. (2009). The first year of practice: New graduate nurses' transition and learning needs. *Journal of Continuing Education in Nursing, 40*(9), 403–410. Retrieved from http://vnweb.hwwilsonweb.com
22. Myers, S., Reidy, P., French, B., et al. (2010). Safety concerns of hospital-based new-to-practice registered nurses and their preceptors. *Journal of Continuing Education in Nursing, 41*(4), 163–171.
23. Spector, N. (2015). The National Council of State Boards of Nursing's Transition to Practice Study: Implications for Educators. *J Nursing Education, 54*(3); 119–120.
24. Hyrkas, K., & Shoemaker, M. (2007). Changes in the preceptor role: Re-visiting preceptors' perceptions of benefits, rewards, support and commitment to the role. *Journal of Advanced Nursing, 60*(5), 513–524.
25. Beecroft, P. C., Dorey, F., & Wenten, M. (2008). Turnover intention in new graduate nurses: A multivariate analysis. *Journal of Advanced Nursing, 62*(1), 41–52.
26. Casey, K., Fink, R., Krugman, M., et al. (2004). The graduate nurse experience. *Journal of Nursing Administration, 34*(6), 303–311.
27. JCAHO. (2004). Sentinel event alert. www.jcaho.org/about+us/news+letters/sentinel+event+alert/sea_30.htm. Accessed July 3, 2007.
28. Miller, L. A. (2005). Patient safety and teamwork in perinatal care, resources for clinicians. *The Journal of Perinatal & Neonatal Nursing, 19,* 46–51.

abnormal placentation refers to patients with placenta accreta, increta, or percreta
- **placenta accreta** placenta abnormally adhered to the myometrium of the uterus
- **placenta increta** placental attachment and growth into the myometrium
- **placenta percreta** placental attachment and growth through the myometrium; may grow onto other organs

ABO incompatibility a lack of compatibility between two groups of blood cells having different antigens because of the presence of one of the types of antigens (A, B, or both) and its absence in the other. When maternal and fetal blood cell types differ and the differing blood cells are exchanged, it can cause an immune response and breakdown of red blood cells (ABO hemolytic disease of the newborn)

abruptio placentae (placental abruption) premature separation of a normally implanted placenta; the separation can be partial or complete

abuse physical, sexual, emotional, or threatened violence against another

accelerations, fetal an increase in the fetal heart rate (FHR; onset to peak in less than 30 seconds) from the most recently calculated baseline. The duration of the acceleration is defined as the time from the initial change in FHR from the baseline to the return of the FHR to the baseline
- **At 32 weeks' gestation and beyond** an acceleration has an acme of 15 beats per minute (bpm) above the baseline with a duration of 15 seconds or more, but less than 2 minutes
- **Before 32 weeks' gestation** an acceleration has an acme of 10 bpm above the baseline and with a duration of 10 seconds or more, but less than 2 minutes
- **Prolonged accelerations** last 2 minutes or more but less than 10 minutes

NOTE: If an acceleration lasts 10 minutes or longer, it is a baseline change.

accreta (see abnormal placentation)

acidemia buildup of acid in the blood

acidosis condition in which there is a disturbance in the acid–base balance of the body, resulting in an accumulation of acids or an excessive loss of bicarbonate

acquired immunodeficiency syndrome (AIDS) a disease caused by the human immunodeficiency virus (HIV) with severe loss of cellular immunity resulting in lowered resistance to infection and malignancy

active-directed pushing coached pushing during the second stage of labor
- **closed glottis** the woman holds her breath and uses the Valsalva maneuver to push
- **open glottis** forced exhalation of air or very brief periods of breath holding for 3 to 5 seconds; may use an expiratory grunt accompanying the push

active immunity protection from a disease resulting from the development within the body of substances that keep a person immune; this could result from having the disease or by the injection of an organism or products of an organism

active management of labor protocol for the augmentation of labor that includes strict criteria for inclusion, early amniotomy, high-dose oxytocin infusion for ineffective contraction patterns

active phase of labor (see stages of labor)

acupressure an alternative medicine technique; physical pressure is applied to acupuncture points to relieve pain, nausea, and other symptoms of labor

acute violence stage (see cycle of violence)

addendum statements added to the chart after the original documentation of an event; may contain additional facts about the situation or correct misinformation in the first entry

adult learning theory (Andragogy) a model of assumptions that characterizes adult learners from learning in childhood; Malcom Knowles presented the adult learner as one who is autonomous, free, and growth oriented with basic assumptions: self-concept, experience, readiness to learn, orientation to learning, motivation to learn, and relevance

advanced directive legal document(s) that allows a person to make decisions about end-of-life care ahead of time

alanine aminotransferase (ALT) an enzyme that contributes to protein metabolism; specifically, it catalyzes the reversible transfer of an amino group from glutamic acid to pyruvic acid to form alanine; the old term for this enzyme was *serum glutamic–pyruvic transaminase* (SGPT); this enzyme is present in the liver; during viral hepatitis and in cases of hepatocellular necrosis, marked elevations are seen

algorithm a logical progression that, for example, outlines sequential steps to be taken in the diagnosis and management of a disease

alpha-fetoprotein (AFP) test determination of fetal antigen levels during pregnancy; elevated levels in amniotic fluid are associated with neural tube defects, and low levels may be associated with Down syndrome

17-alpha hydroxyprogesterone caproate (17P) a naturally occurring metabolite of progesterone and is sometimes used to treat women with a history of preterm birth

amniocentesis puncturing the amniotic sac using a needle so that amniotic fluid can be obtained for testing

amnion the innermost fetal membrane that encloses the fetus and fills with amniotic fluid

amniotic fluid embolus (AFE) entrance of amniotic fluid, fetal cells, hair, or other debris into the maternal circulation initiating a series of rapid, complex events that lead to life-threatening maternal symptoms

amniotic fluid index (AFI) a method of reporting amniotic fluid volume

amniotic phosphatidylglycerol (PG) a class of compounds found in amniotic fluid that can be analyzed to determine fetal pulmonary maturity

amniotomy puncturing the amniotic sac, allowing amniotic fluid to escape; this is sometimes done during active labor

anaphylactoid syndrome proposed term for **amniotic fluid embolus**

angiogenesis the development of new blood vessels

anoxia deficiency of oxygen; *see also* **hypoxia**

antiangiogenic proteins block the angiogenesis signaling molecules

antibody protein substances developed in response to the presence of an antigen; antibodies, which the body produces to inhibit or destroy the antigen, are part of the body's defense against foreign substances such as bacteria and viruses

antigen a substance that, when introduced into a host, is capable of producing antibodies; an antigen can be introduced into the host body, or it can be formed within the body; bacteria and viruses are examples of antigens

antiphospholipid antibodies antibodies directed against phosphorated polysaccharides of fatty acids; associated with immune-mediated illnesses such as lupus and rheumatoid arthritis

antiretroviral therapy treatment with drugs designed to prevent the HIV virus from replicating in HIV-infected persons

anxiolytic medication or other intervention that inhibits anxiety

Apgar score assessment tool used to determine a newborn's adaptation to the extrauterine environment

arborization fern-like appearance

arrest of descent failure of the presenting fetal part to continue to descend during the second stage of labor despite uterine contractions and maternal pushing efforts

arrest of dilation failure to continue cervical dilation during active labor

arterial embolization procedure to obstruct a blood vessel. May be used to control hemorrhage

aspartate aminotransferase (AST) an enzyme that contributes to protein metabolism; specifically, it is important in the biosynthesis of amino acids because it catalyzes the reversible transfer of an amino group between glutamic and aspartic acid; the old term for this enzyme was *serum glutamic-oxaloacetic transaminase* (SGOT); when cell damage occurs (e.g., in the liver), AST is released into the tissues and bloodstream

asphyxia decrease in the body's oxygen along with an increase in the carbon dioxide content caused by interference with respiration

atony (see uterine atony)

augmentation increasing contractions by chemical stimulation to help labor progress

auscultation method of assessment of the FHR, accomplished by listening and counting the rate

avulsion a forced tearing of tissues

AZT azidothymide (chemical name), ZVD (zidovudine, generic name), and Retrovir (brand name); a nucleoside analog reverse transcriptase inhibitor drug commonly used to treat HIV infection; special precautions are recommended for dentistry

bacterial vaginosis a bacterial infection of the vagina, characterized by a foul-smelling, grayish vaginal discharge that exhibits a characteristic fishy odor when 10% potassium hydroxide is added

ballottement a sign that can be determined during abdominal examination of the pregnant woman; when the fingers tap lightly over a fetal part, it "bounces" back under the fingers; this sign can also be felt during a vaginal examination

baroreceptors specialized tissue located in the carotid arch and aortic sinus; cells in these areas are sensitive to stretching of surrounding tissues caused by increased blood pressure; when pressure is increased, these areas communicate this change to the brain, which responds by reducing the heart rate and cardiac output in an attempt to reduce blood pressure

base deficit (BD) the amount of bases used by the body in an attempt to normalize a reduced pH (neutralize the acid); illustrates the degree of change in the bicarbonate concentration of the body

baseline fetal heart rate the mean FHR rounded to increments of 5 bpm during a 10-minute segment, excluding periodic and episodic changes, periods of marked variability and segments of the baseline that differ more than 25 bpm; baseline must be for a minimum of 2 minutes in any 10-minute segment; normal range is between 110 and 160 bpm

baseline uterine tone amount of tone remaining in the uterus between contractions, usually between 5 and 15 mm Hg; can be measured only by an intrauterine pressure catheter

baseline variability fluctuations of the FHR of 2 cycles/min or more; visually quantified as the amplitude from peak to trough in bpm; the categories of variability are as follows:
- **absent** amplitude range is undetectable (appears as straight line)
- **minimal** amplitude range is detectable, but 5 bpm or fewer
- **moderate** (normal) amplitude range is 6 to 25 bpm
- **marked** amplitude range is more than 25 bpm

β-adrenergic agonist substance that attaches to specific receptor sites in the smooth muscle and this inhibits the chemical reaction necessary for smooth muscle to contract

β-adrenergic receptors specific sites on smooth muscle cells (e.g., the cells of the myometrium) where chemicals (agonists) can couple to produce a chemical reaction

β-mimetic drugs unique chemical substances that are able to bind to β-receptor sites on smooth muscle cells, causing a depressant or relaxing effect on the contracting ability of that cell; such cells are found in the myometrium of the uterus; β-mimetic drugs belong to a group of chemicals called "agonists"

biparietal diameter (BPD) the largest transverse diameter of the fetal head; measures the distance between the parietal bones

Bishop's score a pre-labor cervical score to assist in predicting whether induction of labor will be required; also has been used to predict the odds of preterm birth

bloody show the passage of a small amount of blood or blood-tinged mucus through the vagina near the end of pregnancy or during labor

Braxton–Hicks contractions intermittent painless contractions of the uterus; occur more frequently toward the end of the pregnancy and can sometimes be mistaken for true labor

calcium channel blocker medication that inhibits the influx of calcium ions into cardiac and smooth muscle cells

capacity the age and competence of an individual required for giving informed consent

caput succedaneum swelling produced on the presenting part of the fetal head during labor

carrier individual who is capable of transmitting a disease to another person; many times, carriers are not sick and have no idea that they are capable of spreading a disease

catecholamines group of chemicals that mediate physiologic and metabolic responses associated with sympathetic nervous system functioning

CD4⁺ T cell critical subpopulation of regulatory T lymphocytes involved in the induction of most immunologic functions; depletion of this subset of T lymphocytes is the key element in profound immunosuppression seen in HIV infection

cephalic replacement (Zavanelli maneuver) rotation of the fetal head back to occiput anterior, flexing of the fetal head, and firm pressure to push the fetal head back into the vagina. A cesarean section is then performed to deliver the baby

cephalopelvic disproportion (CPD) a condition that develops when the fetus' head is of size, shape, or position that it cannot pass through the woman's pelvis

cervical ripening softening of the cervix, occurs normally as physiologic process before labor or can be accomplished artificially by use of dilators and medications.

cervix the "neck," or lowest part, of the uterus that extends into the vagina; during labor, the cervix dilates, allowing the fetus to pass through it

cesarean birth manual removal of the fetus, placenta, and membranes through an abdominal incision
- **primary cesarean** a woman's first cesarean birth
- **emergency cesarean** emergency operative birth in the setting of life-threatening complications for either mother or fetus
- **cesarean birth on maternal request** cesarean birth in the absence of any obstetric or maternal medical indications, *also* **elective cesarean delivery**
- **repeat cesarean** subsequent cesarean births
- **cesarean hysterectomy** removal of the uterus during a cesarean birth; the cervix, fallopian tubes, and ovaries may also be removed

cesarean incision the abdominal incision created to remove the fetus, placenta, and membranes
- **classic** incision on upper part of the uterus in the vertical midline
- **low-segment transverse** transverse incision made on the lower part of the uterus, just above the symphysis pubis
- **low-segment vertical** vertical incision made on the lower part of the uterus

chancroid lesions that appear as red and ulcerated papules; may be associated with syphilis

chemoreceptors specialized tissue, located in the aortic and carotid bodies and in the medulla, that are sensitive to decreases in oxygen, carbon dioxide content, and pH in the blood; they recognize these changes, initiating responses that assist the body in compensating for these problems

chorioamnionitis infection of one of the membranes forming the amniotic sac, which holds the fetus during the pregnancy

chorion the outermost fetal membrane; contributes to the formation of the placenta

cleft palate congenital defect in which an opening is left in the roof of the mouth (the palate); during fetal development, this area fails to close and a communicating passageway between the mouth and nasal cavities is left

clonus spasmodic alteration of contraction and relaxation of a foot or hand

collusion secret agreement or cooperation between or among individuals for illegal or deceitful actions

competence the ability to do something successfully or efficiently

confidentiality protection of patient information in all forms

confirmatory test a highly specific test designed to confirm the results of an earlier screening test

conservator person appointed by a court to manage the personal and legal affairs of an incompetent adult

continuous glucose monitoring system (CGMS) made up of three technologies: a sensor, transmitter, and receiver; the sensor is a small wire that goes just under the skin to read interstitial glucose levels; the transmitter is usually part of the sensor and wirelessly sends glucose levels to the receiver every 5 minutes; the receiver can be an insulin pump, a small separate device, a smartphone, or I Watch upon which glucose levels and trends are displayed

contraction(s) shortening or tightening of a muscle; often used to describe the activity of the uterus that brings about dilatation of the cervix and descent of the fetus during labor

corticosteroid synthetic hormone, such as betamethasone or dexamethasone, given to women in preterm labor or to whom preterm birth is anticipated to enhance fetal lung maturity

corticotropin-releasing factor (CRF) neuropeptide released by the hypothalamus to stimulate the release of corticotrophin by the anterior pituitary

corticotrophin-releasing hormone chemical released by the cortex response to stress; may play a role in determining the length of gestation

counterpressure direct pressure applied gradually and steadily over boney areas of the body

cultural competence conscious motivation to develop cultural awareness, knowledge, skill in encounters with those from other cultures

cycle of violence describes three phases of violence, including
- **tension-building phase** the victim is compliant, but the abuser becomes angry with increasing frequency and intensity, with increased frequency of threats of harm, humiliation and intimidation
- **acute violence phase** intentional use of force which may increase in severity with each cycle; characterized by outbursts of violent, abusive incidents; may be preceded by verbal abuse and include psychological abuse
- **honeymoon or reconciliation phase** victim is showered with apologies and affection by the abuser, abuser gives assurances that the behavior will never happen again, makes excuses for the behavior, or even denies that violence occurred

cytokines substances produced by the immune system in response to infection; also, recent findings indicate that cytokines (e.g., interleukin-1β seems to play a role in labor initiation

debriefing a structured learning process of (1) receiving an explanation, (2) receiving information, (3) reporting of measures of performance, and/or (4) identifying opportunities to improve processes, systems, or outcomes

decelerations, fetal heart rate
- **early decelerations** in association with a uterine contraction, a visually apparent, gradual (onset to nadir 30 seconds or greater) decrease in the FHR with return to baseline; the nadir or low point of the deceleration occurs at the same time as the peak of the contraction
- **late decelerations** in association with a uterine contraction, a visually apparent, gradual (onset to nadir 30 seconds or greater) decrease in the FHR with return to baseline; the onset, nadir, and recovery of the deceleration occur after the beginning, peak, and end of the contraction, respectively
- **variable decelerations** abrupt (onset to nadir less than 30 seconds), visually apparent decrease in the FHR below the baseline; the decrease in FHR is 15 bpm or more, with a duration of 15 seconds or more, but less than 3 minutes
- **prolonged decelerations** visually apparent decrease in the FHR below baseline; deceleration is 15 bpm or more, lasing 2 minutes or more but less than 10 minutes from onset to return to baseline; if the deceleration lasts longer than 10 minutes, it is a baseline change

decidua the lining of the uterus that envelopes the impregnated ovum to form part of the placenta

dehiscence separation of a surgical wound

dermatome the area of skin supplied with afferent nerve fibers by a single posterior spinal root

diabetes a heterogeneous set of metabolic diseases all characterized by impaired glucose utilization and resulting in hyperglycemia
- **T1DM (Type 1 diabetes mellitus)** accounts for ~5% of all diabetes, Characterized by absolute deficiency of insulin. An autoimmune.

characterized by absolute deficiency of insulin. An autoimmune response destroys the insulin-producing pancreatic beta cells resulting in a need for exogenous insulin for survival and to prevent ketoacidosis
- **T2DM (Type 2 diabetes mellitus)** accounts for ~95% of all diabetes, characterized by insulin resistance and relative insulin deficiency often associated with obesity and sedentary life style. Sometimes can be managed by diet and exercise alone, but more often requires oral agents, or injectable particularly insulin to gain BG control. Almost all need insulin for optimum control during pregnancy
  - **gestational diabetes mellitus (GDMA1)** controlled with diet and exercise
  - **gestational diabetes mellitus (GDMA2)** controlled with diet, exercise, and requiring the addition of oral meds and/or insulin

diabetic ketoacidosis (DKA) an acute, life-threatening complication of diabetes from hyperglycemia, a shortage of insulin, inability of glucose to enter the cells, and production of ketone bodies from fat breakdown

diabetogenic producing diabetes symptoms

dipping when the presenting part has descended into the false pelvis but is not through the pelvic inlet

direct fetal monitoring *see* internal fetal monitoring

disseminated intravascular coagulation (DIC) a secondary disorder in blood clotting resulting from the overstimulation of the body's clotting processes; initially, generalized intravascular clotting occurs, succeeded by a deficiency in clotting factors and subsequent hemorrhaging; signs of hemorrhage may appear beneath the skin or mucous membranes, as evidenced by ecchymosis or petechiae

dizygotic pertaining to or derived from two separate zygotes (fertilized ova), as in a twin gestation resulting from two different fertilized ova

documentation recording, in written or electronic format, actions and decisions regarding patient care

domestic violence actual or threatened abuse of an intimate partner; *also* intimate partner violence, partner abuse, spousal abuse, wife abuse

doula supportive companion who accompanies a laboring woman to provide emotional, physical, and informational support and acts as an advocate for the woman and her family

Down syndrome congenital condition accompanied by moderate to severe mental retardation

durable power of attorney a written document in which one person (the principle) appoints another person to act as an agent on his/her behalf

duress threats, violence, constraints, or other action brought to bear on someone to do something against their will or better judgment

dysrhythmia irregularity in the heart rate that can be a result of an electrical abnormality, congenital anomaly, or injury; can be a transient and benign problem or a continuous and serious condition; most fetal dysrhythmias are benign

dystocia abnormal labor as seen in very slow cervical dilatation or fetal descent or a complete halt in progress, which can be due to maternal or fetal conditions

early decelerations *see* decelerations, FHR

eclampsia pregnancy-related hypertensive disease accompanied by hypertension, proteinuria, edema, tonic and clonic convulsions, and coma; can occur during pregnancy or shortly after delivery

effleurage a form of massage involving a circular, stroking motion made with the palm of the hand

EIA an enzyme immunoassay test for HIV infection; has 99% sensitivity when performed under optimal laboratory conditions

on serum specimens from persons infected for 12 weeks or more (formerly called *ELISA*)

elective birth making a choice to have a baby prior to labor

emancipated released from parental care and responsibility; freed from the power of another individual

embolism obstruction of a blood vessel by foreign substances or a blood clot (as in erythroblastosis fetalis)

endemic a disease that is indigenous to a geographic area or population

end-of-life care care of patients with a terminal illness/condition that has become advanced, progressive and incurable

endogenous originating within the body

endogenous insulin insulin that is secreted from the pancreas (within the body)

endothelin-derived releasing factor (EDRF) substance that acts as a vasorelaxor in the vascular smooth muscle

endothelium layer of epithelial cells that lines the cavities of the heart and of the blood and lymph vessels

endothelium (endothelial lining) a type of epithelium that lines the interior surface of blood and lymphatic vessels

en face face to face

engagement the entrance of the largest diameter of the fetal head into the smallest diameter of the maternal pelvis; the first movement made by the fetal head in preparation for birth

Engerix-B currently licensed hepatitis B vaccine that is the result of genetic engineering; the usual schedule of doses is at birth, and then at 1 and 6 months of age; may be given in an alternate four-dose schedule at birth, 1, 2, and 12 months; a recent CDC advisory also recommends administration before 2 months of age, at 2 to 4 months, and at 6 to 18 months

enteric precautions procedures followed in the care of certain patients that are intended to reduce the risk of contamination of personnel or other patients from potentially infected intestinal waste

epigastric pain pain occurring in the right upper quadrant of the abdomen and that is the result of hepatic edema and hemorrhages in the liver capsule

epinephrine a substance produced by the adrenal medulla gland predominantly; it is produced synthetically and is used therapeutically as a vasoconstrictor, cardiac stimulant, and bronchiole relaxant

episodic fetal heart rate changes those that do not occur in relation to a contraction

erythroblastosis condition of hemolytic disease of the newborn characterized by anemia, jaundice, and enlargement of the liver and spleen

esophageal atresia closure or absence of the esophagus

euglycemia normal level of glucose in the blood

exogenous insulin insulin that comes from a source outside the body

external fetal monitoring *also* "indirect or noninvasive fetal monitoring"; this method involves the use of an ultrasonic transducer and tocodynamometer to monitor fetal heart tones and contractions, respectively; these are held in place by belts

feather blow a breathing technique used to avoid pushing; uses visualization of a feather and blowing just enough to keep the feather bouncing up and down in the air above the lips

fetal anencephaly condition in the fetus in which there is an absence of the brain and spinal cord

fetal attitude relation of fetal parts to each other; the basic attitudes are flexion and extension; for example, when the baby's head is bent toward its chest, the head is in an attitude of flexion

fetal bradycardia baseline FHR less than 110 bpm for 10 minutes or more

fetal fibronectin (fFN) glycoprotein produced by the chorion, found at the junction of the membrane and the uterus

fetal hydrocephaly condition in the fetus in which there is an increased accumulation of cerebrospinal fluid within the ventricles of the fetus' brain; this leads to rapid head growth; it is a result of interference with normal circulation and absorption of the fluid

fetal inflammatory response syndrome (FIRS) condition characterized by systemic inflammation and an elevation of fetal plasma interleukin-6

fetal karyotype chromosomal contents found in the cell nucleus of the fetus

fetal lie relationship of the body of the fetus to the body of the mother; fetal lies are longitudinal or transverse
- **longitudinal lie** fetal body from head to toe is parallel to the length of the mother
- **transverse lie** fetal body lies at right angles to the mother's body

fetal monitoring type of electronic monitoring in which information about the FHR and the contraction pattern are continually assessed; *see also* external fetal monitoring

fetal position position of the fetus within the uterus in relation to the maternal pelvis

fetal presentation within the uterus, the lowest part of the fetus that comes first, either the head, buttocks, or, rarely, the shoulders

fetal reserve amount of oxygen provided to the fetus above that which is needed; oxygen supplied minus the oxygen needed

fetal scalp electrode spiral electrode attached directly to the presenting part of the fetus; determines the FHR by counting R waves in the fetal ECG; this results in a tracing that allows variability to be assessed; part of the internal monitoring system

fetal station the location of the fetal presenting part in relation to the maternal ischial spines

fetal tachycardia increase in the baseline FHR to greater than 160 bpm

first stage of labor (see stages of labor)

floating when the fetal presenting part is entirely out of the pelvis and can be moved by the examiner

fontanelle spaces where the sutures of the skull bones meet; "soft spots" on the baby's head

forceps assisted birth *see* assisted delivery

fraud intentional deception of an individual to gain that person's cooperation in surrendering their property or legal rights

fulminant occurring with great rapidity

funisitis inflammation of the umbilical cord

gap junctions intracellular channels that allow movement of small molecules or ions for communication between cells

Gaskin maneuver positioning of a laboring woman on her hands and knees or "all fours" to reduce a shoulder dystocia. Named after Ina May Gaskin, MA, CPM, founder and director of the Farm Midwifery Center

gestational hypertension blood pressure elevation detected for the first time after midpregnancy (20 weeks); elevated pressures are transient, there is no progression to preeclampsia and the woman is normotensive by 12 weeks postpartum

gluconeogenesis synthesis of glucose from noncarbohydrate sources, such as amino acids and glycerol; occurs primarily with the liver and kidneys when carbohydrate supply is low

glycogenolysis the splitting up of glycogen in the liver, which yields glucose

grand multipara woman who has had five or more live births

group B streptococcus (GBS) gram-positive bacteria that can be a cause of both meningitis and sepsis in the neonate

HAART highly active antiretroviral therapy; a combination of antiretroviral medications that work well against HIV

hematoma localized collection of clotted or partially clotted blood

hemoglobin A_{1c} (HbA_{1c}) measurement of the percent of glycosylation (linkage of hemoglobin to glucose) that occurs in red blood cells

hepatitis B immune globulin (HBIG) substance that supplies antibodies needed to provide immediate protection against hepatitis B

herpes simplex virus (HSV) type 1 serologic subtype of the herpes virus strain that primarily infects nongenital areas of the body, mainly mucocutaneous tissue of the mouth; however, HSV-1 can cause genital herpes infections as well

herpes simplex virus (HSV) type 2 virus that causes infections in the genital organs

HIV the human immunodeficiency virus that causes AIDS
- **HIV-1** one of five known retroviruses; discovered in 1984 and once called human T-cell lymphotrophic virus type III
- **HIV-2** one of five known retroviruses; discovered in 1986 and once called human T-cell lymphotrophic virus type IV

HIV DNA PCR preferred virologic method for diagnosing HIV infection in infants

HIV infection acquiring of HIV in the blood and other body fluids and tissues; the individual may have no symptoms whatsoever

HIV RNA test *also* viral load or just RNA; a blood test that measures the amount of HIV virus in a person's blood plasma

homeopathy alternative, natural system of healing and symptom relief

honeymoon phase (see cycle of violence)

horizontal transmission transmission of microscopic organisms (e.g., viruses) from one sexual partner to another

HTLV-III a retrovirus known as human T-cell lymphotropic virus type III; a more specific name for HIV-1

hydatidiform mole result of a degeneration of the early developing placenta; multiple grape-like cysts develop, along with rapid growth of the uterus and bleeding

hydralazine (Apresoline) an arterial vasodilator used as an antihypertensive agent

hydramnios (polyhydramnios) presence of excessive amounts of amniotic fluid (2,000 mL or more) in the uterus

hydrops edema in the fetus

hyperbilirubinemia excessive amounts of bilirubin in the blood; prenatal conditions in the mother such as diabetes, infections, drug ingestion, and blood incompatibility between mother and fetus can predispose the newborn to hyperbilirubinemia; certain neonatal conditions such as obstruction of the biliary duct or the lower bowel can also predispose the newborn to this condition; treatment to lower and stabilize bilirubin levels is necessary because excessive levels can lead to brain injury

hyperglycemia excessive glucose in the blood stream

hyperglycemic hyperosmolar nonketotic syndrome (HHNS) occurs in type 2 diabetes and is characterized by extreme hyperglycemia, absence of ketones, severe dehydration, and decreased consciousness

hyperinsulinemia excessive insulin in the blood stream; in a fetus it is associated with increased abdominal fat and hypoglycemia at birth; at puberty and adulthood it is associated with damage to blood vessels, high blood pressure, heart disease, obesity, osteoporosis, and cancer

hyperpnea breathing that is deeper and more rapid than expected

hyperventilation increased inspiration and expiration of air as a result of rapid or deep breathing, which leads to the reduction of carbon dioxide in the blood; symptoms include dizziness, light headedness, and tingling in the fingers and around the mouth

hypocalcemia abnormally low levels of calcium in the blood

hypoglycemia abnormally low levels of glucose in the blood

hypoglycemia unawareness an autonomic neuropathy in which the sympathetic response to low blood sugar does not occur and alert the patient to low blood sugar—usually a result of frequent episodes of hypoglycemia

hypopharynx laryngopharynx, the bottom part of the pharynx that connects the throat to the esophagus

hypothermia having a body temperature below normal

hypoxemia decreased oxygen content in the blood

hypoxia insufficient availability of oxygen to meet the body's metabolic needs

iatrogenic caused by treatment or diagnostic procedures

idiosyncratic abnormal susceptibility to an agent, such as a drug, which is peculiar or unique to the individual

IgM immunoglobulin M; special proteins produced by the lymphatic system against foreign substances shortly after their invasion; they are larger in size than IgG molecules and incapable of crossing the placenta to any great extent; blood levels rise within days of an infection and fall to a nondetectable level within a few months

ileus intestinal obstruction

immune serum globulin (ISG) substance that contains proteins capable of acting as antibodies and thus potentially confers some passive immunity to the individual receiving it

immunization becoming immune or the process of rendering a patient immune

immunoassay a biochemical test that measures the presence of a macromolecule in a solution through the use of an antibody or antigen; the macromolecule detected is often referred to as an "analyte" and is in many cases a protein

immunogenicity ability to stimulate the formation of antibodies

inborn neonate infant whose birth occurred within the birth center or hospital

increta (see abnormal placentation)

indirect fetal monitoring *see* external fetal monitoring

induction of labor artificially starting labor and ensuring ongoing labor, usually through oxytocin administration

information as a legal term, refers to the content of the explanation given to the patient

informed consent legal term describing a process by which patients are given specific information regarding procedures, may be written or verbal

inoculate introduce a substance (the inoculum) into the body that can produce a disease or an immunity to the disease, depending on the circumstances and the substance; inoculate is sometimes a cultured substance

insulin sensitivity refers to how well someone responds to insulin individuals) that are sensitive to insulin (often but not always—T1DM) utilize it efficiently and, therefore, require less insulin than those who have T2DM

insulin resistance cells are unable to use insulin effectively resulting in glucose remaining in the blood stream. The presence of glucose in the blood stream stimulates the pancreas to secrete more insulin resulting in excess insulin in the blood stream (T2DM)

internal fetal monitoring *also* called direct and invasive fetal monitoring; type of electronic monitoring in which the FHR is monitored by the use of a helix electrode and the laboring woman's contraction pattern is monitored by the use of an intrauterine pressure catheter

intimate partner abuse (see domestic violence)

intimate partner violence (see domestic violence)

intrauterine pressure catheter catheter inserted into the uterine cavity alongside the presenting part of the fetus, allowing baseline uterine tonus and contraction intensity to be assessed in mm Hg

involution (uterine) the decrease in uterine size after childbirth

ischemia inadequate blood supply to an organ or tissue in the body

ketosis excess of ketone bodies in the blood; in uncontrolled diabetes mellitus, there is a great increase in fatty acid metabolism and impaired or absent carbohydrate metabolism, resulting in the increased production of ketone bodies

labetalol (Normodyne, Trandate) a selective alpha$_1$ and nonselective beta-adrenergic receptor blocking medication; used in pregnancy to treat hypertension

labor down allows uterine contractions (the power) to bring the fetus further down the birth canal and rotate the fetal presenting part for birth

lactobacilli lactic acid producing bacteria normally found in the vagina, mouth, and intestine

late deceleration *see* deceleration, fetal

late preterm birth infants delivered between 34 and 36 weeks' gestation

latent phase (see stages of labor)

lecithin:sphingomyelin ratio (L/S ratio) complex and fairly lengthy test used to assess lung maturity in the fetus; a ratio of 2.0 or higher usually indicates mature lungs

leptin (Greek: "thin") a hormone secreted by adipose tissue that travels to the brain to signal satiety thus preserving "energy" balance. The placenta produces leptin—it's role is not well understood except that it is increased in diabetes and preeclampsia

leukocytosis increased white blood cell count

lithotomy position in which the woman lies on her back with her thighs drawn up toward her chest, her knees flexed, and her legs extended out to the side

living will an advanced directive that outlines the patient's wishes for end-of-life care

lochia discharge of blood, mucus, and tissue from the uterus during the post delivery period; types of lochia are described by color and include **rubra, serosa,** and **alba**

low birth weight newborns weighing

L/S ratio *see* lecithin:sphingomyelin ratio

macrophages type of white blood cell involved in the immune response by destroying/ingesting foreign material, debris, or dead cells

macrosomia large body size, including enlargement of organs such as the liver and spleen

malpractice failure of a professional person to act in accordance with current accepted professional standards or failure to foresee possibilities and consequences that a professional person, having the necessary skills and training to act professionally, should foresee no matter what the motivation

maturity-onset diabetes of youth (MODY) relatively mild, non–insulin-requiring form of diabetes mellitus beginning at a younger age than usual

McRobert's maneuver positioning of the mother's thighs on her abdomen to straighten the sacrum and decrease angle of incline of the symphysis pubis making it easier to deliver the anterior shoulder in the case of shoulder dystocia

meconium dark green or black material present in the large intestine of the near-term or term fetus; also the first stool passed by the newborn

meconium aspiration syndrome (MAS) syndrome caused by the inhalation of meconium or meconium-stained amniotic fluid into the lungs

mentum chin

microangiopathy disease of small blood vessels in which the basement membrane of the capillaries thickens or thrombi form in the arterioles and capillaries

microcephaly congenital deformity in the fetus in which the head is abnormally small in relation to the body; mental retardation is often associated with this condition

midpelvis most important plane of the pelvis because it has the least room

molding normal overlapping of skull bones of the baby so that the head will fit through the pelvis during labor

monozygotic pertaining to or derived from a single zygote (fertilized ovum), as in a twin gestation occurring from a single fertilization ovum

Montevideo units measurement of uterine activity made when an intrauterine pressure catheter is in place

morbidity state of disease; cases of disease in relation to a specific group or population

mortality death rate; ratio of number of deaths to a specific group or population

multipara woman who is in other than her first labor

multiple gestation pregnancy with more than one fetus; an example is twins

nasopharynx part of the pharynx situated above the soft palate (postnasal space)

necrotizing enterocolitis a serious illness involving necrotic lesions of the intestines; occurs primarily in preterm or low–birth-weight neonates

negligence failure to exercise the care that a reasonably prudent person would exercise in like circumstances

neonatal resuscitation actions to restore or enhance breathing and circulation in the newborn

nephropathy disease of the kidney caused by microvascular changes and resulting in a loss of protein in the urine

neuraxial anesthesia (regional anesthesia) form of anesthesia that is given centrally (i.e., in the spinal canal) or peripherally (i.e., in the skin) to block pain impulses without causing a loss of consciousness

neuropathy disease of the nervous system involving peripheral nerve dysfunction such as numbness or change in sensation

neuroprotection mechanisms and strategies used to protect against neuronal injury or degeneration in the central nervous system

newly born refers to an infant during the brief period of the first few minutes to hours of life

nifedipine (Procardia) a calcium channel blocking medication; used in pregnancy to treat hypertension and as a tocolytic agent

nitrous oxide (laughing gas) non-flammable, colorless, short-acting gas with analgesic and anxiolytic properties

noninvasive fetal monitoring *see* external fetal monitoring

nonpharmacologic nondrug therapies

nosocomial infections that are hospital acquired, in contrast with community-acquired infections

nuchal cord umbilical cord with one or more loops around the neck of the infant; commonly present and ordinarily does no harm

nullipara woman in labor for the first time

nulliparous having never given birth to a child

obstetric hemorrhage significant loss of blood during the antepartum, intrapartum, or antepartum periods

occiput back of the fetal skull, below and behind the posterior fontanelle

oligohydramnios abnormally small amount of amniotic fluid; an AFI of 5 cm or less

oliguria severely decreased urinary output (less than 400 mL in 24 hours or 30 mL per hour for two consecutive hours)

operative vaginal birth manual extraction of the fetus with a vacuum device or forceps

opportunistic infection infection developing in the host organism because of a lowered immune capability

organogenesis time of organ development, which occurs (during the second to eighth week in gestation)

oropharynx central portion of the pharynx lying between the soft palate and upper portion of the epiglottis

outborn neonate infant whose birth occurred outside the birth center or hospital and who is then admitted

oxytocin hormone that stimulates the uterus to contract or a drug (Syntocinon or Pitocin) that imitates the natural hormone

palliative care *also called* comfort care; care aimed at prevention and relief of suffering, support for best possible quality of life for patients and their families

paracrine type of hormone function in which the hormone synthesized and released from endocrine cells binds to receptors in nearby cells, affecting their function

parous having had at least one child, either alive or dead at birth

partner abuse *see* domestic violence

partogram a graphic record of assessment data used during labor

parturition the act or process of giving birth

passive immunity immunity to a disease produced by injection of material containing the antibodies against a specific disease

pathogen microorganism or substance capable of producing disease

Pco$_2$ partial pressure of carbon dioxide (quantity of CO_2 in the blood)

pelvic planes imaginary flat surfaces passing across parts of the true pelvis at different levels; used to describe dimensions of various parts of the pelvis

percreta (see abnormal placentation)

perinatal time between 20 weeks' gestational age and 28 days after birth

perinatal morbidity frequency or rate of disease among fetuses or infants between 20 weeks' gestational age and 28 days after birth

perinatal mortality death of a fetus or infant between 20 weeks gestational age and 28 days after birth

perinatal transmission transmission of diseased blood elements that occurs during the perinatal period or during birth

periodic fetal heart rate changes transient FHR changes associated with contractions

physiologic care characterized by spontaneous onset and progression of labor that includes biological and psychological conditions that promote effective labor, birth, and newborn transition

placenta the spongy structure attached to the wall of the uterus throughout pregnancy through which nutrients and oxygen pass from the woman's blood to the fetus and through which waste products from the fetus pass into the woman's blood

placenta battledore placenta with the umbilical cord inserted at the edge

placenta circumvallate placenta encircled with a dense, raised, white nodular ring

placenta previa abnormal implantation of the placenta in the lower uterine segment; classification of the type of previa is based on how close the placenta lies to the cervical opening (os)
- **total placenta previa** completely covers the os
- **partial placenta previa** covers a portion of the os
- **marginal placenta previa** close to the os

plasma fluid component of blood

plasma-derived vaccines vaccines that are produced from the pooled serum of infected individuals

PO$_2$ partial pressure of oxygen (quantity of O_2 in the blood)

polycystic ovary syndrome (PCOS) a hormonal imbalance in which the ovaries make more androgens than normal; women with PCOS have insulin resistance and hyperinsulinemia

polydipsia excessive thirst; may be caused by dehydration

polyphagia excessive hunger, caused by tissue loss and the state of starvation that occurs with the inability of the cells to utilize glucose

polyuria frequent urination seen in diabetes because water is not reabsorbed by the renal tubules owing to the osmotic activity of glucose

postmortem care care of a body after death

postprandial after eating

postterm gestational age of more than 42 weeks; *also* postterm infant

precipitous suddenly

preeclampsia disease occurring during pregnancy (after 20 weeks or during the first week after delivery) with the development of high blood pressure in addition to protein in the urine, edema, or both

preexisting diabetes (overt diabetes) refers to diabetes which existed prior to pregnancy—T1DM or T2DM

premature rupture of membranes (PROM) spontaneous rupture of membranes before the onset of labor, regardless of gestational age

preterm infant with a gestational age of less than 37 weeks; the term *premature* is sometimes used (*see also* late preterm birth and very preterm birth)

preterm birth delivery of an infant at less than 37 weeks' gestation

preterm premature rupture of membranes (PPROM) rupture of membranes before term (37 completed weeks gestation) with or without the onset of labor

prevalence proportion of individuals in a population having a disease

primigravida woman who is pregnant for the first time

primipara woman who has given birth to her first child, whether or not the child is living or was alive at birth

prodromal time in which a symptom indicates the onset of a state (e.g., labor or a disease)

progesterone hormone produced by the ovaries when a woman is not pregnant and by the placenta during pregnancy; it has many important functions, including preventing the uterus from contracting during pregnancy

prolapsed cord condition in which the umbilical cord slips down along the side of the fetal presenting part or comes ahead of the presenting part

proliferative retinopathy new blood vessel formation near the optic disk that can extend to growth in the vitreous chamber, rupture, and vitreous hemorrhage; in addition, fibrous tissue is generated and adheres to the posterior vitreous membrane and can lead to retinal detachment

prolonged acceleration *see* acceleration, fetal

prolonged deceleration *see* deceleration, fetal

prophylaxis observing procedures or steps to prevent a disease or harmful effect

prostacyclin hormone synthesized in the endothelial lining of the blood vessels; a potent vasodilator and inhibitor of platelet aggregation

prostaglandins group of chemical substances (derivatives of fatty acids) present in many tissues; stimulate the uterus to contract

protease inhibitor class of antiviral medications used to treat HIV/AIDS and hepatitis caused by hepatitis C virus

proteinuria presence in the urine of abnormally large quantities of protein, usually albumin; by definition, occurs with a reading of 2+ on a random urine specimen or when there is 500 mg of protein in a 24-hour specimen (less than 250 mg of protein per day is excreted in the healthy adult)

pyelonephritis inflammation of the kidney caused by an infective process

pyloric stenosis condition found in the infant in which the opening from the stomach to the small intestines is narrowed so much that partially digested food cannot pass in a normal manner; a characteristic sign of this is highly forceful vomiting

Recombivax B synthetic, genetically engineered vaccine for hepatitis B

reconciliation phase (see cycle of violence)

relaxin hormone secreted by the corpus luteum; acts on smooth muscle of the uterus to produce relaxation of muscle fibers

replication process of duplicating or reproducing (e.g., replication of an exact copy of a polynucleotide strand of DNA or RNA)

restitution movement of the newborn head once it is born wherein the neck untwists and the head turns approximately 45 degrees to resume its normal relationship with the shoulders, which are in an anteroposterior position at the pelvic outlet

retinopathy damage to the retina of the eye caused by the microvascular deterioration from elevated blood glucose levels

retrovirus unique virus form that contains an enzyme, reverse transcriptase, enabling it to synthesize DNA in the cells of a host; this DNA then enters the nucleus of that cell and becomes part of it; the viral DNA (genes) therefore becomes duplicated along with the host's cell genes, and new generations of cells are produced; these new generations contain the virus's genetic material

Rh incompatibility lack of compatibility between two groups of blood cells having different antigens; caused by the presence of the Rh factor in one group and its absence in the other

rubra (see lochia)

safety plan plan giving a victim of abuse steps to follow in a dangerous situation, including detailed information about defensive measures

scotomata presence of specks or spots in the vision disturbing vision temporarily; suggestive of lesions in the retina or visual pathway

second stage of labor (see stages of labor)

semi-Fowler's position semi-sitting position in which the patient is positioned at approximately 45 degrees

sensitivity probability that a test will be positive when infection or a specific condition is present

seroconversion process of blood serum developing an antibody response to a specific antigen (e.g., a virus or bacteria)

seronegative the absence of a primary infection with a specific agent, or the disappearance of antibodies after treatment or absence of antibodies usually found in a given disease/syndrome

seropositive producing a positive reaction to serologic tests

seroprotective level of antibody response that indicates protection (immunity) after exposure or vaccination

serous exudate accumulation of a fluid, having the nature of serum, in a cavity or on a surface

serum that part of blood that remains after clotting has occurred

shoulder dystocia difficult delivery of the shoulders of the fetus

simulation imitation or representation of a real process/situation

sinciput brow or forehead of the fetus

sinusoidal pattern baseline pattern that demonstrates a regular undulating pattern above and below the fetal heart baseline; can be a sign of severe fetal anemia or fetal asphyxia or may be the effect of certain medications

spaces used in conduction anesthesia the spinal cord is covered by three layers; the outermost layer is the dura, the middle layer is the arachnoid, and the inner layer is the pia
- **arachnoid space** between the middle and inner layer covering the spinal cord and contains the spinal fluid
- **extradural space (epidural, peridural)** space found outside the outermost covering of the spinal cord into which chemicals may be injected for the purpose of inducing anesthesia
- **subdural space** space found between the outermost and the middle layer of the spinal cord

spina bifida congenital defect in the walls of the spinal canal caused by lack of union between parts of the vertebrae; as a result, the membranes of the spinal cord are pushed through the opening, forming a tumor

spiral electrode *see* fetal scalp electrode

spousal abuse (see domestic violence)

stages of labor * Stage I onset of labor until the woman is fully dilated; divided into latent and active labor phases
* Stage 1 latent phase (early, preparatory phase) from the onset of regular uterine contractions that cause cervical change until the woman enters the active phase of labor.
* Stage I active phase (dilational phase) begins when the laboring woman has accelerated cervical dilation; usually beginning at 5 cm for multiparous and at 6 cm for nulliparous women
* Stage II full dilation of the cervix until birth
* Stage III birth of the baby until placental delivery
* Stage IV after the delivery of placenta through stabilization of the mother (usually 2 hours)

standards of practice accepted published professional levels of care for which the individual professional is held accountable; the legal profession and courts use these in malpractice cases

steroids chemical compounds that make up, among other things, hormones found in humans; many drugs are composed of steroids

STI sexually transmitted infection

strip graph tracing produced on graph paper by the electronic fetal monitor; allows FHR and contraction patterns to be continually assessed

sugaleal potential space between the periosteum (skull) and the epicranial aponeurosis (scalp). A subgaleal hemorrhage is a potential complication of vacuum assisted birth; can be associated with intracranial hemorrhage or skull fracture and must be distinguished from caput succadaneum and cephalohematoma.

suprapubic pressure pressure applied above the maternal symphysis pubis with a hand over anterior fetal shoulder with downward and lateral motion to relieve shoulder dystocia

surfactant mixture of phospholipids (primarily lecithin and sphingomyelin) secreted by alveolar cells into the alveoli and respiratory air passages, which reduces the surface tension of pulmonary fluids and contributes to the elastic properties of pulmonary tissue

sutures spaces between the bones of the fetal skull, which are covered by membranes

symphysiotomy transection of the firm ligaments between the left and right symphyseal bones, may be used in the event of a shoulder dystocia to gain pelvic circumference and facilitate of the baby's anterior shoulder. The procedure can be done rapidly, under local anesthesia

tension-building phase (see cycle of violence)

term gestational age of 38 to 42 weeks; *also term infant*

therapeutic privilege withholding information about a treatment or medication when the individual's health would be significantly jeopardized by full disclosure of the information

thermoregulation regulation of temperature, especially body temperature

thrombocytopenia abnormal decrease in the number of blood platelets; bleeding disorders are a consequence

thrombophlebitis inflammation of a vein; associated with the formation of a blood clot

thromboxane produced primarily by the platelets; potent vasoconstrictor; stimulates platelet aggregation

tocodynamometer part of an external monitoring system that provides information about the laboring woman's contraction

pattern by detecting changes in the shape of her abdominal wall directly above the uterine fundus

tocolytic effect of quieting or inhibiting smooth muscle activity; the myometrium of the uterus is composed of smooth muscle

tocolytic therapy process of administering medications for the purpose of inhibiting uterine contractions

transplacental transmission passage of a pathogen from the woman to the fetus through the placental vasculature

trial of labor (TOLAC) labor after a previous cesarean birth

trophoblastic disease disease resulting from degeneration in the early development of the placenta; a hydatidiform mole results

tubal ligation operative procedure using ligation, surgical closure, and/or cauterization to render the fallopian tubes incapable of sperm or ova transport

tumor necrosis factor-a a cell signaling *cytokine* involved in systemic *inflammation* and insulin resistance. TNF puts residues on the cell's insulin receptor blocking it at the cell surface inhibiting insulin's action. The placenta secretes TNF-α

turtle sign the sudden retraction of the fetal head back against the woman's perineum after emerging from the vagina

ultrasonic transducer part of the external monitoring system that monitors FHR by detecting movement within the fetal heart as the heart valves open and close; similar to sonar

uterine atony loss of normal tone of the muscles of the uterus; results in relaxation of the muscles that normally control postpartum uterine bleeding

uterine dystocia abnormal labor or difficult labor

uterine rupture disruption of the layers of the uterus

uterine tachysystole greater than five uterine contractions in 10 minutes averaged over 30 minutes

uterine tonus degree of muscle tone within the uterus; *see also* baseline uterine tonus

vacuum-assisted birth (vacuum extraction) birth of infant assisted by the placement of vacuum device to provide gentle traction and guidance of the fetal head

vagal stimulation stimulation of the vagus nerve; can be caused by intubation of neonate

vaginal birth after cesarean (VBAC) vaginal birth after a previous cesarean birth

variability *see* baseline FHR variability

variable deceleration *see* deceleration, fetal

vasa previa fetal umbilical vessels cross or come near the cervical os

vasopressor substance or medication that causes vasoconstriction

velamentous cord insertion major vessels found in the cord separate in the membranes at a distance from the edge of the placenta where they are surrounded only by a fold of amnion

vertex top of the skull between the anterior and posterior fontanelles

vertical transmission transmission of microscopic organisms (e.g., viruses) to the fetus and newborn either through breaks in the placental barrier during pregnancy or at the time of birth

very preterm birth infants delivered before 32 weeks' gestation

vibroacoustic stimulation process of fetal stimulation using sound; objective is to elicit a fetal startle or movement that is then used to evaluate fetal status

viral load (viral titer) a numerical expression of the quantity of virus in a given volume

viral replication process of a virus reproducing itself

viral suppression a very low level of detectable virus

viremia (viremic) state of having viruses in the blood

virulent very poisonous; infectious

voluntariness circumstances surrounding an individual's giving consent

Western blot test supplemental laboratory test that detects specific antibodies to components of a virus; mainly used to validate repeatedly reactive enzyme immunoassays (EIA) or enzyme-linked immunoassays (ELISA) for HIV infection; is highly specific when strict criteria are used to interpret the results; when a repeatedly reactive EIA or ELISA and a positive Western blot test occur, it is highly predictive of HIV infection, even in a population with a low prevalence of infection

wife abuse *see* domestic violence

zidovudine zidovudine (Retrovir) used along with other medications to prevent women from passing HIV to the fetus during pregnancy

INDEX

Note: Page numbers followed by f indicate figures; those followed by t indicate tables.

A

Abdomen
- of newborn, 493t
- physical examination of laboring woman, 53
- signs of abruptio placentae, 48
- systematic search for fetal heart tones, 87f

Abdominal dressing, 477

Abdominal emergencies, acute, 505

Abdominal muscles, 81

Abdominal trauma, maternal, 418

Abruption, 254

Abruptio placentae, 48
- defined, 453, 453f
- grading of, 455t
- nursing care, 455–457
- predisposing factors, 48
- risk factors for, 454, 454t
- signs and symptoms, 455
- signs of, 48

Accelerated starvation of pregnancy, 377

Accelerations, 157, 157f

ACE inhibitors. *See* Angiotensin converting enzyme (ACE) inhibitors

Acetaminophen, 321

Acidemia, 178

Acidosis
- definition of, 178
- respiratory *vs.* metabolic, 179

Acme, 5, 5f

ACNM. *See* American College of Nurse-Midwives (ACNM); Association of Certified Nurse Midwives (ACNM)

ACOG. *See* American College of Obstetricians and Gynecologists (ACOG); American Congress of Obstetrics and Gynecology (ACOG)

Acquired immunodeficiency syndrome (AIDS), 329. *See also* Human immunodeficiency virus (HIV)

Acromial process, 31, 31f

Active management of labor (AML), 217

Active management of third stage of labor (AMTSL), 107–108
- delayed cord clamping, 108
- gentle cord traction, 107
- uterotonic medication administration, 107

Acupressure, for labor pain, 124–125

Acupuncture, for labor pain, 124–125

Acute HIV infection and seroconversion, 328

Acute respiratory distress syndrome (ARDS), 451

Acute violence phase, 417

Acyclovir, 351

Adaptation, newborn, 490

Adefovir dipivoxil, 361

Admission, laboring woman, 41
- critical information, identification of, 41–46
- high-risk mother and fetus, identification of, 43–44
- history taking, guidelines for, 42–43
- key questions to be asked, 42
- physical examination, 50–54
- presence of high-risk factors, identification of, 44–45
- status of membranes, evaluation of, 46–49
- testing for ruptured membranes, 55–60
  - fern test, 61–62
- true labor *vs.* false labor, 45–46
- vaginal examination, 62–67

Admission for birth, 406

Adult learning theory. *See* Perinatal education program implementation

Advanced maternal age (35 years or older)
- factors, 400
- intrapartum and postpartum care, differences, 401
- risks with, 400–401

Aerobic metabolism, 178

AFE. *See* Amniotic fluid embolism; Amniotic fluid embolism (AFE)

Afebrile pneumonia, 346

Age-related pregnancy
- advanced maternal age (35 years or older), 400–401
- birth control, 400
- breastfeeding, 400
- depression, 400
- teen pregnancy, 399–400

Agitation, 550

AHA. *See* American Heart Association (AHA)

17-a-Hydroxyprogesterone caproate (17P), 263

AIDS. *See* Acquired immunodeficiency syndrome (AIDS)

Airway complications, 408

Alanine transaminase (ALT), 282

Alcohol, 412–413. *See also* Substance use and abuse

Alcohol wipes, 382

Aldrete Scoring System, 479, 480t

Allergic or anaphylactic reaction, 133t

Alpha-adrenergic agonists, 304

ALT. *See* Alanine transaminase (ALT)

Ambulances, 508

Ambulation, 118–119

American Academy of Pediatrics (AAP), 323

American College of Nurse-Midwives (ACNM), 142

American Congress of Obstetrics and Gynecology (ACOG), 142, 323
- Task Force on Hypertensive in Pregnancy, 277

American Heart Association (AHA), 290

American Society of Anesthesiologists, 121

AML. *See* Active management of labor (AML)

Amniocentesis, 361
- transabdominal, 318

Amnioinfusion, 175

Amnion, 46

Amniotic fluid, 46
- benefits to fetus from, 46
- hydramnios, 48–49

CCS0416